T0306047

VIRAL PANDEMICS

This new edition of *Viral Pandemics* illuminates how the increasing emergence of novel viruses has combined with intensifying global interconnectedness to create an escalating spiral of viral disease. It includes an introduction to the key characteristics of viral pathogens that make them so dangerous followed by a comprehensive survey of epidemic viral disease from 1900 to the present.

Now featuring new chapters on COVID-19 and mpox, the book uses a historical narrative to follow the path of each virus from its original detection to its emergence as an explosive pandemic. This allows readers to appreciate the biologic potential of the virus, the dynamics of epidemic disease spread, and the contemporaneous abilities of medicine and science to contend with the pathogen. In parallel, the book discusses those elements of connectedness that enable a localized disease outbreak to become a global pandemic, allowing readers to appreciate the increasingly critical role that human activity plays in global disease. In the last two chapters, the authors take a different approach. *A Look Back* critically evaluates the response to COVID-19 against the history of the emergence of public health in response to several other modern global pandemics and identifies some lessons we can still learn to improve our response to future pandemics. *A Way Forward* integrates the biologic and environmental factors that emerged as critical in the analysis of all the pandemics in the book and then uses this composite picture to propose ways to interrupt the escalating cycle of viral pandemic disease.

Written in a straightforward and accessible style, this book is ideal reading for students of public health and its history, the history of medicine and medical anthropology, as well as general readers keen to understand how viral pandemics have shaped, and continue to shape, millions of lives.

Rae-Ellen W. Kavey, MD, MPH, is a pediatric cardiologist and public health practitioner who retired as Professor of Pediatrics from the University of Rochester School of Medicine. Her career in academic medicine combined care of children with congenital heart disease and a public health approach to prevention of heart disease beginning in childhood. She is currently an adjunct history professor at CUNY John Jay College of Criminal Justice.

Allison B. Kavey, PhD, is a history professor at CUNY John Jay College of Criminal Justice and CUNY Graduate Center. She works in the early modern history of science and medicine.

VIRAL PANDEMICS

From Smallpox to COVID-19 & Mpox

2nd Edition

Rae-Ellen W. Kavey and Allison B. Kavey

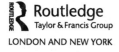
Routledge
Taylor & Francis Group

LONDON AND NEW YORK

Designed cover image: © Getty Images

Second edition published 2025
by Routledge
4 Park Square, Milton Park, Abingdon, Oxon OX14 4RN

and by Routledge
605 Third Avenue, New York, NY 10158

Routledge is an imprint of the Taylor & Francis Group, an informa business

© 2025 Rae-Ellen W. Kavey and Allison B. Kavey

First edition published by Routledge 2020

British Library Cataloguing-in-Publication Data
A catalogue record for this book is available from the British Library

ISBN: 978-1-032-54823-4 (hbk)
ISBN: 978-1-032-54822-7 (pbk)
ISBN: 978-1-003-42766-7 (ebk)

DOI: 10.4324/9781003427667

Typeset in Bembo
by Newgen Publishing UK

Dedications

REK

For Les, whose unfailing support made this book possible.
For Molly, faithful companion from first page to last.

ABK

For all those whose lives have been upended by viruses:
"We work in the dark, we do what we can, we give what we have."
Henry James

CONTENTS

FIGURES

Chapter 1

Chapter 2

Chapter 3

Chapter 4

Chapter 9

Chapter 10

Chapter 11

AUTHOR BIOGRAPHIES

Rae-Ellen W. Kavey, MD, MPH is a pediatric cardiologist and public health practitioner who retired as Professor of Pediatrics from the University of Rochester School of Medicine. Her career in academic medicine combined care of children with congenital heart disease and a public health approach to prevention of heart disease beginning in childhood. She is currently an adjunct history professor at CUNY John Jay College of Criminal Justice.

Allison B. Kavey, PhD, is a history professor at CUNY John Jay College of Criminal Justice and CUNY Graduate Center. She works in the early modern history of science and medicine.

PREFACE

When I volunteered to join the US response to Ebola in West Africa, I knew very little about the virus. It was the late fall of 2014. Newly retired from 40 years in academic medical practice, I was inspired by President Obama's call to action and challenged by the idea of using my medical training in a new situation. After almost 40 years as a practicing physician with a master's degree in Public Health, epidemics were part of both my training and my experience. But as a pediatric cardiologist, they were never a top-of-mind issue. I was rejected as an Ebola volunteer but by then I was completely engaged in the study of viruses and eventually that led to the first edition of this book, co-written with my daughter Allison who is a historian of medicine.

Learning about Ebola exposed me to the extraordinary variety of emerging and re-emerging viruses whose remarkable capacities make them formidable public health adversaries. All the major epidemics since the turn of the last century have been caused by viruses. Every year, the World Health Organization develops a list of dangerous pathogens with the potential to cause future outbreaks and pandemics for prioritization of research and development. Any type of pathogen can be selected but for the last 10 years, all were viruses. It was appreciation of the increasing danger inherent in emerging viral pathogens and recognition of the enormous associated public health risk that suggested viral pandemics as the focus of this book.

Two critical vantage points are integrated in the book: mine, as an experienced physician with an extensive public health background; and my daughter Allison's, as an academic historian of science and medicine. In the first edition of the book, we combined our experience as clinician and historian with extensive research to create a new approach to the evolving history of viral pandemics and its implications. From smallpox and yellow fever, through influenza, polio, HIV/AIDS, West Nile virus and SARS, Ebola and Zika, we presented a comprehensive survey of epidemic viral disease from 1900 through 2019. In each chapter, the narrative follows the path of a virus from its original detection through its initial appearance as the cause of disease to its emergence as an explosive pandemic. In parallel, we identify the elements of connectedness that allowed a local disease outbreak to become a global pandemic, examining the increasingly critical role that human encroachment plays in that process. In creating this historic narrative, it was increasingly clear that serious viral disease outbreaks were occurring at shorter and shorter intervals and were more and more likely to expand and become global pandemics. We had already concluded that it was only a matter of time until a new virus emerged in a globally connected area with the right combination of high infectivity, ready transmissibility and high mortality to cause a new pandemic disaster.

That conclusion was only slightly premature: as we were finalizing the first edition of the book in January 2020, we began to read reports of a new virus emerging in Wuhan, China. Totally immersed in viral pandemic study, we followed the new disease outbreak breathlessly in news reports in the media and in just-released scientific papers, from its first appearance as a cluster of atypical pneumonia cases caused by a novel coronavirus in a single Chinese city. By the end of January 2020 when there was conjecture about how far this outbreak would spread, we were already convinced that here was the global pandemic we had been anticipating. With permission from our editor, we were able to extend the book to report the early spread of SARS-CoV-2 through the end of April 2020, as COVID-19 case numbers and deaths rose all over the world.

In this second edition, we continue the story of the still-ongoing global SARS-CoV-2/COVID-19 pandemic, one of the deadliest pandemics in modern history. The final trajectory is still evolving as the book is being written but its enormous global impact is already apparent with more than 774,075,000 cases and 7,000,000 deaths. This second edition traces the course of that pandemic and its ramifications for medicine, science, public health and history. And while COVID-19 is still winding down, we have already experienced a multi-nation pandemic of Mpox, described in Chapter 9. This new edition also updates the story of every virus in the first edition with an inescapable conclusion: the world is engaged in an era of more complex and more frequent viral epidemics exacerbated by all the factors that drive twenty-first-century civilization. More and worse are still to come.

The book ends with two new chapters: in Chapter 10, Allison examines COVID-19 and our public health response to it through the lens of the history of responses to previous, historic pandemics. By reviewing the development of public health as a field and learning why it continues to rely on just a few, traditional approaches to tackle epidemics, we can see where we went wrong with COVID and how we can do better when we face the next viral outbreak. In the final chapter, Rae-Ellen creates a composite picture of the state of viral disease by integrating the factors that emerged as critical in the analysis of all the pandemics in this book and evaluates this biologic/environmental combination against the medical and scientific measures that have emerged in response. As with the first edition, it remains our hope that by elucidating the lessons of these viral pandemics, we can see how best to achieve a more timely and effective response in the future.

ACKNOWLEDGMENT

Special thanks to Chris George, an unmatched research associate.

1

A BRIEF INTRODUCTION TO VIROLOGY

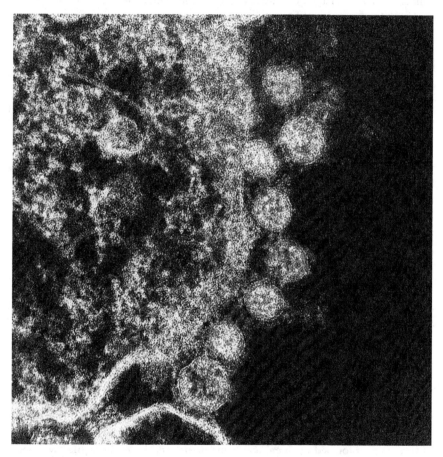

FIGURE 1.1 Scanning electron micrograph of a cell heavily infected with SARS-COV-2 virus particles, isolated from a patient sample.

Source: Image captured at the National Institute of Allergy and Infectious Disease, National Institutes of Health, Integrated Research Facility (IRF) in Fort Detrick, Maryland. NIAID.gov

DOI: 10.4324/9781003427667-1

Global health in the twenty-first century faces unprecedented challenges from highly pathogenic viruses. These invisible but enormously powerful agents have already caused a series of terrifying disease outbreaks: since just the turn of the century, we have faced the emergence of West Nile virus in North America, the continuing global spread of HIV/AIDS, SARS (Severe Acute Respiratory Syndrome), the 2009 H1N1 influenza pandemic, MERS (Middle Eastern Respiratory Syndrome), an overwhelming Ebola pandemic, the global spread of Zika with its devastating pre-natal consequences, the overwhelming SARS-CoV-2/COVID-19 pandemic (whose virus is shown in Figure 1.1) and mpox/monkeypox as a multi-nation disease outbreak. In each case, the unique abilities of the causative virus were critical elements in determining the outcome of the pandemic. To understand the intrinsic factors that determine viral pathogenicity, we begin by tracing the history of virus discovery.

The story begins in the sixteenth century with Girolamo Fracastoro, a Renaissance scholar of philosophy, poetry and medicine who studied with Copernicus at the University of Padua. At the tender age of 19, he was appointed as a professor at the University and elected the official physician of the ecumenical council of the Roman Catholic Church. From his earliest days, he adopted a scientific approach to the study of nature and this may have led to his absorption in understanding the causes of disease. In his 1546 work, *De Contagione et Contagiosis Morbis (On Contagion and Contagious Diseases)*, he described his theory that infection results from "tiny, self-multiplying bodies that can be spread by direct or indirect contact, through infected objects, or even through the air over long distances."[1] This idea of infectious "contagion" had been suggested by others since antiquity but Fracastoro's explanation was the first clear articulation of the concept. At the time, his views were completely ignored in favor of the erroneous "miasma theory": that lethal disease-causing agents arose spontaneously from decomposing material in the earth that traveled by air as a poisonous, foul-smelling vapor. Given the ghastly stench that arose above communities in the Middle Ages without any form of sewage management, it is easy to understand how this theory persisted. It was the mid-1800s before the French microbiologist, Louis Pasteur, determined that it was microscopic bacteria that caused disease and Robert Koch defined the procedure for proving that specific diseases are caused by specific bacteria, essentially formalizing Fracastoro's theory as the germ theory of disease.[2]

Bacteria are the smallest microbes which can survive independently because they carry all the necessary cellular machinery and genetic material to produce energy and reproduce within a single cell. Confirmation of bacteria as the cause of disease transformed the practice of medicine, and by early in the twentieth century, practical extension of the germ theory led to many improved public health sanitation practices like water treatment and sewage disposal. Public education increased awareness of the ways in which bacteria thrive and this supported improved personal hygiene practices like handwashing and safe food preparation. While antibiotics as specific treatments for bacterial infections did not appear until much later in the twentieth century, public health improvements introduced and reinforced by comprehension of the germ theory of disease significantly decreased deaths from infectious diseases from the early 1900s.

Within this context of increasing scientific knowledge and improving public health, viruses were virtually unknown. Bacteria which could be recognized and identified with a light microscope were established as the "germs" of the germ theory. However, despite all the progress linking pathogenic bacteria with disease, a significant number of clearly infectious diseases remained for which no causative bacteria could be identified. It was the late nineteenth century before any progress was made with this dilemma. Scientists who were unable to identify a bacterial cause for a well-recognized disease of tobacco plants called tobacco mosaic disease (TMD) found that an extract of crushed leaves from infected plants passed through a filter that removed all bacteria still caused the disease: they theorized that the filtrate must contain a sub-microscopic infectious agent.[3] This filterable agent was found to multiply only in an environment that included tobacco leaf cells, not in a cell-free environment. This demonstration, confirmed subsequently for all these tiny submicroscopic agents, led ultimately to the conclusion that they were parasites, obligate intracellular organisms which could replicate only in a plant, animal or human host. The term *virus* comes from the Latin word for poison and during the eighteenth and nineteenth centuries, it was used to describe all forms of infectious agents. Over time, *virus* became the specific term for these submicroscopic infectious agents. When the 1918 influenza pandemic occurred, viruses were known only as a mysterious group of tiny microbes that were infectious, filterable and required living cells for replication but their structure and function remained unknown.[3]

While not specifically identified, viruses had caused disease as long as there had been life on earth and outbreaks of viral disease were recorded for centuries, ever since humans began living together in communities. Smallpox was first reported in approximately 10,000 BC and it is still considered to be among the most lethal viral infections. At around that same time, mumps, measles and polio, all caused by viral pathogens, were first described in ancient Egypt. While not necessarily identified as influenza, major flu outbreaks occurred throughout recorded history, beginning as early as 412 BC and extending right through the nineteenth century. The yellow fever virus – the first virus specifically identified as causing human disease – was identified in 1900. In 1909, poliomyelitis was definitively shown to be caused by a virus. By the early twentieth century, viruses had a long and tragic record of causing serious pandemic disease.

It was at this time that the effort to understand viruses became inextricably linked with the devastating 1918 influenza pandemic (more to follow on this pandemic in Chapter 4). Faced with a terrifying disease outbreak for which they had no treatment, doctors and scientists struggled to find a comprehensible bacterial cause, a search which continued long after the pandemic ended. At that time, a viral etiology could only be identified indirectly, by using an ultrafiltrate from a diseased subject to induce disease in a susceptible human, plant or animal host, or by detecting the presence of antibodies against the disease in survivors of the illness in question. Using these indirect methods, viruses had been confirmed as the cause of a number of important human and animal diseases including smallpox, yellow fever, rabies and measles. In 1919, a year after the primary 1918 pandemic ended, scientists from Japan and from France reported separately that a bacteria-free emulsion of mucous or blood from influenza patients produced classical flu symptoms of varying severity when given to monkeys and to human medical volunteers.[4,5] These results strongly suggested that influenza was caused by a virus but scientists were unconvinced, perhaps because at the time, so little was known about the basic nature of viruses.

It was not until ten years after the influenza epidemic that a young American scientist named Richard Shope began studying swine flu, an influenza-like illness that had sickened millions of pigs in the Midwest in the fall of 1918, just as the lethal stage of the influenza pandemic began, and has continued as a seasonal illness in pigs since that time. Shope found that a filtrate of mucous from a pig with swine flu would produce a similar flu-like illness in a healthy pig – conclusion: the cause of swine flu was a virus.[6] By this time, Wilson Smith, Christopher Andrewes and Patrick Laidlaw, three young British researchers had identified the ferret as a good model for influenza, since the animals developed a classic flu-like illness described by the researchers as "fever, sneezing, mucopurulent nasal discharge and sticky encrustation around the nose" within 48 hours after instillation of nasal washings from human volunteers with the flu (I cannot help but picture cages full of miserable, congested ferrets!). Nasal washings from these infected ferrets were then shown to transmit the disease to other ferrets. In addition, injection of serum from ferrets who had recovered from the flu blocked development of the clinical disease. In 1933, these scientists published their work in Lancet, confirming for all that human influenza was caused by a virus.[7] Shope and the British team then collaborated and showed that ferrets inoculated with swine flu filtrate developed an illness indistinguishable from the experimental flu caused by the human flu virus. Did humans give influenza to pigs? Was the swine flu virus actually the human flu virus? Using serum from survivors of the 1918 pandemic, the team showed incomplete blocking of swine flu virus infection, suggesting that the swine flu virus and the human influenza virus were closely related but not identical.[8] Since there was no virus from the 1918 pandemic available for investigation, this swine flu connection could not be further evaluated at the time.

The next important discovery – and this was very important – occurred with attempts to develop an effective influenza vaccine: recognition of the capacity of the influenza virus for spontaneous mutation. Originally, all influenza disease was thought to be caused by the single virus identified in 1933 so vaccines were developed to prevent infection with this specific virus. The concept of immunity was well-established by the early 1900s, based on the historic observation that for many diseases, a single episode conferred lifelong resistance to recurrent infection. With the dawn of bacteriology, antitoxins and vaccines against several important bacterial pathogens including diphtheria, tetanus, anthrax, cholera, plague and typhoid had already been developed. In Britain, Smith and Fellowes developed an experimental influenza vaccine using the 1933 virus strain in a mouse lung model with the virus inactivated by formaldehyde. Tests with the vaccine in ferrets showed that it prevented influenza symptoms with an associated increase in neutralizing antibody levels. On this basis, they conducted a small trial in 30 soldiers in 1936; there was no flu outbreak for clinical comparison that year, but the vaccine did increase antibody levels. The next year, they gave the vaccine to 500 military men with 500 unvaccinated men as controls. The trial was a complete disaster! There was a major flu outbreak but the vaccine proved completely useless, with no difference in influenza cases between the vaccinated and unvaccinated soldiers. The team looked at all the available evidence that could explain the failure of their vaccine. They had already recognized that flu viruses from different years and from other parts of the world evaluated in their lab differed.[9] This evidence of antigenic variation between strains was also recognized by American researchers, Thomas Francis and T.P. Magill in 1936 using cross-neutralization tests.[10] Putting all this information together, Andrewes and his team concluded that the complete failure of their vaccine prepared with the 1933 virus to prevent infection with the 1937 virus strain indicated that significant variation in the virus must have occurred between flu seasons. Recognition of spontaneous mutation of the influenza virus was a critically important revelation that explained a significant part of the dangerous potential of viruses but, at the time, it was seen as a perplexing problem with no solution.

By this time, viruses were recognized as having many of the characteristics already identified for infectious disease pathogens in general. In particular, transmission and infection – the processes by which viruses spread to and infect new hosts – were found to follow the patterns already described for bacteria. Since viruses cannot replicate without using the machinery of a host cell, transmission and infection of new hosts are of primary importance. After contact, viral pathogens can enter our bodies through the mucous membranes of the mouth, eyes, nose, or genital tract; or, through breaks in the skin barrier. There are multiple routes of pathogen transmission to these potential entry sites – aerosol, airborne, direct contact, fomite, oral and vector – and viruses use them all. Aerosol transmission involves the spread of droplets from the nose, mouth or respiratory tract of an infected person via sneezing, coughing, or talking – this is the primary mode of transmission for all the viruses that cause the common cold. Airborne transmission means inhalation of virus carried in the air, potentially remote from the source of infection. Transmission by direct contact requires that infected skin, mucous membranes or body fluids contact the mucous membranes or a break in the skin of the new host – sexually transmitted diseases are primarily spread this way. Fomite transmission occurs when items used by infected individuals transfer the virus from one individual to another – counter-tops, clothing and bedding are all potential surfaces for viral contamination and transmission.

Fomite infection involves a secondary exposure route such as direct contact for the pathogen from the contaminated object to enter the new host. Oral infection involves ingestion of food or water contaminated by the virus but it can also occur by fecal-oral transmission, from the hands of an infected individual with poor hygiene to the hands – and then the mouth – of a new host. Infected insects or animals – called vectors– can also transmit viral disease: the most common vector for human viral disease is the mosquito. Finally, viruses can be vertically transmitted from mother to baby during pregnancy and in the peri-partum period, across the placenta or through direct contact during or immediately after birth, and during breast-feeding. This is an important mode of transmission for viruses that are carried in the blood and other body fluids. Many viruses use multiple modes of transmission – another way they maximize their potential to infect.[11,12]

Between the 1930s and the 1950s, progressive understanding of viruses was inextricably linked to progress in imaging, genetics and molecular biology. Invention of the electron microscope (EM) in 1931 gave scientists the first images of viruses which were seen to be extremely small, roughly 100 to 300 times smaller than bacteria, ranging from 20 to 400 nanometers in diameter.[13] In 1935, examination of the infamous tobacco mosaic virus revealed the very simple basic structure of all viruses as shown in Figure 1.2: a protective protein shell or

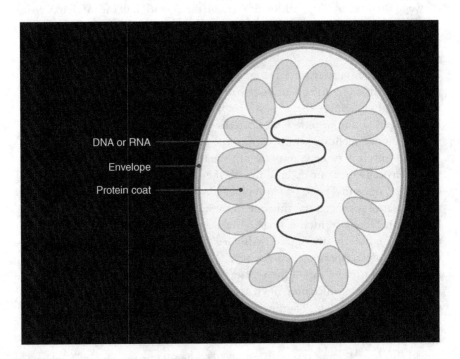

FIGURE 1.2 Basic virus diagram.

Source: https://en.wikipedia.org/wiki/en:Creative_Commons

capsid around a nucleic-acid core of either DNA or RNA, the viral genome.[14] This work showed that viruses were actually particles, not cells, with the capsid composed of protein subunits called capsomeres; the arrangement of capsomeres around the viral genome determined the shape of the virion. In some viruses, an outer layer was seen to envelope the capsid.[15] As the smallest and simplest of known infectious agents, viruses were famously described as "a piece of bad news wrapped up in protein."[16]

As early as the mid-1930s, researchers began studying bacteriophage, a type of virus which only infects bacteria. Bacteriophage do not cause disease in humans and they multiply rapidly in large numbers so they are ideal subjects for the study of viruses. Beginning with EM visualization, Max Delbruck and Salvador Luria, young researchers at the Marine Biological Lab in Woods Hole, described the process of viral replication.[17] Outside of a host cell, they showed that a virus was metabolically inert but when contact was made, the virus inserted its genetic material and took over the cell's functions. Newly created virus components were assembled into thousands of new viruses – called virions – which left the host cell, either by bursting through the call membrane and killing the host cell, or by budding through the cell membrane in which case, the cell survived and could function as a viral reservoir.[18,19] In either case, the released virions then went on to infect new host cells.

In 1945, the Delbruck-Luria team made another critically important discovery when they described genetic recombination: two virus particles simultaneously infecting the same cell could exchange parts of their strings of genes resulting in new, hybrid forms of the original viruses.[20] Along with Alfred Hershey, Delbruck and Lurai received the 1969 Nobel Prize for medicine because of their "discoveries concerning the replication mechanism and the genetic structure of viruses."[21]

Viral studies were critical to the new and important field of molecular genetics. Beginning in the mid-1940s, scientists focused on identifying the exact nature of the biomolecule that carries hereditary information. Although the five nucleotide bases – adenine, cytosine, guanine, thymine and uracil – had originally been described back in 1910, it was not until 1950 that Erwin Chargaff and his team discovered that within deoxyribonucleic acid or DNA, thymine(T) is always paired with adenine(A) and cytosine(C) is always paired with guanine(G).[22,23] In 1952, working again with bacteriophage, Alfred Hershey and Martha Chase showed that DNA is the molecule that carries all of the genetic instructions for cell growth and replication.[24] In 1953, Watson and Crick famously identified the double helix structure of DNA, based on work in viruses, and crystallographic and x-ray diffraction images obtained by Rosalind Franklin and Maurice Wilkins.[25] They showed that human cells contain two strands of DNA, each composed of sequences of the four nucleotide bases. The nucleotide bases in one strand are paired with their complementary partners in the opposite strand – A with T, C with G – to form the connecting rungs of the DNA ladder. Viruses use the same system of matching base pairs in their DNA but they have a very simple genome, averaging only 3 to 400 genes, compared with 20,000 to 25,000 genes in the human genome.[26] In 1956, a series of experiments culminated in the demonstration that ribonucleic acid or RNA could also be the carrier of genetic information when this was shown to be the case for the infamous tobacco mosaic virus.[27] However, the adenine-thymine base pairing in DNA is replaced with adenine-uracil pairing in RNA. In 1984 – more than 60 years after the Great Influenza Pandemic – the influenza virus was found to be a single-stranded RNA virus with eight segments.[28] Among so-called "medical" viruses – those identified as associated with disease – 70% are RNA viruses.[29]

Understanding of the structure of genetic material led to recognition that point mutations – spontaneous changes in a single nucleotide – were common to all cells, bacteria and viruses and this was identified as an explanation for ongoing variation, like that recognized with the influenza virus back in the 1930s. With point mutation, these small, subtle changes are incorporated into the viral genome, a process called *genetic drift* which can result in literally thousands of viral lineages and sub-lineages. Mutation rates differ significantly between DNA and RNA viruses because the process of DNA division is highly regulated with specific checkpoints to detect miscopied DNA and eliminate major mutations. RNA viruses have no such system and therefore have much higher mutation rates, approximately one mutation per genome copy.[29] Only mutations that do not interfere with essential viral function survive but the high mutation rate in RNA viruses leading to a veritable cloud of mutant descendants provides many opportunities for this to occur.

The process of recombination identified by the Cold Spring Harbor team – two virus particles simultaneously infecting the same cell exchanging parts of their genetic material to produce new hybrid forms of the original viruses – was found to occur primarily in DNA viruses and was recognized as resulting in new viral strains which could infect previously resistant hosts, an important part of the infectivity of viruses. A particular form of recombination called "reassortment" occurred only in RNA viruses with segmented RNA. In this setting, whole segments of genetic material are exchanged resulting in progeny with immediate and major antigenic change, a process called *genetic shift*.[30,31] Based on findings like these, it was recognized that reassortment could yield an entirely new and antigenically novel virus strain. In the time needed for a virus replication cycle, an infinitesimal killer virus could emerge, highly infectious, easily transmittable and lethal. It was molecular genetic work that identified this most important characteristic of RNA viruses: endless evolution by both spontaneous nucleotide substitution and genetic reassortment leading to continuous emergence of new, antigenically novel strains. Faced with an entirely new virus strain, hosts have little if any resistance so these emerging strains have high infectivity. This is especially true when reassortment occurs between an animal virus and a human virus.

In addition to the capacity for reassortment, some viruses have an unexpectedly wide host range with natural hosts that are infected in a primary transmission cycle and alternative hosts which can be infected by spillover from that original species to another. This species cross-over was recognized by Richard Swope when he found the human influenza virus from the 1918 pandemic had crossed over to infect pigs.[6] An important part of the dangerous potential of viruses emerges when a virus is transmitted directly from animals to humans. Spillover of a virus across the species barrier to infect a human exposes an immunologically naïve subject to a potentially devastating new pathogen. Such zoonotic transmission requires intimate contact between animals and people so historically, it was identified in domestic animals.[32] As rising global population density has brought wild animals and human populations into increasingly close contact, new infectious disease threats are often found to have wildlife origins. Zoonotic viruses are the most frequent newly emerging human pathogens, constituting 85% of all pathogens discovered since 1980.[33] With their high rates of nucleotide substitution, poor mutation error-correction ability and therefore higher capacity to attack new hosts, RNA viruses have been identified as a major threat for cross-species infection. Reservoir infections are a final and important source of viral survival and infectious potential. Viruses cannot survive independently but they can be sustained in animal or human hosts who have no apparent signs of disease but serve as an ongoing source of infection and of genetic material for the emergence of unique and dangerous new pathogens.[34]

It was not until the 1970s that progress was made in understanding the complex process of virus cell entry into host cells, the mandatory initiation of cell infection. The critical first step is bonding of an invading virus to a host cell's plasma membrane receptors. Virus-specific surface proteins bind with a large range of cell surface proteins, lipids and glycans including optionally, multiple receptors.[34] Only rarely do viruses fuse directly with the host cell plasma membranes; the majority of viruses are transported by the endocytotic mechanisms of the new host cell before penetrating the cytosol, the liquid phase of the cytoplasm in an intact cell.[35] After penetration, invading viruses move to sites of replication in the cytosol, for RNA viruses, or the nucleus, for DNA viruses. Uncoating of the viral genome is the final step in the entry process. The development of cryo-electron microscopy has resulted in multiple new imaging techniques based on the principle of imaging radiation-sensitive specimens in a transmission electron microscope under cryogenic conditions.[36,37] This powerful new technology is being applied to virus-specific identification of the cell entry process, an important contemporary research target focused on development of new, effective antiviral treatment and prevention strategies.[38]

Development of techniques for gene sequencing led to phylogenetic evolutionary analysis, an important tool for describing the interconnected evolutionary histories of living organisms based on their molecular sequences. This is actually a derivation of the concept first described explicitly by Charles Darwin who used morphological characteristics to determine the degree of similarity between organisms and thereby imply an evolutionary relationship.[39] As molecular techniques became available providing detailed, unambiguous identifiers in the form of DNA or RNA sequences, these replaced the old, indirect, observational methods.[40] DNA or RNA sequence analyses provide explicit information about the entire genome of an organism. Comparison of sequencing data from different organisms allows construction of a tree-like pattern that depicts the evolutionary relationships among the group. Because of the number and complexity of nucleotide sequences in most comparisons, computer programs are used to perform the analyses. These techniques allow visualization of the origin of changes in disease severity and transmissibility of specific pathogens.

A secondary goal of phylogenetic analysis is to determine the *timing* of ancestral sequence divergence. In RNA viruses where spontaneous mutation (i.e., divergence) is common, phylogenetic analysis can determine when separate genetic lineages arose relative to each other. This concept gave rise to the idea of a *molecular clock* – using the mutation rate of biomolecules to determine the time in prehistory when two or more biomolecules diverged, with the benchmark time before divergence based on fossil or archeological dates.[41–43] Timing the emergence of new mutations is important in analysis of viral epidemics because it allows us to infer the pattern and order of evolutionary change, especially when correlated with historic data and this can identify the origin of a pandemic virus.

The Infinite – and Infinitely Powerful – Virosphere

Early viral research focused on the identification of pathogenic viruses as the cause of specific diseases. Scientists developed a relatively simple system of viral classification based on the type of nucleic acid (DNA or RNA); the shape of the virus capsid; the capsid diameter and/or the number of capsomeres; and the presence or absence of an envelope. Over time, we have recognized that disease etiology is an exceptionally narrow lens with which to view the vast world of viruses which are the most abundant entities on the planet. By focusing on viruses that cause disease, we have identified only a tiny fraction of the earth's virus population. Viruses are the most abundant life forms in the ocean with "10 billion viruses per liter of sea water."[44] They play a role in all the earth's ecosystems but our understanding of this is still largely unexplored. Within the human microbiome – the ecological community of commensal, symbiotic, and pathogenic microorganisms that share our body space – there are literally millions of stable viral communities which scientists are only beginning to study via recent advances in sequencing and bio-informatic technologies.[45] And the number of virions in the virosphere – the universe of viruses on the planet – is almost beyond comprehension: a study in the Sierra Nevada mountains found 800 million viruses cascade onto every square meter of the earth's surface every day![46]

Viruses are formidable enemies. Despite their tiny size and minimal structure, their inertia and inability to independently replicate or produce energy, viruses have remarkable capabilities. Their extraordinary diversity, their remarkable capacity for rapid evolution and their ability to infect multiple species, allow

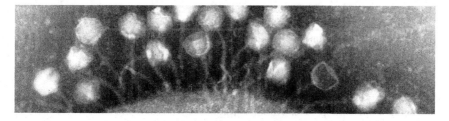

FIGURE 1.3 Electron micrograph of viral bacteriophage infecting a cell.
Source: Dr. Graham Beards. WikiMedia. Fair use.

them to endlessly evolve into novel forms that can cause new diseases, capable of sweeping through whole populations and leaving utter devastation behind. Multiple modes of transmission like the airborne method shown in Figure 1.3 amplify the ability of viruses to cause infection. When a virus infects a living cell, it can rapidly multiply and destroy its host; it can lie dormant, emerging to multiply or reassort at some later date; or it can co-exist within that reservoir host for generations. It is these unique capabilities which identify viruses as a major threat to human existence. In the following chapters, each dedicated to a specific viral epidemic, we will analyze the characteristics of the causative virus to identify the factors that allowed a local disease outbreak to explode into a global pandemic. In so doing, we will also explore a tiny fraction of the enormously diverse population of the earth's vast virosphere.

References

[1] Magner LM. *A History of Medicine.* Second edition. New York, NY. Informa Healthcare. 2005; p.496–497.
[2] Magner LM. *A History of Medicine.* Second edition. New York, NY. Informa Healthcare. 2005; p.502, 516.
[3] Levine AJ. *Viruses.* New York, NY. Scientific American Library. Distributed by W.H. Freeman and Company. 1992; Chapter 1.
[4] Nicolle C, LeBailly C. Recherches experimentale sur la grippe. *Annales de l'Institut Pasteur* 1919; 33:395–402.
[5] Yamanouchi T. Skakami K, Iwashima S. The infecting agent in Influenza. *Lancet* 1919; 193: 971.
[6] Shope RE. Swine influenza, Experimental transmission and pathology. *J Exp Med* 1931; 54: 349–373.
[7] Smith W, Andrewes CH, Laidlaw PP. A virus obtained from influenza patients. *Lancet* 1933; 2:66–8.
[8] Wood JM, Williams MS. History of inactivated Influenza vaccines. In: *Textbook of Influenza.* Oxford: Blackwell Science 1998: pp. 317–323.
[9] Glover RE, Andrewes CH. The antigenic structure of British strains of influenza virus. *J Comp Path Ther* 1943; 53:32–41.
[10] Francis T, Magill TP. The antibody response of human subjects vaccinated with the virus of human influenza. *J Exp Med* 1938; 68:147–60.

[11] Barreto ML, Teixeira MG, Carmo EH. Infectious diseases epidemiology. *J Epidemiol Comm Health* 2006;60(3): 192–195.

[12] Antonovics J, Wilson AJ, Forbes MR, et al. The evolution of transmission mode. *Philos Trans R Soc Lond B Biol Sci* 2017; 372(1719): 20160083.

[13] Crawford DH. *Viruses. A Very Short Introduction.* Oxford University Press Inc., New York, N.Y. 2011. Pg. 4.

[14] Kausche GA, Pfankuch E, Ruska H. Die Sichtbarmachung von pflanzlichem Virus im Übermikroskop. *Naturwissenschaften*. 1939; 27(18): 292–299.

[15] Crawford. 2011. Pg. 5.

[16] Medawar PB, Medawar JS. Aristotle to Zoos. *A Philosophical Dictionary of Biology.* 1983. Harvard University Press. Cambridge, Massachusetts, USA. 1983.

[17] Luria SE, Delbruck M, Anderson TF. Electron microscope studies of bacterial viruses. *J Bacteriol* 1943; 46: 57–76.

[18] Crawford. 2011. Pg. 9.

[19] Casasnovas JM. Virus-receptor interactions and receptor-mediated virus entry into host cells. *Subcell Biochem* 2013; 68:441–466.

[20] Luria SE. Mutations of bacterial viruses affecting their host range. *Genetics* 1945; 30:84–99.

[21] The Nobel Prize in Physiology or Medicine 1969. Nobel Media AB 2013, Nobelprize.org, Web access October 12, 2016.

[22] Mathews AP. Professor Albrecht Kossel. *Science*. 1927 Sep 30;66(1709):293–293.

[23] Chargaff E, Zamenhof S, Green C. Composition of human desoxypentose nucleic acid. *Nature* 1950; 165(4202): 756–7.

[24] Hershey A, Chase M. Independent functions of viral protein and nucleic acid in growth of bacteriophage. *J Gen Physiol.* 1952; 36(1): 39–56.

[25] Crick F, Watson JD. Molecular structure of nucleic acids: A structure for deoxyribose nucleic acid. *Nature* 1953; 171:737–738.

[26] Willyard C. New human genome tally reignites debate. *Nature* 2018; 558:354–355.

[27] Pennazio S, Roggero P. Tobacco mosaic virus RNA as genetic determinant: genesis of a discovery. *Riv Biol.* 2000; 93(3):431–55.

[28] McCauley JW, Mahy BWJ. Structure and function of the influenza virus genome. *Biochem J* 1983; 211: 281–294.

[29] Gelderblom HR. *Structure and Classification of Viruses. In Medical Microbiology, Eighth Edition. Chapter 41.* Edited by Patrick R. Murray, Ken S. Rosenthal, Michael A. Pfaller. Elsevier. Philadelphia, PA. 2016.

[30] Steinhauer DA, Holland JJ. Rapid evolution of RNA viruses. *Ann Rev Microbiol* 1987; 41: 409–433.

[31] Burnet FM, Lind PE. A genetic approach to variation in influenza viruses: recombination of characters in influenza virus strains used in mixed infections. *J Gen Microbiol* 1951; 5(1): 67–82.

[32] Parrish CR, Holmes EC, Morens DM, et al. Cross-species virus transmission and the emergence of new epidemic diseases. *Microbiol Mol Biol Rev* 2008; 72(3):457–470.

[33] Woodhouse M, Gaunt E. Ecological origins of novel human pathogens. *Crit Rev Microbiol* 2007; 33: 231–242.

[34] Haydon HT. Identifying Reservoirs of Infection: A Conceptual and Practical Challenge. *Emerg Inf Dis* 2002; 8(12): 1468–1473.

[35] Yamauchi Y, Helenius A. Virus entry at a glance. *J Cell Science* 2013; 126(6): 1289–1295.

[36] Lozach P-Y. Early virus-host cell interactions. *J Mol Biol* 2018; 430: 2555–2556.

[37] Milne JLS, Borgnia MJ, Bartesaghi A, et al. Cryo-electron microscopy: a primer for the non-microscopist. *FEBS* 2013; 280(1): 28–45.

[38] Caston JR. Conventional electron microscopy, cryo-electron microscopy and cryo-electron tomography of viruses. *Subcell Biochem* 2013; 68: 79–115.

[39] Helenius A. Virus entry: Looking back and moving forward. *J Mol Biol* 2018; 430: 1853–1862.

[40] Futuyma DJ, Agrawal AA. Evolutionary history and species interactions. *PNAS* 2009; 106(43): 18043–18044.

[41] Heather HM, Chain B. The sequence of sequencers: the history of sequencing DNA. *Genomics* 2016; 107:1–8.

[42] Morgan GJ, Zuckerkandl E. Linus Pauling, and the molecular evolutionary clock, 1959–1965. *J Hist Biol* 1998; 31(2): 155–178.

[43] Ho S. The molecular clock and estimating species divergence. *Nature Education* 2008; 1(1): 168–169.

[44] Crawford. 2005. Pg. 17.

[45] Prescott SL. History of medicine: Origin of the term microbiome and why it matters. *Human Microbiome J* 2017; 4:24–25.

[46] Reche I, D'Orta G, Mladenov N, Winget DM, Suttle CA. Deposition rates of viruses and bacteria above the atmospheric boundary layer. *ISME J* 2018; 12: 1154–1162.

Suggested Reading

Anthony Peter, Lise Wilkinson. *An Introduction to the History of Virology.* Cambridge University Press. Cambridge, London, New York. 1978.

Arnold J. Levine. *Viruses. Scientific American Library.* W.H. Freeman and Company. New York. 1992.

Dorothy H. Crawford. *The Invisible Enemy. A Natural History of Viruses.* Oxford University Press. Oxford, UK, New York. 2000.

Dorothy H. Crawford. *Viruses. A Very Short Introduction.* Oxford University Press Inc. New York. 2011.

Ed Yong. *I Contain Multitudes: The Microbes Within Us and a Grander View of Life.* Harper Collins Publishers. New York. 2016.

Patrick R. Murray, Ken S. Rosenthal, Michael A. Pfaller. *Medical Microbiology,* Eighth Edition. Elsevier. Philadelphia, PA. 2016.

2

THE SMALLPOX STORY

Gone but Not Forgotten

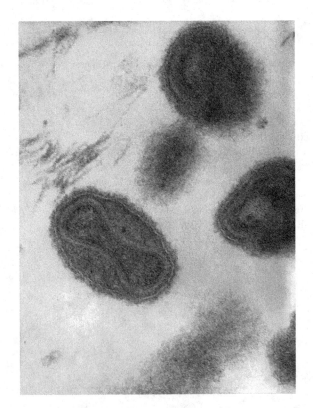

FIGURE 2.1 Electron micrograph of smallpox virus.

Source: Photograph courtesy of US Public Health Image Library. PHIL.CDC.gov

DOI: 10.4324/9781003427667-2

A SMALL REMINDER

Everybody remembers where they were when they first learned about the attacks on the World Trade Center. Like the assassination of JFK and the death of John Lennon, these events mark our hearts and our memories forever. But I'm guessing that many fewer will remember the other act of terrorism that occurred in that same month – a bioweapons attack that on this occasion took many fewer lives but had the potential to end the world as we know it.

On October 2, 2001, three weeks after 9/11, an infectious disease specialist recognized a possible case of inhalational anthrax in a critically ill man in Palm Beach County, Florida. On October 4, the diagnosis was confirmed when Bacillus anthracis was identified and Florida Department of Health and the Centers for Disease Control and Prevention (CDC) launched emergent epidemiologic and environmental investigations to determine the source of the patient's anthrax exposure. Bacillus anthracis spores were found at American Media Inc. in Boca Raton where the patient worked as a photo editor. On October 5, this first victim of the anthrax attacks died and subsequently it was determined that the spores that infected him had been contained in one of five letters with Trenton, New Jersey postmarks, mailed September 18, 2001, exactly one week after the World Trade Center attacks. The letters were mailed to ABC, CBS and NBC News and the *New York Post* newspaper, all in New York City, and the National Inquirer in Boca Raton, Florida – the site of the first victim's infection. Three weeks after the first mailing, two more letters containing anthrax with the same New Jersey postmark, were mailed, addressed to two Democratic Senators, Tom Daschle and Patrick Leahy. At the time, Daschle was the Senate Majority leader and Leahy was head of the Senate Judiciary Committee. Ultimately, the letters infected 22 people with anthrax and five died.

The attacks on the World Trade Center were an unprecedented tragedy. But as a physician with a public health background, the 2001 anthrax attacks were an important personal wake-up call: at the time, I was only minimally aware of existing American biodefense efforts and the major thing I could recall about anthrax was that the bacteria causes pneumonia and creates spores which can survive for extremely long periods of time. I learned quickly: anthrax is a serious infectious disease caused by contact with the spores of the bacteria, Bacillus anthracis. The most critical disease presentation is caused by inhalation of the spores as occurred in the Florida case in this outbreak, associated with a mortality rate of more than 80%. Anthrax can be treated with antibiotics but its non-specific presentation often delays diagnosis until disease is far advanced. It is a well-known agent of bioterrorism.

It was sometime after 9/11, in those first weeks of fear and confusion and passionate patriotism, when the Department of Homeland Security was established and when American flags flew from every possible vantage point, that I first heard the term "weapons of mass destruction" or WMD, defined by the United Nations as a "nuclear, radiological, chemical or biological weapon that can harm and/or kill a large number of humans or cause great damage to man-made structures, natural structures or the biosphere." The first recorded use of the term is by the Archbishop of Canterbury in 1937 in reference to the aerial bombardment of Guernica, Spain:

> Who can think at this present time without a sickening of the heart of the appalling slaughter, the suffering, the manifold misery brought by war to Spain and then China? Who can think without horror of what another widespread war would mean, waged as it would be with all the new weapons of mass destruction?

For most, I think WMD denotes nuclear weapons but it is at least as likely that the next major terrorist attack will be chemical or biological. Multiple sources make it clear that anthrax and smallpox were critical components of the American biological warfare program initiated by FDR in 1942, in response to reports that the Germans were preparing a biological weapon for use against the Allies. A new American bioweapons team was working with Canada and Britain to create biological cluster bombs when the United States dropped the atomic bomb on Hiroshima, effectively ending the war. But during the Cold War, the American biological warfare program expanded, focused on methods for dissemination of biological agents like smallpox and anthrax in multiple settings. By 1968, we had developed effective techniques for mass delivery of biological WMD when unexpectedly, President Nixon announced the unconditional end of all US offensive biological weapons programs. In 1972, the United States signed the Biological and Toxin Weapons Convention, along with the United Kingdom, the Soviet Union and more than a hundred other countries. The signers agreed that all offensive biological weapons research would end and all existing biological arsenals would be destroyed. Subsequently, the United States focused its bioweapons research on defense but attacks with biological agents and intelligence reports indicate that most other signatories neither stopped manufacturing new bioweapons nor destroyed their arsenals. According to Russian defectors, the Soviet bioweapons program actually accelerated after 1972 with both smallpox and anthrax as major components. Biological WMD are a critical international concern.

The investigation of the 2001 anthrax attacks was a long, complex narrative of intrigue and ignorance. At the outset, the FBI focused on determining whether there was any connection with the World Trade Center attacks, eventually concluding that the anthrax attacks were an independent act of domestic bioterrorism. A critical early error was made in October 2001, when the FBI and the CDC agreed to the destruction of a large collection of anthrax spores collected over more than seven decades and stored at Iowa State University, eliminating the possibility of matching the strain of anthrax used in the attacks and a strain in the collection which might have allowed early identification of the perpetrator. As it happened, the FBI "Amerithrax" Task Force – which consisted of investigators from the FBI, the US Postal Inspection Service, and other law enforcement agencies, as well as federal prosecutors from the District of Columbia and the Justice Department's Counterterrorism Section – expended hundreds of thousands of investigator work hours on the case which included collection of 5730 environmental samples from 60 locations. New genetic methods were even developed for analysis of anthrax to trace the origin of the anthrax spores. Ultimately, the attacks were attributed to an American government scientist with a history of mental illness who was a longtime anthrax researcher. He committed suicide in 2008, just as the FBI was preparing to charge him. The case was finally declared closed in 2012 but there are still doubts about the conclusion of the investigation. It *is* clear that in the anthrax letter attacks of 9/11, we escaped a potentially devastating epidemic since it is estimated that under ideal weather conditions, release of just one kilogram of anthrax spores over Washington DC could infect up to 50,000 people.

The 9/11 attack and the anthrax attacks precipitated a complete overhaul and escalation of the American biodefense program which had been relatively untouched since 1972. New guidelines for preparedness against bioweapons were developed and disseminated by the CDC focused on diseases that can be directly transmitted between people and have high mortality rates, especially smallpox and anthrax. Despite its complete eradication in 1980, smallpox is still considered a first-line potential biological weapon. Whether the many, diverse defense efforts that were initiated following 9/11 are in any way effective remains to be seen. But everything I read about biological weapons of mass destruction raised the specter of smallpox as a key component in that armamentarium. And that led me to the two opposing stories in this chapter: the history of smallpox and its eradication as a clinical disease and its ongoing role as a potential WMD ...

The Smallpox Story: Gone but Not Forgotten

On May 8, 1980, the World Health Organization announced that after a 10-year campaign, smallpox had been eradicated from the face of the earth.[1] This has been hailed as the greatest public health achievement in medical history. It has certainly been effective in limiting contemporary medical experience with this dreaded disease: in almost 40 years of practice, my only exposure to smallpox was my own vaccination scar. So in a book focused on illuminating the progressive threat of emerging viral pandemics, where is the place for an eradicated disease like smallpox? The answers are clear: first, the campaign stands as a model for how application of epidemiologic and pathogen-specific knowledge plus sheer human persistence can alter the course of even the deadliest diseases; – and study of how smallpox eradication was accomplished provides important lessons for current and future disease eradication efforts. Second, the story of smallpox as a potential bioterrorist weapon shows us that with powerful viral pathogens, we are never safe.

The Disease

Smallpox is a ghastly disease. Infection occurs through inhalation of the airborne *Variola major* virus (shown in Figure 2.1) via droplets from the nose or mouth of an actively infected individual, from face-to-face contact with an infected individual or by direct contact with contaminated objects such as bedding or clothing. The virus is highly infectious – susceptible persons have up to a 90% chance of contracting the disease if they are exposed to someone who is infected. There is a 12–14 day incubation period before symptoms begin. Once inhaled, the virus invades the lining of the mouth and throat, migrates to regional lymph nodes in the neck and begins to multiply. During the incubation period, the infected individual is asymptomatic and non-infective. Around the 12th day, lysis of infected cells occurs and the virus explodes into the bloodstream in large quantities with further viral multiplication in the spleen, bone marrow and lymph nodes. Initial symptoms at this time are non-specific and include fever, myalgia, malaise, headache, nausea, vomiting and backache followed by the appearance of the first visible lesions, small reddish spots in the mouth and throat. These lesions rapidly enlarge and ulcerate, releasing large amounts of virus into the saliva at which point the individual becomes very highly infectious. In 90% of patients, the characteristic skin rash begins 24–48 hours later, first on the face with rapid spread to proximal portions of extremities, the trunk, and lastly the distal extremities including the palms and soles. The ultimate distribution is worst on the face and extremities. The virus invades the lowest levels of the skin, the dermis, via the capillary blood supply. By the second day of the rash, the macules become raised papules and by the third or fourth day, these become vesicular, filled with an opalescent fluid which becomes turbid within 24–48 hours as the pustules fill with tissue debris. This stage lasts 24–36 hours, after which no new lesions appear. Over the next 5 days, the pustules enlarge so that in most cases, the entire surface of the face is covered with sharply raised, tensely distended and extremely painful vesicles which are deeply embedded in the skin, literally tearing the dermis from its underlying support (Figure 2.2). In the typical case, fluid slowly leaks from the pustules over the next week after which they progressively dry up and crust over. By the end of the third week of the illness, scabs have formed over all the lesions, which

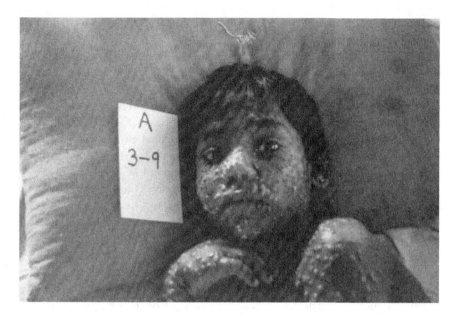

FIGURE 2.2 Unidentified child with classic smallpox rash.

Source: Archives of the US Centers for Disease Control and Prevention (cdc.gov).

then flake off leaving depressed, depigmented, disfiguring scars. As terrible as smallpox looked, the suffering it caused was even worse as the pox lesions were intensely painful, making eating very difficult, every movement agony and sleep impossible.[2]

The virus can be transmitted throughout the course of clinical illness, but this is most intense during the first week of the rash, when mouth lesions have ulcerated but most skin lesions are intact. Infectivity decreases as scabs form over the lesions, but the infected person is contagious until the last smallpox scab falls off. If stored in cool, dry, and dark conditions, the variola virus can survive in lesion crusts or tissues for months or even years.[3] Infection from fomites – nonliving objects or substances carrying infectious organisms and therefore capable of transferring them from one individual to another – was recognized during epidemics in the 1500s and this led to the practice of burning all the bedding and personal items associated with a smallpox patient.

With classic smallpox, death occurred in ~30% of patients due to a massive immune response that caused severe disruption of the clotting system with development of disseminated intravascular coagulation (diffuse clotting throughout the body, a common endpoint of severe systemic infection) and multiple organ failure. In eighteenth-century Europe, 400,000 people died annually of smallpox, and one third of the survivors were blind.[4] The case-fatality rate varied from 20–60% and left most survivors with disfiguring scars. The case-fatality rate in infants was even higher, approaching 80% in London and 98% in Berlin during the late 1800s.[4,5] No wonder smallpox was viewed as "... the most terrible of all the ministers of death."[4]

Historically, there were some variations in the clinical presentation. Sometimes, the pustules merged into sheets, forming a confluent rash, which could begin to detach the outer layers of skin from the underlying flesh – a ghastly, incredibly painful variation. Patients with confluent smallpox often remained ill even after scabs formed over all the lesions. In 5–10% of cases, a malignant form of the disease developed where the skin lesions remained almost flush with the skin. Historically, this was much more common in children and was associated with prolonged high fever, extensive rash of the mouth and throat and severe symptoms of systemic illness. Skin lesions matured slowly and by the seventh or eighth day were still flat and appeared to be buried in the skin. Finally, in ~2% of adult cases, a hemorrhagic form of the disease developed with subconjunctival bleeding in the eyes and internal hemorrhage in the spleen, kidney, muscle, and other organs accompanied by derangements of the clotting system. Death often occurred suddenly between the fifth and seventh days of illness, when only a few insignificant skin lesions were present. With each of these variations, the fatality rate was higher than with classic smallpox, ranging from 60–90%.[2]

Late in the nineteenth century, a milder form of smallpox appeared, originally in South Africa, South America, Europe, and Australia and subsequently, in the United States. This much less serious disease was called *Variola minor* or *Variola alastrim* in contrast to *Variola major*, the classic form of the disease. Although individuals infected with *Variola minor* did develop characteristic pox lesions, the pox were widely separated and victims generally felt well throughout the illness, with no disfiguring scars after recovery and no risk of blindness. The mortality rate was only 1%. But importantly, surviving either *Variola major* or *Variola minor* provided lifelong immunity to both forms of smallpox.[2]

★★★★★★★★★

From the earliest descriptions, the marks of smallpox determined how it was defined. The word "variola" was applied to smallpox beginning in 570 BCE, as a term derived from the Latin "varius" which means stained, or "varus" which means mark on the skin.[4] Smallpox was the full name given to the disease to differentiate it from syphilis (the "great pox") and other diseases with rashes that also left residual scars. The date of first appearance of smallpox is unclear. Historical records suggest it evolved from a virus affecting animals – most likely rodents – and made the leap to humans in about 10,000 BCE, when the river valleys of Egypt and the Middle East were first settled. The smallpox virus only survived within the body of humans, so from that point onwards, it passed in a chain of infection from the ancient world right into the modern age. Historically, what are considered to be signs of smallpox infection have been found on skeletal remains from Africa as early as 10,000 BCE.[6] Mummies recovered from 1570–1085 BCE in ancient Egypt are thought to demonstrate smallpox scars, most famously, the mummy of Ramses V.[4,5] In 430 BC, a major epidemic is thought to have occurred in Athens, Greece, chronicled by Thucydides. This was the first time it was recorded that those who survived smallpox were subsequently immune, an observation confirmed by Abu Bakr Mohammad Ibn Zakariya al-Razi, known in the West as Rhazes, the leading scholar of the early Islamic world.[7] Traders are thought to have carried the disease from the Mediterranean to India during the 1st millennium BC.[6,8] Smallpox may even have contributed to the decline of the Roman empire, when in 108 AD, it is thought to have been the cause of an acute illness in the city of Antonine which killed as many as 7 million people.[4,9] However, this early history is unconfirmed as smallpox is never described in the Bible and it is absent from the literature of the Greeks and Romans with no description in the works of Hippocrates.[10] From India, smallpox spread into China in the first century AD and reached Japan in the sixth century.

It is clear that smallpox appeared in Europe during the Middle Ages, apparently coming from both Asia and Africa following trade and migration routes and the paths of the crusaders. We know that "pox houses" were built in the era of the Crusades, along the routes from Europe to the Holy Land. Some historians believe smallpox in the medieval period was a much less severe form of the disease and that over time, smallpox grew more and more deadly. By the sixteenth century it was endemic throughout Europe with cyclical epidemics causing severe mortality. Smallpox continued to ravage Europe, Asia, and Africa from the 1600s into the 1900s. By the eighteenth century, smallpox in Britain was at its height. It was at this time that the great Victorian historian Lord Macaulay wrote:

> The smallpox was always present, filling the churchyards with corpses, tormenting with constant fear all who it had not yet stricken, leaving on those whose lives it spared the hideous traces of its power, turning the babe into a changeling at which the mother shuddered, and making the eyes and cheeks of the betrothed maiden the objects of horror to the lover.[4]

In the last half of the 1700s, smallpox accounted for 10–20% of all deaths in England and Scotland. It was famously described as a disease of "princes and paupers', and the royal dynasties of Europe were particularly badly hit. In the first eight decades of the eighteenth century, smallpox killed an Austrian emperor, a king of Spain, a tsar of Russia, a queen of Sweden, and a king of France. Smallpox also had a devastating effect on England's ruling elite: Charles II's brother and sister were both killed by smallpox; his nephew, King William III, suffered smallpox; and William's wife, Queen Mary, died of it. William's successor Queen Anne caught smallpox and survived, but her son, Prince William, the heir to the throne, died – and this ended the Stuart line.[4] The worldwide death toll was staggering well into the twentieth century, with total global mortality estimated at 300 to 500 million, vastly exceeding the combined total of all deaths in all world wars.

Spanish and Portuguese explorers introduced smallpox to the New World, where it devastated the native populations of the Americas who, having never encountered it before, had no immunity to it. The fate of the New World and the Caribbean was in many ways determined by this disease, which ravaged indigenous populations from the fifteenth century onwards into the twentieth century.[11-13] Half the native population of Puerto Rico died of smallpox within a few months in 1519. When Spanish explorers encountered the Aztec civilization of Mexico, they carried the smallpox virus with them: within a few months, half the Aztec population died, allowing a few hundred Spanish conquistadors to conquer this ancient civilization.

In North America, too, smallpox eliminated native tribes: in the three years before the Mayflower landed on the coast of New England, 90% of the native population of Massachusetts reportedly died of the disease. This tragedy continued well into the nineteenth century: as American pioneers expanded westwards across the continent, they brought smallpox epidemics to decimate naïve, aboriginal populations wherever they were encountered. In the United States, more than 100,000 cases of smallpox were recorded as late as 1921.[14]

★★★★★★★★★★★

With such a dreaded and ubiquitous disease, it is perhaps not surprising that historically, doctors and scientists turned their efforts towards prevention. From the time of the Athenian plague in 430 BC, it had been recognized that smallpox survivors were immune to further infection. Based on this observation, multiple techniques developed to allow deliberate exposure to tiny doses of smallpox in the hope that immunity would occur without severe illness.[15] An early effort in China involved blowing powdered smallpox scabs through a tube into the nostrils of a healthy person.[16] Most popular and most effective was the variolation technique of inoculation: infected matter was taken from a pox of an infected person and spread into a fresh cut made on the skin of someone who had never had the disease. In the best case scenario, the inoculated person developed a very mild case of the disease, was left unscarred and able to see, and could never be infected again. This process was developed in Africa, India, and China sometime before the tenth century, and was introduced to the Ottoman Empire by Circassian traders around 1670.[17,18] They had good reason to do so – they sold slave girls into sultan's harems, and rather than having their merchandise scarred by smallpox and thereby rendered valueless, they inoculated them before sending them to court. These women introduced the practice into the Ottoman Empire, where Europeans first encountered it.

The variolation technique was described by an English ambassador to Turkey in 1714 in a letter home, and it became an accepted part of English aristocratic culture due to the efforts of Lady Mary Wortley Montague.[19] Lady Montague was an aristocratic beauty who was infected with smallpox in 1715 and left horribly scarred; she lost her twenty year old brother to the virus in 1717. Despite her scars, she married the diplomat Edward Montague who was posted to Istanbul as ambassador to the central government of the Ottoman Empire. There, she learned about inoculation and began writing about its amazing efficacy to her friends in

London. By inoculating her own children (her 5-year-old son in Istanbul and her 4-year-old daughter upon their return to London) in front of members of the royal court and urging her social circle to do so as well, she led the first public health inoculation effort in England.[20] That effort was picked up by the king, who commissioned a study by Charles Maitland, the physician who inoculated Lady Montague's children. Prisoners from Newgate Prison (in which residence had a higher mortality rate than smallpox!) were chosen to be inoculated. In exchange for their participation, they were pardoned. This trial proved successful – the prisoners survived and later proved immune to exposure to smallpox. Maitland moved on to orphanages for his next trial and when those children also survived and were smallpox resistant, he was called upon to inoculate the two daughters of the Princess of Wales. Their survival and subsequent immunity resulted in widespread acceptance across England, and variolation became standard practice for institutionalized children and adults, and for those who could afford it.[21] Performed correctly – with a tiny dose of smallpox material, administered just under the skin – variolation was very effective, and the most skillful variolators in the eighteenth century achieved impressive results in the fight against smallpox.

There were two significant problems with variolation: first, by introducing smallpox matter into the body, there was always the risk that the patient would contract a full-blown case of the disease. And indeed, approximately two out of every hundred patients variolated against smallpox in the eighteenth century died: this was significant, but a far lower mortality rate than among those who were naturally infected.[2] The second problem was that, after the procedure, the patient was transiently contagious, and could spread smallpox to others. Nonetheless, variolation spread across Europe through the mid-1700s, based on the success in England, the support of the Royal Society of Physicians and the English royal family.[22]

In 1721, inoculation reached America, and with the support of Cotton Mather, a Protestant minister and Harvard-trained physician, and his colleague Zabdiel Boylston, it became broadly accepted in New England after a significant epidemic hit the colony there.[23] Religion was a powerful force in the world at that time and Cotton Mather's enthusiasm for inoculation was especially interesting because he couched it in religious terms. (For more on this, see the Historic Perspective section at the end of this chapter.) Religious questions aside, the practice of inoculation spread throughout the American colonies, supported by Benjamin Franklin who wrote in his autobiography:

> In 1736 I lost one of my sons, a fine boy of four years old, by the small-pox, taken in the common way. I long regretted bitterly, and still regret that I had not given it to him by inoculation. This I mention for the sake of parents who omit that operation, on the supposition that they should never forgive themselves if a child died under it; my example showing that the regret may be the same either way, and that, therefore, the safer should be chosen.[24]

George Washington had all his soldiers inoculated by variation during the Revolutionary War and attributed at least some of his ultimate success to the absence of smallpox among the troops.[25]

Edward Jenner and the Development of Smallpox Vaccine

In the late 1700s in England, it was common knowledge that milkmaids who had developed cowpox were immune to smallpox and there were scattered reports of effective vaccination with cowpox material in England. Edward Jenner, a young British physician and scientist, took up this concept scientifically and used extracted fluid from a cowpox lesion to inoculate a young child. In a completely uncontrolled study, when the boy was injected with smallpox material 6 weeks later, there was no reaction. Although Jenner's original report of this case was rejected for publication by the Royal Society of Physicians, he persisted, adding new material and eventually, he self-published this work. The report describes 10 cases of "vaccination," his new term for the process to prevent smallpox, the word derived from vacca, the Latin word for cow.[26] Of note, Jenner also described inoculation with horsepox to prevent smallpox infection, a process called equination. Recent genetic analyses of extant vaccinia viruses have revealed horsepox virus genes in some strains, supporting the validity of this history.[27]

Jenner's paper received mixed reviews and vaccination did not immediately take off, but within a few months, many of his physician friends began asking for the vaccine. Vaccination spread as physicians adopted it and convinced their patients to try it instead of inoculation. They championed the procedure because vaccination was far safer: side effects were rare and there was no risk of developing smallpox disease. Jenner's findings were confirmed by William Woodville, from the Smallpox and Inoculation Hospital in London, and by 1800, vaccination had reached most European countries and been adopted in the New World: Jenner was well on his way to becoming an international scientific superstar. In 1802, his place in history was guaranteed when the English Parliament granted him a patent on the smallpox vaccine. Because he was not part of the inner circle of the Royal College of Physicians, he still faced scorn and ridicule from some in the English medical community but by 1810, vaccination had won the day in England and was fast spreading across Europe. Jenner was the first person to make a scientifically based attempt to control an infectious disease. He established the practice of vaccination and understood the important implications of his work. As early as 1801, he wrote of vaccination "... the annihilation of the smallpox, the most dreadful scourge of the human species, must be the final result of this practice."[28] In Jenner's honor, Louis Pasteur changed the definition of the term "vaccine" to refer to any inoculated material that produces disease immunity.[29]

Originally, the pox material used for vaccination was kept alive by being transferred from arm to arm, including serial infection of children as a way to transport the virus across the ocean from Europe to the Spanish colonies in the Americas early in the nineteenth century.[30] Contamination as a result of this arm-to-arm procedure led to inadvertent transmission of other serious diseases, including syphilis and tuberculosis, so the vaccine was subsequently produced on the skin of animals, primarily calves but also rabbits and horses.[31] Somewhere in this process, the original cowpox vaccine agent was replaced by a brand new, previously unknown virus which was called "vaccinia." *Vaccinia* was subsequently found to be an immunologically distinct strain, thought to possibly be derived from the cowpox virus by repeated serial passage in animals.[30] Alternatively, *Vaccinia*, cowpox virus, and *Variola* are thought to all be derivatives of a common ancestral virus with cross-immunity insuring that infection with one provides protection against all. Whatever the origin, *Vaccinia* became the consistent agent used in vaccines against smallpox from the early 1900s.[31,32]

The vaccination technique evolved from multiple scratches of the skin with diffuse application of cowpox fluid to a standardized procedure using a bifurcated needle holding a droplet of manufactured vaccine. With either technique, a red papule appears at the site after about 3 days and by 7 days, this has the classical appearance of a mature pox lesion – an umbilicated vesicle containing turbid fluid surrounded by an inflamed halo that may continue to expand over the next 3 days. Swollen lymph nodes and fever are common but resolve as the pustule dries up and crusts over. The scab falls off within ~3 weeks leaving a small round scar, the mark of successful smallpox vaccination which conveys full immunity to smallpox in more than 95% of persons for at least 5–10 years. Successful revaccination provides protection for more than 20 additional years.[2]

Historically, a range of remedies were used to "treat" smallpox, with no effect. Once vaccination against smallpox was established and available, vaccination within three days of exposure was shown to prevent or significantly lessen the severity of smallpox symptoms in the vast majority of people. Even if performed later – four to seven days after exposure – vaccination modified the severity of disease. Other than vaccination, treatment of smallpox was primarily supportive, including wound care, prevention of super-infection, and fluid therapy. People with semi-confluent and confluent types of smallpox had therapeutic issues similar to patients with extensive skin burns and required intensive fluid management because of this – this would still be a primary focus of treatment in this setting today. Flat and hemorrhagic types of smallpox would be treated with the same therapies used to treat shock, including fluid resuscitation, inotropes to maintain blood pressure and respiratory support.[33]

Smallpox represents the first disease that primarily challenged the medical community to develop a strategy for preventing its spread rather than treating its symptoms. With the help of inoculation and then vaccination, smallpox came to be a much less common part of life across the globe. It would take another century before religious ideology and cultural practice would overcome the many lingering anxieties about whether it was acceptable to God to prevent a natural disease or how to weigh the relative risks of deliberately infecting someone with a potentially deadly infectious agent.

****

The Virus

How the smallpox agent was identified as a virus is somewhat confusing because much of the early research thought to be about *Variola major* actually involved *Vaccinia*, the cowpox-derived/mutated agent used in vaccination, rather than the smallpox virus itself. The assumption appears to have been that since the vaccinia-based vaccine caused immunity to develop, *Vaccinia* must be very similar to *Variola*, the agent that caused smallpox – and smallpox was obviously much more dangerous to the investigator. Even before the first definition of viruses as filterable infectious agents not retained by standard bacteriologic filters and not visible by light microscopy, *Vaccinia* had actually been visualized by light micros- copy as "inclusion bodies" in vaccine material, as had *Variola* in human cells and lymph of individuals infected with smallpox.[34] In 1906, Paschen introduced the idea that these "inclusions" seen by light microscopy were in fact, infective smallpox virions.[35] At the time, potential visualization of the organism by light microscopy did not advance the theory that Vaccinia and Variola were viruses since failure to be seen with standard techniques was one way that viruses had originally been recognized. Viruses could only be further identified indirectly, by inducing disease in a susceptible host with a bacteria-free filtrate from a dis- eased subject, or by proven prevention of re-infection in survivors of the illness in question.

Then, Adelchi Negri, an Italian microbiologist, showed that the infectivity of vaccine lymph persisted after the lymph had been passed through a filter that held back bacteria: this was the first strong evidence that *Vaccinia* – and by inference, therefore, the smallpox agent, *Variola* – was a virus.[36] It was not until 1932 that Ledingham showed that antisera against *Vaccinia* specifically neutralized infect- ivity, a second step in the identification of *Vaccinia* – and therefore the smallpox agent, *Variola* – as viruses.[37] Deliberately infecting a person with smallpox to induce disease was dangerous and unethical, but when injection of the *Variola* agent onto the chorio- allantoic membrane of a developing chick embryo resulted in characteristic pox, *Variola major* – the cause of smallpox – was at last confirmed to be a virus.[38]

Variola has been classified as a member of the Orthopox group. Four orthopox viruses cause infection in humans: *Variola (major and minor)*, *Vaccinia,* cowpox, and monkeypox. The *Variola* virus infects only humans in nature, although primates and other animals have been infected in a laboratory setting. *Vaccinia*, cowpox, and monkeypox viruses can infect both humans and other animals. *Variola minor, Variola major* and *Vaccinia* share common amino acid sequences: this explains the immunity to all three diseases that develops after infection with any one of them and the effectiveness of a vaccine based on Vaccinia in preventing development of Variola.[39]

With the advent of electron microscopy and molecular genetics, *Variola* was seen to be a large brick-shaped virus (Figure 2.1).[40] In 1940, the viral genome was demonstrated to contain DNA, and subsequently, this was shown to be a single linear, double stranded DNA genome of 186 kilobase pairs with a hairpin loop at each end connecting the two DNA strands.[39] The DNA is bound to proteins in a nucleoprotein complex called the core, shaped like a dumbbell in the center of the virus, surrounded by a lipid and protein membrane. The pox virion is the largest of all virions and its genetic material is among the largest of all viral genomes. The highly accurate poxviral DNA polymerase has conserved the sequences of these genes among all orthopoxviruses. Genes in the central region encode proteins involved in replication and virion structure while the flanking areas contain genes encoding proteins that modify the intra- and extracellular environment to favor viral replication and spread.[41,42]

Poxviruses differ from most other DNA viruses in that they replicate in the cytoplasm rather than in the nucleus of susceptible cells. To accomplish this, they have a battery of enzymes including DNA-dependent RNA polymerase which are used to transform basic building materials − amino acids, nucleotides and lipids parasitized from the infected cell − into components of the new virion. The DNA-dependent RNA polymerase transcribes messenger RNA into DNA. The virus also has an inner and outer membrane envelope; the outer envelope contains viral-specific polypeptides, including hemagglutinin, which are involved in virus attachment to host cell surface membranes. Finally, the extreme virulence of the variola virus is derived from a set of genes that reduce the multiple defense mechanisms of host organisms. A complement-regulatory protein inactivates the host complement system and prevents the host cell from engaging the immune complement cascade. The virus can also use fusion proteins to expose the host cell to extracellular material thereby promoting degradation.[43,44]

Nucleotide sequencing of variola fragments began in the 1980s and ultimately, complete genome sequencing of variola strains collected between 1944 and 1977 was accomplished. Historic strains that affected European and American populations between the thirteenth and eighteenth centuries were all eradicated following the initiation of widespread vaccination. Comparative genomic analysis of 45 epidemiologically varied variola virus isolates from the last 30 years indicates low sequence diversity, suggesting little if any spontaneous mutation and therefore, no difference in functional genes. Analysis of viral linear DNA suggests that variola evolution involved direct descent and DNA end-region recombination events.[42]

Phylogenetic analysis − nucleotide and/or amino acid sequencing of individual virus strains − allows measurement of molecular divergence between strains and can be used to construct a theoretical evolutionary tree. With smallpox, this kind of analysis has been limited because the only available viral strains have come from twentieth-century specimens obtained before eradication of the disease in 1980. Analysis of the *Variola* isolates from the WHO Collaborating Center Repository collected between the mid-1940s and the 1970s show very high nucleotide sequence similarity to two pox viruses that infect animals, the taterapox virus from West Africa and the camel pox virus from central Asia, supporting the idea that the human virus arose from an animal strain. There was minimal diversity between the *Variola* virus isolates indicating a very low spontaneous mutation rate with the greatest variation related to site of geographic origin.[45,46] Evolutionary clock analyses can predict the time to the most recent common ancestor and for *Variola*, the branches have shown widely divergent results, ranging from 1374 years ago up to 50,000 years ago; this difference indicates either a recent or an ancient origin and reflects the incomplete molecular genetic evidence at the time.

Then in 2016, excavation of the crypt of a seventeenth-century Lithuanian church recovered the mummified body of a child. Radiocarbon dating yielded an estimated date of death between 1643 and 1665 AD. Analysis of genetic material allowed development of a complete *Variola* genome.[47] The lineage was found to have the same pattern of gene degradation as twentieth-century *Variola* strains but the gene sequence recovered from the mummified body was shown to be the predecessor of all the known *Variola* genomes. This important finding strongly suggests that genetic diversification of the smallpox virus is a relatively recent phenomenon with the major known viral lineages appearing between the seventeenth and nineteenth centuries. The researchers concluded that the smallpox lineages which caused disease in the twentieth century had only been in existence for approximately 200 years. These findings do not preclude an ancient history for smallpox, since earlier viral lineages could have disappeared because of natural selection, host resistance to older variants or random chance.[48] They do mean, however, that the exact origin of the smallpox virus remains a mystery.

Edward Jenner could hardly have made a more fortuitous choice for effective vaccine development and ultimately for disease eradication than the highly stable DNA virus, *Variola*. Humans are the only hosts and the only victims – there is no other disease reservoir; and, there is no sub-clinical disease – every infected person displays the characteristic rash and therefore every case can be identified. With established, sustained immunity after vaccination with a widely available, safe and effective vaccine, the stage was set for disease eradication.

Smallpox Eradication

Despite an effective vaccine, smallpox remained a serious worldwide problem well into the twentieth century. Recurrent smallpox epidemics were usually followed by short-term intensive vaccination efforts, but these were complicated by minimal public health infrastructure in many parts of the world and by problems with vaccine quality, preservation and delivery. During WWI, there were massive smallpox epidemics in Russia, Germany and Austria with ~250,000 deaths per year across Europe. In the United States and Canada, the last major smallpox epidemics occurred in the early 1920s. In the United States, rates of smallpox infection decreased steadily as mandatory vaccination of schoolchildren was put in place throughout the first half of the twentieth century and the invention of the ice box made vaccine storage efficient. There has been no endemic smallpox disease in the USA since 1926.

While the United States and European countries were getting smallpox under control, the developing world still suffered from it. Infection rates were high in Africa, South America, and Asia, where vaccination was not as widespread as in the West. During the Second World War, cases of smallpox infection increased. Previously unexposed regions were overtaken by variola carried by foreigners, or by soldiers who brought the virus home from foreign lands. From 1941 to 1946, the percentage of countries in which smallpox was endemic rose from 69–87%. During that period, smallpox killed three to four million people annually.

In 1947, there was an outbreak of smallpox in NYC when a man who had recently visited Mexico became ill, was hospitalized, and died; after his death, he was found to have had smallpox.[49] A second case and then a third appeared and concern about epidemic spread surged. When the first case was recognized, the NYC Health Commissioner encouraged all New Yorkers who had not been vaccinated since childhood to be re-vaccinated. Free vaccine clinics were established throughout the city and vaccine was provided to private physicians for administration. After the second death, the mayor urged all 7.8 million New York residents to receive the vaccine. In support, police, fire, departments and hospitals were mobilized to provide space for the effort. Two days later, epidemiologic investigation indicated that all 3 patients with diagnosed cases were related indicating that, in all likelihood, the outbreak had been successfully halted through vaccination of known contacts. Despite this evidence that the outbreak had been contained, the city pushed forward with its "Be sure, be safe, get vaccinated!" program. Ultimately, 5–6 million people were vaccinated over a two month period. This was the largest mass vaccination effort ever conducted for smallpox to that time and marked the last outbreak of smallpox in America.[49]

Globally, smallpox outbreaks decreased through the 1940s and 1950s in industrialized countries with established health services and an insured vaccine supply. According to the CDC:

> By 1959, … smallpox in the Americas was endemic (only) throughout South America. Smallpox had been eliminated in Europe and most of the North African countries as well as Japan, the Philippines, Malaysia and French Indo-China. However, major epidemics continued to occur throughout densely populated India, Pakistan, Bangladesh, and Indonesia. Most countries in sub-Saharan Africa were effectively without control programs. In all, at least fifty-nine countries with 1.7 billion people – 60% of the world's population – still lived in smallpox endemic countries of the world.[50]

Two important preliminary steps towards smallpox eradication were the 1950s development of a method for production of an inexpensive freeze-dried vaccine that was heat-stable for a month at body temperature; and improvements in vaccination technique with confirmation that a single vaccination provided immunity for at least 10 years.[51] Beginning in 1950, international efforts were made to establish smallpox eradication programs, initially confined to the Western Hemisphere and then expanded to address the entire world.[52] From 1953 onwards, there were annual proposals to the World Health Organization (WHO) to undertake global smallpox eradication but none were successful until 1958 when the delegate from the Union of Soviet Socialist Republics (USSR) presented a lengthy report about smallpox, prompted by frequent outbreaks in Russia caused by cases coming from neighboring countries in Asia. To encourage an eradication campaign, the USSR even pledged to supply large amounts of the heat-stable, freeze-dried vaccine.[53] In response, the WHO director-general presented a report later in 1959 recommending national smallpox eradication campaigns in every country with endemic smallpox, aimed at vaccinating 80% of the population. There was unanimous agreement with the intent of this proposal but only minimal funding, far below the level needed to launch this kind of effort. One reason for this was the widespread conviction that eradication would require 100% vaccination, a practical impossibility in many ways, including chronic inaccuracy and under-reporting of smallpox cases. For example, in 1959, 96,571 cases of smallpox were reported but this was later found to represent less than 1% of actual cases. Beginning that year, the WHO director-general wrote annually to each country with known endemic smallpox announcing the planned eradication program and requesting accurate reporting of cases as a preliminary to an eradication program. However, financing and staffing in support of this program remained limited and accordingly, so was progress. Years passed with the smallpox eradication program proposal bogged down in budgetary limitations and Cold War politics.[54]

Then in 1965, President Lyndon Johnson unexpectedly announced US funding for a 5-year program to eradicate smallpox and measles in West Africa, to be administered by the CDC. At that time, measles was a leading cause of death among children in Africa. The announcement was precipitated by the development of a new and effective measles vaccine which was first tested in Burkina Faso by the US Agency for International Development (USAID). The measles vaccine proved so successful that other West African countries requested similar programs and in response, Johnson funded a new 5-year CDC-administered program. This signaled a definite shift in US support for a campaign against smallpox. In fact, US delegates to the WHO were instructed to pledge support for an international program to completely eradicate smallpox within the next decade. In response, after years of debate, consideration and re-consideration, a special budget was approved by the World Health Assembly in May 1966 to fund a 10-year global program to eradicate smallpox.[54]

Dr. D.A. Henderson, a young epidemiologist at the CDC who had headed up the USAID program in West Africa, was appointed Director of the Smallpox Eradication Unit, based at WHO headquarters in Geneva and administered through that bureaucracy. A small staff of four(!) undertook this formidable task, given the estimated annual number of smallpox cases at 10 to 15 million with 2 million deaths in 43 countries that spanned the globe (see Figure 2.3).[55]

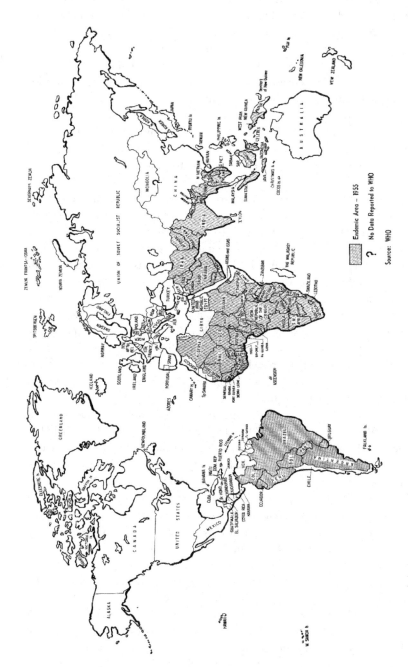

FIGURE 2.3 Global map showing distribution of smallpox in 1955.

Source: Public Health Image Library. CDC. PHIL/cdc.gov

Henderson developed a two-component strategy based on epidemiologic principles: mass vaccination of all available subjects to directly reduce the number of susceptible people and prevent disease spread; and isolation of victims and vaccination of all of their known contacts by development of a reporting-surveillance system with response teams who would investigate disease reports, identify victims and thereby contain outbreaks – an approach now known as ring vaccination. Specific characteristics of the smallpox virus made this eradication strategy plausible: humans are the only victims and there is no sub-clinical disease – every infected person displays the characteristic rash and therefore every case can be identified. In addition, 80% of those who have been vaccinated have a permanent scar and can also be readily identified. In addition, the freeze-dried vaccine can be stored without refrigeration for up to a month, a critical factor for eradication teams in tropical countries.[56]

The program began in January 1967 using mobile vaccination and surveillance teams because of inadequate existing infrastructure in most countries with endemic disease. The use of surveillance to identify smallpox cases and initiate the containment strategy was a new approach to smallpox eradication efforts and fortuitously, it proved to be dramatically successful just as the program began. Right out of the box, a test case occurred in East Nigeria in late January 1967 when initial vaccine supplies were limited so the mass vaccination approach was impossible. The team shifted to the surveillance-containment approach, using an existing missionary reporting system to identify areas with active cases, isolate victims and prioritize vaccination to contacts in those places. Amazingly, smallpox transmission was completely interrupted within 6 months. With this dramatic success, the surveillance-containment approach was validated and became the major strategy of the eradication program. This early success in Nigeria heralded a series of successful programs culminating in eradication of smallpox in West Africa in May 1970.[57] Despite a long list of problems including recruitment and training of completely inexperienced teams, variable vaccine supplies, country-specific political demands, repair and maintenance of mobile unit vehicles, substandard vaccine quality, diplomatic challenges, monsoon floods and devastating drought, war, political corruption and communication barriers, the Smallpox Eradication Unit forged ahead, establishing teams in every one of the countries with endemic disease by 1971. The next successes were in South America and Indonesia where smallpox was eradicated by March 1971 and April 1974, respectively.[58]

India, Pakistan and Bangladesh proved to be especially challenging. At the beginning of the program, they accounted for more than half of all reported smallpox cases. The disease was so pervasive that India even had its own Hindu goddess of smallpox, Sital Mara. Despite substantial national effort and international leadership and support, smallpox persisted unabated in central India. Special field teams were created to aggressively implement the surveillance-containment program, using village-by-village and then house-by-house searches. Ultimately, a veritable army of public health workers was deployed to identify and quarantine every case of smallpox and vaccinate every contact. After a formidable team effort, smallpox was eventually eradicated from India by June 1975 and Bangladesh by January 1976.[59]

Ethiopia and Somalia were the last smallpox strongholds. Fueled by public rejection of vaccination, severe drought and famine, and civil disorder in a large country with roads and bridges in terrible condition, an effective attack on smallpox eventually required the use of helicopters which ultimately eliminated the disease in Ethiopia by July 1976. Somalia shared a long open border with Ethiopia and its highly mobile nomadic population made disease detection extremely difficult. In addition, the Somali government was actively obstructive. Despite these obstacles, the last case of naturally acquired smallpox in Somalia – and in the world – occurred in October 1977. The Smallpox Eradication Program was ultimately declared successful at the end of December 1977. Remarkably, the Smallpox Eradication Unit, led by their extraordinary director, D.A. Henderson, had achieved what many thought to be an impossible goal in only 10 years.[59,60]

The Post-Eradication Era: Smallpox as a Biological Weapon

The world's last case of smallpox actually occurred after the international campaign ended. In August 1978, a medical photographer named Janet Parker at the University of Birmingham in England fell ill with fever and a hideous rash. Two weeks later when she was already critically ill, she was diagnosed with smallpox. She contracted the virus via an air duct from a smallpox research lab on the floor below her own office. Ms. Parker died and the director of the smallpox research lab committed suicide. This incident reinforced the deadly capacity of smallpox at a time when there were smallpox virus stocks in at least 75 research labs around the world. After this incident, many countries called for destruction of all stocks of the virus. In 1980, as part of the declaration of eradication, WHO mandated that only the CDC Centers in the United States and the Research Institute for Viral Preparations in the USSR be allowed to retain a limited supply of the virus in high-security labs.[61]

To this day, debate continues over whether the American smallpox virus reserve should be retained for theoretical research purposes or destroyed because of the threat posed by possible escape of the virus. Scientists continue to call for complete destruction of the virus. When gene sequencing techniques developed, it was proposed that all smallpox virus stocks be destroyed once several different strains of the viral genome were sequenced – this proposal was endorsed by the United States and Russia but when the sequencing goal was reached in 1994, the US Department of Defense objected. Despite continuing recommendations from the global scientific community and formal review every 3–4 years by a WHO Advisory Group of Independent Experts, the American smallpox virus stock has never been destroyed.[62]

★★★★★★★★★

The smallpox reserve introduces the second chapter of the smallpox story: smallpox as a potential biological weapon. A biological weapon is defined as a harmful biological agent such as a pathogenic microorganism or a neurotoxin used as a weapon to cause death or disease, usually on a large scale. Since the declaration of smallpox eradication in 1980, the general population has not been vaccinated against smallpox – and this means that accidental or deliberate release of the smallpox virus could have devastating consequences for our now unprotected and highly mobile global population.[63]

Historically, smallpox has already been used as a biological weapon, perhaps most famously in 1768 during the French and Indian Wars when invading British soldiers under the direction of Lord Jeffery Amherst, gave blankets from smallpox victims to North American Indian tribes, initiating massive disease outbreaks with high mortality.[11] Smallpox was also used very effectively by the British Military during the US Revolutionary War until George Washington had all of his troops vaccinated. No doubt there were many other instances when bioweapons like smallpox were used without historic documentation. In 1928, use of biological weapons was formally addressed by the Geneva Protocol which was drawn up and signed by all participants under the auspices of the League of Nations, with explicit prohibition of the use of chemical and/or biological weapons in war.[64] Despite this prohibition, there were active bioweapons programs in many countries including Japan, the Soviet Union and the United States dating from as early as the 1930s.

Japan was the first country known to be considering germ warfare when it initiated a massive program after the First World War. Led by Major General Ishii Shiro and by decree of Emperor Hirohito, multiple biological warfare sites were established by the late 1930s. Using established pathogens like smallpox, anthrax and the plague, the Japanese focused their research on methods for mass exposure. Their most famous bioweapons site, Unit 731, developed balloon bombs for dispersion of pathogens by airplane and plague bombs to be transported by submarine. According to news reports in 1939, Shiro's team actually dispatched an airplane to spread *Yersinea pestis*, the bacteria that causes the bubonic plague, during the Japanese–Soviet war using infected fleas – the dispersal caused a localized outbreak of the plague that killed 22 Chinese citizens.[65] Among other techniques, the Japanese biowarfare team developed a bomb to inject anthrax-coated shrapnel and a radio-controlled bomb cluster designed to create a cloud of bacteria just above the ground.[66] After the surrender of Japan that led to the end of the Second World War, Shiro and members of his Unit 731 were investigated by US scientists and their research and manufacture of germ bombs, techniques of mass production of bacteria and their bio-warfare experiments were discovered. Their records included horrific descriptions of testing on human subjects.[67] Incredibly, the Japanese scientists were reportedly exonerated from being sued for war crimes in exchange for their "human experimentation" data which was considered valuable information for microbiology and disease pathogenesis. Regardless of the ethics of this decision, the Japanese bioweapons program is thought to have ended at the end of the Second World War although it is impossible to be sure of this.

From Russian defectors, we know that the Soviet Union also initiated its biological weapons program in the 1920s despite the fact that the USSR was a signa-
tory to the 1925 Geneva Convention.[64] Original efforts focused on weaponization
of known pathogens and according to Colonel Kanatzhan Alibekov, known in
the USA as Ken Alibek, a colonel in the Russian bioweapons program who
defected to the United States in 1992, the Soviet Union aerosolized *Francisella
tularensis*, the bacteria that causes tularemia, and used it against German troops
in 1942; details of this effort and of the entire program are contained in Alibek's
book.[68] As he describes it, the Soviet program accelerated during the Cold War,
and ultimately, there were reportedly more than 50 different research facilities
which weaponized and stockpiled multiple bio-agents. These included smallpox,
for which a specific factory was created near Moscow in 1947. According to
Alibek, the smallpox program used a highly virulent strain of smallpox from
India which they developed for delivery in an aerosolized form. A production
line to manufacture smallpox on an industrial scale was launched with the *Variola
major* virus stockpiled in large quantities throughout the 1970s and 1980s.[69] This
effort occurred despite the apparent wholehearted participation of the USSR in
the WHO global campaign to eradicate smallpox. To our knowledge, the Soviet
weaponized smallpox was never released, but its destination remains uncertain.
Over time, the Soviet bioweapons effort grew into an enormous program, combining multiple institutions under different ministries with commercial facilities,
collectively known as the Biopreparat after 1973. Biopreparat pursued offensive
research, development, and production of biological agents as if it was legit-
imate biotechnology research. Annualized production capacity for weaponized
smallpox, rabies and typhus combined was reported to be 90–100 tons.[70]

By the 1980s, the Cold War was at its height. According to Alibek, the
USSR believed that war between the superpowers was likely and the work
of the Biopreparat was focused on that inevitability. The massive clandestine
bioweapons program developed an exceptionally dangerous aerosolized form of
anthrax which was accidentally released from a secret bioweapons facility in the
Soviet city of Sverdlovsk in April 1979. Propelled by a slow wind, the anthrax
cloud drifted southeast, producing a 50-kilometer trail of disease and death.
At least 66 people died, making this the deadliest recorded human outbreak
of inhalation anthrax. A study published subsequently in the journal *Science* in
1994 concluded that the geographic pattern of the outbreak clearly showed that
it was caused by an aerosolized form of anthrax released from the local Soviet
bioweapons facility.[71] When Ken Alibek was a bio-weaponeer – his own term –
in the Soviet Union, he was involved in development of a method to produce
anthrax in huge quantities in a form that could be loaded onto cruise missiles and
delivered to targets in the United States without advance warning. He reports
this had been accomplished by 1987.

The fall of the Berlin Wall, the shredding of the Iron Curtain and the end
of the Cold War were followed by the dissolution of the Soviet Union. In
September 1992, Russia signed an agreement with the United States and Great

Britain, promising to end its bioweapons program and to convert its facilities for benevolent scientific and medical purposes.[72] Compliance with the agreement and the fate of the former Soviet bio-agents and facilities are, however, still largely undocumented with no visible campaign to dismantle the residual elements of the program. US security analysts have raised the possibility that Soviet bioweapons could have fallen into the wrong hands. Ken Alibek believes that, following the collapse of the Soviet Union in 1991, disaffected scientists could have clandestinely sold samples of biological agents like smallpox or moved the program to rogue states to continue illicit biological weapons development. In their comprehensive book, Leitenberg and Zilinskas describe the full scope of the USSR's offensive biological weapons research and report that the means for waging biological warfare could well persist in Russia today.[73]

Meanwhile, the United States developed its own extensive bioweapons program beginning as early as the First World War when tests of two methods for dissemination of ricin, the deadly byproduct of castor beans, were conducted; neither delivery method was perfected before the war in Europe ended. To this day, there is no antidote for ricin toxicity. Although this early American effort was unsuccessful, it signaled the serious early intent of the military to develop bioweapons. When the Second World War erupted, the official US government position was that biological weapons were impractical and as late as 1941, the USA had no biological weapons capability despite knowledge of the growing offensive programs in Russia and Japan. President Franklin Roosevelt approved development of a biological warfare program in November 1942 and in response, the US Army Biological Warfare Labs were established at Fort Detrick, Maryland in the spring of 1943. Within 6 months, a high-security biological weapons facility was completed, followed by construction of multiple satellites. Galvanized by reports that the Germans were preparing a pilotless biological weapon for use against the Allies, the American team coordinated with Canada and Britain to develop bombs to be filled with anthrax spores that could be dropped from planes. While safety testing was still going on, the United States dropped the atomic bomb on Hiroshima and that ultimately led to the end of the war. Germany was subsequently found to have no weapons systems for delivery of biological weapons.[74]

During the Cold War, the United States biological warfare program expanded into a military-driven research program with the focus on delivery of biological weapons in multiple settings. The Detrick team established a Special Operations unit to evaluate the contamination of clouds with biological weapons. Working with the British, they conducted simulated open-air germ raids in the Caribbean using anthrax spores and *Pasturella tularensis* as agents, and monkeys and guinea pigs as experimental victims. Over the next decade, right through the Korean War, the American bioweapons program continued to investigate delivery of airborne pathogens. The program included the use of human subjects, Seventh-Day Adventist soldier volunteers who were sprayed with the agents that cause "Q fever, tularemia, typhoid fever, Eastern, Western and Venezuelan equine encephalitis, Rocky Mountain spotted fever and Rift Valley fever," either after vaccination or with treatment to prevent development of the disease.[75] In 1956, as the deployment of a biological weapon appeared more and more feasible, the National Security Council adopted a special directive stating that the United States was prepared "to use bacteriological weapons in general war" under the direct orders of the President.[76] When Kennedy became president, a major new biological weapons program began, with a shift in approach from biological agents aimed to kill to those that would incapacitate. Throughout, research focused on dissemination of known disease agents like smallpox via options like spray generators hidden in briefcases for use in crowded public areas, and aerosol sprays delivered by military jet planes. By the summer of 1968, field trials established that the United States had proven technology for effective delivery of biological weapons.[77]

The controversial Vietnam War brought public awareness of the US biological weapons program. The use of chemicals, riot-control agents, and herbicides like Agent Orange drew national and international criticism. Information about the American bioweapons research program was released to overwhelmingly negative public opinion. In response, then President Nixon issued his "Statement on Chemical and Biological Defense Policies and Programs" on November 25, 1969 in a speech from Fort Detrick:

> The United States shall renounce the use of lethal biological agents and weapons, and all other methods of biological warfare. The United States will confine its biological research to defensive measures such as immunization and safety measures.[72]

The statement ended, unconditionally, all US offensive biological weapons programs and led to signing of the Biological and Toxin Weapons Convention by the United States, the United Kingdom and the Soviet Union in 1972. Nixon ordered all US biological weapons research to be confined to defensive purposes and the destruction of the existing biological arsenal; this is thought to have been accomplished over the next several years, with the notable exception of the smallpox reserve.[78] Ultimately, despite more than 30 years of research and billions of dollars in funding, the United States has never been known to employ offensive biological weapons.

Over the next two decades, American efforts focused on bioweapon defense. The United States is said to have believed that all other international bioweapons programs had been eliminated. As we know from the reports of defectors, however, far from abandoning its bioweapons program, the Soviet Union had intensified it with their "civilian" pharmaceutical company Biopreparat, functioning as a front for a massive offensive bioweapons program well into the 1990s.[70] As part of Operation Desert Storm, the US war with Iraq in 1990–1991, intelligence reports revealed that Iraq had a biological warfare program that had begun in the 1970s. By 1991, Saddam Hussein was reported to regard his biological warfare program as a critical part of his arsenal of WMD, authorized for use against the USA. No biological weapons were utilized during Desert Storm but covert bioweapons research continued in Iraq after the war until 1995 when the program was reportedly abandoned.[79] Over time, evidence that bio-warfare efforts were alive and well around the world has accumulated. According to a 1995 report by the US Office of Technological Assessment, there were at least 17 nations known to possess biological weapons at that time: Libya, North Korea, South Korea, Iraq, Taiwan Syria, Israel, Iran, China, Egypt, Vietnam, Las, Cuba, Bulgaria, India South Africa and – last but not least – Russia.[80] Under President Clinton, attempts were made to increase the American biodefense program, including plans to vaccinate all military personnel against anthrax, increase surveillance for bioweapons, augment public health readiness against bioweapons attack and stockpile vaccines and disease antidotes but a coherent biodefense program never developed.[81]

9/11/2001

The terrorist attacks on the United States on September 11, 2001 followed by the delivery of anthrax powder to American journalists and politicians associated with 22 infections and 5 deaths described in the introduction to this chapter initiated a new era of intense American concern about bioterrorism. Smallpox is in the highest risk category along with anthrax, botulism, plague, tularemia, and viral hemorrhagic fever viruses like Ebola. The threat of an aerosol release of smallpox is considered a clear and present danger, with a single case of smallpox designated as a WHO "public health emergency of international concern."[82]

In the immediate post 9/11 atmosphere, the 2002 White House budget requested $11 billion over 2 years to "enhance national protections against biological terrorists."[83] Former President George W. Bush signed the Project BioShield Act in 2004 to accelerate research, development, purchase and availability of medical countermeasures against chemical, biological, radiological and nuclear agents. With specific reference to smallpox, the Advisory Committee on Immunization Practices (ACIP) of the CDC developed new recommendations for smallpox pre-vaccination of designated health care teams at every acute care hospital in the country. In the event of a bioweapons attack with smallpox, these teams of vaccinated individuals were designated to provide continuous care of suspected smallpox cases for the first 48 hours until additional health care workers could be vaccinated. The ACIP recommendations, published in 2003, provided detailed instructions on the composition of the smallpox care teams and the prevention of disease transmission.[84] After 2008, the recommendations were updated with the freeze-dried vaccine, Dryvax, replacing the live smallpox vaccinia vaccine, ACAM2000, for protection of at risk individuals.[85] Between December 2002 and October 2009, more than 1.8 million US service members received smallpox vaccinations.

Globally, emergency supplies of smallpox vaccine were dramatically increased after 9/11. There is a physical stockpile of smallpox vaccine held at WHO Headquarters in Switzerland, composed of calf-lymph smallpox vaccines from a variety of sources dating from the final years of the eradication program, estimated to consist of ~2.4 million doses. In addition, there is a pledged stock-pile held by multiple donor countries in their respective national stockpiles for use in time of international need. In the United States, the Advisory Committee on Immunization Practices recommends routine smallpox vaccination for specific populations at high risk of occupational exposure to orthopoxviruses. The FDA has approved two new vaccines for stockpiling based on safety profile and proof of generated immune response to be used for such individuals.[86] ACAM is a replication-competent vaccine which contains *Vaccinia Ankara*; the vaccine does not contain the variola virus and cannot cause smallpox but it can cause a vaccine-related infection which is usually mild. The live, infectious vaccinia virus can also be transmitted from the vaccine recipient to unvaccinated persons who have close contact with the inoculation site. The risk of side effects in contacts is the same as those for the vaccine recipient so the vaccination site requires special care to prevent virus spreading. In 2019, the FDA licensed a new vaccine, trademarked JYNNEOS, but also known by the brand names Imvamune and Imvanex. This is an attenuated live vaccine for the prevention of smallpox and monkeypox. As a replication-deficient vaccine, it cannot cause infection and can be used for vaccination of people with immune deficiencies.[86]

After 9/11, the subject of treatment for smallpox was revisited. Animal studies suggested that the antiviral drug cidofovir might be a useful therapeutic agent. Cidofovir was the first nucleotide analogue approved for clinical use and has demonstrated in vitro activity against poxviruses; its clinical utility is unknown. It is given intravenously with careful monitoring of kidney function. Specific application in smallpox infection has not been investigated.[87] The US government has stockpiled 2 million doses of the anti-viral medication Arestvyr, an egress inhibitor which prevents the formation of extracellular enveloped forms of orthopoxviruses to be used in exposed individuals in combination with the smallpox vaccine in the event of a smallpox bioterrorist attack. Tecovirimat is an oral antiviral drug for orthopox viruses which inhibits the function of a major envelope protein required for the production of extracellular virus.[88,89] Theoretically, it could be combined with smallpox vaccine to maximize disease suppression after exposure to the virus. For obvious reasons, it has never been tested in humans but more than 90% of monkeys and rabbits that were infected with a virus similar to smallpox and then given the drug survived. In August of 2018, the FDA approved TPOXX, a commercially developed version of tecovirimat to treat smallpox. TPOXX has now been added to the American emergency stockpile for biodefense against smallpox with 2 million doses delivered to the US government to be added to the stockpile as part of the emergency biodefense reserve.[89]

Looking Back :: Moving Forward

In the rush of concern about bioterrorism, it is easy to forget the early history of smallpox – how this dreaded disease haunted populations all over the world with disfigurement and death for more than five centuries, well into the 1900s. Richard Preston reports that "In the last hundred years of its existence, smallpox ... killed at least a half a billion people."[90] It is easy to forget the efforts of ordinary citizens like Lady Jane Montague and of scientists like Edward Jenner which resulted in development and acceptance of an effective vaccine. The struggle to prevent the disease – first with variolation and then with vaccination – was dramatically successful, the first completely effective disease prevention program in world history. There are critical characteristics of the smallpox virus that made eradication possible and that bear repeating in terms of future eradication efforts: the virus is stable with little spontaneous mutation over time; humans are the only victims and there are no subclinical cases of smallpox meaning no infected individuals will be missed; the existing vaccine, available in a freeze-dried form, is safe and highly effective. And the Smallpox Eradication Program was a model of how a knowledgeable and determined leader can empower thousands of committed workers all over the world to complete a single critical task. D.A. Henderson used his knowledge of epidemiology to design the technique of ring vaccination in which every known contact of each smallpox case was sought out and vaccinated. Effectively, this technique created a wall of immunity around areas of active disease, preventing the spread of smallpox and allowing the virus to die off – this technique has since been used to effectively vaccinate against Ebola. By eliminating layers of bureaucracy and authorizing teams of local village health workers to perform the critical work of searching for and reporting smallpox cases, Henderson created superbly effective surveillance teams all over the world. Inspired by his tireless dedication and flexible leadership, smallpox was eradicated from the face of the earth – a singular, remarkable triumph. There is still much to be learned from the history of smallpox eradication.

That should have been the end of the smallpox story. It could have been the end of the smallpox story. But instead of destruction of all existing *Variola* virus reserves, the World Health Organization recommended that special collaborating centers be created to "hold and handle stocks of *Variola* virus."[91] Per that recommendation, we know of at least two remaining stocks of the live smallpox virus, one at the CDC in Atlanta and one at the Research Institute for Viral Preparations in Moscow. These two reserves are being maintained despite the enormous risk inherent in accidental release of the smallpox virus, and subsequent sequencing of the virus allowing the genetic blueprint to be safely preserved indefinitely. There is persistent concern about the deliberate use of smallpox as a bioweapon – the Russian defector, Ken Alibek, describes 40 years of Soviet research that included a production line capable of manufacturing eighty to one hundred tons of liquid, weapons-grade smallpox virus per year: one teaspoon of this smallpox preparation could in theory infect every person on the planet.[92,93] The Russian bioweapons program reportedly even had plans to develop a more deadly hybrid virus, a combined smallpox/Ebola agent using molecular genetic techniques.

Internationally, there is evidence that development of biological weapons is ongoing. According to the US Department of Defense, countries including

China, Egypt, Iran, Israel, North Korea, Russia and Syria continue to develop biological weapons, despite the fact that most are signatories of the 1972 Biological Weapons and Toxins Convention treaty.[94] Assumed possessors of biological weapons like Iran, North Korea, and Syria are suspected of sponsoring and harboring terrorist groups like Al-Qaeda and the splinter groups that comprise ISIS, where development of biological weapons represents a terrifying potential source for terrorism.

There are no records documenting the use of biological weapons in warfare since 1972, but their use as a tool of terror emerged dramatically after 9/11 when the USA was threatened by the spread of anthrax spores. This incident put the threat of biological weapons at the top of national and international security agendas and emphasized the need for contemporary reinforcement of the Biological Weapons and Toxins Convention treaty. Interviewed in 2016, Tom Ridge, the first US Secretary of Homeland Security said:

> ... one of the most significant gaps, in my judgment is bio-defense. I mean, face it, (9/11) was 15 years ago, and yet we still don't have a (consistent bioweapons) strategy. I think that one of the most serious, long-term threats from any source, is in the biological area. And 15 years after anthrax, we're still struggling to have a strategy and to operationalize a capability to respond quickly with a vaccine and recover from an incident ... with a contagious pathogen. It's a real problem.[95]

In this age of terrorism, when the threat of biological weapons hangs over our increasingly vulnerable planet, the history of smallpox is both a major success story and a powerful cautionary tale.

HISTORIC PERSPECTIVE: VACCINATION – RACE AND RELIGION

The eradication of smallpox in 1980, with the exception of two known stores maintained in government laboratories in the United States and Russia, is considered one of the greatest public health victories of the modern world. Smallpox devastated populations beginning in the ancient world, where skeletons entombed in Egypt still show the scars left by this vicious virus. It has a relatively high mortality rate of 30% with higher rates of long-term disability, including blindness and scarring. It is also highly contagious, so the fact that it was eliminated from the world through the concerted application of vaccination reflects the tenacity of public health efforts in the face of even the most aggressive viruses. While it seems logical to use vaccination to end a disease that cost billions of lives between the first ancient outbreak and the final recorded case in 1977, it actually caused serious debates in the early modern world when inoculation (which preceded vaccination) first proved to be effective. This box focuses on the seventeenth century religious debates that occurred in the United States and in other Protestant countries over the relationship between divine will and disease. While this might seem like a uniquely early modern debate, its echoes are heard today in the refusal by people of some faiths to accept some forms of medical treatment, such as Jehovah's Witnesses who will not accept transfusions, and those who reject vaccinations on religious grounds, such as Christian Scientists and the Dutch Reformed Church. The issue of refusing vaccination on religious grounds has never been more relevant: increasingly parents are opting out of vaccinating their children, and they are using religious grounds for that refusal. 47 states allow this practice, and parents are not required to provide proof that their basis for refusing vaccination is, in fact, religious.[96] While anti-vaccination propaganda inaccurately portrays vaccinations as the cause for autism and other developmental disorders, it simultaneously ignores the reality that vaccinating less than a high proportion of a population will permit epidemics to re-emerge. The rise of small outbreaks of measles, mumps, and other previously eradicated (in North America) childhood killers demonstrates the critical importance of vaccination. Perhaps a look at early modern religious debates over smallpox immunization will help to clarify our current situation.

Inoculation is the practice of taking pus from the pox of an infected patient, scoring an uninfected person's arm, and placing the pus directly over the scoring. The practice was widely used in China and the Middle East before being imported to England and then North America through the efforts of Lady Mary Wortley Montague, an English aristocrat who had been badly disfigured by smallpox and lost her brother to it. She was married to the English ambassador to Turkey, where she encountered the procedure and observed that it caused a much less severe case of smallpox to occur in the recipient individual but still conferred immunity. She inoculated her own children and was a major force in introducing the practice to the English aristocracy upon her return home. Inoculation carried risks, including the potential for starting a new epidemic and the death of the inoculated patient, but it was a far more effective solution than any other available before Edward Jenner's vaccine. The debate over whether or not to inoculate rested not in any question about whether inoculation was successful in preventing smallpox or on its potential dangers. Instead, it lay in the interpretation of disease as part of divine will. For some Protestants, if God sent a virus to assail his followers but there was a known preventative or cure available, it was immoral not to use it. For others, accepting suffering was a means of demonstrating faith, and disease was a test of faith given by God. In 1583, for example, a physician wrote to magistrates about the use of natural remedies to protect against or treat the plague during an epidemic warned against trying to protect oneself in opposition to divine will, stating if anyone of "conscience and religion shall be persuaded to think that he resisteth the will of God, [or] if by the help of man he labor to avoid his punishment, he must suffer himself to be better taught."[97] Susan Emlen, a Quaker woman in 1814 Philadelphia afflicted by breast cancer who chose to have a mastectomy (a rare procedure at that time, done without anesthesia and having significant complications), wrote of her spiritual understanding of her cancer in letters to her father and husband. She repeatedly referred to her cancer as a trial for her soul sent, in a quote from Lamentations, by a gracious power "who afflicts not willingly."[98] Note that despite her deep religious calling and spiritual comprehension of her cancer, Emlen sought the most aggressive treatment possible, perhaps in part because her brother in law was "the father of American surgery," Phillip Physick, who held a medical degree from Edinburgh and had practiced for three years under the renowned London surgeon John Hunter.[99] Emlen, supported by her surgeon and husband, saw no conflict between seeking every possible solution for her cancer and experiencing her spiritual trial. But a century before Emlen was diagnosed, Boston saw a heated contest between religious and medical authority and different interpretations of Protestantism in the context of a debate over smallpox inoculation.

The Reverend Cotton Mather was the proponent of smallpox inoculation in this case, which occurred during the smallpox outbreak of 1721. It was a major outbreak, in which 6,000 cases were reported in a city of 11,000 people, and the mortality rate was 14%. This was the deadliest smallpox outbreak in New England of the seven that occurred during the first half of the eighteenth century.[100] Mather was a member of the Royal Society with a strong interest in natural philosophy and the traditional understanding that clergy are responsible for the health of their flock's bodies as well as their minds. As a result, he maintained a healthy interest in medicine, though he had no formal training in it. In 1716, he wrote the Royal Society to indicate that he had read the article in the *Transactions* discussing smallpox inoculation in Turkey, but he also asserted that he had already heard of this procedure through a discussion with his African servant, Onesimus, who had been inoculated before being transported to the Americas. Mather confirmed Onesimus's account by querying other Africans about the practice, and upon learning that it was effective, became a strong proponent of the procedure. When smallpox hit Boston again, he found a doctor, Zabdiel Boylston, to help him inoculate volunteers. Mather believed inoculation was a divine gift sent to help save lives and ignoring it would be tantamount to rejecting divine assistance, but he also seemed very interested in the practical applications of the practice. His efforts were most vociferously countered by the physician

William Douglass, who remained convinced that inoculation was ridiculous on two fronts: first, because Mather's trials were based on the report of an African servant and a Royal Society article about a practice in the Middle East, and he did not value knowledge generated in non-European contexts, and second because he feared it would only hasten the spread of smallpox by exposing more people to it and creating more cases. Douglass was one of the few practicing medical men in Boston who actually held a medical degree, and historians have attributed some of his resistance to the inoculation trial to an effort to establish authority over medical practice at a time when the profession was dominated by people without university training. Douglass's racialized perspective on which people could produce valuable knowledge were typical for his time, as was his urge to defend his professional territory.[101] Mather, on the other hand, was a bit of a maverick, as he combined his traditional area of knowledge with his deep passion for natural philosophy and medicine. While Mather and Boylston were brave for putting their reputations on the line to defend inoculation, however, it is the volunteers who truly deserve recognition. 287 individuals chose to be inoculated, and not much is known about their backgrounds or what drove their decision. What is known, however, is that the mortality rate among those who were inoculated was 2%, a remarkable relative risk reduction of 86%, compared with the overall mortality rate for that outbreak.[102] Mather and Boylston's use of the most sophisticated study design available, employing control and experimental groups, underlined the validity of their results and encouraged other practitioners in New England to adopt inoculation. It also damaged the ongoing argument that all diseases occurred differently in people of different races, putting an early nail in the coffin of racial medicine. Mather and Boylston's efforts were perhaps the first North American clinical trial, and they proved critical to the adoption of inoculation in the colonies.

References

1. World Health Organization. *Global Commission for the Certification of Smallpox Eradication. The Global Eradication of Smallpox: Final Report of the Global Commission for the Certification of Smallpox Eradication.* Geneva: World Health Organization; 1980.
2. Breman JG, Henderson DA. Diagnosis and management of smallpox. *N Engl J Med* 2002; 346: 1300–1308.
3. Milton DK. What was the primary mode of smallpox transmission? Implications for biodefense. *Front Cell Infect Microbiol* 2012; 2: 2150–156.
4. Barquet N, Domingo P. Smallpox: the triumph over the most terrible of the ministers of death. *Ann Intern Med* 1997; 127: 635–642.
5. Riedel S. Edward Jenner and the history of smallpox and vaccination. *BUMC Proc* 2005; 18: 21–25

6. Ruffer MA, Ferguson AR. Note on an eruption resembling that of variola in the skin of a mummy of the Twentieth Dynasty (1200–1100 BC). *J Pathol Bacteriol* 1911; 15: 1–4.

7. Littman RJ, Littman ML. The Athenian plague: smallpox. *Proceedings of the American Philological Association* 1969; 100: 261–75.

8. Rhazes (Abu Bakr Muhammad Ibn Zakariya al-Razi). *De variolis et morbillis arvardes.* London: G Bowyer; 1766.

9. Littman RJ, Littman ML. Galen and the Antonine plague. *American Journal of Philology* 1973; 94: 243–255.

10. Dixon CW, *Smallpox.* London, England. J. & A. Churchill, Ltd.; 1962. Pp.188.

11. Stearn EW, Stearn AE. *The Effect of Smallpox on the Destiny of the Amerindian.* Boston: Humphries; 1945.

12. Duffy J. *Epidemics in Colonial America.* Baton Rouge, LA: Louisiana State University Press; 1953.

13. Kavey AB. A Brief History of Love: A Rationale for the History of Epidemics. *Health and Humanities Reader.* Edited by Therese Jones, Delese Wear, Lester D. Friedman. Rutgers University Press; 2014. Pg. 430–442.

14. Duffy J. Smallpox and the Indians in the American colonies. *Bull Hist Med.* 1951; 25: 324–41.

15. Hume EH. *The Chinese Way in Medicine.* Baltimore: Johns Hopkins Univ Pr; 1940.

16. Holwell JZ. *An Account of the Manner of Inoculating the Small Pox in the East Indies.* London: Royal College of Physicians; 1767.

17. Plotkin SL, Plotkin SA. A short history of vaccination. In: Plotkin SA, Mortimer EA Jr, eds. *Vaccines.* 2d ed. Philadelphia: WB Saunders; 1994:1–11.

18. Timoni E. An account, or history, of the procuring of the smallpox by incision or inoculation, as it has for some time been arvard at Constantinople. *Philosophical Transactions of the Royal Society* 1714–1716; 29: 72–82.

19. Halsband R. *The Life of Lady Mary Wortley Montague.* Oxford: Clarendon Pr; 1956.

20. Stearns RP. Remarks upon the introduction of inoculation for smallpox in England. *Bull Hist Med* 1950; 24: 103–22.

21. Maitland C. *Mr. Maitland's account of inoculating the small pox.* London: J Downing; 1722.

22. Klebs AC. The historic evolution of variolation. *Bulletin of the Johns Hopkins Hospital.* 1913; 24:69–83.

23. Mather C, Dummer J, Tumain W. *An Account of the Method and Success of Inoculating the Small-Pox in Boston in New England.* London: J Peele; 1722.

24. Franklin, B. *The Autobiography of Benjamin Franklin: 1706–1757.* London: The Floating Press; 2009.

25. Thursfield H. Smallpox in the American War of Independence. *Annals of Medical History* 1940; 2: 312–318.

26. Jenner E. *An inquiry into the causes and effects of the variolae vaccinae, a disease discovered in some of the western counties of England, particularly Gloucestershire, and known by the name of the cow pox.* London: S Low; 1798.

27. Esparza J, Schrick L, Damaso CR, Nitsche A. Wequination (inoculation of horsepox): an early alternative to vaccination(inoculation of cowpox) and the potential role of horsepox virus in the origin of the smallpox vaccine. *Vaccine* 2017; 35(52): 222–7230.

28. Jenner E. *The origin of the vaccine inoculation.* London: Printed for the author by DN Shury; 1801.

29. Henderson DA. *Smallpox – The Death of a Disease: The Inside Story of Eradicating a Worldwide Killer.* Amherst, NY: Prometheus Books; 2009. Pg. 47.

30. Sanchez-Sampedro L, Perdiguero B, Mejias-Perez E, et al. The evolution of poxvirus vaccines. *Viruses* 2015; 7: 1726–1803.

31. Huygelen C. Jenner's cowpox vaccine in light of current vaccinology. *Verh K Acad Geneeskd Belg* 1996; 58(5): 479–536; discussion 537–8.

32. Downie AW. The immunological relationship of the virus of spontaneous cowpox to vaccinia virus. *Br J Exp Pathol* 1939; 20(2): 158–176.

33. Bennett JE, Dolin R, Blaser MJ. *Principles and Practice of Infectious Diseases*, 8th edition. Philadelphia, PA: Churchill Livingstone, Elsevier; 2015.. pg.1396.

34. Gordon M. Virus bodies. John Buist and the elementary bodies of vaccinia. *Edinburgh Med* 1937; 44: 65–71.

35. Paschen E. Was wissen wir uber den Vakzineereger? *Munch Med Woeachr* 1906; 53: 2391–2393.

36. Negri A. Ueber Filtration des Vaccinevirus', *Z. Hyg. InfektKrankh.* 1906; 54: 327–346.

37. Ledingham, JCG. The aetiological importance of the elementary bodies in vaccinia and fowl-pox. *Lancet* 1931; 2: 525–526.

38. Goodpasture EW, Woodruff AM, Buddingh GJ. Variola Infection of the Chorio-Allantoic Membrane of the Chick Embryo. *Am J Pathol* 1932; 8: 271–282.7.

39. Wittek R. Organization and expression of the poxvirus genome. *Experientia* 1982; 38(3): 285–410.

40. Nagler FPO, Rake G. The use of the electron microscope in diagnosis of variola, vaccinia and varicella. *J Bacteriol.* 1948; 55(1): 45–51.

41. Shchelkunov SN1, Totmenin AV, Loparev VN, et al. Alastrim smallpox variola minor virus genome DNA sequences. *Virol* 2000 Jan 20; 266(2): 361–86.

42. Theves C, Biagini P, Crubezy E. The rediscovery of smallpox. *Clin Microbiol Infect* 2014; 20: 210–218.

43. Haig DM. Poxvirus interference with the host cytokine response. *Vet Immunol Immunopathol* 1998; 63(1–2): 149–156.

44. Shchelkunov SN. Orthopoxvirus genes that mediate disease virulence and host tropism. *Adv Virol* 2012; 2012: 524–573.

45. Li Y, Carroll DS, Gardner SN, et al. On the origin of smallpox: correlating variola phylogenics with historical smallpox records. *Proc Nat Acad Sci* 2007; 104: 15787–15792.

46. Esposito JJ, Sammons SA, Frace AM, et al. Genome sequence diversity and clues to the evolution of Variola (smallpox) virus. *Science* 2006; 313: 807–812.

47. Duggan AT, Perdomo MF, Piombino-Mascali D, et al. 17th Century Variola virus reveals the recent history of smallpox. *Curr Biol.* 2016; 26: 3407–3412.

48. Wertheim JO. Viral evolution: mummy virus challenges presumed history of smallpox. *Curr Biol* 2017; 27: R119–R120.

49. Sepkowitz KA. The 1947 smallpox vaccination campaign in New York City, revisited. *Emerg Infect Dis* 2004; 10 (5): 960–961.

50. Henderson DA. *Smallpox – The Death of a Disease: The Inside Story of Eradicating a Worldwide Killer.* Amherst, NY: Prometheus Books; 2009.pg. 63–64.

51. Henderson. 2009. Pg. 53.

52. Henderson. 2009. Pg. 57,60.

53. Henderson. 2009. Pg. 61.

54. Henderson. 2009. Pg. 62–73.

55. Henderson. 2009. Pg. 81.

56. Henderson. 2009. Pg. 79–95.
57. Henderson. 2009. Chapter 4.
58. Henderson. 2009. Chapters 6–7.
59. Henderson. 2009. Chapter 8.
60. Fenner F, Henderson DA, Arita I, et al. *Smallpox and its Eradication. Geneva, Switzerland.* World Health Organization, 1988. www.who.int/emc/diseases/small pox/Smallpoxeradication.html. Accessed Feb. 2, 2017.
61. Henderson. 2009. Pg. 256–257.
62. Henderson DA. Smallpox virus destruction and the implications of a new vaccine. *Biosecur Bioterr* 2011; 9: 163–168.
63. Henderson DA, Inglesby TV, Bartlett JG, et al. Smallpox as a biological weapon: medical and public health management. *JAMA* 1999; 281: 2127–2137.
64. League Of Nations Treaty Series. Publication of Treaties and International Engagements registered with the Secretariat of the League of Nations. Volume 94, pp. 66–74. Registered Sept. 7, 1929.
65. Regis. 1999. Pg. 17–19.
66. Regis. 1999. Pg. 85–93.
67. Regis. 1999. Pg. 107–111.
68. Alibek K, Handelman S. *Biohazard: The Chilling True Story of the Largest Covert Biological Weapons Program in the World.* New York, NY: Dell Publishing, Random House; 1999. Pg. 29–31.
69. Alibek. 1999. Pg. 107–112.
70. Miller J, Engelberg S, Broad W. *Germs: Biological Weapons and America's Secret War.* New York, NY: Touchstone Press.; 2001. Pg. 254.
71. Meselson M, Guillemin J, Hugh-Jones M, et al. The Sverdlovsk anthrax outbreak of 1979. *Science* 1994; 266: 1202–1208.
72. Miller. 2001. Pg. 134–135.
73. Leitenberg M, Zilinskas RA. *The Soviet Biological Weapons Program: A History.* Cambridge, MA: Harvard University Press; 2012.
74. Regis E. *The Biology of Doom: The History of America's Secret Germ Warfare Project.* New York, NY: Henry Holt & Company LLC; 1999. Pg. 68–74.
75. Regis. 1999. Pg. 168.
76. Regis. 1999. Pg. 177.
77. Regis. 1999. Pg. 185–206.
78. Regis. 1999. Pg. 207.
79. Miller. 2001. Pg.183–188.
80. Alibek. 1999. Pg. 277.
81. Miller. 2001. Pg. 250.
82. National Institute for Allergies and Infectious Diseases, NIH. NIAID Emerging Infectious Diseases/Pathogens: Emerging Pathogens.
83. Miller. 2001. Pg. 340.
84. Sato H. Countermeasures and vaccination against terrorism using smallpox: pre-event and post-event smallpox vaccination and its contraindications. *Environ Health Prev Med* 2011; 16(5): 281–289. www.ncbi.nlm.nih.gov/pmc/articles/PMC3156838/
85. FDA. 2013. ACAM2000 (Smallpox Vaccine) Questions and Answers. www.fda.gov/BiologicsBloodVaccines/Vaccines/QuestionsaboutVaccines/ucm078041.htm
86. Vaccines | Smallpox | CDC. Available at: www.cdc.gov › smallpox › clinicians › vaccines. Accessed on Feb.6, 2020.

87. Bavarian Nordic. 2013. Bavarian Nordic Complete Delivery of 20 Million Doses of IMVAMUNE Smallpox Vaccine to the US Strategic National Stockpile. Press Release. www.bavarian-nordic.com/investor/news.aspx?news=3051

88. De Clercq E. Clinical potential of the acyclic nucleoside phosphonates cidofovir, adefovir, and tenofovir in treatment of DNA virus and retrovirus infections. *Clin Microbiol Rev* 2003; 16: 569.

89. Mucker EM, Goff AJ, Shamblin JD, et al. Efficacy of Tecovirimat (ST-246) in Nonhuman Primates Infected with Variola Virus (Smallpox). *Antimicrob Agents and Chemother* 2013; 57(12):6246–6253.

90. FDA News Release. FDA approves the first drug with an indication for treatment of smallpox. www.fda.gov/NewsEvents/Newsroom/PressAnnouncements/ucm613 496.htm

91. Henderson. 2009. Pg. 255.

92. Alibek. 1999. Pg. 122.

93. Henderson. 2009. Pg. 16.

94. 2010 Report on Adherence to and Compliance with Arms Control, Nonproliferation and Disarmament Agreements and Commitments, U.S. Department of State, July 2010. Accessed April 18. 2017.

95. Tom Ridge: 15 Years after Anthrax Letters, "We Still Don't Have a Strategy". P/J Media. September 9, 2016. Accessed April 16, 2017.

96. Sandstrom A. Nearly all states allow religious exemptions for vaccinations. July 16, 2016; www.pewresearch.org/fact-tank/2015/07/16/nearly-all-states-allow-religious-exemptions-for-vaccinations/. (West Virginia became the 47th state to provide religious exemption in 2017 when it passed Senate Bill No. 286. "States with Religious and Philosophical Exemptions from School Immunization Requirements," National Conference of State Legislatures webpage, December 20, 2017. Available at: www.ncsl.org/research/health/school-immunization-exempt ion-state-laws.aspx

97. von Ewich J. *The Duetie of a Faithfull and Wise Magistrate, in Preseruing and Deliuering of the Eommon [sic] Wealth from Infection, in the Time of the Plague or Pestilence Two Bookes. Written in Latine by Iohn Ewich, Ordinary Phisition of the Woorthie Common Wealth of Breame, and Newlie Turned into English by Iohn Stockwood Schoolemaister of Tunbridge.* Early English Books Online (London: Imprinted at the three Cranes in the Vintree by Thomas Dawson, 1583), f. 112v–r.

98. Garflinkel S. "This Trial Was Sent in Love and Mercy for my Refinement: A Quaker Woman's Experience of Breast Cancer Surgery in 1814," p. 68–90 in Judith Walzer Leavitt (Ed), *Women and Health in America* (second edition), Madison: University of Wisconsin Press; 1999. P.83.

99. Garfinkel, 71.

100. Minardi M. The Boston Inoculation Controversy of 1721–1722: An incident in the History of Race. *William and Mary Quarterly* 2004; Third Series; 62(1): 47–76.

101. The fight over inoculation during the 1721 Boston smallpox epidemic. Available at: http://sitn.hms.harvard.edu/flash/special-edition-on-infectious-disease/2014/ the-fight-over-inoculation-during-the-1721-boston-smallpox-epidemic/

102. Boylston, Z. *An Historical Account of the Small-pox Inoculated in New England, Upon All Sorts of Persons, Whites, Blacks, and of All Ages and Constitutions: With Some Account of the Nature of the Infection in the Natural and Inoculated Way, and Their Different Effects on Human Bodies: with Some Short Directions to the Unexperienced in this Method of Practice /* Humbly Dedicated to Her Royal Highness the Princess of Wales. Boston: 1730.

Suggested Reading

Brian WJ Mahy, Marc HV van Regenmortel (Eds.) *Desk Encyclopedia of Human and Medical Virology.* Elsevier Academic Press. Oxford, UK, San Diego, CA. 2010.

Donald A Henderson. *Smallpox – The Death of a Disease: The Inside Story of Eradicating a Worldwide Killer.* Prometheus Books. Amherst, NY. 2009.

Edward Regis. *The Biology of Doom: The History of America's Secret Germ Warfare Project.* Henry Holt & Company LLC. New York. 1999.

Gerald Geison. *The Private Science of Louis Pasteur.* Princeton University Press. Princeton, NJ. 1995.

Jefferey R Ryan. *Biosecurity and Bioterrorism: Containing and Preventing Biological Threats.* Second Edition. Butterworth-Heineman, Oxford UK, Cambridge, MA. 2016.

Judith Miller, Stephen Engelberg, William Broad. *Germs: Biological Weapons and America's Secret War.* Touchstone Press. New York. 2001.

Ken Alibek, Stephen Handelman. *Biohazard: The Chilling True Story of the Largest Covert Biological Weapons Program in the World.* Dell Publishing. Random House. New York. 1999.

Randall M Packard. *A History of Global Health: Interventions into the Lives of Other Peoples.* Johns Hopkins University Press. Baltimore, MD. 2016.

3

YELLOW FEVER

A Jungle Story

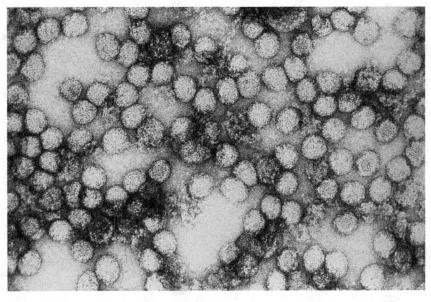

FIGURE 3.1 Electron micrograph of yellow fever virus.

Source: Alamy / CDC / BSIP. Public Health Image Library. CDC.gov

DOI: 10.4324/9781003427667-3

MOSQUITOES LOVE ME

Mosquitoes love me. A huge group can be sitting around at dusk having a lovely time but only I will be surrounded by a swarm of happy mosquitoes. This was never such a big deal until my sister Sarah moved to Venezuela and invited us to visit. Sarah has been an adventurous traveler since she was a teenager. She and her husband first moved first to Ethiopia when he joined CIDA, the Canadian International Development Agency, the federal agency that administers the official government program for developing countries. Originally it was just the two of them moving from one post to another but by the time they moved to Venezuela, they had two young daughters, a 5-year-old and a newborn. The 5-year-old is the closest thing my own daughter has to a sister and the move to South America had been a painful separation so we excitedly planned a trip over winter break.

It was 1986. Allison was 8 years old and this was her first passport: I still have it, that sweet innocent face with a superimposed official cancellation stamp. Sarah warned us about travel requirements so we went to the Travel Clinic at the university medical center where I worked. Reams of material from the CDC outlined an alarming list of dangers. There was no safe drinking water so bottled water was recommended for all intake. Malaria was prevalent so we needed drug prophylaxis plus insect repellant and mosquito nets. No vaccinations were required and I don't recall any mention of yellow fever. However, even then, the State Department warned "violent crime ... is pervasive in Venezuela, both in the capital Caracas and throughout the country. Heavily armed criminals are known to use assault rifles to commit crimes at banks, shopping malls, public transportation stations, and universities." Assault rifles! I was shocked: Caracas was the site of the Canadian embassy where my brother-in-law worked and the destination of our flight. I called my sister. She agreed that crime was an issue but assured me that their community was completely safe. Reassured – after all, she and the girls *were* living there! – we arrived in Caracas in the middle of February, pre-loaded with quinine.

We landed at night at the Simon Bolivar International Airport outside the city, with the runways paralleling the ocean front. Caracas is in a river valley about 10 miles away with low mountain peaks on all sides. The family Volvo 4 X 4 climbed up and up and then down into the city. It was much grander than I expected with blocks and blocks of skyscrapers interspersed with patches of luxuriant vegetation. There was no sign of crime on the streets and absolutely no sign of mosquitoes. Their townhouse was gorgeous with dark Brazil wood floors, huge tropical plants and white upholstered furniture throughout. But there *was* evidence of insect life: that first night, I went down to the kitchen for a bottle of water and when I turned on the light, a dozen huge cockroaches as big as dinner plates scuttled for cover. If there are mosquitoes, I thought, they are going to be massive. The next day, we swam at the Caracas Country Club and then had lunch on the terrace of a hotel, all very posh – but around the perimeter, security guards with machine guns paraded throughout our meal. I thought: Danger: Check; Security: Check.

The next day we headed east to Playa Cumana, a beach resort east of Caracas. Once out of the city, we were driving in dense jungle over very rudimentary roads. The car pitched from one turn to the next, lurching upright only to dive into another corner. An hour or so into the trip, I heard a small voice from the back of the car: "Mummy?" I looked back to see Allison's white, agonized face. "Are you car sick?" The car jerked to a stop and we jumped out, literally on the edge of the jungle. I was holding Allison's hair out of the way and patting her back when the mosquitoes found us. A dense, black swarm of huge mosquitoes whined and whizzed around our heads, landing on every inch of exposed skin. Swatting and slapping, we scrambled back into the car carrying several dozen mosquitoes with us. The car was pandemonium as we tried to eliminate every one. Moving on at last, I thought, Mosquitoes: Check; and then – this could be a disaster.

But the beach resort was incredible – a row of small cottages at the edge of the most beautiful beach I have ever seen: soft, pure white sand and turquoise-green waves drifting towards the shore. Standing at the edge of the ocean, the beach stretched out as far as you could see in either direction with not a single thing in sight. We ate at a big picnic table shaded by pairs of giant coconut palms. The ocean off the shore was shallow and the girls ran in and out of the waves while the grown-ups took turns as lifeguard. At night, we fell asleep to the sound of the waves. And there were no mosquitoes. Yes, Allison and I were studded with itchy bumps, especially on our arms and legs and the backs of our necks but there were no new mosquitoes – and by the time we left, the bites were starting to recede. All these years later, I still remember that as a perfect, golden time.

From there, we flew to Angel Falls, the world's highest uninterrupted waterfall, dropping almost 1000 feet from a table-top mountain in southeast Venezuela. Considered the eighth wonder of the world, Angel Falls are not easy to reach, requiring a special flight from Caracas to a tiny airport in Canaima. On the way in, the pilot zoomed in close and tilted the plane way over so we could glimpse the spectacular fall of water from the air before we landed. Canaima itself perches on the edge of a base camp, the starting point for river trips to the falls. We travelled up river by motorboat and then hiked up to where we could see the falls, a narrow cascade of water shooting out from a cleft at the top of the mountain and falling straight down a vertical cliff face. At the bottom, the water strikes with such force that it sounds like a continuous thunder roll and the base is continuously shrouded in a cloud of water vapor. It is beyond spectacular.

But it's the night I remember most. We were all staying together in a basic concrete shelter with no electricity. There were screens on the windows but we were told to also use mosquito nets which hung from the ceiling over each cot. Lying under my net in absolute blackness, the sound of the jungle was overwhelming, a palpable force filling the room. There was a loud constant hum composed of many sounds – chirps, rustles, knocks, warbles. And over everything, there was the continuous electric whine of mosquitoes. The noise was so intense I did not fall asleep for many hours. But in the morning with the bright sun hot overhead, the jungle sounds were hardly noticeable. On our way to breakfast, we saw gorgeous parrots in the trees around the compound and orchids growing wild. I saw no mosquitoes. But back in the jeep headed for the airport, I realized in a way I never had before that mosquitoes can be a formidable force.

Historically, mosquitoes date back to Aristotle in the second century bc. Called variously gnats or little flies or midges, they are described exactly as we experience them today: a small insect with long legs and delicate wings that make a persistent, whining buzz in flight and whose bites draw blood and leave itchy welts behind. Insects very similar to modern mosquito species have been found preserved in amber dating back more than 100 million years but contemporary phylogenetic studies suggest diversion of different species more than 200 million years ago. Mosquitoes have a complex life-cycle characterized by dramatic short-term changes in shape and function. Female mosquitoes lay their eggs along the edge of small pools of stagnant water – even a bottle cap filled with rain water will do. Larvae hatch with their heads down, breathing through a siphon or a pore called a spiracle in the tail. Within days, the pupa emerges and then transforms into the adult insect. Completion of all three stages can take as little as 5 days. Adult mosquitoes mate only a few days after emerging from the pupal stage, the males attracted by the characteristic whine of females. After mating, the females of most species require a blood meal to provide nutrition for their eggs to mature, typically in a period of days. Once the eggs are fully developed, the female lays them in stagnant water and the process begins again.

The mosquito's head is specialized for feeding and for receiving sensory information through its long, segmented antennae which identify appropriate host odors, as well as potential breeding sites where females can lay eggs. In all mosquito species, the male antennae also contain auditory receptors to detect the whine of females. A large part of the female mosquito's sense of smell is devoted to sniffing out blood sources but more than a third of 72 odor receptors on the antennae are actually tuned to detect chemicals found in perspiration. Many studies have attempted to define exactly why some individuals like me are so attractive to mosquitoes. A prime attractant is 1-Octen-3-ol or octanol, a byproduct of linoleic acid metabolism in humans which is contained in expired breath and sweat. Apparently, female mosquitoes find certain proportions of octanol and carbon dioxide in sweat irresistible. Mosquitoes also carry a specific protein called Or4 that allows detection of sulcatone, another by-product of human metabolism. Sulcatone is a volatile odorant that exists as a miasma around us, again more prominently in some humans than others: mosquitoes and other blood-feeding insects use the scent of sulcatone to hunt us down. Apparently, use of this miasma as a tracking device is especially true for certain mosquito species.

During blood feeding, mosquitoes inject saliva containing any pathogens they are carrying along with an anticoagulant to prevent blood clotting. Mosquito-borne diseases cause millions of deaths worldwide every year with a disproportionate effect on children and the elderly in developing countries. Three mosquito species bear primary responsibility for the spread of human diseases: Anopheles mosquitoes are the only species known to carry malaria as well as filariasis/ elephantiasis and the viral encephalitides; Culex mosquitoes also carry filariasis and the encephalitides plus the West Nile virus; and Aedes mosquitoes carry dengue, chikungunya, Zika, encephalitis and yellow fever …

Yellow Fever: A Jungle Story

For more than four centuries, right into the early twentieth century, coastal populations in Europe and in North, Central and South America, suffered repeated outbreaks of a dreaded illness known variously as yellow jack, vomito negro, Barbados distemper, bilious fever, the American Plague or just yellow fever.[1] The origin of the disease, its specific cause, the mode of transmission: all were unknown; but its frequent recurrences and high fatality rate – as high as 50% in some summers – were well established. As soon as summer arrived, port cities in Europe as far north as Ireland, Central America and the Caribbean, and the United States as far north as Boston, experienced recurrent, life-threatening outbreaks of yellow fever. The disease was first recognizably described in a Mayan manuscript in 1648 and designated formally as yellow fever (YF) in 1750, but for coastal dwellers from Spain to Northern Ireland, from the Caribbean to Boston, it was the scourge of summer.[2] Yellow fever was and remains an international problem but unravelling the historiography of yellow fever is an American story …

Yellow Fever: The Disease

Yellow fever can be recognized from historic texts stretching back hundreds of years because of its classical symptoms.[3] The initial presentation is like many viral illnesses, beginning with abrupt onset of fever, headache, chills, fatigue, muscle pain especially in the neck and back, nausea and loss of appetite. In addition, the yellow fever virus has a specific property called "viscerotropism" which reflects a predilection to preferentially infect the organs of the body, especially the liver, heart and kidneys. This is evident even at this early stage where subclinical findings of liver involve ment appear as a rise in hepatic enzymes. The virus is also neurotropic – meaning attracted to the nervous system – but actual brain infection is extremely rare. In most infected individuals, disease symptoms resolve in 3 to 5 days but in 15–25% of cases there is a one- or two-day hiatus when symptoms improve before a second, toxic phase of the disease begins, characterized by recurrence of high fever, abdominal pain and jaundice (visible yellowing of the eyes and the skin), relative bradycardia (slow heart rate), low urine output and hematemesis (vomiting blood). These severe symptoms reflect the involvement of the liver, kidneys and heart. At this stage, liver enzymes are markedly elevated and liver function is affected, resulting in evidence of coagulopathy (clotting problems) with bleeding ranging from bruising to nosebleeds to severe hemorrhage. Multisystem involvement can occur with failure of the liver, kidneys and heart plus delirium, seizures and coma. Despite these last signs of central nervous system involvement, autopsies have not revealed infection or inflammation of the brain. After 5 to 10 days, this toxic progression is fatal in 20–50% of manifest cases giving an overall YF fatality rate of 3–8%. Older age, higher neutrophil (white cell) count, greater evidence of liver dysfunction (higher liver enzymes, bilirubin and clotting times), higher creatinine levels indicating kidney failure, and higher RNA plasma viral load all correlate significantly with a fatal outcome.[4] Because the diagnosis of uncomplicated YF is not made in the majority of cases, the mortality rate based on manifest infection has often been overestimated. Even now, there is no specific treatment but intensive supportive care can decrease mortality in patients with the severe form of the disease. In those who survive, recovery can be very prolonged but there is usually no permanent organ damage.

Only after antibody studies became available was it realized that at least half of individuals infected with the yellow fever virus are completely asymptomatic and 35% have the mild form of the disease with complete recovery in only a few days. Only 15% of infected individuals develop the classic, severe form of the disease which is the historic yellow fever picture.[5] The reasons for variation among patients infected with the same virus stem from a complex system of virus-host interactions, including intrinsic and acquired host resistance factors and differences in pathogenicity of different virus strains. Surviving the infection – whether asymptomatic, mild or severe – provides lifelong immunity.

Yellow fever was the first recognized viral hemorrhagic fever and is the prototype for this group of life-threatening diseases, represented most prominently at this time by Ebola. These pathogens combine multiple mechanisms to produce symptoms related to damage to the walls of small blood vessels and to the liver, interfering with the body's ability to clot. The internal bleeding that results can range from relatively minor to life-threatening. Each hemorrhagic fever virus acts on the body in pathogen-specific ways, resulting in a variety of symptoms in association with bleeding.

★★★★★★★★★★

Yellow fever brought devastating morbidity and mortality from at least the 1500s right into the early twentieth century when major outbreaks in the port cities of Europe and North, South and Central America recurred. One exceptionally well-documented epidemic occurred in Philadelphia in the long, hot summer of 1793.[6,7] At that time, Philadelphia was the nation's capital and the largest city in North America; trade with the Caribbean islands was common, primarily for sugar and coffee. In the first week of August, a ship from Santo Domingo was unloaded at the port. As vividly described by Murphy in *An American Plague: The True and Terrifying Story of the Yellow Fever Epidemic of 1793*, a young sailor from the ship fell violently ill with fever and died within a few days in a boarding house in the city.[6] Within 2 weeks, there were 7 more deaths on that same block, all associated with severe fever. By the third week of August, Philadelphia doctors were seeing many cases of this "bilious fever," clustered in the streets around the dock area. A massive exodus of panicked citizens began: ultimately, as many as 20,000 citizens of the total population of 55,000 are reported to have abandoned the city during the outbreak. The exodus included George Washington and his family who moved temporarily to Germantown, MD. Doctors struggled to deal with the increasing numbers of desperately ill people. The famous physician Benjamin Rush lived in Philadelphia at the time but even he had nothing to offer except the useless bleeding and purging that he had established as standard of care for almost every illness at that time.[7] Between illness, death and departure, the city was increasingly deserted but the epidemic raged on through September and into October. It was only after the weather turned decisively colder at the end of October that the epidemic ended. It is estimated that 5,000 people, 10% of the population, died during the Philadelphia yellow fever epidemic of 1793.

This was the pattern of the long series of yellow fever outbreaks that descended on port cities – when summer came and ships from the Caribbean and Central America arrived, yellow fever emerged again and again.[1] At least 25 major epidemics were recorded in the United States alone with repeated summer outbreaks in Philadelphia, Baltimore and New York through the eighteenth and nineteenth centuries. In the American south, there were annual outbreaks with especially deadly epidemics described along the Gulf Coast in New Orleans in 1853 and in the whole lower Mississippi Valley in 1878 – 20,000 people died in that single epidemic. The last major outbreak in the United States occurred in 1905 in New Orleans. Europe was not spared, with repeated epidemics – also in port cities – recorded as far north as Northern Ireland. It is no exaggeration to say that yellow fever was among the most dreaded diseases of that time.[3]

The Vector

At the time, the prevailing theory of disease causation was still the "miasma theory" – lethal disease-causing agents were thought to arise spontaneously from decomposing material in the earth and travel by air as a poisonous, foul-smelling vapor, leaving disease in its path. The often-observed association between hot weather and increasing stench with the outbreak of diseases like malaria and yellow fever certainly supported this theory. Another less widely accepted concept was that disease was transmitted by fomites which clung to the bedding and clothes of victims – this was closer to the idea of a contagious agent as the cause of disease proposed most clearly by Fracastero in 1546 but previously by others since ancient times, as described in Chapter 1.[8] It was not until 1796 that John Crawford, an Irish-American physician, promoted a new concept of disease causation in a series of essays about malaria which directly contradicted the miasma theory. He thought that malaria was "occasioned by eggs … laid during a mosquito bite, hatched in the wound and migrated through the host's body," producing the manifestations of the disease.[9] While rejected entirely by the scientific community, this was the first expression of an insect vector for disease. In 1850, Josiah Nott, an American physician living in Alabama took up the idea that insects – including mosquitoes – were also the disease vector for yellow fever. Although a detailed exploration of his writings suggests that this was not a fully formulated idea, Nott is credited with the concept of mosquitoes as the agent for dissemination of yellow fever.[10,11] The mosquito as vector of both yellow fever and malaria was clearly described by Dr. Louis-Daniel Beauperthuy, a physician from Guadalupe, in 1854 when he wrote that they are "produced by venomous fluid injected under the skin by mosquitoes, like poison injected by snakes."[12] Then, in 1860, the French microbiologist, Louis Pasteur, determined that bacteria cause disease and Robert Koch subsequently defined the procedure for proving that specific diseases are caused by specific bacteria.[13] Together, they formalized the germ theory of disease and transformed the concept of disease causation, with subsequent, significant impact on the understanding of yellow fever.

The yellow fever story then shifts to Havana, Cuba where repeated outbreaks of yellow fever occurred, beginning in 1620 after the arrival of a Spanish fleet from Panama. Two centuries later, phylogenetic studies using gene sequencing like those used to try to track the origin of the smallpox virus show that the yellow fever agent first appeared in East Africa approximately 3000 years ago and then spread to West Africa.[14] Analysis of viral isolates from outbreaks in Africa and Central and South America, and an outbreak in the Canary Islands in 1494 have been used to develop the evolutionary history of yellow fever in the Americas.[15] These studies demonstrate that the spread of yellow fever to North and South America corresponded closely with the timing and the routes of the slave trade, from West Africa to Central America and the Caribbean Islands.[16,17] Once introduced, YF spread widely wherever mosquito populations supported it: from port cities in Central America and the Caribbean Islands, to North America as far north as Massachusetts, and South America along the coast of Brazil. In Cuba, a continuous yellow fever epidemic raged between 1649 and 1655, wiping out one third of the population. By the end of the nineteenth century, yellow fever had been continuously present in Havana for more than 100 years.

In response to this ongoing epidemic and the recurrent outbreaks at home, especially a very severe epidemic in the Mississippi River valley in 1878, the United States National Health Board sent an official commission, the Havana Yellow Fever Commission, to Cuba to study yellow fever in 1879.[18] The group worked cooperatively with a similar commission from Spain addressing the same problem and described the epidemiology of yellow fever but made no other major discoveries. Perhaps their greatest accomplishment was to engage a young Cuban physician in the study of yellow fever: Dr. Carlos Finlay was designated as the official Cuban liaison to both commissions. Always inquisitive, Dr. Finlay saw microscopic evidence that the disease attacked small blood vessels and raised the possibility of a vector. He became convinced that mosquitoes, an abundant and ubiquitous presence in Cuba at that time, might be that vector. From his writings:

> It occurred to me that to inoculate yellow fever (into blood vessels) it would be necessary to pick out the infectious material from within the blood vessels of a yellow fever patient and to carry it likewise into the blood vessel of (another) person. All of which conditions the mosquito satisfied most admirably through its bite.[19]

Finlay then identified the *Culex cubensis* mosquito – now called *Aedes Aegyptii* – as the most likely vector because of the two prevalent mosquito species in Havana at that time, it preferred to live in proximity to humans. He then tried to use *Culex* mosquitoes infected by biting yellow fever patients to infect military volunteers with a dramatic initial result: the very first subject developed classic symptoms of yellow fever nine days after being bitten. Although subsequent findings were variable (very likely because infection is asymptomatic in more than half of people), Dr. Findlay presented the results of his investigations to the Academy of Sciences in Havana in 1881 in a report entitled, "The Mosquito Hypothetically Considered as the Agent of Transmission of Yellow Fever."[20] His audience was unimpressed but, undaunted, Finlay continued his work. By 1900, he had inoculated 102 volunteers using a single bite from an infected mosquito with mixed results in terms of classic yellow fever episodes but impressive long-term immunity in almost half of his subjects.

During the Spanish-American war (April to August, 1898), more American soldiers died from yellow fever and malaria than from combat. After the war, yellow fever continued to ravage both the Cubans and the Americans in Cuba as an occupying force. In response, the US military sent a new Yellow Fever Commission led by Major Walter Reed, accompanied by James Carroll, Jesse William Lazear and Aristides Agramonte.[21] Unable to identify any other convincing cause, the Commission met with Carlos Finlay who described his experiments and gave the group a sample of eggs from mosquitoes he believed were contaminated with yellow fever to initiate their investigations. Reed tested the mosquito theory by hatching the eggs from Finlay's collection and then allowing the mosquitoes that emerged to bite several volunteers, including Lazear and Carroll from the commission team. Both Carroll and Lazear developed yellow fever and Lazear died of the disease, providing tragic proof to Major Reed that mosquitoes transmitted yellow fever. After Lazear's death, the team developed a systematic series of experiments based on his notes which described critical timing issues in both the acquisition of the yellow fever agent by a mosquito and the mosquito's ability to transmit the infection.[22] These experiments proved that mosquitoes can only acquire the yellow fever agent if they feed on an infected person during the first 3 to 5 days after they are infected and that mosquitoes cannot pass on the infection to another human until after a 10–12 day period of incubation. The team also conclusively eliminated the theory that yellow fever was transmitted by fomites: volunteers were isolated in separate buildings, one containing clothing and bed linens from yellow fever patients and the other containing infected mosquitoes. Only volunteers in the building containing mosquitoes developed yellow fever.[23] Finally, James Carroll, an expert in bacteriology, showed that yellow fever was caused by a filterable agent found in the blood of infected patients which caused yellow fever when injected into non-immune volunteers.[24] Remember that at that time, viruses were defined by two negative characteristics: they were not retained by standard bacteriologic filters and they were not visible by light microscopy. They could only be further identified indirectly, by inducing disease in a susceptible host with a bacteria-free filtrate from a diseased subject, or by proven prevention of re-infection in survivors of the illness in question. Carroll's demonstration that a filterable agent in the blood of yellow fever victims induced the disease in non-immune volunteers was the very first demonstration that a virus could cause a specific disease in humans. The Fourth Yellow Fever Commission team definitively proved that the *Culex cubensis* mosquito – now *Aedes Aegyptii* – was the mode of transmission for the yellow fever agent and that this agent was a virus, shown in Figure 3.1. [This work is documented in remarkable detail in the *Philip S. Hench Walter Reed Yellow Fever Collection (circa 1800–circa 1998)*, located in "A Collection in Historical Collections" in the Claude Moore Health Sciences Library in the University of Virginia.]

As a result of the findings of the Reed Commission, Major William C. Gorgas, the Army's chief sanitation officer in Cuba, was ordered to implement a program of mosquito eradication. Gorgas first isolated yellow fever patients with screens to prevent mosquitoes from feeding on them and acquiring the virus. He then attacked the mosquito population, ordering his team to fumigate every building in Havana with insecticides and eliminate all sources of standing water. As a result of these efforts, the number of yellow fever cases fell precipitously and, by 1902, no new cases were reported in Havana. With Gorgas's practical application of the Reed commission's findings, the Army was able to curb and (by the evidence of the time), eradicate yellow fever in Havana, paving the way for future operations in any environment where yellow fever was prevalent. Gorgas implemented a similar program during the building of the Panama Canal in 1905 after roughly 85% of workers in the initial attempt had been hospitalized with either malaria or yellow fever. He convinced President Theodore Roosevelt to fund a mosquito eradication effort in Panama and then led a team of 4,000 workers, his "mosquito brigade." The team fumigated all the homes in the area and aggressively eliminated all standing water. Within a year, new cases of yellow fever had been virtually eliminated, a critical factor in completion of the Canal in 1914.[25] (For more on this fascinating story, see the historical perspective at the end of this chapter.)

★★★★★★★★★★

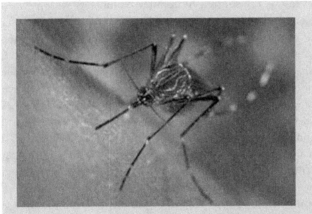

FIGURE 3.2 *Aedes aegyptii* mosquito

Source: Mosquito Bites: Everyone is at Risk! https://media@cdc.gov.CDC.gov

The adult *Aedes Aegypticus* mosquito is a supremely elegant insect, approximately 4 to 7 millimeters long. As seen in Figure 3.2, the insect is dark brown to black in color with silvery-white pattern on the top of the thorax in the shape of a harp and white basal stripes on each segment of the hind legs. With their long delicate wings, they are the divas of the mosquito world. In his comprehensive study of this mosquito, Sir Richard Christophers describes "blood as the natural food of the female," while both males and females survive on nectar or sap from plants and flowers for nutrition.[26] The blood meal is essential for the development of eggs so females seek out a warm-blooded animal, usually a human, within a few days after breeding. The insect is so quiet and so light that its landing is usually entirely undetected. From close observation of feeding behavior, the female mosquito lands on exposed skin, shifts its proboscis into a nearly vertical position and quickly punctures the skin. The insect then crouches down, sinks the fascicle to its full depth and, it uninterrupted, feeds for up to three minutes until the abdomen is greatly distended before withdrawing the fascicle. More often, multiple bites on several different people are needed to take in enough blood. After feeding, flight is difficult because the weight of blood taken can actually exceed the weight of the unfed insect. The fully engorged mosquito can remain sitting on the skin for as much as 15 minutes. The female then rests for a period of days during which digestion occurs followed by egg maturation. This can take three days to three weeks, depending on the temperature, with faster maturation at higher temperatures, before the eggs are laid on the surface of small collections of fresh water and the life cycle begins again. If the female mosquito bites an individual with yellow fever during the first 5 days of the illness, she acquires lifelong yellow fever infectivity. After approximately 10–12 days for virus incubation, an infected female will inoculate approximately 1000–100,000 virus particles with each subsequent bite. Female mosquitoes can lay a set of up to 100 eggs about every third night after mating only once. They typically lay as many as three sets before dying, requiring a blood meal to provide protein for each set.[26]

Aedes aegyptii is the perfect urban vector of yellow fever because it is rarely found more than 100 yards from human habitation. It is active in the daytime and early evening and prefers heavy shade. It freely enters homes and other buildings and has even been shown to readily move vertically in high rise buildings.[27] Within homes, the largest numbers are found in bedrooms, in secluded places like closets and under beds.[28] In short, humans are the perfect hosts providing comfortable, safe shelter and a plentiful source of blood, all under one roof.

Though the mosquito is now widely established throughout the tropical and sub-tropical regions of the world, it was located solely in Africa until the fifteenth century.[29] At that time, *Aedes aegyptii* is thought to have adapted to breeding in small water collections in response to a profound drought. Such breeding sites were often man-made objects that contained water, from buckets to saucers to the water-storage jars on ships – thought to be the genesis of the described close connection between the mosquito and human habitation. This "human-adapted" behavior explains the mosquito's spread across Africa and the introduction to the new world on slave trade ships between the fifteenth and eighteenth centuries. Slave ships carrying thousands of West Africans together with the domesticated *Aedes aegyptii* mosquito allowed breeding and disease transmission cycles to be established en route.[16,17] Arrival in Central America delivered a critical mass of viremic hosts and active vectors into a receptive environment. This allowed rapid dissemination of yellow fever across the tropical regions of Central and South America, where it caused the recurrent yellow fever epidemics of the next three centuries.

As described in the Philadelphia epidemic,[6] the mosquitoes then travelled from their natural tropical habitat to temperate harbor cities in Europe and North America on trade ships carrying sugar and coffee. The ships had all the mosquito's requirements: cisterns of water, humans in crowded conditions and concealed spaces. The recurrent yellow fever epidemics in port cities in the eighteenth and nineteenth centuries where the population was largely non-immune were the consequence of transportation of the *Aedes Aegyptii* mosquito in conjunction with human migration and trade.[16,17]

★★★★★★★★

With the dramatic successes of Reed and Gorgas, it was believed that the *Aedes Aegyptii* mosquito was the sole vector responsible for transmission of yellow fever and that man was the only susceptible host. Mosquito eradication efforts carried out in many large Central and South American cities appeared to lead to the disappearance of yellow fever and at the time, scientists felt that mosquito control was all that was needed to completely eradicate the disease. This conviction was held so strongly that in 1915, the Rockefeller Foundation felt confident enough to pledge the eradication of yellow fever from the face of the earth.[30] Unfortunately, sustained mosquito eradication efforts proved unsuccessful in eliminating YF in South America suggesting the underlying epidemiology of the disease was more complicated.

Following reports that yellow fever was prevalent in West Africa, the West African Yellow Fever Commission was organized by the Rockefeller Foundation in 1925. Led by retired Colonel Henry Beeuwkes, the commission was charged with isolating the organism causing the disease, confirming the method of transmission and identifying those areas in which the disease is continually present. Attempting to establish an animal model, Beeuwkes imported monkeys and chimpanzees to the lab in West Africa which was already stocked with guinea pigs. Adrian Stokes, a pathologist with the Commission, injected blood from a West African man with yellow fever into the group of lab animals. Neither guinea pigs nor marmosets had any reaction, but a rhesus monkey became sick and died with autopsy findings consistent with yellow fever: an animal model was born.[31] Unfortunately, Stokes himself developed yellow fever. Despite his illness, he insisted that his blood be injected into rhesus monkeys and that *Aedes aegyptii* mosquitoes be allowed to feed on him. Both his blood and the infected mosquitoes caused fatal yellow fever in the lab monkeys, thus fulfilling Koch's postulates for disease causality. Subsequent, successful isolation of the virus and its confirmation as the cause of yellow fever came at a heavy price, as 32 lab-associated cases of the disease occurred between 1927 and 1931, with five deaths including that of Adrian Stokes. The isolated virus was named the *Asibi* strain after the 28-year-old West African yellow fever survivor who provided the blood sample.

Epidemiology of Yellow Fever

Continued work of the West African Yellow Fever Commission began to untangle the complex epidemiology of yellow fever. Once the virus had been isolated, a team from the Rockefeller headed by Max Theiler developed a test to demonstrate immunity to yellow fever when white mice were found to be susceptible to the virus. This "mouse protection test" could be used to test for the presence of antibodies to the virus and was utilized to conduct an immunity survey, testing serum collected from multiple animals.[32] These results revealed a broad band of yellow fever immunity stretching across Africa, from the West Coast through Central Africa to Uganda in East Africa, from approximately 15 degrees north to 15 degrees south of the equator.[33] However, while clinical outbreaks of yellow fever were common in West Africa, they were rare in East Africa. This led to the concept that yellow fever arose in East Africa and was potentially endemic there with such ubiquitous immunity that no yellow fever cases could develop. After intensive epidemiologic work, this concept was confirmed when multiple monkey species in the jungle forests of Uganda in East Africa were found to have immunity to yellow fever.[33] In 1941, Alexander Mahaffy and his team from the Commission isolated the yellow fever virus from wild-caught *Aedes simpsoni* mosquitoes and from a human with clinical yellow fever during a local epidemic in Uganda in East Africa.[34] Multiple additional *Aedes* mosquito species found in the tropical forest canopy like *Africanus* and *Aldopictus* were also found to carry the virus. The YF virus was maintained in the jungle by transmission from female mosquitoes to their offspring and to lower primate vertebrate hosts, primarily monkeys. Outbreaks in humans in this situation occurred only with contact with the forest. In towns and cities, the virus was found to be primarily transmitted by the highly domesticated *Aedes aegyptii* while in the forest, the virus was transmitted by several other jungle mosquito species. In all settings, the infected hosts – monkeys or humans – greatly increased the number of circulating viruses, a process called amplification. The virus was shown to be carried from one host to another by the biting mosquito vector, a horizontal transmission pattern. Mosquitoes also passed the virus via infected eggs to their offspring by vertical transmission. The eggs produced were resistant to drying, lying dormant through drought conditions and hatching when rain began. The mosquito was therefore recognized as the true reservoir of the virus, ensuring transmission from one host to another and from one year to the next.

These observations ultimately led to description of three separate yellow fever transmission cycles.[33] The *jungle or sylvatic cycle* of yellow fever involves endemic disease in tropical rain forests in para-equatorial Africa and South America where multiple *Aedes* tree-hole mosquito species that inhabit the forest canopy are the reservoir for the yellow fever virus. These mosquitoes transmit the virus to monkeys and other small mammals. There are only occasional human cases of yellow fever in this setting because contact between jungle mosquitoes and man is rare, but when the disease occurs, it is identical both clinically and serologically to classic urban yellow fever. The *intermediate or savannah cycle* occurs in areas with sparse human habitation bordering jungle areas, in Africa and South America. Multiple mosquito species which inhabit the jungle borders are involved in viral transmission including *Aedes furcifer, Aedes luteocephalus,*and *Aedes simpsoni*. It is these mosquitoes from the forest canopy that Allison and I encountered on our trip to Venezuela. Human cases of yellow fever occur in response to bites by these mosquitoes but because contact with humans is infrequent, large outbreaks are rare and are usually associated with movement of groups of people into the area during periods of social unrest. The *urban cycle* is the already described classic form of the disease which occurred as recurrent epidemics in West Africa, Europe, Central, South and North America from the eighteenth into the twentieth centuries. In this setting, the yellow fever virus is transmitted from human to human by the *Aedes aegyptii* mosquito. Because of the preference of this species for human habitation and human blood, the urban pattern of transmission has the potential to cause explosive epidemics of disease when the virus is newly introduced into areas with high human population density.

****

The Vaccine

Discovery of the extent of endemic yellow fever in the jungle mosquitoes and monkeys of Africa and South America led to a clear understanding of why insect eradication in urban centers would not eliminate the disease so attempts at vaccine development began as early as the late 1920s. True isolation of the virus in 1928 was followed by several critical observations: serum from humans and monkeys that had survived yellow fever protected monkeys against experimental yellow fever; a preliminary vaccine based on a killed virus did not confer immunity; and serum from disease survivors in South America protected against the YF virus in Africa.[35,36] These findings suggested that a live vaccine was needed and if developed, would be globally protective against yellow fever.

In 1930, the Rockefeller Institute in New York was already the world's most important center of experimental yellow fever research. Conditions for experimenting with monkeys had been established and the basic properties of the virus had been analyzed. It was here that Max Theiler developed the test that demonstrated the presence of yellow fever antibodies in humans that was used to map the epidemiology of yellow fever in Africa, and here that he began work on a yellow fever vaccine.[32] The Rockefeller team used the technique that Louis Pasteur developed to create the first lab-produced human vaccine for rabies in 1879, by creating a weakened or attenuated live virus. The attenuated form was created by passing the attenuated disease-causing virus through a series of cell cultures from animal or chick embryos. With each passage, the virus improved its ability to replicate in the new setting, but decreased its ability to replicate in humans. A virus targeted for use in a vaccine may be "passaged" through as many as 200 different cultures before it will no longer multiply in humans. The goal is to create a weakened virus that will be unable to cause illness but will still provoke an immune response that will protect against future infection.[37]

Initially, Theiler and his colleagues struggled to grow the yellow fever virus in tissue cultures. Eventually, based on Pasteur's work, they demonstrated growth in a mouse brain model.[38] After serial passage of the yellow fever virus through this model, Theiler found that the weakened virus conferred immunity in Rhesus monkeys. Unfortunately, while the attenuated virus had diminished ability to attack the liver (its natural, viscerotropic property), the capacity of the virus to attack the brain – its latent neurotropic property – had increased.[39] To address this, Theiler and his team performed a series of experiments, passaging the virus multiple times in different kinds of tissue cultures and repeatedly testing for neurotropic activity. A major breakthrough came in 1937 when the *Asibi* strain of virus – the first ever isolated – was passaged repeatedly in minced chicken embryos from which the central nervous system had been removed. After more than 100 passages, a virus variant spontaneously emerged that lacked both the viscerotropic and the neurotropic properties of the native virus – a very fortuitous example of spontaneous mutation. Fortunately, the properties of this new attenuated virus strain were stable, and virulence for the central nervous system did not recur on repeated testing. The Theiler team named this strain "17D." Animal tests showed the attenuated 17D mutant was both safe and immunizing, allowing Theiler's team to rapidly complete the development of a 17D vaccine.[40] For this work, Max Theiler received the Nobel Prize for Medicine and Physiology in 1951, at that time, the only Nobel ever given for development of a vaccine.

The new vaccine was not harmless – from the outset, there were severe neurological reactions in a very small number of people – but on balance, the 1937 field trials with the new 17D vaccine in Brazil, directed by the Rockefeller Foundation, were highly successful. Following these, the Foundation funded large-scale manufacture of the vaccine. During the Second World War, the Foundation coordinated the vaccination of all American and British military personnel. Some adverse reactions related to batch manufacture had to be addressed but overall, this massive campaign was successful. By war's end, millions of vaccine doses had been given with effective protection of active military personnel from yellow fever. Following the war, the manufacture and distribution of the yellow fever vaccine passed from the Rockefeller Foundation to the United States Public Health Service and to other international institutions and government agencies.[41] Severe adverse events after vaccination are rare, but very rarely, severe hypersensitivity or anaphylactic reactions, YF vaccine-associated neurologic disease, and YF vaccine-associated viscerotropic disease can occur.[42] The original YF vaccine is still the gold standard, contra-indicated only in individuals with immune suppression and in babies less than 9 months of age; in individuals over 60 years of age, the vaccine is given electively, with agreement of the clinician and patient.

The Virus

Against the backdrop of ongoing vaccination programs, characterization of the yellow fever virus itself continued, albeit at a leisurely pace.[43] In 1953, the virus was first visualized by electron microscopy and was seen to be small and round with a slightly irregular contour.[44] By the 1960s, antibodies against yellow fever could be identified by simplified lab tests and these results led to the realization that the YFV was antigenically related to a group of viruses called the *Arboviruses* because they were all carried by arthropods – mosquitoes or ticks. This terminology was formally adopted by the WHO in 1963.[45] The yellow fever virus is a single-stranded positive-sense RNA virus. Ultimately, reverse transcription-polymerase chain reaction (RT-PCR), the genetic test that identifies nucleotide sequences, was applied to the yellow fever virus and complete sequencing of the virus was first reported in 1985.[46] Based on this nucleotide sequencing, a new taxonomic classification, the *Flavivirus* genus, was created in 1994. The first mammalian viruses to be assigned to this classification included the yellow fever virus which lent its Latin name, "flavus," for the characteristic yellow color of its victims, to the group. The yellow fever virus is the prototype member of the *Flavivirus* genus which includes more than 70 taxonomically recognized, globally-distributed species and is constantly being updated to reflect newly-identified viruses and advances in analytical methods.[47]

The family *Flaviviridae* contains 3 genera: the above-described flaviviruses, which include yellow fever (YFV), West Nile virus (WNV), dengue virus (DENV) and Zika virus (ZKV); the hepaci-viruses, which include hepatitis B and C viruses; and the pesti-viruses, which infect hoofed mammals. The vector-borne arboviruses are grouped as a clade within the *Flavivirus* genus and this is subdivided into a mosquito-borne clade and a tick-borne clade. The mosquito clade is divided into two branches: one branch contains the neurotropic viruses, often associated with encephalitic disease in humans or livestock. This branch tends to be spread by the Culex mosquito species and to have bird reservoirs – an example is the West Nile virus. The second branch is the group associated with hemorrhagic disease in humans. These tend to have Aedes species as vectors and primate hosts – the yellow fever virus is emblematic of this group.[46]

The yellow fever virus is now known to be a small (40 to 60 nm), enveloped virus harboring a single positive-strand RNA genome of 11 kb that, like the smallpox virus, replicates in the cytoplasm of infected cells. The genome encodes a polyprotein that is cleaved into three structural proteins and seven nonstructural proteins. Surface macromolecules of the YF virus are its main virulence factors and contribute to the entry, signaling and cell-cell interactions of the virus. During virus replication, the structural proteins are incorporated into progeny virions, while the non-structural proteins remain in infected cells where they coordinate RNA replication and viral assembly, and modulate innate immune responses.[46] The synthesis of yellow fever virus RNA is detectable within 3 to 6 hours after infection and progeny virions created in the host cell are released after about 12 hours.

Patterns of antigenic conservation and divergence differ widely between viruses: the yellow fever virus is a single antigenic serotype which is highly conserved and this is why the 17D vaccine protects against all strains of the virus. At the nucleotide sequence level, it is possible to distinguish seven major genotypes of yellow fever representing West Africa (two genotypes), Central-East Africa and Angola (three genotypes), and South America (two genotypes). Spontaneous mutation is not a common feature of the yellow fever virus.[47]

Laboratory confirmation of YF is required for complete diagnosis but is rarely accomplished since the majority of infected individuals are asymptomatic and testing requires highly trained laboratory staff and specialized equipment and materials. There are multiple laboratory criteria for diagnosis but the most frequently used is detection of YFV genomic sequences in blood or organs by PCR. Frequently, clinical YF is not diagnosed until the patient has either recovered or succumbed, if a confirmed diagnosis is ever made. Case definitions state that a *suspected* case is characterized by acute onset of fever followed by jaundice within 2 weeks of the onset of the first symptoms, while a *confirmed* YF case requires laboratory confirmation or an epidemiologic link to a laboratory-confirmed case or outbreak.[48]

Several studies investigating the immune response in healthy subjects receiving the vaccine have shown that 17D vaccination leads to an integrated immune response that includes several effector arms of the innate immune response as well as rapid activation of T cell immunity and production of neutralizing antibodies within 10 days of vaccination; antibodies have been confirmed as persisting for up to 40 years.[49] Practically speaking, immunity after vaccination is lifelong.

★★★★★★★★★★★

The fascinating and beautiful *Aedes Aegypti* mosquito has been shown to play a critical role in disease transmission for multiple members of the Flaviviridae family. It is the primary vector for yellow fever but also one of the main transmitters of dengue, chikungunya and Zika, all increasingly important global public health concerns. Dengue alone is responsible for 50–100 million annual infections including major outbreaks in the Caribbean, South America and the southern United States. Since 2013, the chikungunya virus has caused large global disease outbreaks in India, Southeast Asia, the Caribbean islands, Latin America, South America and the southern United States. Finally, beginning in 2015, the Zika virus (ZKV) – described in depth in Chapter 7 – has caused a major pandemic affecting more than 15 million people. Centered in Brazil, ZKV infection in most patients causes no symptoms but in pregnant women in the first and second trimesters, ZKV infection is associated with significant risk for severe congenital brain abnormalities in the developing fetus. In summary, the easy co-existence of humans and *Aedes aegyptii* has major health consequences. The struggle to control *Aedes Aegyptii* is reflected in an ongoing global struggle with all these diseases.

★★★★★★★★

Public Health Management of Yellow Fever

Between the 1930s and the 1960s, mass YF vaccination campaigns were carried out in South America and in multiple West African countries resulting in a progressive disappearance of the disease in those locations. However, the range of yellow fever virus transmission in the Americas expanded with cases reported in Panama in the 1950s, the first in 43 years. Before the end of the decade, the disease had spread throughout Central America, finally stopping near the southern border of Mexico. From the 1960s forward, low or absent vaccination levels globally, combined with the births of subsequently unvaccinated children and the deaths of older, protected individuals resulted in increasing yellow fever outbreaks in Africa and in Central and South America. Thousands of cases were reported annually in West Africa, where vaccination coverage had waned or was absent, and in Ethiopia where the disease had never been reported previously.[47]

Since the 1940s, the International Sanitary Regulations drafted by WHO have stipulated that "vaccination against yellow fever shall be required of any person leaving an infected local area on an international voyage and proceeding to a yellow fever receptive area." This was the first regulatory language that overtly mandated yellow fever vaccination requirements for country entry. Modified and renamed the International Health Regulations in 1969 and then completely revised in 2005; the most current iteration stipulates, "Vaccination against yellow fever may be required of any traveler leaving an area where the Organization has determined that a risk of yellow fever transmission is present."[50] The WHO also asked countries to establish entry regulations, requiring travelers to show official proof of vaccination against the disease. Despite these regulatory efforts, vaccination programs anywhere in Africa between 1960 and 1980 were almost exclusively in reaction to disease outbreaks.

Since the 1980s, there has been an exponential increase in yellow fever cases in both sub-Saharan Africa and tropical South America. Between 1987 and 1991, a total of 18,735 yellow fever cases and 4522 deaths were reported to the World Health Organization – this was the highest level of yellow fever activity for any 5-year period since 1948; given the very high prevalence of clinically asymptomatic infection, the true number of cases will have been vastly greater.[43,47] Ecological surveillance of jungle mosquitoes and monkeys suggested that these outbreaks occurred because of amplification of the virus in non-human primates combined with an increasing population of unvaccinated individuals in progressively closer proximity – in other words, the increasing impact of human encroachment on previously remote jungle areas.[43] Globally, WHO now estimates there are between 84,000 to 170,000 cases and 60,000 deaths from yellow fever each year; as always, there is significant under-reporting, due to asymptomatic infections and lack of effective surveillance systems so the actual disease burden is much higher. Based on the distribution of *Aedes aegyptii* as shown in Figure 3.3, yellow fever is an annual risk to *900 million(!)* individuals

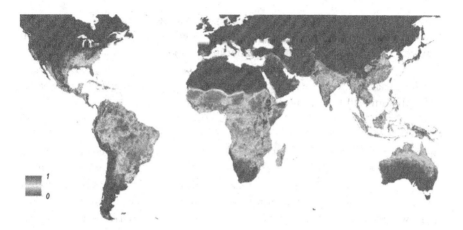

FIGURE 3.3 Global map of the predicted distribution of *Aedes aegyptii*.

Source: "The global distribution of the arbovirus vectors Aedes aegypti and Ae. aldopictus." Kraemer MUG, Sinka ME, Duda KA et al. *eLIFE* 2015;4:e08347. American Public Health Service. APHC.gov. National Institutes of Health, USA.

and travelers in the 44 known endemic countries of Africa and Latin/South America with West Africa as the region most affected; a large proportion of cases occur in children.

Since 1988, the WHO, the United Nations Children's Fund (UNICEF), and the World Bank have recommended that 33 African countries add the vaccine to the routine immunization program in infants and children after studies showed that this would be highly cost-effective.[51,52] In 2001, the Global Alliance for Vaccines (GAVI) began to fund a program to include the yellow fever vaccine in routine immunization programs and analyses show that 22 of the 33 countries had adopted the program by 2006. Immunizing children, however, will not prevent disease outbreaks when the rest of the population remains vulnerable. In response, the Yellow Fever Initiative was launched in 2005 as a partnership among the WHO, GAVI, UNICEF and the ministries of health in each country to begin a catch-up immunization campaign across West Africa and to secure a large, stable vaccine supply. By 2012, 69 million people in 13 countries had received the yellow fever vaccine.[53]

Unfortunately, the demand for the yellow fever vaccine for preventive campaigns consistently exceeds availability. The limited global production capacity cannot meet increasing demand for several reasons. The manufacturing process for the vaccine is slow and cumbersome, essentially unchanged from Theiler's method back in the 1930s, using 7- to 9-day-old chick embryos in specific pathogen-free eggs which are infected with the virus and then incubated. The infected embryos are then harvested under aseptic conditions after which homogenization and centrifugation produces a surface liquid that is preserved for use in vaccines. The vaccine supply is limited because each embryo can produce only 100–300 vaccine doses and the supply of pathogen-free eggs is restricted.[54] The emergency vaccine stockpile, administered by a WHO committee in Geneva, holds only six million doses. Because profits are low, many pharmaceutical companies have dropped production of the yellow fever vaccine. In 1970, 14 private or national vaccine factories made yellow fever vaccine; now only six do, and only four sell the vaccine to the World Health Organization.

★★★★★★★★★★

In December 2015, a new sustained yellow fever epidemic began in Angola and spread to the Democratic Republic of the Congo (DRC) with almost 1000 confirmed cases and 7300 suspected cases in those two countries by the fall of 2016.[55] With an at-risk population in Africa alone of over 500 million people, there was immediate concern about a massive epidemic with the potential for global spread. Ultimately, this outbreak developed into the largest and most widespread epidemic of YF in more than 20 years. The crisis initiated an emergency mass immunization campaign aimed to end disease transmission before the rainy season started in September 2016, a peak time for YF-carrying mosquitoes. The logistical details were daunting, requiring almost 20 million syringes and over 40,000 health workers and volunteers. The vaccine requires refrigeration and an unreliable energy supply made this a major challenge with ultimately, more than 100,000 ice packs used to deliver the vaccine.

The vaccines used came from the global stockpile co-managed by Médecins Sans Frontières (MSF), the International Federation of the Red Cross and Red Crescent Societies (IFRC), UNICEF and the WHO. In the first 6 months of 2016 alone, these partners delivered more than 19 million doses of the vaccine – more than three times the 6 million doses usually put aside for a possible outbreak. GAVI, the Vaccine Alliance, financed a significant proportion of the vaccines. Because the vaccine supply was so limited, WHO used a fractional dose strategy based on studies showing that one fifth of the usual dose of the yellow fever vaccine will provide immunity for at least a year – enough time to achieve the critical level of resistance needed to stop the outbreak.[56] A massive training and community engagement effort resulted in 30 million people being vaccinated across the 2 countries. The campaign was at least temporarily successful with no reports of suspected cases in Angola or the DRC after September of 2016.[57]

Experts state that outbreaks like these in Angola and the Democratic Republic of the Congo will become more frequent in many parts of the world unless coordinated measures are taken to protect people most at risk. Recent years have seen global changes in the epidemiology of yellow fever, with outbreaks occurring in areas that were not previously assessed as being at high risk. Climate change, increasing population density, the mobility of people within and across borders, and the resurgence of the *Aedes aegyptii* mosquito, have combined to increase the likelihood of yellow fever epidemics. Awareness of this increased global risk brought together a broad coalition of partners in Geneva, Switzerland, in September 2016 to develop a new global strategy for the "Elimination of

Yellow Fever Epidemics"(EYE). Planned key components of the strategy include preventive vaccination (both in routine immunization schedules and mass campaigns), an expanded global vaccine stockpile for outbreak response and support for greater preparedness in the most at-risk countries.[58]

****

Increasing global connectedness plays a major part in the expansion of *Aedes aegyptii* territory: exponential growth in population density. urbanization and international trade and travel, plus global warming each contribute to the increasing distribution of this mosquito. Incorporating climate and environmental data with land-cover variables and occurrence records in a complex model predicts the current distribution of this mosquito to be concentrated in tropical and sub-tropical areas across the globe, especially sub-Saharan Africa, northern Brazil and southeast Asia, northern Australia, Spain and Greece. The model predicts *Ae. Aegypti* will be distributed throughout Central America and on both coasts of Mexico; in the United States, it will be concentrated in the southeastern states, especially those along the Gulf Coast. As shown in Figure 3.3, this predicted distribution includes all five non-polar continents.[59]

Cases of yellow fever imported from countries with endemic and/or epidemic disease are an important factor in the potential for future epidemics. As an example, on September 28, 1999, a previously healthy 48-year-old Californian presented to a local ER with a 2-day history of fever, chills, headache, photophobia, muscle and joint pain, nausea, vomiting and generalized weakness. Two days earlier, he had returned from a 10-day trip to Venezuela. His physical exam was positive for icteric sclerae (yellowing of the whites of the eyes), tenderness in the upper abdomen and multiple, red, excoriated mosquito bites on the lower legs and feet. His liver function tests were all markedly abnormal and he had biochemical evidence of acute kidney failure – all significant risk factors for a fatal outcome. Despite intensive management, his condition deteriorated rapidly and he died 6 days after presentation. Autopsy findings confirmed the clinical diagnosis of fulminant yellow fever. [60] Had he had a less symptomatic infection, he could have been the reservoir for infection of *A. aegypti* mosquitoes in mainland USA. This was a vaccine-preventable death as proof of yellow fever vaccination was required for travel to Venezuela by 1990, only a few years after Allison and I experienced our mass mosquito attack. At present, a high proportion of travelers to at-risk areas are reported to be immunized, presumably reflecting widespread knowledge about the International Health Regulations. However, with *Aedes aegypti* mosquitoes present in new areas including the coastal United States, there is concern that the yellow fever virus imported by unvaccinated travelers like these could erupt into explosive outbreaks in *Ae. Aegypti*-infested areas now free of the disease.[61]

The 2015–16 epidemic in Angola is a case in point. Angola is one of China's biggest energy investment targets; in 2009, China bought almost one-third of Angola's crude oil. There are reportedly 100,000 Chinese construction workers and business people in Angola and an untold number in the DRC. In early March 2016, three months into the epidemic described above, a previously healthy Chinese man who had worked in Angola since 2009, developed fever and chills. He flew home to Beijing, arriving on day 3 of his illness and was immediately admitted to hospital. Despite intensive efforts, he died on day 9 with fulminant liver and kidney failure. Yellow fever virus was detected in his serum and viral gene sequencing showed the infecting virus belonged to the Angolan subtype.[62] After this case, the Chinese government notified the WHO of 11 additional cases of yellow fever imported from Angola. Despite Chinese, Angolan and WHO-IHR regulations, none of these individuals had received vaccination against yellow fever in China before going to Angola, nor in Angola before returning to China.

These are the first cases of yellow fever ever documented in China. One of the mysteries of yellow fever epidemiology has been its failure to emerge as an established pathogen in Asia despite appropriate tropical and sub-tropical environmental conditions, a susceptible urban population and the established presence of the *Ae. aegypti* vector. In addition, the dengue virus, also transmitted by *A. aegypti*, is now an established disease in China. There are a number of theories to explain this phenomenon including the possibility that Asian strains of *Ae. aegypti* may be less competent yellow fever vectors; limited introduction of a sustained volume of infected men or mosquitoes; and potential cross-protective immunity in individuals infected with other flaviviruses like dengue.[63] By contrast, there are contemporary factors that represent optimal conditions for an Asian epidemic. The volume of travelers entering the region on commercial airlines is very high: the Asian-Pacific region was the largest regional market for air transport in 2016, accounting for one-third of all global passengers. This allows for easy introduction of a large number of individuals carrying the virus into a country with the known mosquito vectors, as well as the potential for rapid dissemination to other high-risk regions in India or Southeast Asia. Most importantly, there appears to be low effective vaccination coverage of Chinese workers in Angola. The risk of illness for an unimmunized person spending 2 weeks in an area of epidemic activity is high, estimated at one in 267. This translates into a substantial number of potential cases among returning workers, with the potential of sustained regional YF exposure. Finally, there is a strong possibility that widespread epidemic transmission could occur in Asia before it is recognized given the similarity of the early clinical presentation to that of other endemic diseases and the lack of clinical experience with YF.[63] Fortunately, the infected Chinese workers who returned from Angola in 2016 all arrived in locations where *Ae. Aegypti* is not established and no known secondary cases resulted.[64] The current scenario of a YF outbreak in Angola, where there is a large community of non-immune foreign nationals, coupled with high volumes of air travel to an environment conducive to transmission in Asia, is unprecedented in history. These conditions raise the alarming possibility of a YF outbreak in a region with a susceptible population of *2 billion(!)* people and a limited infrastructure for effective response. Imported cases like these show how critical it is to recognize this risk now and initiate adequate pre-emptive action to avert a global catastrophe.

Yellow fever is also endo-epidemic in Brazil with seasonal increases in human cases occurring annually in coastal areas between December and May but since 2016, massive outbreaks have taken place in Brazil, reaching YF–free zones and causing thousands of deaths. The 2016–2022 YF epidemics have been the most significant outbreaks of the last 70 years and the number of human cases was 2.8 times higher than total cases in the previous 36 years.[65] A new YFV lineage was associated with the recent outbreaks, with persistent circulation in Southeast Brazil. The typical jungle transmission cycle occurs between forest mosquitoes and forest-dwelling nonhuman primates, with humans serving only as incidental hosts. However, deforestation, which has reduced monkey habitats, combined with expanding urban sprawl have brought yellow fever-carrying primates and mosquitoes closer to human populations in this part of Brazil. In early 2016, the yellow fever virus broke out of its usual jungle transmission pattern and began moving south and east, following forest corridors inhabited by monkeys toward the big coastal cities with huge populations of non-vaccinated, YF-naive individuals, triggering a potential public health emergency.[66] In previous seasons, human YF cases were rare but from 2016 through 2018, there were more than 2000 cases with 745 deaths. All cases were related to sylvatic transmission by *Haemagogus* mosquitoes, a jungle species, but there is significant concern that a person infected with yellow fever in the jungle could easily travel to an urban area and be bitten by an *Aedes aegypti* mosquito, initiating an urban chain of human infections.[66] Yellow fever can spread explosively among unvaccinated people in this situation and international travel means many areas of the world where *Ae. aegypti* are ubiquitous are at risk. As the epizootic waves of the 1916–1919 seasons drifted closer and closer to the large, southern cities in the states of Sao Paulo, Rio de Janeiro and Bahia, the risk of urbanization of the virus led to a mass vaccination campaign. This was initiated in 2018 and in 2020, the country expanded the yellow fever vaccination area to the entire country and adopted a single-dose schedule starting at 9 months of age to protect younger generations for life. In response to this vaccination campaign, Brazil has controlled the outbreak, recording only nine cases and three deaths between 2020 and 2021.[67]

New YF cases were reported again in Uganda in November of 2019. Uganda is classified as a high-risk country in the EYE initiative, with a history of recurrent outbreaks in 2011, 2016 and 2018. The YF virus is endo-epidemic in Uganda meaning repeated disease outbreaks can be anticipated. Risk of epidemic spread is high as the estimated overall population immunity is very low. The affected districts in Uganda share international borders with both DRC and South Sudan, both countries with enormous, unvaccinated populations that are marked by frequent population movement and high interconnectivity. There is significant risk of international spread with low population immunity in the cross-border areas and the continuous forest biome between countries. From 2020–2022, Uganda was one of 14 countries in Africa reporting confirmed cases of yellow fever. With the support of the EYE Strategy and its key partners, including the World Health Organization, UNICEF and Gavi, the Vaccine Alliance, a multi-country outbreak response was organized in neighboring countries that faced more serious yellow fever transmission and YF vaccination became a standard part of routine immunization in children.

In response to recurrent and increasingly large, ongoing epidemics like these on two continents, the WHO recommends aggressive implementation of the traditional triad of surveillance, vaccination, and vector control. However, the global emergency YF vaccine stockpile is depleted, with not enough vaccine to even cover Angola's population during that recent epidemic. As described, the production of new vaccine using the current method of embryonated chicken eggs is slow and limits the capability to rapidly produce large vaccine quantities in response to an outbreak. It is therefore highly unlikely that sufficient YF doses would be available for an effective emergency YF outbreak response anywhere in the world. Any vaccination program must be coupled with the development of systems that can support a rapid outbreak response. These include strengthening laboratory capacity, the ability to carry out epidemiological and entomological investigations, and emergency measures to interrupt transmission. Vector control will require destruction of urban mosquito breeding sites and public education about mosquito avoidance and elimination of domestic breeding sites. Clearly, new options are also required to address the threat of yellow fever infection in non-immunized travelers returning from a country with endemic or epidemic disease.

Preventive mass vaccination campaigns (PMVCs) have been ongoing since the EYE strategy was launched in 2017 in response to the resurgence of yellow fever in Africa and the Americas. To assess the impact of PMVCs in the African endemic region, investigators compared the incidence of outbreaks before and after the implementation of a PMVC and derived the number of yellow fever outbreaks that had been prevented in 33 provinces from 11 African countries. At the province level, the analysis found that implementation of PMVCs was associated with a mean 86% reduction in the risk of a yellow fever outbreak. Overall, PMVCs conducted between 2006 and 2018 were calculated to have reduced the total number of yellow fever outbreaks in Africa by an average of 34%, important empirical evidence of the preventive impact of mass vaccination efforts on yellow fever outbreaks.[67]

★★★★★★★★★★★

Looking Back :: Moving Forward

The yellow fever virus was the first disease-specific pathogen identified as a virus. The story of this discovery, the recognition of the *A. aegypti* mosquito as the virus vector, the first epidemiologic description of the origin of the disease in

East Africa and its transport to Europe and the Americas, recognition of the epidemiology of the disease, identification of the clinical pattern and the development of a highly effective vaccine conveying lifelong immunity are all dramatic successes. However, despite this early progress – most importantly, the existence of an effective vaccine providing lifelong immunity since 1937 – large yellow fever outbreaks remain omnipresent in sub-Saharan Africa and in tropical South America, promoted by increasing global connectedness – specifically, increasing population density and urbanization, human encroachment on jungle habitats due to deforestation and urban sprawl, and climate changes including prolonged increases in rainfall and sustained higher temperatures enhancing spread of the *Ae. Aegypti* vector. The stage is set for introduction of the yellow fever virus into *A. aegypti*-infested but YF-naive areas resulting in a potential global YF pandemic.

Through his blog, Bill Gates, the Microsoft inventor and international philanthropist, has designated one week a year as "Mosquito Week," trying to raise consciousness about the critical role the mosquito plays in global disease transmission. On his October 2016 blog he asks, "What would you say is the most dangerous animal on Earth? Sharks? Snakes? Humans? Of course, the answer depends on how you define dangerous. Personally, I've had a thing about sharks since the first time I saw 'Jaws.' But if you're judging by how many people are killed by an animal every year, then the answer isn't any of the above. It's mosquitoes." He includes a stunning graphic, displaying the number of people killed by different animals in 2015: "The shark only gets credit for 6 worldwide deaths, while the mosquito notches an impressive 830,000."[68] Gates has been involved in attempts to eradicate malaria – also transmitted by mosquitoes – for more than 2 decades. He is especially impressed with a new molecular biology technology called a gene drive. Using CRISPR-Cas9 DNA-editing technology, scientists have created genes that aggressively integrate themselves into a subject's genome so that all offspring will inherit that gene. If, as some researchers have tried, the gene is one that keeps female mosquitoes from reproducing, the mosquito species in question will become extinct. The gene change cannot spread to other species of mosquitoes, so advocates say that it will not endanger the environment, or harm people.[68,69]

To address the limited vaccine supply and questions about vaccine safety, new options for yellow fever vaccine are in development, including a new vaccine based on the mRNA methodology used to create the SARS-CoV-2 vaccines. [70,71] Several of these new vaccines are proceeding through clinical trials but no new safe and effective vaccine has been released to this time.

The other major component of yellow fever control is the management of mosquitoes which currently relies on either insecticides or the destruction of larval breeding sites. However, widespread insecticide resistance and the impracticality of eliminating standing pools of water on a global scale have made this approach ineffective. Two novel approaches that have shown considerable promise in recent years are the genetic control of *A aegypti* mosquitoes and the development of mosquitoes that are resistant to arbovirus infection. The first field-trialed genetic control strategy is known as RIDL (the Release of Insects carrying Dominant Lethal genes) and involves rearing *Ae aegypti* that have been genetically modified to express a repressible lethal gene. During their rearing in insectaries, the mosquitoes are provided with a dietary supplement not present in nature that represses the lethal gene activation. Only male mosquitoes are released and these compete with wild males to mate with wild females. Offspring do not survive to the adult stage because they do not receive the dietary additive in the wild.[72] Lines of RIDL males have been shown to be competitive with wild males and a field release in Bahia, Brazil, reportedly achieved a 95% reduction in local mosquito populations.[73]

An alternative approach is the use of endosymbiotic bacteria to prevent arbovirus replication in the mosquito. The "Eliminate Dengue Project" has demonstrated that infection of the dengue virus(DENV) with *Wolbachia* bacteria prevents transmission of the virus to *Ae.aegypti* mosquitoes.[74] While developed to address dengue, *Wolbachia* also inhibits the replication of the virus that causes yellow fever and chikungunya. *Wolbachia*-infected *A aegypti* mosquitoes have been released in Australia and have been shown to successfully invade wild populations and stop dengue transmission at the community level.[75,76] This approach would be equally effective in reducing yellow fever transmission. Releases are ongoing in DENV-endemic countries such as Indonesia, Vietnam, and – a major site for recurrent yellow fever outbreaks – Brazil. What effect either RIDL or *Wolbachia* will have on arboviral transmission in the wild is unknown. Mathematical models predict that one strain of *Wolbachia* could reduce the basic reproduction number of DENV transmission by 70%. The World Mosquito Program uses field teams in multiple sites to release male and female *Aedes aegypti* mosquitoes with Wolbachia over a number of weeks. These mosquitoes then breed with the wild mosquito population. Over time, the percentage of mosquitoes carrying Wolbachia grows until it remains high without the need for further releases. Mosquitoes with Wolbachia have a reduced ability to transmit viruses to people, decreasing the risk of Zika, dengue, chikungunya and yellow fever outbreaks. The WMP's Wolbachia method helps to protect communities from mosquito-borne viruses without posing a risk to natural ecosystems or human health. In addition, suppressing the mosquito population, or making it arbovirus-resistant, holds great potential for simultaneous control of multiple viruses. Models of DENV transmission control with RIDL also project high efficacy in reducing disease burden. These predictions suggest that such strategies could have a direct impact on transmission of arboviruses like the yellow fever virus where *Ae aegypti* is the principle vector.

It is likely that RIDL, Wolbachia or CRISPR-Cas9 gene-editing will eventually prove conclusively effective and become widely available – they may even be the YF answer the world is looking for. But to this time, the mosquito still prevails. Despite all that we have learned about the antigenically stable yellow fever virus, despite development of a highly effective vaccine that conveys lifelong immunity with a single shot and ongoing mass vaccination efforts, human-aided forces sustain global spread of the yellow fever virus carried by the *Aedes aegyptii* mosquito. Increasing global connectedness plays a major role: our exponentially increasing population brings humans and jungle breeding sites for sylvan transmission closer every year; deforestation concentrates the areas where both the virus and the mosquito vector can survive, closer to sites of human habitation; increasing urbanization creates ever larger, crowded habitats for *Ae. Aegyptii* to thrive; exponentially increasing worldwide air travel transports human virus carriers to enormous naive populations where the mosquito vector already thrives. Global warming also increases the areas where *Ae. aegypti* can breed and multiply. And failure to aggressively deliver effective human vaccination campaigns and establish emergency outbreak infrastructure in vulnerable areas sustains the cycle of disease transmission from mosquitoes to humans and humans to mosquitoes. From the fifteenth century right up to the present, the vector mosquito *Ae. aegypti*, well-adapted to humans and our habits, has caused recurrent, explosive outbreaks of yellow fever. Introduction of the yellow fever virus from Angola into China exemplifies the ongoing threat of these fragile but deadly disease carriers.

HISTORIC PERSPECTIVE: YELLOW FEVER AS AN AGENT OF COLONIALISM

The story of yellow fever intersects in important ways with the history of globalization and, particularly, public health as an agent of colonialism. It is likely that without the globalization of trade and the drive to find more efficient means of transporting goods around the world, yellow fever would have remained an obscure tropical disease. It is certainly true that the means of controlling yellow fever would not have been achieved so rapidly without the efforts of physicians, researchers, and public health experts from all over the world. It is a story that features the emergence of a new nation, marks a sharp loss for one of the great colonial powers and a big opportunity for an emerging power, and demonstrates the ways in which medical knowledge and public health strategies were to become important currencies on the larger and increasingly complex world stage. This box concentrates on these themes as a means of providing historical context for yellow fever and better understanding the influence it commanded in the early twentieth century.

The Panama Canal is a tremendous feat of engineering that took thirty three years to complete but was part of the global imagination for three preceding centuries. The goal was to create an artificial waterway across the Isthmus of Panama to connect the Atlantic and Pacific Oceans and cut both the time and the risk for ships forced to circumnavigate the Straits of Magellan or Cape Horn. The idea of a canal began circulating as early as the 1530s and multiple proposals were made before the end of the nineteenth century. While Panama was not the only place where a canal was considered, its geography made it a logical solution to the problem. Charles V, the King of Spain and Holy Roman Emperor, was the first to propose a canal be cut there to ease the route of ships traveling from Spain to Peru. His primary concern was gaining a trading edge over Spain's great rival in colonialism and trade, Portugal. He ordered a survey of the area, but no construction was undertaken. In 1668 the English physicians and natural philosopher Thomas Browne noted the advantage to be gained by the country with the means and zeal to undertake building a canal where nature had failed to conveniently place a river. He speculated that it would be an ideal site for a manmade water lane connecting the oceans, which would open up trade for his own native country, an emerging imperial power, to access the rich trade in the East: "some Isthmus have been eat through by the Sea, and others cut by the spade: And if policy would permit, that of Panama in America were most worthy the attempt: it being but few miles over, and would open a shorter cut unto the East Indies and China."[77] Thomas Jefferson sided with the Spanish and proposed, in 1788, that they invest in it to expand their hold over trade in the Americas, and several years later, Spanish naval officer Alejandro Malaspina investigated the possibility, along with looking for the Northwest Passage, during his trip around the world to gather scientific specimens and further geographic knowledge (1789–1794). Nothing further came of it, as he was arrested for treason relatively soon after his return to Spain and imprisoned for 6 years, then banned from the country. In 1843, the British took an active interest in building the canal and entered into a contract with the republic of New Granada to build it. Plans were drafted and a construction calendar established, but nothing came of that effort either, nor of another proposal to build a similar canal in Mexico.

The United States formally entered the race in 1846, when it signed the Mallarino-Bidlack Treaty transferring transit rights and military intervention in the Isthmus from Columbia to it.[78] The treaty was ratified in 1848, just as the need for an efficient transit route from the Atlantic to the Pacific increased with the California Gold Rush, with its attendant rise in global trade and labor immigration. In the absence of a viable plan to build the canal, the United States supported the construction of the Panama Railway, which provided an overland means of transporting goods across the territory and established the route the canal would later take. It opened in 1855, the same year the American engineer William Kennish proposed a plan to build a canal across the isthmus. Two French engineers, Armand Reclus and Lucien Napoleon Bonaparte Wyse, next surveyed the land, capitalizing on their recent success building the Suez Canal. The job was finally awarded in 1881 to the engineer who designed the Suez Canal, Ferdinand de Lesseps.

The story of the plans to make the canal, to this point, mirrors the great powers of the early modern world and their emergence into the new era of the nineteenth century: Spain, then Great Britain, France, and finally the United States entered the fray to determine who would gain the upper hand in the lucrative trade to be found in the "New World" of the Americas and the Far East. New only to Europeans, these areas became the arena in which the great colonial powers played out their attempts to dominate trade and transportation in an increasingly complex world. The complexity, and the unexpected challenge of new geographies, would be demonstrated in dazzling clarity by the struggles experienced by the attempts to build the Canal.

Ferdinand de Lesseps made two big errors in his proposal to build the Panama Canal, both of which were based on his poor understanding of the landscape and his lack of experience in tropical environments. The first, his commitment to building the canal at sea level, reflected the fact that he only visited the site a few times and never during the rainy season. Thus, he was not aware that the Chagres River, which was the canal's water source, became much more powerful in the 8 month long rainy season during which it rose about 10 meters: there was no way it could be channeled into a sea level canal. He was caught off guard by the mudslides that accompanied the rains and forced workers to keep changing the angles of the slopes surrounding the canal to prevent it constantly being filled in with slide material. And he was consistently frustrated by the challenges that rain and constant humidity posed to steel equipment and electronics. He was also not familiar with the significant changes in jungle fauna that accompanied the rains, such as the proliferation of venomous snakes, insects, and spiders. His second mistake was also related to his ignorance of the tropics: he did not know that the rainy season brought with it massive epidemics of malaria and yellow fever.[79] By 1884, approximately 200 workers were dying per month, and there was no clear understanding of how to prevent the deaths since the link to mosquitoes had not yet been established. The French effort went bankrupt in 1889, despite de Lesseps' best efforts to keep it alive, and lawsuits ensued surrounding the "Panama Affair." The project had cost 22,000 lives and lost the savings of 80,000 investors, costing approximately US$284 million. While de Lesseps and his son were found guilty of misappropriation of funds, the sentences were later overturned and de Lesseps remained the engineering consultant for the new company that acquired the rights to the Canal and kept the construction site viable while also overseeing the railroad. The French manager of that company finally persuaded him that a sea level canal was not viable, and that a lock and lake strategy was more practical.

The canal site stagnated as the new century began, but the United States began showing interest in purchasing the site or potentially establishing a new canal path in Nicaragua. The French management company dropped the price of the Panama Canal site considerably in the face of competition from Nicaragua, and in June 1902, the United States' Senate passed the Spooner Act, establishing the precedent for pursuing the canal across the isthmus if the necessary rights could be purchased. The project was threatened, however, by a civil war between the controlling Colombian troops and Panamanian rebels. The United States interceded in 1903, partially spurred by the French manager Bunau-Varilla's urging that the USA support the Panamanian rebels and recognize their drive for independence. Roosevelt did so and ordered American warships to block sea lanes that would have permitted Colombian troops to put down the Panamanian rebels. Panama declared independence on November 3, 1903 and the United States was among the first to recognize it as an independent nation. Roosevelt quickly negotiated terms with the new ambassador to build and indefinitely manage and defend the Panama Canal Zone. The treaty was later condemned by many Colombians and Panamanians as infringing on the new nation's sovereignty, a fact that was underlined when Panama remained a US protectorate until 1939. In 1904, the United States officially purchased the French equipment, existing infrastructure, and control over the railroad for $40 million, and paid $10 million to Panama plus a guaranteed payment of $250,000 in subsequent years.

American construction began immediately in 1904, and two big challenges faced the new engineering team: rebuilding the crumbling infrastructure to build the canal and house the workforce; and attracting and maintaining a healthy workforce in the tropics. Both problems resulted from the brutally difficult – and, for many Europeans and North Americans – alien natural environment. The reality facing workers moving into the Canal Zone was harsh. Worker quarters frequently flooded, food was monotonous nearly impossible to keep fresh, and insects were everywhere. Tropical diseases were a daily reality, and keeping workers healthy was nearly impossible. The first effort to understand yellow fever was drawn from observations made by colonial physicians in other areas where the disease was endemic, such as French controlled Senegal and Spanish colonies in the Americas. In both places, it was observed that native adults rarely suffered from severe versions of the disease, while newcomers had very high rates of morbidity and mortality. This reflected the fact that those infected with the virus as children who survived were provided with immunity against severe forms of repeat infection. At the time, however, theories circulated that native people might be genetically capable of withstanding the disease, but there was no clear understanding of how it was transmitted.[80]

The Cuban physician Carlos Findlay proposed that vector for this disease was the mosquito, but that theory was not confirmed until 1900
and the virus itself was not discovered until 1901. This period of time
also saw a proliferation of knowledge about tropical medicine, partially
coming from investment in research by colonial powers and partially
from the publication of research by western physicians working in tropical colonies. In 1898 and 1899, the British Colonial Office opened the
Colonial Medical Service, Patrick Manson's book on tropical disease
was published, and by the turn of the century, American and European
labs had confirmed the vectors and modes of transmission of many
tropical diseases, most notably yellow fever.[81] Thus the French effort
to build the Canal took place with no strong direction for efforts to
control yellow fever, while the American effort inherited an important
piece of knowledge and combined it with existing public health efforts
to control yellow fever. That said, it took the winning combination of
American public health and Latin American knowledge about tropical diseases to keep the imported workforce healthy enough to build
the canal.

The Public Health Service was the organization tasked with managing sanitation and public health in the Canal Zone, a significant
challenge given the environment and the lack of existing sanitation
infrastructure. Among the tasks PHS officers undertook were quarantine of sick workers, the eradication of mosquito larvae and other pests,
management of hospitals, and care of patients. Notable officers included
Henry Rose Carter, whose advanced understanding of mosquito-borne
diseases, proposed means to eradicate them, and was appointed Surgeon
General in 1915, and James Perry, whose work in quarantine in Panama
led to some of the first American reports on health conditions in
Panamanian cities.[82] PHS officers worked alongside the medical wing of
the Isthmian Canal Commission, which held responsibility for the entire
canal project. They were led by William Gorgas, whose career highlights
included establishing sanitation in Havana, Cuba where he managed
first a typhoid and then a yellow fever outbreak during his service there
from 1900–1902. He had firsthand experience demonstrating that sanitary control consistently correlated with political stability, and he set
about establishing the former in the Canal Zone. The strict regulation of
public health in the Canal Zone by ICC and PHS officers "transformed
the Canal Zone and environs into a working laboratory where US health
officials had an enormous amount of power to study disease and enforce
strategies of containment and eradication."[83] The lack of sanitation in
Panama City, especially in the poorest neighborhoods, made it into
PHS reports, as did the lack of access to clean water and the prevalence
of standing water providing breeding grounds for mosquitos. These
reports provided important impetus to improve conditions in Panama's

cities, especially those for which the United States was suddenly responsible, but they also reflect the superior attitude of wealthy, educated,
white Americans toward those they encountered with less education and
darker skin, whether in the United States or outside of it. Many public
health officers remained convinced that willful ignorance, rather than
lack of access to better conditions, kept the poor struggling in terrible
conditions. Thus, American efforts in Panama combined hygiene education with the installation and maintenance of sanitation infrastructure.[84] Mosquito brigades were an important part of this effort, since
their primary job was to eradicate the pests carrying malaria and yellow
fever, the two great killers of the Canal Zone. These brigades often
combined American and Latin American public health workers, providing an important site of knowledge exchange in the fight against
tropical disease.

The Panama Canal could not have been built without the mosquito
vector theory proposed by the Cuban physician Carlos Findlay and
confirmed by British and American laboratory scientists and public
health workers. The success of this massive undertaking rested in
the hands of Public Health Service and ICC medical wing staff who
managed the day to day care of workers, established and maintained
sewage systems and provided clean water, and eliminated pests. Finally,
there could be no canal without the thousands of workers imported
from the Caribbean to do the hard manual labor required to build
a locks canal across mosquito-infested terrain. Paid in silver while
American laborers, usually engineers, were paid in gold, housed in
dismal structures with attention paid to their health only as it applied
to their ability to work, these laborers' bodies provided the data that
became the basis for tropical medicine in the twentieth century. Seen
simultaneously as valuable for their labor and their status as medical subjects, these laborers – imported primarily from Jamaica and
Bermuda – also became symbols of the racial and class biases embedded
in colonial public health. Long after disease vectors were brought under
control, vaccines were developed, and public sanitation in tropical cities
established, these biases remained.

References

(1) Strode GK, Bugher JC, et al. eds. *Yellow Fever.* New York, NY. McGraw-Hill Book Co. 1951.
(2) Tomori O. Yellow fever: the recurring plague. *Crit Rev Clin Lab Sciences* 2004; 41(4): 391–427.
(3) Marfin AA, Monath TP. *Yellow Fever Virus.* In "Desk Encyclopedia of Human and Medical Virology." Edited by Brian W. J. Mahy, Marc H.V. Van Regenmortel. Elsevier Academic Press. 2010. pg.515.

(4) Kallas EG, Gonzaga L, Castineiras ACP, et al. Predictors of mortality in patients with yellow fever: an observational study. *Lancet Inf Dis* 2019; 19(7):750–758.

(5) Johansson MA, Vascoccelos PFC, Staples JE. The whole iceberg: estimating the incidence of yellow fever virus infection from the number of severe cases. *Trans R Soc Trop Med Hyg*. 2014; 108(8): 482–487.

(6) Murphy J. An American Plague. *The True and Terrifying Story of the Yellow Fever Epidemic of 1793.* New York, NY. Scholastic Inc. First edition. 2003. p. 8–9.

(7) Magner LM. *A History of Medicine. Second edition.* New York, NY. Informa Healthcare. 2005. pg. 307,308.

(8) Magner, LM. 2005. pg.496,497.

(9) Lehrer S. *Explorers of the Body.* Second edition. New York, NY. University Inc. 2006. pp. 253–264. (First published by Doubleday, 1979).

(10) Nott JC. Yellow fever contrasted with bilious fever. *New Orleans Med Surg J* 1848; 4:563–601.

(11) Chernin E. Josiah Clark Nott. Insects and yellow fever. *Bull NY Acad Med* 1983; 9: 790–801.

(12) Agramonte A. An account of Dr. Louis-Daniel Beauperthuy – A pioneer in yellow fever research. *Boston Med Surg J* 1908; 158:927–930.

(13) Ullmann A. Pasteur-Koch: Distinctive ways of thinking about infectious diseases. *Microbe* 2005; 2 (8): 383–387.

(14) Mutebi J-P, Wang H, Li L, et al. Phylogenetic and evolutionary relationships among yellow fever isolates in Africa. *J Virol* 2001; 6999–7008.

(15) Bryant JE, Holmes EC, Barrett ADT. Out of Africa: a molecular perspective on the introduction of the yellow fever virus into the Americas. *PloS Pathog* 2007: 3(5):e75.

(16) Lounibos LP. Invasions by insect vectors of human disease. *Ann Rev Ent* 2002; 47: 233–266.

(17) Brown JE, Evans BR, Zheng W, et al. Human impacts have shaped historical and recent evolution in *Aedes Aegypti*, the dengue and yellow fever mosquito. *Evolution* 2014; 68(2): 514–525.

(18) U.S. National Health Board Yellow Fever Commission. The Great Fever. www.pbs. org/wgbh/amex/fever/peopleevents/e_science.html

(19) Chaves-Carballo E. Carlos Finlay and yellow fever: triumph over adversity. *Mil Med.* 2005; 170: 881–885.

(20) Finlay CJ. The mosquito hypothetically considered as the agent of transmission of yellow fever. *Annales de la Real Academia* 1881; 18:147–169.

(21) Holt J. The Proposed Yellow Fever Commission. Editorial. *Boston Med Surg J* 1897; 137: 633–637.

(22) Reed W, Carroll J, Agramonte A. Experimental yellow fever. 1901. *Mil Med* 2001; 166(Suppl 9): 55–60.

(23) Reed W, Carroll J, Agramonte A, Lazear JW. The etiology of yellow fever: an additional note. *JAMA* 1901; 36: 431–440.

(24) Bryan CS. Discovery of the yellow fever virus. *Int J Inf Dis* 1997; 2(1): 52–54.

(25) Stern AM. The Public Health Service in the Panama Canal: A Forgotten Chapter of U.S. *Public Health. Public Health Reports* 2005; 120: 675–679.

(26) Christophers SR. *Aedes Aegypti. The Yellow Fever Mosquito: Its Life History, Bionomics and Structure.* Cambridge University Press. New York, NY; 1960.

(27) Chadee DD. Observations on the seasonal prevalence and vertical distribution patterns of oviposition by Aedes aegypti (L.) (Diptera: Culicidae) in urban high-rise apartments in Trinidad, West Indies. *J Vector Ecol* 2004; 29 (2): 323–330.

(28) De Moura Rodrigues M, Monteiro Marques GRA, Nunes Serpa LL, et al. Density of *Aedes aegypti* and *Aedes albopictus* and its association with number of residents and meteorological variables in the home environment of dengue endemic area, São Paulo, Brazil. *Parasit Vectors* 2015; 8: 115.

(29) Carter HR. *Yellow Fever: An Epidemiological and Historical Study of Its Place of Origin.* Baltimore, MD. Williams & Wilkins; 1931.

(30) Rose W. "Yellow Fever: Feasibility of its Eradication," October 27, 1914, Hench-Reed Collection, Historical Collections, CMHSL, University of Virginia. http://etext.lib.virginia.edu/etcbin/fever-browse?id=00757001

(31) Stokes A, Bauer JH, Hudson NP. Experimental transmission of yellow fever virus to laboratory animals. *Amer J Trop Med* 1928; 8: 103–164.

(32) Theiler M. A yellow fever protection test in mice by intracerebral injection. *Ann Trop Med. Parasit* 1933; 27:57–77.

(33) Mutebi J-P, Barrett ADT. The epidemiology of yellow fever in Africa. *Microbes Infect* 2002; 4: 1459–1468.

(34) Mahaffy AF, Smithburn KC, Jacobs HR, Gillett JD. Yellow fever in Western Uganda. *Trans R Soc Trop Med Hygiene* 1942; 36: 9–20.

(35) Frierson JG. The yellow fever vaccine: a history. *Yale J Biol Med* 2010; 83: 77–85.

(36) Theiler M, Sellards AW. The immunological relationship of yellow fever as it occurs in West Africa and in South America. *Ann Trop Med Parasitol* 1928; 22: 449–460.

(37) Plotkin S. History of vaccination. *PNAS* 2014; 111(34): 12284–12287.

(38) Theiler M, Haagen E. Studies of yellow fever virus in tissue culture. *Proc. Soc. Exp. Biol. Med.* 1932; 29: 435–436.

(39) Theiler M, Whitman L. The danger with vaccination with neurotropic yellow fever virus alone. *Bull. Mens. de l'Offic. Inst. Hyg. Publ.* 1935; 27: 1342–1347.

(40) Theiler M, Smith HH. The use of yellow fever virus modified by in vitro cultivation for human immunization. *J. Exp. Med.* 1937; 65:787–800.

(41) The Rockefeller Foundation, *Annual Report 1947.* New York. The Rockefeller Foundation, 1947.

(42) Staples JE, Monath TP. Yellow fever: 100 years of discovery. *JAMA* 2008; 300(8): 960–962.

(43) Monath TP, Vasconcelos PFC. Yellow fever. *J Clin Virol* 2015; 64: 160–173.

(44) Reagan RL, Brueckner AL. Electron microscopy of yellow fever virus (17D strain). *Am J Pathol* 1953; 29(6): 1157–1159.

(45) Reeves WC. Partners: Serendipity in arbovirus research. *J Vector Ecol* 2001; 26(1): 1–6.

(46) Rice CM, et al. Nucleotide sequence of yellow fever virus: implications for flavivirus gene expression and evolution. *Science* 1985; 229: 726–733.

(47) Tomori O. Yellow fever: the recurring plague. *Crit Rev Clin Lab Sciences* 2004; 41(4): 391–427.

(48) Diagnostic Testing | Yellow Fever | CDC; www.cdc.gov/yellowfever/healthcareproviders/healthcareproviders-diagnostic.html. Accessed, 12/21/2016.

(49) Pulendran B. Learning immunology from the yellow fever vaccine: innate immunity to systems vaccinology. *Nature Rev (Immun)* 2009: 741–747.

(50) WHO International Health Regulations(2005), Second edition, 2008. Available at: www.who.int/ihr/publications/9789241596664/en/

(51) Jonker EFF, Visser LG, Roukens AH. Advances and controversies in yellow fever vaccination. *Ther Adv Vaccines* 2013; 1(4): 144–152.

(52) Monath TP, Nasidi A. Should yellow fever vaccine be included in the expanded program of immunization in Africa? A cost-effectiveness analysis for Nigeria. *Amer J Trop Med Hygiene* 1993; 48(2):274–299.

(53) The Yellow Fever Initiative: An Introduction. World Health Organization, 2007. www.who.int/csr/disease/yellowfev/introduction/en/. Accessed 11/6/2016.

(54) Barrett ADT. Yellow fever in Angola and beyond – The problem of vaccine supply and demand. *N Engl J Med* 2016; 375:301–303.

(55) World Health Organization Yellow Fever – Angola (14 June 2016). Geneva. WHO, 2016. www.who.int/csr/don/14-june-2016-yellow-fever-angola/en/ (Accessed January 31,2016).

(56) Wu JT, Peak CM, Leung GM, Lipsitch M. Fractional dosing of yellow fever vaccine to extend supply: a modelling study. *Lancet* 2016; Nov 9. [Epub ahead of print]

(57) WHO | Yellow Fever Situation Report. [News release] 28 October 2016. Millions protected in Africa's largest-ever emergency vaccination program. www.who.int/entity/mediacentre/news/releases/2016/africa-yellowfever-vaccination/en/ - 45k. Accessed Nov 6, 2016.

(58) WHO / Emergencies preparedness, response/ Pandemic and Epidemic Diseases (PED)/Yellow fever. Resetting the yellow fever strategy. Sept. 16, 2016.

(59) Kraemer MUG, Sinka ME, Duda KA, et al. The global distribution of the arbovirus vectors Aedes aegypti and Ae. aldopictus. *eLIFE* 2015; 4:e08347. Accessed Nov. 7, 2016.

(60) Schwartz F, Drach F, Olson J, et al. Fatal yellow fever in a traveler returning from Venezuela, 1999. *MMWR* 2000; 49(14):303–305.

(61) Paules CI, Fauci AS. Yellow fever – Once again on the radar screen in the Americas. *N Engl J Med* 2017; 376:1397–1399.

(62) Chen Z, Liu L, Lv Y, et al. A fatal yellow fever virus infection in China: description and lessons. *Emerg Microbes Inf* 2016; 5: e69. Published online, 13 July 2016. Accessed, Nov 7, 2016.

(63) Wasserman S, Tambyah PA, Lim PL. Yellow fever cases in Asia: primed for an epidemic. *Int J Inf Dis* 2016; 48: 98–103.

(64) World Health Organization (WHO): Yellow Fever – China. Disease Outbreak News. 22 April 2016. Accessed from WHO website, Nov 8, 2016.

(65) WHO. Yellow fever – Brazil. Accessed August 16, 2019. www.who.int/csr/don/18-april-2019-yellow-fever-brazil/en/

(66) Darlington S, McNeil Jr, DG. *Yellow Fever Circles Brazil's Huge Cities.* The New York Times. March 5, 2018.

(67) Jean K, Raad H, Gaythorpe KAM, et al. Assessing the impact of preventive mass vaccination campaigns on yellow fever outbreaks in Africa: A population-level self-controlled case series study. *PLoS Med* 18(2): e1003523. Published: February 18, 2021. https://doi.org/10.1371/journal.pmed.1003523

(68) The Deadliest Animal in the World | Bill Gates - Gates Notes October, 2016 www.gatesnotes.com/Health/Most-Lethal-Animal-Mosquito-Week

(69) NIH Begins Yellow Fever Vaccine Trial. Technology Networks. July 28,2016. www.technologynetworks.com/Biologics/news.aspx?id=193690. Accessed Dec. 14, 2016.

(70) Zurbia-Flores GM, Rollier CS, Reyes-Sandoval A. Re-thinking yellow fever vaccines: fighting old foes with new generation vaccines, *Human Vaccines & Immunotherapeutics*, 2022; 18:1, doi: 10.1080/21645515.2021.1895644

(71) Medina-Magües LG, Mühe J, Jasny E, et al. Immunogenicity and protective activity of mRNA vaccine candidates against yellow fever virus in animal models. *npj Vaccines* 2023; 8: 31. https://doi.org/10.1038/s41541-023-00629-7

(72) Phuc HK, Andreasen MH, Burton RS, et al. Late-acting dominant lethal genetic systems and mosquito control. *BMC Biology* 2007; 5: 1–11.

(73) Carvalho DO, McKemey AR, Garziera L, et al. Suppression of a field population of *Aedes aegypti* in Brazil by sustained release of transgenic male mosquitoes. *PLoS Neglect Trop Dis* 2015; 9:e0003864.

(74) Walker T, Johnson PH, Moreira LA, et al. The wMel *Wolbachia* strain blocks dengue and invades caged *Aedes aegypti* populations. *Nature* 2011; 476: 450–453.

(75) Hoffmann AA, Montgomery BL, Popovici J, et al. Successful establishment of *Wolbachia* in *Aedes* populations to suppress dengue transmission. *Nature* 2011; 476: 454–457.

(76) O'Neill SL, Ryan PA, Turley AP, et al. Scaled deployment of Wolbachia to protect the community from Aedes-transmitted arboviruses. *Gates Open Res* 2018; 2:36–51.

(77) Browne T. *Pseudoxia Epidemica* 1668; 6:8. Available at: https://books.google.co.uk/books?id=aOI_AQAAMAAJ&printsec=frontcover&dq=pseudodoxia+epidemica&hl=en&sa=X&ved=0ahUKEwj43rT8h9bRAhUCuhoKHdbkB34Q6AEIGjAA#v=onepage&q=pseudodoxia%20epidemica&f=false

(78) Malaspina A. Available at: www.biographi.ca/en/bio/malaspina_alejandro_5E.html

(79) "Mallarino-Bidlack Treaty" accessed from the Library of Congress; www.loc.gov/law/helo/us-treaties/bevans/b-co-ust000006-0868.pdf

(80) Tropical diseases: a manual of the diseases of warm climates. NY, NY: Patrick Manson. William Wood & Company. Originally published, 1898.

(81) Ngalamulume K. Keeping the city totally clean: Yellow fever and the Politics of Prevention in Colonial St Louis de Senegal, 1850–1914. *J African History* 2004; 45(2): 183–202, 188.

(82) Minna Stern A. The public health service in the Panama Canal: A forgotten chapter of U.S. Public Health. *Public Health Rep* Nov–Dec 2005; 120(6): 675–679.

(83) Stern, 676.

(84) Perry JC. *Public Health Reports*. Washington: GPO; 1904. Apr 15, A study of the vital statistics as regards the prevailing diseases and mortality of the city of Panama for the year 1903; pp. 657–64.

Bibliography

Francois Delaporte. *The History of Yellow Fever. An Essay on the Birth of Tropical Medicine.* The MIT Press. Cambridge, MA, London. 1991.

Patrick R Murray, Ken S Rosenthal, Michael A Pfaller. *Medical Microbiology.* 8th Edition. Elsevier. Philadelphia. 2016.

Timothy C. Winegard. *The Mosquito: A Human History of Our Deadliest Predator.* Dutton/Penguin Random House. New York. 2019.

4

THE GREAT INFLUENZA

A Virus for All Time

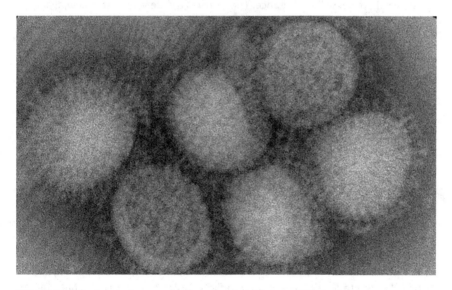

FIGURE 4.1 Electron micrograph of pandemic influenza H1N1 virus.

Source: www.cdc.gov

DOI: 10.4324/9781003427667-4

CANADA GEESE: VIRAL RESERVOIRS IN FLIGHT

I grew up in western Canada in a family of readers and the public library was like a second home from the time I was in grade school. I loved browsing the shelves, choosing the books I would lug home every 2 weeks. The fall that I turned 12, I was finally allowed to go to the library on my own, and I was walking home alone for the first time with my new stash of books. We lived in Saskatchewan then, on the edge of a new subdivision and our street backed up to a wheat field. For the last few days, we had seen a large flock of Canada geese from our backyard, picking their way among the severed stalks, honking, grouping and regrouping, small clusters running forward and taking off for short flights before circling back to the ground. They were huge birds with their distinctive black heads and white chin straps, and they were loud, constantly calling back and forth. Our mum told us that the Canada goose mates for life and that the birds live in large family flocks. I'm sure she told us about migration but I was completely awe-struck when I turned onto our street and saw the entire field of geese lift off at once. They formed a wide V above the field, flying higher and higher until all I could hear was the faint distant sound of honking. High against the pale blue sky, they powered away, finally disappearing into the horizon. The haunting sound of Canada geese in flight still fills me with awe.

Since that long ago day, I've been fascinated with bird migration, one of the most complex events in animal biology. It turns out that the pattern of regular seasonal movement between summer breeding and wintering grounds occurs in many species, prompted by decreasing food supplies as summer ends. The dwindling daylight photoperiod initiates endocrine changes which result in a massive increase in appetite and this leads to huge fat stores throughout the body, even around the eyes in geese. Then some critical combination of decreasing daylight and falling temperature prompts the beginning of the seasonal flight. Canada geese typically fly about 3000 feet above the ground at an average speed of about 40 mph but they can fly much higher and have been clocked at speeds as high as 70 mph. During migration, they usually fly in the V formation that I witnessed, with each bird in line flying a little bit higher than the goose in front of it. The lead goose breaks the headwind, allowing the birds behind to "draft" along, making flight easier. Canada geese honk continuously during flight, and take turns as the leader, reducing fatigue for the flock as a whole. Migrations can be as long as 3000 miles, up to 1500 miles in a single day, navigating by a combination of inherent abilities including sensing the direction of polarized light from the sun and stars, detection of magnetic fields and visual and olfactory landmarks.

It is more than 50 years since my first sight of Canada geese in flight and there have been many reasons to change my feeling of unadulterated awe for these magnificent creatures. The Canada goose has experienced major population explosions in areas throughout North America due in part to the success of wildlife management programs and in part to climate change which has led birds to stay year-round in areas once too cold for wintering. If goslings do not experience migration in the first year of life, they never migrate, so enormous – and ever increasing – flocks of geese have become permanent inhabitants of North American parks and golf courses in temperate areas that provide manicured lawns and ponds and lakes, the perfect landscape for comfortable Canada goose habitation. Alas, large numbers of geese means enormous amounts of goose droppings, almost 2 pounds per day for each adult bird, apparently a delicious treat for dogs but a source of frustration and disgust for human beings. In addition, nesting pairs are very protective and can be quite vicious in defending what they feel is their territory. And if all these issues were not enough, there is the problem of bird strikes, the collision of an aircraft with an airborne bird. Canada geese are among the birds known to be sucked into a jet engine where they can strike an engine fan blade, initiating a cascade which can result in engine failure. A 12-pound Canada goose striking an aircraft going 150 mph at lift-off generates the force of a 1000-pound weight dropped from a height of 10 feet, according to Bird Strike Committee USA. In 2009, a flock of Canada geese caused the crash of a US Airways flight just after take-off from LaGuardia airport. As documented in the 2016 film "Sully," the pilot heroically guided the powerless plane to a safe landing on the Hudson River. Forensic analysis of remains in both engines confirmed that the birds were Canada geese. Although rare, the Federal Aviation Administration estimates bird strikes cost US aviation more than $400 million annually and have resulted in over 200 worldwide deaths since 1988. I know these are all important issues – but they have never been enough to dent my devotion.

It wasn't until I started to seriously study epidemics that I learned that Canada geese and other migratory waterfowl are the natural reservoir for the influenza virus. Somehow, knowledge that my Canada geese could have been the source of the virus that caused the infamous 1918 pandemic, the worst viral pandemic in known history, has given me a different perspective. Contemporary surveillance of geese along North American migratory routes has confirmed genetic virus diversity within birds in the migratory corridor. This means the birds can disperse new and potentially highly virulent influenza gene lineages all along their migratory route. Epidemiologists are terrified that this could be the source of a new pandemic strain ...

The Great Influenza: A Virus for All Time

Viral infections are the bread and butter of pediatrics since viruses cause the most frequent complaints that bring children in to see us: colds, ear infections and gastroenteritis, the unpleasant combination of vomiting and diarrhea, known as the "stomach flu." Since these are usually not serious and no specific treatment is available, we reassure the parent and prescribe a variety of remedies to improve symptoms while the illness runs its course. I can hear myself now, cheerfully reassuring the exhausted mother of a cranky, sick child, "It's only a virus." The history of the deadly influenza pandemic of 1918 and the extended struggle science and medicine have waged to control the influenza virus reveal a much more complex and nuanced story.

By the early 1900s, knowledge of the germ theory of disease had already begun to transform public health sanitation practices like water treatment and sewage disposal, and improved personal hygiene practices like handwashing and safe food preparation. While antibiotics as specific treatments for bacterial infections did not appear until much later in the twentieth century, comprehension of the germ theory had already resulted in major public health improvements that significantly decreased deaths from infectious diseases.[1] In this setting of increasing scientific knowledge and improving public health, viruses were still virtually unknown. *Bacteria* were the "germs" of the germ theory and their identification as the specific causes of infectious diseases was a major focus of science and medicine.[2] In the late 1800s, viruses had been identified as infectious, sub-microscopic organisms that were obligate intracellular parasites, capable of replication only in a plant, animal or human host. By the time the 1918 influenza pandemic occurred, very little more was known: viruses were a mysterious group of tiny microbes that were infectious, filterable and required living cells for replication but their structure and function remained unknown.[3]

Influenza, however, was well known. Major outbreaks of influenza had occurred throughout recorded history, beginning as early as 412 BC. There were increasing reports of flu epidemics and pandemics from the late fifteenth and early sixteenth centuries into the eighteenth century, with at least three pandemics in the nineteenth century, the last of which occurred from 1889 to 1893 and extended from Russia to Europe, England and ultimately the Americas. This pandemic, called the Russian flu, was the first to be rapidly spread by people travelling on trains and steamships, an early example of the important roles of transportation and interconnection in disease transmission. By the time of the deadly influenza pandemic in 1918, the unidentified influenza pathogen had a long history of causing devastating disease.

The Disease

Even in the early 1900s, the typical influenza or "flu" infection was well recognized, characterized by nasal and airway congestion, cough, fever, chills, joint and muscle pain, conjunctivitis, headache and extreme fatigue. It is highly contagious, spread from one person to another in three main ways: by direct transmission, when an infected person coughs or sneezes into the face of another person – a route that is highly favored by children; the airborne route via inhalation of virus-contaminated air; and through hand-to-eye, nose, or mouth transmission, from contaminated surfaces or direct personal contact. The airborne route is the most important since the average sneeze or cough can send ~100,000 contagious germs into the air at speeds up to 100 miles per hour to a distance of 6 feet.[4] Surfaces can be contaminated and small droplets like the tiny influenza virus – shown in Figure 4.1 – can remain suspended for hours to days so the opportunities for infection from a single unprotected sneeze are substantial!

Symptoms begin one to two days after infection and usually last one to two weeks; they can be very mild but most adults can remember experiencing a bad flu attack when they were so achy and weak and sick that they had to stay in bed for days. Infected individuals – even those without symptoms – shed the virus for 7 to 8 days. Even in uncomplicated cases, cough and fatigue can last as long as two weeks. Influenza is much more serious in those with underlying lung or heart problems and a small but significant number of people develop a secondary pneumonia which can be very serious.[5]

Influenza viruses infect the epithelial cell lining of the entire respiratory tract – from the nose, through the throat, into the trachea and bronchi to both lungs – and begin replicating immediately after arrival, peaking after 48 hours. Mild cases show pathological changes only in the upper and lower respiratory tracts, but severe cases show clear evidence of air space disease/pneumonia in the lungs. Not surprisingly, most pathologic information comes from severe cases with direct pulmonary involvement. In typical, self-limited disease, the tracheobronchial changes of influenza infection can be summarized as redness and inflammation with mucopurulent mucous discharge; microscopically, there is destruction and shedding of the pseudostratified epithelium of the inflamed trachea and bronchi, leaving just the basal layer intact. As the infection subsides, the epithelium is regenerated, a process that can take up to a month.[6]

The symptoms of influenza reflect a combination of direct effects of the virus on respiratory epithelial cells and systemic symptoms from the elaboration of cytokines, cell signaling molecules that aid cell-to-cell communication in immune responses and stimulate the movement of cells towards sites of infection. Following primary exposure, cytokine inflammatory responses are triggered when infected cells die, increasing blood flow, and bringing plasma and leukocytes (white blood cells) to the site of injury, elevating local temperatures, and causing pain. The acute inflammatory response is also marked by the activation of pro-inflammatory cytokines including interleukin-6 (IL-6), type 1 interferons, and tumor necrosis factors (TNF) like TNF-alpha; a combination of these factors is considered to be responsible for the respiratory tract symptoms of pain, congestion and cough plus systemic symptoms of fever, muscle pain, headache and exhaustion. Increasing inflammation is accompanied by immune cell infiltration and tissue damage. As the infection subsides, the epithelium is regenerated; in most cases, function can be completely restored by this reparative process.[6]

Cytokines are central to the induction of the body's immune response to viral infection via activation of specialized white cells including natural killer (NK) cells, white cells which are part of the innate immune system, mediating the initial response to infection by responding quickly to detect and kill virally infected cells. The innate immune system attempts to limit a viral infection immediately, before the adaptive antigen-specific immune response is engaged. The antigen-specific response to infection is mediated by T cells (thymus-derived cells) and B cells (bone marrow- or bursa-derived cells), the major cellular components of the adaptive immune response. T cells are responsible for cellular immunity, a protective immune response that involves activation of phagocytic white cells and the release of cytokines and chemokines in response to a viral invader. B cells proliferate and secrete large amounts of virus-specific antibodies. These antibodies bind to the surface of the viral antigen which is then identified for elimination. Once virus-specific antibodies are created, they can persist and will bind to the surface whenever that specific virus is re-introduced, preventing future infection.[7,8]

These days, mortality from the flu averages less than 1%, usually in the elderly or those with underlying lung disease. Based on autopsy studies, about one third of people who die from flu-related causes expire because the virus overwhelms the immune system; another third die from the immune response to secondary bacterial infections, usually in the lungs; and the remaining third perish due to the failure of one or more other organs. According to the World Health Organization: "Every winter, influenza occurs globally with an annual attack rate estimated at 5–10% in adults and 20–30% in children. Worldwide, these annual epidemics are estimated to result in about 3 to 5 million cases of severe illness, and about 250,000 to 500,000 deaths."[9] Attack rate is defined as the proportion of those who become ill after a specified exposure: for the influenza virus, the true asymptomatic fraction is difficult to define, varying from a low mean of 16% in outbreak investigations to as high as 85% in longitudinal studies where infection was defined using serology.[10] It is safe to say that significant proportions of those who are infected with the influenza virus develop a symptomatic illness while an important fraction remain asymptomatic.

The flu occurs in the cold season in both hemispheres, in the Northern Hemisphere, from October through April and in the Southern Hemisphere, from April to September. Why influenza appears primarily in winter conditions is still not entirely understood. The virus does survive longer in cold, dry conditions and, in light of airborne and direct person-to-person transmission, clustering of people indoors in the winter is also thought to be a factor but the complete explanation for seasonality of influenza remains obscure.[11] Historically, one of the most challenging features of influenza is that the expression of the disease is highly variable between seasons. In many years, the flu can be little more than a bad cold, but intermittent pandemics with severe morbidity and much higher mortality have swept the globe in every century since recorded time.

The Great Influenza: The Global Influenza Pandemic of 1918

There are three essential requirements for a global pandemic to occur: emergence of a new agent that infects humans; little or no population immunity to that agent; and easy pathogen transmission from one person to another – typically, this means airborne transmission. In 1918, a new hyper-virulent strain of influenza with all these characteristics emerged and the subsequent pandemic that it caused was one of the worst natural disasters in history. The exact site of origin of the pandemic is unknown but two commonly cited countries are the United States and China. The American story reflects the time when the United States entered the First World War in the spring of 1917. Mobilization ultimately included a military draft of all men aged 18–35 years who were shipped over to Europe as fast as they could be trained. More than 4,000,000 military personnel were in frequent, close contact during training in the USA and transport to and from the battlefields of Europe, a perfect setting for person-to-person disease transmission. As described in detail by John Barry in his excellent book *The Great Influenza*[12] and summarized here, there was a sudden outbreak of severe influenza in Haskell County, Kansas, reported by a local physician to the US Public Health Service. With a constant flow of traffic between Haskell County and Camp Funston, a nearby major military training facility, it was only a month before the first case of influenza was reported there. Within 3 weeks, more than 1100 men were hospitalized on the military base with influenza, and thousands more were treated as outpatients, confirming the ease of human-to-human pathogen transmission and the general absence of immunity to this virus. In Kansan civilians, the first wave of influenza ended by mid-March but the military outbreak – fueled by incoming recruits – continued at Camp Funston into the late spring. When American soldiers began arriving in large numbers on the Western front in Europe early in the summer of 1918, the theory is that they carried the influenza virus from this first wave of disease with them.

The story of a Chinese origin for the virus is also very intriguing. In November 1917, a severe, contagious respiratory disease of unknown origin was reported in Northern China. Characterized by fever, cough, congestion, headache and muscle pain, it was variably diagnosed as "pneumonic plague" and "winter sickness" and was reported to have high mortality. Despite efforts by Western doctors, no diagnosis was confirmed before the outbreak ended in the spring of 1918. Meanwhile, during the winter of 1917–1918 on the Western Front in Europe, manpower among the British troops was critically low so arrangements were made to mobilize men from the Chinese Labor Corps (CLC). Desperate for manpower, the British Government recruited nearly 100,000 Chinese laborers to support their troops on the Western Front. Recruitment took place in the interior of northern China, in the area where the strange respiratory disease had been reported and there were newspaper reports of "pneumonic plague" in the transport camps of the CLC. Ultimately 25,000 Chinese workers were transported to the front around this time, either by ship directly to Europe around the horn of Africa, or by ship to Vancouver, across Canada by train, and then across the Atlantic to France.[13,14] Based on British and Canadian War Diary reports from January through to September 1918, many of the Chinese men had to be hospitalized with "purulent bronchitis" and there was a high mortality rate associated with this illness.

Meanwhile, back in China, the respiratory disease seen in the winter of 1917–1918 recurred the following autumn, and this time it was diagnosed as "Spanish Influenza," the name given to influenza in Europe. While influenza was subsequently widespread in China in 1918–19, the disease was mild in many places compared with elsewhere in the world with a much lower mortality rate, suggesting that population immunity may have been higher.[13] This raises the possibility that the 1918–19 influenza virus originated in China in the winter of 1917 and was carried to France by Chinese migrant workers. Given what we know now about how often new highly virulent viruses arise in China, this is a compelling theory.

Regardless of the country of origin, the next wave of influenza was disastrous and involved multiple sites.[15] It began in the mid-summer of 1918 with sporadic reports of clusters of very severe influenza cases from England, Europe and the United States, characterized by sudden onset, often progressing rapidly to severe respiratory distress with hemorrhage from the lungs, nose and ears. While death from usual seasonal influenza was (and is) rare, mortality from this outbreak was high from the outset. At autopsy in these cases, the normal architecture of the airways and the lungs was found to be destroyed in a pattern never seen before with influenza. The excess influenza deaths involved two overlapping clinical pictures: one pattern was the rapidly evolving severe respiratory distress pattern associated with acute airway destruction; the second pattern was an aggressive secondary bacterial pneumonia which began a few days after the onset of the flu.[6]

Among European countries, Spain was one of the earliest to be hit hard by the disease and one of the few with open reporting, leading to the designation of the disease as the "Spanish flu." In early August, there was a report from Switzerland of an epidemic of influenza in Switzerland called "the Spanish sickness." At that same time, army training sites in the USA were reporting flu outbreaks of increasing severity and number, and several outbreaks occurred on naval steamships docking in Canada and the United States.

Then, in late August, major outbreaks were reported simultaneously in multiple military transport sites: in western France in the major harbor city of Brest where multiple naval ships dropped new recruits from the USA; in Freetown, Sierra Leone, a major coaling center for military ships on the western coast of Africa; and in Boston harbor, on board a massive receiving ship where military personnel in transit were housed.[15] In each of these sites, the disease struck suddenly and severely and the number of influenza cases rose exponentially. In Boston, by the first week of September, the outbreak had spread beyond the military ship with influenza cases reported in civilians, and this was followed by an overwhelming outbreak at Camp Devens, a military camp which housed 40,000 men just outside the city.

Barry reports that in a single day, more than 1500 men reported ill with influenza.[12] The disease followed the pattern of sudden onset and for most patients, went on to an influenza-like illness that was transiently very debilitating but not usually fatal. However, despite the best efforts of military medical teams supported by the Red Cross, more than 100 men died each day, so many that a special barracks was set aside as a morgue. The hospital was overwhelmed with hundreds of young soldiers packed together on makeshift cots along with stricken doctors and nurses. The hospital was designed to treat 1200 patients but at the peak of the outbreak, more than 6000 soldiers were crammed in, coughing, bleeding and dying. Influenza cases were quarantined at their military camps but this did nothing: the disease exploded in cities and towns all over the country.[15]

In the civilian US population, the epidemic swept up and down along the east coast from Maine to New Orleans, inland into the Midwest and eventually, the west coast. Thousands were desperately ill and hundreds in each town and city died as federal, state and municipal governments struggled to find ways to help the sick and take care of the bodies of the dead. Doctors and scientists put all their efforts into finding some way – any way – to treat this terrifying version of a disease they thought they understood. The virus ultimately sickened tens of millions of people in the USA. After a week to 10 days of misery, most recovered but 10–20% of victims suffered from the intensely virulent, fatal form of the disease with extreme fever and chills, bleeding from the lungs, nose and ears, profound shortness of breath and cyanosis of the face and extremities due to hypoxia, with pockets of air under the skin due to rupture of the lungs. As in the fatal cases earlier in the outbreak, autopsies showed that the architecture of the airways and the lungs was destroyed.[6,16]

Strikingly, the death toll was worst in three age groups – infants and the elderly, as usually seen with virulent pneumonia – but mystifyingly, also in previously healthy young adults. In those who survived the acute onslaught of the virus, the disruption of the airways and lung tissue allowed invasion by colonizing strains of bacteria. In subsequent clinical and immunologic studies of severe influenza, an excessive inflammatory reaction has been described with markedly higher levels of the proinflammatory cytokines including interferons, tumor necrosis factors, interleukins and chemokines that are part of the typical immune response in all influenza cases. Called "cytokine storm," these dramatically elevated cytokine levels have been shown to correlate directly with tissue injury and an unfavorable prognosis in severe influenza cases.[17,18] Overall, the synergistic direct effects of aggressive primary infection with the virus, secondary opportunistic bacterial pneumonias and the induction of cytokine storm are felt to be responsible for the high mortality. Because the immune response is maximal in healthy young adults, the excessive inflammatory reaction is thought to be the reason for the high mortality in that age group. The number of deaths worldwide was estimated to be at least 50 million with approximately 675,000 occurring in the United States. More Americans died from influenza than during all of the First World War.

As influenza ravaged the United States, it appeared simultaneously all over the world. From Alaska through Mexico to South America, from Iceland across all of Europe into the Middle East and down through all of Africa, from the Mediterranean to India and the Far East: the death toll was at least 10% overall, far above the usual 1%, but dramatically higher, as high as 25%, in native populations whose immune systems had presumably never been exposed to influenza viruses of any kind: Eskimos, Native Americans, Pacific Islanders and Africans. A very few isolated settlements who were able to maintain isolation were spared but overall, virtually all of civilization was threatened. In India alone, there were at least 20 million deaths and worldwide, more than 50 million people died. More people died of influenza in a single year than in the infamous "Black Death" bubonic plague from 1347 to 1351. It is still one of the worst pandemics in recorded history.[19]

However, the virus appeared to become spontaneously less lethal as the epidemic continued and this was seen in the lower death rates in American cities which presented with disease later in the course of the pandemic. At the same time, survivors of the disease had developed immunity and without new hosts, the virus – and therefore, the pandemic – died out. In general, the cycle from the first case of influenza to the final case lasted 6 to 8 weeks. By late November 1918, the pandemic second wave was over. There was a weak third wave in the winter of 1919 and again in 1920 but the terrifying influenza pandemic of 1918 was effectively over within 3 months of its precipitous onset. The pandemic contributed significantly to the ultimate collapse of an already weakened Germany and thereby to the end of the war, with peace declared on November 11, 1918, just as the pandemic began to wind down.[15]

The First World War presents a unique opportunity to observe the impact of globalization on the spread of an infectious disease, beginning with the critical role of travel. Never before had so many people traveled so rapidly and so widely around the world to a common site. Both the major theories of influenza introduction featured international travel from remote sites – middle America or northern China – to the battlegrounds of Europe via trains and crowded transport ships. Never before had the population density been higher than in the European conflict zones, where men from all over the world were brought together. In numbers alone, more than 10 million men had been mobilized to the battlegrounds of Europe by the end of the war, primarily from colonies of the British Empire but also including 4 million Americans. Troops were packed together in trenches, bunkers and tents and consequent overcrowding mandated close interpersonal contact among whole battalions of men. With an airborne virus like influenza, rapid pathogen transmission was almost guaranteed. And never before had a pathogen had such a wonderful opportunity to hitch international global rides on people, boats and trains. As the war wound down, soldiers who were transported home on crowded transport ships and trains carried the virus with them and transmitted the infection virtually all over the world. The

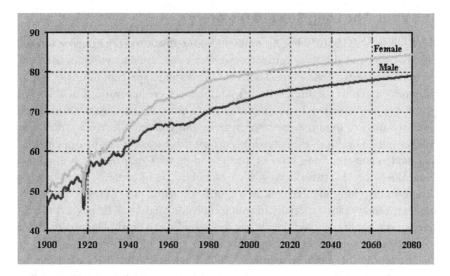

FIGURE 4.2 Median age at death by gender and calendar year: 1900–2100.

Source: US Social Security Administration, SSA.gov. www.ssa.gov › oact › NOTES › as116_V.

extensive global spread of the 1918 influenza virus dramatically exemplifies the critical roles of travel and global interconnectedness in pandemic disease spread.

The impact of the epidemic in the USA is shown dramatically by considering the average life span in the United States between 1900 and 2000. Life span is a reasonable measure of the overall health of a population and is a primary indicator of the effect of disease and health care on mortality but it also reflects the state of nutrition, housing and health education. The importance of these other factors is apparent when we look at the difference in lifespan between whites and blacks: in 1900, the average life span in the United States was 47 years in white men and 33 years in black men; for women, the average life span was 49 years in white women compared with 34 years in black women. The dramatic increase in average life expectancy in the USA during the twentieth century is shown graphically in Figure 4.2.[20]

The sharp decrease in life expectancy in 1918 and 1919 reflects the large number of young people who died of influenza, a large enough number to decrease average life expectancy for the whole population by almost 10 years! You can also see that as the century progressed, average life expectancy increased dramatically. By 1950, the average age at death for white men and women was 67 and 72 years respectively, a mean increase of 43%. The gain was even greater in blacks, to 59 years in black men and 63 in black women, a mean increase of 79%. There were further gains in the second half of the century, overall a mean 61% increase for whites and 106%(!) for blacks.

The Virus: The Long Road to Discovery

As the twentieth century began, more and more diseases were linked with specific bacteria and although antibiotics were not yet available, vaccines had been created for selected infections. There was increasing appreciation of the role of immunity and tests for disease-specific antibodies were becoming available. The practice of medicine was beginning to rest on a scientific base. At the same time, understanding of the importance of hygiene and sanitation led to an increasing role for public health in everyday life. Against this backdrop, influenza emerged as a sudden and terrifying wave of disease and death. Compared with usual seasonal flu outbreaks, this illness was characterized by its acute, severe onset, by progression to lung involvement in a significant subset of cases and by a much higher mortality rate, especially in young adults. In fatal cases, there was progressive respiratory distress and then septic shock leading to death. Doctors had little to offer except oxygen, fluids, rest and prayer.

During the influenza epidemic of 1892, a scientist named Richard Pfeiffer isolated a small rod-shaped bacteria from the noses of flu-infected patients; he believed this was the cause of influenza.[21] The bacteria was named *Bacillus influenzae* but became known as Pfeiffer's bacillus and when the influenza pandemic began in 1918, most physicians and scientists believed this bacteria was the cause of influenza, in line with the germ theory that specific bacteria cause specific diseases. Because of the gravity of the illness and the severe lung involvement, there was an intense focus on confirming the cause for influenza, with doctors collecting blood and sputum cultures on every patient, hoping to identify Pfeiffer's bacillus or another known bacteria since this would potentially allow development of antisera and vaccines that could protect against the infection; anti-pneumococcal serotherapy was in its infancy but this technique could theoretically have been employed if a type-specific bacteria was identified.[22] Despite these efforts, neither Pfeiffer's bacillus nor any other bacteria was consistently identified in flu victims – more commonly, multiple known bacteria including streptococcus and pneumococcus were found in the lungs of patients with secondary pneumonia complicating the flu.[9] Despite the enormous number of cases and the extensive efforts of doctors and scientists, no cause for the 1918 influenza pandemic was discovered at the time.

The search for a cause continued after the pandemic ended. In 1919, scientists from Japan and from France reported separately that a bacteria-free emulsion of mucous or blood from influenza patients produced classical flu symptoms of varying severity when given to monkeys and to human medical volunteers.[23,24] These results strongly suggested that influenza was caused by a virus but scientists were unconvinced, perhaps because at the time, so little was known about the basic nature of viruses. Viruses were defined by two negative characteristics: they were not retained by standard bacteriologic filters and they were not visible by light microscopy. They could only be identified by inducing disease in a susceptible plant or animal with a bacteria-free filtrate from a diseased subject, or indirectly, by detecting the presence of serum antibodies against the disease in survivors of the illness in question. Using these methods, viruses had been confirmed as the cause of a number of human and animal diseases including smallpox, rabies, measles and polio.

It was 1933, 15 years after the influenza pandemic ended, before scientists in the United States – Richard Shope, studying swine flu – and in Britain – Wilson Smith, Christopher Andrewes and Patrick Laidlaw, studying flu in ferrets – showed convincingly that influenza was caused by a virus and that this virus infected many different animals. The ability of a single virus to infect both humans and animals was a previously unrecognized feature of the armamentarium of viruses that would prove to be critically important in understanding the ability of viruses to evolve and to infect.[25,26] Confirmation that influenza was caused by a virus was followed immediately by attempts to develop a vaccine against the virus since the concept of immunity was well-developed by the 1900s and antitoxins and vaccines against diseases like smallpox, diphtheria, tetanus, anthrax, cholera, plague and typhoid had already been developed. All influenza was thought to be caused by the single virus identified in 1933 so vaccines were developed to prevent infection with this specific virus. It was these attempts at vaccine development that revealed one of the most important traits of the influenza virus: the capacity for spontaneous mutation. When a vaccine developed by Smith and Andrewes using the 1933 virus that had been effective in lab animals was a complete failure in humans in the 1936 flu season, they and other researchers recognized that significant variation in the virus must have occurred between flu seasons.[27,28] Spontaneous mutation is one of the most powerful weapons of the influenza virus and its identification was a major step forward in understanding its virulence.

The start of the Second World War led to concerns about another wartime pandemic so vaccine development took precedence over pure laboratory investigation. Thomas Francis and Jonas Salk, two of the American scientists whose work ultimately led to creation of the polio vaccine, developed an inactivated influenza vaccine by injecting the virus into chicken eggs where it multiplied, producing high antigen concentrations which they used to induce immunity.[29] This vaccine was shown to be safe but only modestly effective. In 1940, a second type of influenza virus was identified from individuals with what appeared to be typical, seasonal influenza: the original virus was named influenza A and the new virus, influenza B. Ultimately, unlike the type A flu virus strain, type B was found to exist only in humans; it causes a typical flu illness but it does not cause pandemic disease. From 1942 onward, all flu vaccines have contained antigens against both A and B strains. Antibody titers in response to the inactivated vaccine showed good theoretical protection against both viruses but clinical protection against seasonal influenza remained limited, presumably reflecting the spontaneous variation of the virus. Ultimately, four major strains of influenza virus were identified, A, B, C and D. Influenza A and B strains are responsible for seasonal flu outbreaks every winter but only influenza A strains have caused pandemic disease. Influenza type C generally causes only a mild respiratory illness and influenza D viruses do not cause disease in humans. As the cause of pandemic disease, influenza type A is the focus of this chapter.

In 1935, the electron microscope(EM) gave us our first images of viruses, revealing their simple basic structure: a protective protein shell around a nucleic-acid core of genetic material, as described in Chapter 1.[30] Using bacteriophage, a kind of virus that only infects bacteria, a simple description of viral replication was developed. Outside of a host cell, a virus was metabolically inert but once connected to a cell in a new host, the virus inserted its genetic material and took over the cell's functions. New viruses were formed, self-assembled and burst out of the host cell, killing that cell and going on to infect others.[31] A critically important discovery was also made using bacteriophage when two virus particles simultaneously infecting the same cell were seen to exchange parts of their strings of genes resulting in new, hybrid forms of the original viruses – a process called recombination.[32]

In 1945, the influenza A virus was first visualized by electron microscopy and was found to be one of the smallest viruses identified to that time.[33] The virus was described as roughly spherical, and only 80 to 120 nanometers in length. Subsequent more sophisticated EM analyses have clearly shown a degree of pleomorphism, with the native virion morphology including spherical, elliptical and filamentous forms.[34] Early EM examination using negative staining techniques

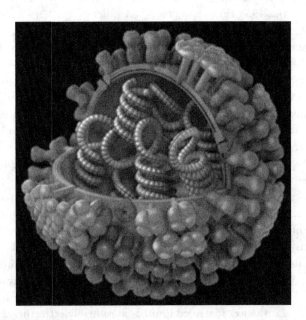

FIGURE 4.3 Graphical image of Influenza A virus with surface glycoproteins and interior displayed.

Source: www.cdc.gov › flu › resource-center › freeresources › graphics › images. cdc-gov revealed the virus to be covered by spiky surface projections of two distinct types – hemagglutinin (HA) and neuraminidase (NA) – and electrophoresis showed these to have different biologic activities.[34] Subsequent imaging by cryo-EM reveals HA to be a membrane glycoprotein shaped like a drumstick with a globular head on a broad stem. Influenza NA is a glycoside hydrolase enzyme seen as a mushroom-shaped projection with the cap composed of four spherical subunits. On the surface of the virus, the ratio of HA to NA is approximately four to one and these two surface proteins are accompanied by a much smaller number of a third membrane protein (M2) which is a matrix ion channel as shown in Figure 4.3.[35,36]

Complete knowledge of the process of cell infection is still evolving but HA and NA were found to be critically important components in the influenza virus. To summarize what is a far more detailed process, HA binds to a sialic acid receptor on the surface of host cells and mediates virus attachment to the cell surface. NA then cleaves sialic acid from the viral receptors allowing the virus to enter the cell by endocytosis. HA mediates release of the genome into the host cell nucleus by pH-dependent membrane fusion. After transcription and replication, a series of steps allows progeny virions to be assembled and NA accelerates their release from the host cells.[34,37]

★★★★★★★★★★★★

After deoxyribonucleic acid (DNA) was identified as the carrier of cellular genetic information and the double helix structure of DNA was recognized, ribonucleic acid (RNA) was also recognized to be a carrier of genetic information.[38-42] In 1986, the influenza virus was found to be a single-stranded RNA virus with eight segments.[43,44] This discovery had major implications for understanding variation in influenza viruses. Spontaneous mutations, including substitutions, deletions and insertions of single nucleotides, were found to be one of the most important mechanisms for producing variation. Such point mutations were a characteristic common to all cells, including bacteria and viruses. With this kind of mutation, small, subtle changes occur randomly and are incorporated into the viral genome, a process called *genetic drift*. Mutation rates differ significantly between DNA and RNA viruses: RNA viruses like the influenza virus have very high mutation rates, approximately one mutation per genome copy, because lack of proofreading by RNA polymerases allows multiple replication errors.[45] (By contrast, there is much higher replication fidelity found among DNA viruses.) Each round of RNA virus replication results in a mixed population with many variants, most of which are not viable, but some of which have potentially advantageous mutations that allow the mutant to survive and even become dominant under the right selective conditions. Only mutations that do not interfere with essential viral function survive but the high mutation rate in RNA viruses provides many opportunities for this to occur. Genetic drift results in literally thousands of lineages and sub-lineages of influenza viruses.

Recombination – the process of two virus particles infecting the same cell exchanging parts of their genetic material to produce new hybrid forms of the original viruses – was first described in 1936 and was subsequently found to occur primarily in DNA viruses; it was recognized as resulting in new viral strains which could infect previously resistant hosts. A particular form of recombination called "reassortment" was found to occur only in segmented RNA viruses, like the influenza virus. Whole segments of genetic material could be exchanged between viruses infecting the same cell, resulting in progeny with immediate and major antigenic change.[46] Based on findings like these, it was recognized that the process of genetic information exchange by reassortment can occur between animal and human strains of a virus and can result in an entirely new and antigenically novel virus strain. In a single influenza virus replication cycle, a potential killer virus can emerge, highly infectious, easily transmittable and lethal. Endless evolution by both spontaneous mutation and by genetic reassortment results in the continuous emergence of new, antigenically novel influenza virus strains to which human hosts can have limited or no resistance.[47] These findings provided powerful insight into the infectious potential of the influenza virus.

It is with the surface proteins HA and NA that the results of continuous mutation in the influenza virus – by drift or by shift – are most powerfully expressed. HA and NA are the major determinants of influenza A infectivity, transmissibility, pathogenicity, host specificity and antigenicity. The receptor binding residues of influenza A are located in the HA head domain. In viral hosts, cell surface receptors vary substantially between host species as well as in target tissues and cell types of the same species, leading to variations in the HA-binding capacity of circulating viruses. Therefore, receptor specificity plays an important role in viral cell and tissue tropism, interspecies transmission and adaptation to a new host. Spontaneous point mutations in HA can alter the sialic acid receptor specificity on potential host cells and thereby alter the antigenicity, host range, replication efficiency and pathogenicity of the virus. Inability of variant strains to bind with surface receptors is an important mechanism limiting the emergence of new pandemic strains. Host range and virulence are also the result of optimized molecular interactions between viral HA, NA and cellular factors. Together, HA receptor-binding mutations and NA activity-enhancing mutations are critically important mediators of influenza A cross-species infection.[48] Using serologic tests with hyperimmune serum, a total of 18 HA subtypes (H1-18) and 11 NA subtypes (N1-11) have been found in nature. Influenza A virus subtypes are classified based on the sequence and antigenic divergence of the HA and NA surface proteins on the surface of the viral envelope. The US Centers for Disease Control and Prevention (CDC) follows an internationally accepted naming convention for influenza viruses beginning with the antigenic type (A,B,C); the geographic site of origin; the strain number and the year of identification. The influenza A virus is identified specifically by description of the hemagglutinin and neuraminidase antigens in parentheses.[36]

★★★★★★★★★★

Return of the Canada Goose

By this time, migratory water birds, including specifically (my beloved) Canada geese, had been shown to harbor a large number of different influenza A virus strains.[49] Ultimately, wild aquatic birds – particularly Canada geese, wild ducks, swans, gulls, shorebirds and terns – were identified as the natural hosts of the influenza virus and the source of all influenza viruses in other species. Enormous pools of influenza virus strains were found to continuously circulate in these wild birds, providing a stable evolutionary reservoir of viral gene sequences available as potential recombinants for introduction into human populations.[50] Genetic analyses reveal that antigenic drift of the influenza A virus takes place at a much lower rate in wild birds than it does in other host species. The strains that exist in wild birds appear to be in relative evolutionary stasis, as shown by the fact that strains collected from wild birds many decades apart were virtually identical. This implies that an optimal host-parasite relation has been reached and that any change in genetic make-up will result in fewer functional strains that will not survive. In these water birds, the virus is non-pathogenic and lives in the gastro-intestinal tract, excreted continuously in the feces. Water sources that are homes for aquatic birds are infected and this is a natural source for virus transmission from one bird or animal to another.

Aside from humans, the influenza A virus has also been found to infect a wide variety of other mammalian species, including all marine mammals, pigs, horses and New World bats. This wide host range is part of the reason that influenza viruses have shown so much genetic diversity over time since extensive spontaneous antigenic mutation occurs continuously in each mammalian host. All 18 HA subtypes (H1-18) and 11 NA subtypes (N1-11) have been found in nature. Viruses of all known subtypes except H17N10 and H18N11 are maintained in aquatic birds but only a subset of HAs (H1, H2, and H3) and NAs (N1 and N2) naturally circulate in humans. Subtypes H17N10 and H18N11 have been found only in bats. New influenza virus subtypes with minor but cumulative antigenic variations emerge constantly by spontaneous mutation from the wide number of animal reservoirs and it is these new subtypes which are responsible for the annual occurrence of new influenza virus strains. By contrast, *major* new influenza strains with pandemic potential arise only rarely from reassortment between a human flu virus and strains from avian reservoirs plus or minus additional animal virus strains, producing an entirely new virus subtype with previously unseen HA and NA antigens.[50] Human and avian strains of the influenza virus both replicate well in pigs which represent an important intermediary in viral mutation: when the same pig cell is infected with multiple avian and human and/or animal viruses, genetic exchange between the strains can reassort to produce antigenically unique and potentially highly virulent offspring which can appear suddenly, in a single infectious cycle.[51] This allows no opportunity for immunity to develop or for preventive vaccines to be created and guarantees accelerated disease spread. All known influenza pandemics in recent human history have been caused by viral subtypes which emerged after reassortment of genes from the H1N1 human virus plus avian and/or other animal sources.

★★★★★★★★★★★★★

Global Influenza Pandemics after 1918

It took many decades for the true infective armamentarium of the influenza A virus to be appreciated. Because it is an RNA virus, there is ongoing continuous mutation by genetic drift. The influenza virus is segmented and infects multiple species – this allows reassortment to occur with unique combinations of animal and human gene segments emerging as highly virulent reassortants. The combination of genetic drift and shift means entirely new strains of the virus that infect humans arise constantly. Because these are entirely new strains, there will be little or no population immunity. And the influenza virus is airborne insuring widespread transmission from one person to another. Little wonder scientists and physicians were – and still are – haunted by the fear that another strain like the one that caused the 1918 pandemic Spanish flu could emerge at any time. In 1947, these concerns prompted the nascent World Health Organization (WHO) to establish an international influenza surveillance program called the World Influenza Center. Originally based in the National Institute for Medical Research in London where Andrewes, Smith and Laidlaw had carried out much of their work, the Center was responsible for coordinating influenza surveillance efforts, carrying out and coordinating laboratory work on influenza, and training new lab workers. By 1952, it was clear that a worldwide network of labs was needed to optimize surveillance and support countries without existing viral lab capacity and the WHO established the Global Influenza Surveillance Network, tasked with determining which influenza strains to include in the next year's vaccine.

And then, in February 1957, a completely new strain of influenza A with previously unknown HA and NA did appear, originally in China. Despite all ongoing surveillance efforts, it was not identified in advance by scientists or viral researchers. The known influenza A virus was re-labelled H1N1 and the new strain as H2N2. Immunity to this new strain was rare in people less than 65 years old and the existing vaccine offered no protection at all: experts predicted a major pandemic of this Asian flu and they were not disappointed. In the first months of 1957, the virus spread throughout China and the Far East and by midsummer reached the United States. Although the concept had already been proven, it was this pandemic that clarified the importance of new hybrid viruses formed by reassortment in cells infected simultaneously with different influenza viruses from different species. The H2N2 virus was ultimately found to be the product of reassortment between an influenza virus from wild ducks and the circulating human influenza virus strain, with 3 gene segments from the avian influenza gene pool combined with five from the human strain.[52] A new vaccine was emergently developed but production took many months while infection rates waxed and waned through the fall and winter. H2N2 influenza-related deaths were maximal between September 1957 and March 1958. Although the Asian flu pandemic was nowhere near as devastating as the 1918 pandemic, more than 1,000,000 people died worldwide, including almost 70,000 in the United States. The emergent development of a vaccine against the H2N2 virus and the availability of antibiotics to treat secondary infections were thought to have significantly limited the spread and mortality of the pandemic. But the sudden, spontaneous appearance of a brand new influenza virus derived from a combination of bird and human virus strains suggested a possible origin for the 1918 influenza pandemic and potentially for new pandemic strains – and this sent shivers of apprehension through scientists and doctors around the globe.

Enhanced appreciation of the continuous evolution of the influenza virus did nothing to prevent two subsequent pandemics. In early 1968, a new flu virus was detected in Hong Kong, found to be an H3N2 virus which arose by reassortment, with two genes from the migratory water bird reservoir combined with six genes from the virus circulating at the time in humans.[52] The first record of the outbreak in Hong Kong appeared on July 13, 1968. Despite the surveillance efforts of the Global Influenza Network, the London Times was actually the first source to sound the alarm about the new, "Hong Kong flu" pandemic This H3N2 virus was highly contagious: within two weeks of its emergence, more than 500,000 cases of influenza had been reported. By the end of July, the virus had spread through all of Southeast Asia and by September, the Hong Kong flu had reached the Philippines, Australia, India, Europe and the Panama Canal Zone. That same month, the virus entered California carried by returning Vietnam War troops and it was widespread in the United States by December. Worldwide, 700,000 people died due to the H3N2 virus with 33,800 deaths in the USA. It was the mildest flu pandemic in the twentieth century, likely because the Hong Kong virus differed from the 1957–58 Asian influenza virus by only the HA antigen and its impact was likely moderated by partial immunity due to prior N2 exposure. Improved medical care and more effective antibiotics for secondary bacterial infections were also available for those who became ill. The H3N2 virus that caused the 1968 pandemic is still in circulation today and is the most prevalent influenza A strain involved in causing seasonal influenza.

Early in the spring of 2009, a new H1N1 flu virus was first detected in influenza cases in Mexico, associated with strikingly high mortality rates in younger individuals. Assessment of what was found to be the H1N1(09) virus was a complex reassortment story. In the late 1990s, a series of reassortment events were recognized to have occurred between North American influenza viruses found in pigs, humans and birds. As a result, "triple reassortant North American swine influenza viruses" with genes from humans, North American pigs and birds had been detected in many parts of the world for around 10 years prior to the

2009 H1N1 flu. Then in 2004, reassortant influenza viruses with genes from North American and Eurasian pigs were found in samples collected from pigs in Hong Kong. Mixing of the "triple reassortant North American swine influenza viruses" with Eurasian swine viruses resulted in the 2009 H1N1 influenza virus, a new, previously unseen strain of influenza which involved genes from *five* different flu viruses: North American swine influenza, North American avian influenza, human influenza A and Eurasian swine influenza viruses.[53] Initially, the epidemic was called the swine flu because all the different gene segments of the virus could be traced back to influenza viruses found in pigs. Once again, the vaccine prepared for the seasonal flu offered no protection and children were found to have no preexisting immunity to the new strain. Again, a major pandemic was predicted. The H1N1(09) flu spread rapidly across the United States, to Europe, and eventually worldwide. In June, the WHO declared the outbreak to be a pandemic, the first in 41 years; ultimately, 74 countries were affected. New vaccines were emergently developed and these became available beginning in the early fall. By November 2009, 48 US states had reported cases of H1N1(09), mostly in young people. That same month, over 61 million vaccine doses were ready, just as reports of flu activity began to decline in parts of the country. Eventually, 80 million Americans were vaccinated against the 2009 strain of H1N1 and although belated, this may have minimized the impact of the illness. Globally, there were estimated to be more than 500,000 H1N1(09) related deaths, 80% in people younger than 65 years of age. The WHO declared the global H1N1 flu pandemic over on August 10, 2010.

The Vaccine

The WHO has been making annual recommendations for which viral strains to include in development of their annual vaccine since 1973 and from 1998 onwards, these have been made twice a year, for the Northern and Southern hemisphere flu seasons. The WHO influenza network, now known as the Global Influenza Surveillance and Response System (GISRS) has grown large and complex from its origin in 1947, with 143 institutions in 113 Member States, 6 Collaborating Centers and 4 Essential Regulatory Laboratories. GISRS monitors trends in circulating influenza strains year-round, collecting genetic data and identifying new mutations. The data are provided remotely by National Influenza Centers (NICs) of the Global Influenza Surveillance and Response System (GISRS) and other national influenza reference laboratories collaborating actively with GISRS, or are uploaded from WHO regional databases.

Since 1997, the system has used a global web-based tool called FluNet for influenza virus surveillance. The virological data entered into FluNet includes the number of influenza viruses detected by subtype and is critical for tracking the movement of viruses globally and interpreting epidemiological data. The data at country level are publicly available and updated weekly, as tables, maps and graphs. Each year, the annual flu vaccine combines antibodies against the viral strains which predominated in epidemiologic surveillance during the preceding year plus the three viral strains circulating most commonly in humans: influenza A (H1N1), (H3N2) and the influenza B virus; plus the three prominent subtypes of avian influenza A viruses known to infect both birds and people: H5, H7 and H9. However, the intricate international reassortment events described for the H1N1(09) virus exemplify the complicated processes that the surveillance networks are trying to track. More than 250 million doses of influenza vaccine are produced annually against the WHO-recommended influenza strains.

The 1957, 1968 and 2009 flu pandemics were not detected in advance and the prepared vaccines offered no protection, suggesting that the surveillance program and the annual flu vaccine development process are essentially ineffective against new viral strains that develop suddenly by reassortment. Because there is a substantial time lag – estimated to be at least 6 months – related to vaccine manufacture time, a vaccine can even become obsolete because of new strains that emerge less rapidly, by spontaneous mutation. When a new, particularly virulent or widespread influenza strain appears – usually a brand new lineage developed by reassortment – a significant proportion of the population will have no resistance so an additional specific vaccine has to be created emergently to prevent onset of a new pandemic. A recent analysis of flu vaccine effectiveness over the last 44 years indicates that the carefully composed annual trivalent inactivated vaccine has an average efficacy of only 59% in adults, 18 to 65 years of age, with no demonstrated efficacy in adults 65 and older nor in children below 17. The live attenuated flu vaccine given as a nasal spray showed 83% efficacy in children 6 months to 7 years old, but no studies supported its efficacy in older children or adults.[54] Just as originally reported back in the 1930s, the flu vaccine is and always has been only modestly effective against seasonal influenza. And against the constant background threat of a new highly infectious and highly virulent virus emerging suddenly by genetic reassortment, this extensive, surveillance process appears to be almost completely ineffective.

Finally: Identification of the 1918 Pandemic Flu Virus

An important piece of understanding the 1918 pandemic – specific identification of the virus which caused the pandemic – eluded investigators for more than 75 years, even as knowledge about the influenza virus increased and techniques for viral investigation advanced. In the years since the basic nucleotide units and the spiral helix structure of DNA were discovered, it was recognized that the order of the paired nucleotides contained all the information necessary for the hereditary and biochemical properties of life. Since that time, the ability to measure or infer these sequences has become a major focus of biologic research, typified more recently by the Human Genome project. In 1977, Frederick Sanger developed the first technique for DNA sequencing, an early method to map the information coded in DNA.[55] This was followed by the development of the polymerase chain reaction technique or PCR. First reported in 1983, PCR is a technique used to reproduce selected sections of DNA or RNA for analysis.[56] It allows isolation of fragments from genomic DNA or RNA by selective amplification of a specific region and can be applied to any nucleic acid sequence, even in samples containing only minute quantities of genetic material. Readers may be most familiar with it through its use in conviction of criminals based on recovery of very small DNA samples from crime scenes. It was not until 1995 that Jeffery Taubenberger, a molecular pathologist in the Armed Forces Institute of Pathology, hit upon the idea of using PCR to examine preserved lung tissue specimens from soldiers who died of the flu in 1918 as a way to reconstruct the genetic code of the virus which caused the influenza pandemic. Among the Institute's archived specimens, he found tiny cubes of preserved lung tissue from two soldiers who succumbed to the flu on the same day in 1918. PCR applied to microscopic sections of these specimens found the virus, but only in fragments. Subsequent PCR evaluation of lung tissue from an Inuit victim whose body had remained frozen in the permafrost from the time of her death during the 1918 pandemic allowed the researchers to sequence the entire genome and conclude that the influenza virus was an H1N1 avian virus.[57] Other researchers used the genome to reconstruct the 1918 H1N1 pandemic strain and test it in mice. All the mice infected with the reconstructed 1918 virus died, while all those exposed to a control strain survived. At autopsy, the researchers found severe inflammation in the lungs and bronchial passages, findings very similar to those in people who died of the 1918 virus. In a separate experiment, the reconstructed 1918 virus was found to be at least 100 times as lethal as an engineered virus that contained only five of the 1918 genes plus three genes from a control H1N1 strain. Subsequent testing in ferrets and monkeys showed similar high virulence for the recovered 1918 virus strain.[58] Based on all of their findings, Taubenberger and his group theorized that the 1918 influenza virus jumped intact, directly from birds to humans.[59]

DNA and RNA sequence analysis provides explicit information about the entire genome of an organism. Phylogenetic analysis compares DNA or RNA sequencing data from different organisms to construct a tree-like pattern that depicts the evolutionary relationships among the group and allows estimation of the time when a new viral mutation arose.[60,61] Application of these phylogenetic techniques has answered critical questions about the 1918 pandemic influenza virus which persisted even after it had been completely sequenced and the virus recreated. What was the evolutionary origin of the virus? What were the origins of swine flu and of the typical, non-lethal H1N1 seasonal flu which emerged subsequently? Using a molecular clock model that explicitly allowed different evolutionary rates in different species, Michael Worobey and his team performed a complete phylogenetic analysis of full-length nucleotide sequences of all available influenza A viruses from humans, birds and pigs encoding the H1, H2 and H5 subtypes of HA (hemagglutinin) and the N1 subtype of NA (neuraminidase) from a repository of stored influenza A viruses in the Viral Genomes Resource at the National Center for Biotechnology Information at the NIH. Published in

2014, the findings of Worobey and his team indicate that genetic components of the H1 portion of the 1918 virus circulated in humans before 1907.[62] The 1918 pandemic virus arose via reassortment between this pre-existing human influenza A H1 lineage and an avian strain, in a human or swine host. The pre-existing human H1 virus acquired avian N1 neuraminidase and internal protein genes. The resulting pandemic virus had seven RNA segments of avian origin plus one segment coding for HA from the pre-existing human virus strain. This novel reassorted strain explains both the virus's impressive ability to infect humans and the absence of immunity. The virus causing classic swine flu – the one discovered by Richard Shope in 1933 after the disease appeared historically in pigs at the time of the 1918 pandemic – appears to have descended directly from the human pandemic virus. The study's findings also suggest that the seasonal H1N1 virus developed by intra-subtype reassortment between the pandemic lineage and a co-circulating antigenically distinct H1 strain. Reassortment is clearly an important key to the pandemic potential of the influenza A virus.

★★★★★★★★★★★

Influenza Treatment

At the time of the 1918 pandemic, the only available treatment for influenza was supportive care. There were no antibiotics to treat secondary bacterial pneumonia, no ventilators to support pulmonary function and allow lung recovery, and no direct antiviral medications. Antibiotics began to appear in the 1930s and 1940s and are frontline treatment of bacterial pneumonia complicating influenza today. Artificial ventilation began with invention of the iron lung to support polio patients in 1929; this was replaced by positive pressure ventilators beginning in the early 1950s. Again, mechanical ventilation is widely used to support patients with respiratory failure in the context of severe influenza infection today. Finally, use of heart-lung bypass to allow the lungs to recover from overwhelming infection is an important element in treatment of individuals with lungs that have been critically compromised by influenza.

Perhaps most importantly, specific antiviral medications have been developed since the 1960s. These medications do not kill the virus directly but rather attack at critical stages of the life cycle. Culture methods to identify the virus responsible for an illness have been available since the mid-1970s, followed by rapid influenza diagnostic tests (RIDT) which detect the influenza viral nucleoprotein antigen. Commercially available RIDTs can provide accurate results within 30 minutes or less and these are an important part of the contemporary management of influenza.[63]

There are currently six licensed prescription influenza antiviral agents available in the United States: three are neuraminidase(NA) inhibitors that block the release of viral progeny in influenza A and B; the best known is oral oseltamivir phosphate, sold as Tamiflu; zanamivir is an inhaled drug marketed as Relenza;

and, intravenous peramivir, is marketed as Rapivab. The fourth recommended drug is oral baloxavir marboxil marketed as Xofluza — it is an endonuclease inhibitor that interferes with viral RNA transcription and blocks virus replication. The majority of currently circulating influenza viruses are susceptible to the neuraminidase inhibitor antiviral medications, oseltamivir(Tamiflu), zanamivir and peramivir. A second category of anti-viral drugs is a class of medications known as adamantanes, which target the M2 ion channel protein of influenza A viruses: amantadine and rimantadine are only active against influenza A. There are high levels of resistance in the circulating influenza A virus population to the adamantanes so they are not currently recommended for treatment of influenza.

Clinical trials and observational studies show that early antiviral treatment shortens the duration of fever and illness symptoms and may reduce the risk of complications, with greatest benefits when started within 48 hours of influenza illness onset. Currently, the CDC specifically recommends initiation of a neuraminidase inhibitor treatment as early as possible for anyone with confirmed or suspected influenza who has severe, complicated, or progressive illness; who requires hospitalization; or who is at greater risk for influenza-related complications.[64] The combination of antibiotics to treat secondary bacterial infections, ascending levels of respiratory support and direct antiviral agents will hopefully decrease complications and mortality in the event of a future influenza pandemic.

Evidence of the excessive and potentially destructive immune response to severe influenza has raised the possibility of immunomodulatory therapy. A wide variety of agents have been assessed in animal and some human studies including corticosteroids, peroxisome proliferator-activated receptor agonists, shingosine-1-phosphate receptor 1 agonists, cyclooxygenase-2 inhibitors, anti-TNF factor therapy, intravenous immunoglobulin therapy and statins.[65] High dose steroids increase morbidity and mortality and are not recommended. Limited data suggests that combinations of antiviral and antibiotic agents may be useful. There is also limited data supporting the use of passive immune therapies like convalescent plasma and hyperimmune globulin.[66] Consistently effective targeting of the immune system in severe influenza is the subject of ongoing research efforts.

The Threat of Pandemic Avian Flu

When my mother explained the way Canada geese fly south for the winter, understanding of bird migration was of a relatively simple north-south transit pattern between known winter and summer nesting sites. More than 100 years of bird-ringing followed by satellite tracking in recent decades have revealed the true immense complexity of bird migration. GPS tracking shows that migration routes and schedules vary with each season based on multiple environmental conditions and individual bird and flock factors. Over time, the flyway concept emerged, defined as the system of migration paths that link resting and nesting sites and ecosystems for different birds in different countries and on different continents.[67] A single flyway is composed of many overlapping migration systems of individual bird populations and species, each with its own intrinsic habitat preferences and migration strategies, and each subject to ongoing modification. Global flyway systems depicted on different map projections illustrate the enormous scope and complexity of bird migration and make obvious the potential for overlap of bird populations across continents. A polar projection like the one shown in Figure 4.4 highlights the fact that all the world's flyways converge over the Arctic. Given what we know about water birds as the natural reservoir of the influenza virus, this global aviation network – depicted in Figure 4.4 – provides a unique opportunity for reassortment between viral strains from different bird and animal populations with subsequent intercontinental disease spread along the migratory flyways.[68]

And this leads us to Avian influenza. Influenza infection in domestic birds has been known to poultry farmers for centuries but was first recorded in Italy in 1878. The disease, originally known as Fowl Plague but now known officially as "avian influenza"; and colloquially as "bird flu," causes intermittent massive outbreaks in poultry, including repeated major outbreaks in the United States but before 1990, infections were sporadic and contained. In the 1990s, the world's poultry population exploded, reflecting the exponential growth in human population and the accompanying increased demand for animal protein. Poultry farmers responded with increasingly intensive poultry production methods including high-density farms and frequent flock movement plus breeding of a single, genetically homogeneous species, a perfect environment for contracting and spreading infection.

The virus causing Fowl Plague was identified as an influenza virus in 1955 but it was not until 1996 that the virus was isolated from a goose in China and found to be an H5N1 sub-lineage of influenza A. The potent flu virus now known as HP (for highly pathogenic) H5N1 was then recognized in Hong Kong in March of 1997, when it suddenly surfaced in chickens.[69] Flocks of infected birds acutely developed progressive difficulty breathing and then died, often within minutes; autopsies showed internal hemorrhage and severe necrosis of the lungs and other internal organs. Hong Kong scientists identified the virus as H5N1 but found it to be highly infectious in birds, much more than the usual influenza virus. Then in May of 1997, a 3-year-old boy was admitted to hospital in Hong Kong with fever and shortness of breath. Over the next several days, he developed respiratory failure and despite intensive support, progressive multi-organ failure led to death 7 days after hospitalization. Viral cultures in Hong Kong evaluated by multiple international labs confirmed infection with H5N1 – the first time an avian influenza virus had caused human disease. Fatal avian influenza in chickens recurred in the fall and in November, a 13-year-old girl presented with fever and pulmonary hemorrhage. Again, cultures were positive for HP H5N1 and again, despite intensive support, multiple organ failure developed and the patient died. When these cases were reported, there was immediate fear around the world that the H5N1 virus had mutated to be able to infect humans directly

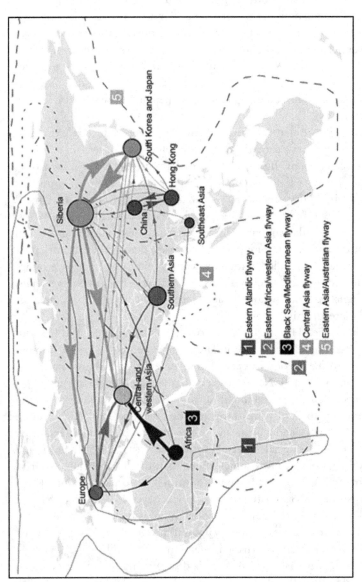

FIGURE 4.4 Global migration patterns of highly pathogenic Avian Influenza A (H5N1) viruses estimated from sequence data sampled during 1996–2012. Arrows represent direction of movement, and arrow width is proportional to the migration rate. Migration rates <0.07 migration events per lineage per year are not shown. The area of each circle is proportional to the region's eigenvector centrality; larger circles indicate crucial nodes in the migration network.

Source: Global and local persistence of Influenza A(H5N1) virus. *Emerging Infectious Disease* 2014; 20(8). CDC.gov

and therefore spread easily – that a new and deadly pandemic was about to begin. The avian epidemic persisted in domestic birds but by the end of December, there had been only 18 identified cases of H5N1 bird flu in people, of whom 6 died; one-half of cases were in adolescents and children less than 13 years old. All occurred in individuals who had contact with live poultry in the days before they fell ill with evidence of very limited human-to-human transmission, only with close, sustained contact. Viral analysis of the avian and human cases showed >99% correlation indicating disease had been caused by the same H5N1 strain, and nucleotide sequencing suggested that the H5N1 strain was a reassortant from co-circulating avian influenza virus strains. Alarmingly, cultures of chickens in Hong Kong markets showed that almost 20% were infected with this virus. In response, the government ordered the slaughter of *all* poultry in Hong Kong, on farms and in markets: over the last 3 days of that December, 1.5 million chickens were killed. At the same time, importation of live chickens from mainland China was suspended. There were no further human cases of H5N1 in 1997 and virologists and infectious disease specialists in Hong Kong and all over the world breathed a sigh of relief.[69] After this alarming outbreak, the Hong Kong government instituted new infection control policies but despite these efforts, the H5N1 virus was detected again in chickens and geese beginning in 1999 and in May 2001, clusters of chicken deaths from avian influenza occurred. The H5N1 virus was again isolated but shown to be a genetically different sub-lineage from the 1997 H5N1 isolate. There was a second territory-wide slaughter of poultry and the import of live birds was again suspended, the beginning of a recurrent pattern of culling and quarantine to attempt to prevent the spread of H5N1 outbreaks.

With what appeared to be a decline in human HP-H5N1 cases, attention shifted from H5N1 to H7N9: avian influenza A, a subtype that had previously been detected only in asymptomatic birds. In March 2013, H7N9 presented for the first time in humans in China and subsequently, annual infections in both humans and birds were observed. The disease was of concern because identified patients became extremely ill with progressive severe respiratory illness after recent exposure to live poultry or poultry-contaminated environments, especially in markets where live birds had been sold. This virus does not transmit easily from person to person, and sustained human-to-human transmission has not been reported. During the fifth epidemic, from October 1, 2016 through September 30, 2017, the WHO reported 766 human infections with Asian H7N9 virus, the largest H7N9 epidemic to date. Throughout the first four epidemics of Asian H7N9 infections, only low pathogenic avian influenza (LPAI) viruses were found but during the fifth epidemic, mutations were detected identifying the emergence of high pathogenic avian influenza (HPA1) viruses with reduced susceptibility to influenza antiviral medications.[70] Because of its pandemic potential, the CDC worked with Chinese partners to enhance surveillance for Asian H7N9 viruses in humans and poultry, to improve laboratory capability to detect and characterize the viruses, and to develop, test and distribute new candidate vaccine viruses that could be used for rapid vaccine production if needed.

Simultaneously, the Chinese government worked to minimize Asian H7N9 spread. Chinese scientists developed a new H7N9 vaccine for chickens which was first used in September 2017. There was a major decrease in H7N9 cases in response, and ultimately, a very aggressive and successful poultry vaccination campaign stopped all human cases.[71]

Despite efforts at containment, however, HP H5N1 variants continued to emerge and spread to wild birds and domestic poultry flocks, at first in Asia and then globally, repeatedly involving multiple countries on 4 continents. China has been identified as the critical epicenter for the emergence of novel avian influenza viruses because of its traditional farming and marketing methods. In China, pigs and domestic waterfowl like chickens, geese and ducks are raised in close proximity to one another, and to the large numbers of humans that tend them. Wetlands used for rice production allow free-grazing migratory water birds to feed in the same areas year-round. This arrangement allows for frequent co-infection of pigs with both human and bird strains of the influenza virus and maximizes the potential for reassortment and the emergence of a novel lethal strain. And the Chinese people prefer to buy freshly killed birds so there are "wet markets" – flash forward here to SARS and SARS-CoV19 – where live birds and other animals from multiple sites are caged to be killed on the spot. Nowhere else on earth is the evolution of influenza viruses to include animal, avian and human strains facilitated to this extent. Studies in China confirm the existence of multiple H5N1 sub-lineages, expressing wide antigenic diversity. And once a novel avian influenza strain like H5N1 develops, migratory waterfowl are easily infected through shared water sources and can then carry the virus around the globe.[72] The HP H5N1 virus already has two of the characteristics necessary to cause a pandemic: new variants are novel microbial agents that can infect humans and there is minimal or no population immunity. Lacking to this time is only easy and sustainable transmission of the virus to humans and efficient human-to-human spread.

Looking at the last two global outbreaks of avian influenza exemplifies the gravity of this growing problem. In December 2014, an epidemic of a new H5 virus strain, HP H5N2, appeared in domestic poultry in the United States, introduced via North American flyways.[73] This highly virulent strain was apparently created when migratory water birds from North America and from Asia intermingled in the Far East. The birds carried the new virus strain over the pole with the first HP H5N2 infections documented in Canada geese in western Canada and the northern US states.[74] Despite extensive existing safety measures to protect domestic bird flocks, the disease spread rapidly involving captive wild birds, free-ranging birds, backyard flocks, and commercial flocks in 21 American states. Ultimately, the virus resulted in the deaths of more than 42 million chickens and 7.5 million turkeys either by direct infection or by culling to prevent disease spread, before the epidemic ended in June of 2015. The disease destroyed 10% of the country's egg-laying chicken population and 3% of its annual turkey production. There were no human cases of H5N2 influenza but this new and serious epidemic in domestic poultry was a reminder that the capacity for rapid mutation which is the hallmark of the influenza virus means the potential to cause new human or animal disease is always present with migratory water birds always available for rapid transport and dissemination.

In the fall of 2020, a highly pathogenic Asian influenza H5N1 variant (HPAI H5N1) caused by reassortment between poultry and wild bird viruses emerged again, first in Europe and then across Europe and into Africa, the Middle East and Asia and finally, North and South America. From late 2021 through 2023, this wild-bird adapted HPAI H5N1 virus has caused poultry outbreaks worldwide involving 5 continents.[75] In January 2022, the first HPAI H5N1 virus infection in wild birds in the United States since 2016 was reported and in February 2022, there was an HPAI H5N1 outbreak in turkeys, the first in a commercial poultry facility in North America. Despite containment efforts, this highly contagious virus has mutated to infect multiple species and has taken a staggering toll on animals around the globe. The H5N1 virus has infected domestic birds in more than 80 countries from big commercial poultry farms to tiny backyard henhouses, affecting 72 million farmed birds in the United States alone. It has struck a wide range of wild bird species, killing gulls and terns by the thousand. And it has turned up repeatedly in mammals, including minks, foxes, skunks, bears, cats, sea lions and dolphins. In the spring of 2024, the virus was found in herds of dairy cows in the USA. Reports of infected wild birds and domestic flocks have continued despite all efforts including quarantine of involved sites and disposal of all the birds in an infected flock, followed by site decontamination.

This most recent avian influenza HP-H5N1 pandemic has been the worst ever global pandemic, with devastating impact on wild and domestic birds and increasing numbers of cases in mammals.[75] Globally, the WHO reports 870 human cases from 2003 to 2022, along with at least 450 deaths – a fatality rate of more than 50% – but almost all cases have been in individuals with extensive contact with birds; there is still no evidence of sustained person-to-person transmission. In response, the United States Department of Agriculture expanded wild bird surveillance for avian influenza to include the Mississippi and Central Flyways and enlarged the existing surveillance program in the Atlantic and Pacific Flyways, to allow surveillance of all birds that may interact with wild birds from Europe and Asia. As of the fall of 2023,, the Eurasian H5 strain of highly pathogenic avian influenza (HPAI) is surging again in Europe and North America and causing mass animal mortality events in South America. It has also appeared for the first time in birds from Antarctica.

Commenting on HP H5N1, Dr. Margaret Chan, then Director-General of WHO, stated:

> The H5N1 virus is treacherous – we know that it can jump the species barrier to infect mammals and humans and that it is prone to mutation. Indeed, every case of human infection increases the probability that the virus will mutate. We don't know if or when the H5N1 virus might evolve

into a pandemic strain that spreads easily among people, or what its lethality might be. We know only that a pandemic is possible, and that's why the world must prepare now for the very real threat of a global public-health H5N1 emergency.[76]

Preparedness efforts against H5N1 have been substantial with an H5N1 vaccine stockpiled for pandemic preparedness by the United States government, to be used if the virus begins transmitting easily to humans and efficiently from person to person. But as we know, reassortment allows a new viral strain to emerge in a very short time and if such a virus does develop easy human-to-human transmission, there will be no time for vaccine development or delivery. Epidemiologists have estimated that in a worst-case scenario, up to one billion people could die with HP-H5N1 influenza within 6 months.

★★★★★★★★★

Looking Back :: Moving Forward

Virtually unknown in 1900, viruses have since caused an ongoing series of terrifying pandemic disease, beginning with the 1918 global influenza pandemic. Unravelling the story of the influenza virus was a nearly century-long voyage of discovery which included development of advanced bio-imaging techniques, invention of molecular biology, major advances in microbiology and pharmacology, an increasingly sophisticated understanding of immunology, unravelling of the structure of DNA, transformation of clinical genetics and integration of human and animal biology, with collaboration of scientists from all those disciplines from all over the world. It is essentially the story of the emergence of modern science and modern medicine. It is now established that when human, avian and/ or other influenza animal host viruses coexist in a single cell, an infinitesimal killer virus can emerge in the time needed for a single viral replication cycle. It was molecular genetic work that identified this most important characteristic of the influenza virus: endless evolution by both spontaneous mutation and by genetic reassortment leading to continuous emergence of new, antigenically novel strains. Faced with an entirely new influenza virus, human hosts have limited or no resistance so these emerging strains have high infectious potential. And the influenza virus is airborne so transmission from one individual to another is remarkably efficient. At the same time, migratory water birds were identified as permanent reservoirs for the influenza virus and their interaction and migration were recognized as an efficient international delivery system for new viral strains.

We know now that constant genetic mutations and multiple hosts ensure that the emergence of dangerous novel influenza strains is inevitable. Since confirmation that the 1918 pandemic was caused by the influenza virus in the 1940s, there has been an intense, long-standing focus on development of an effective vaccine. However, from the outset, the technique for vaccine development was fraught with problems – problems that are intrinsic to the characteristics of the virus itself and to historic techniques of vaccine production. The original influenza vaccines were developed by growing the virus in fertilized chicken eggs, a technique which requires 6 to 8 months from start to finish. Given the success with development of smallpox and yellow fever vaccines, this was a very reasonable approach. However, with a constantly evolving pathogen, in the time required to develop a vaccine based on preventing the most prevalent strains circulating in the *previous* season, an entirely new and dangerous strain can easily emerge. In fact, the pandemics of 1957, 1968 and 2009 confirm that this is not just a theoretical concern. A new method based on mammalian-cell culture technology has been in limited use since 2012 but this cuts only 5 to 6 weeks off the production time. In addition, the FDA requires evaluation of the safety and efficacy of each new vaccine through clinical trials in an appropriate target population – the cost and time required for these trials is also significant. At the same time, the WHO's Global Influenza Surveillance and Response System (GISRS) is now a massive, enormously complex and costly process, involving more than 140 institutions in 100 Member States with multiple Collaborating Centers and Regulatory Laboratories using a global web-based tool for year-round influenza virologic surveillance. The intricate international reassortment events described for the H1N1(09) pandemic virus exemplify the complicated processes that the surveillance networks tried – and failed – to track. The vaccine developed to prevent infection with the pre-identified 2009 seasonal strains was completely ineffective against the pandemic virus which originated when three strains of influenza merged by antigenic shift, reassortment, and recombination, with pigs as the mixing vessel. More than 250 million doses of influenza vaccine are produced annually against the WHO-recommended influenza strains; a 2013 World Health Organization analysis pegged each manufacturers' cost of refreshing the annual vaccine at $5 million to $18 million per year with return of an estimated three billion dollars of profit for the pharmaceutical industry per year.[77] All this time, effort and money produces an inadequate product, only effective in an average 59% of subjects. A new approach is urgently needed.

And while knowledge of the influenza virus was increasing and recognition and management of influenza epidemics was improving, global vulnerability to an infectious pathogen also increased with growing world population density, rapid and frequent global trade and travel, chaotic urbanization, recurrent wars, substandard living conditions, and the effects of global warming. Complete understanding of the emergence of influenza viruses, their variable pathogenicity and their capacity for continuous evolution remains an ongoing effort which must be integrated into the context of ever-increasing global risk. The challenge for science and medicine going forward is rapid detection and elimination of new life-threatening microbes in an increasingly vulnerable world.

A new approach to influenza vaccine development is clearly indicated. In response to this pressure, there have been efforts to develop a universal flu vaccine that would convey durable cross-protective immunity against diverse virus strains dating back many years. Studies in animal models show that using relatively invariant parts of the virus can induce immunity with the most promising approaches based on antibodies specific for the relatively conserved ectodomain of matrix protein 2 and the infra-subunit region of hemagglutinin.[78] Multiple teams have taken up the challenge of developing a safe and effective universal influenza vaccine, using a wide variety of strategies including vaccine-induced antibodies against the HA stem, blockage of interferon evasion genes with a constructed virus, and antibodies that bind to the influenza virus and recruit T-cells to destroy infected cells.[79-87]

The influenza A virus has proven to be a master of evolution, constantly adapting to new environments and evading immune responses and attempts at prevention with vaccines. For the last hundred years, novel antigenic influenza variants have been responsible for annual seasonal flu epidemics and for four devastating global pandemics as well as ongoing pandemics of avian influenza. Since the early years of the twenty-first century after the HP H5N1 virus first presented in people, many public health experts have feared the imminent development of efficient person-to-person transmission leading to a worldwide H5N1 pandemic with very high mortality. That has not happened – not yet, at least. Intervening pandemics with Ebola, Zika and SARS-CoV2 have shifted attention away from influenza. However, according to Dr. José Esparza, president of the Global Virus Network, "Most pandemics can at least theoretically be controlled with well-established measures of case isolation, contact quarantine and good infection control in hospitals. The one major exception is pandemic influenza – public health measures and pharmaceutical interventions have only limited effectiveness and pandemic vaccines take months to develop and deliver."[88] A contemporary, mathematically based simulation estimates that a new lethal influenza strain like the one that caused the 1918 flu could kill 33 million people in 6 months.[89]

In response, new approaches to development of a universal flu vaccine are underway. The Bill and Melinda Gates Foundation and the Page Family have provided strong support for research into development of a universal flu vaccine by launching the "Universal Influenza Vaccine Development Grand Challenge" during the centenary year of the 1918 flu pandemic. The challenge offers up to 2 million dollars to fund research designed to identify "novel, transformative concepts that will lead to development of universal influenza vaccines offering protection from all subtypes of circulating and emerging (drifted and shifted) Influenza A subtype viruses and Influenza B lineage viruses for at least three to five years."[90] As of this writing in May 2024, no universal influenza vaccine has been developed.

Research continues. A novel approach to efficient vaccine development is the synthetic generation of influenza vaccine using recombinant DNA techniques to generate HA and NA gene sequences as a synthetic candidate virus on a standard vaccine backbone. This virus template would allow instantaneous exchange of identified sequence data from a pandemic strain with local gene synthesis. Using this technique, a vaccine tailored specifically to address a new pandemic strain could be developed almost instantaneously and produced locally, eliminating many of the time-consuming steps in the traditional process. Gene synthesis by this cell-free, enzymatic technique has enormous theoretical appeal although there are substantial technical and regulatory hurdles to be addressed. The FDA has approved one vaccine developed using recombinant DNA but it is not yet utilized for routine immunization.[85,86]

One universal vaccine is in a clinical trial after a successful phase II trial. The nasal flu vaccine M2SR (Redee Flu) is based on a novel approach to prevent replication of the influenza virus in humans by introducing a live virus that cannot replicate but triggers a robust immune response ensuring broad protection.[85] M2SR has already been shown to protect against multiple influenza A subtypes in influenza-naïve and previously infected ferrets. In a first-in-human, randomized, dose-escalation, placebo-controlled study of safety and immunogenicity, the M2SR vaccine was safe and well tolerated and generated dose-dependent durable serum antibody responses against diverse H3N2 influenza strains.[91]

Seasonal influenza vaccines offer little protection against pandemic influenza virus strains and it is difficult to create effective pre-pandemic vaccines because it is uncertain which influenza virus subtype will cause the next pandemic. Based on recent advances in mRNA technology which led to the effective vaccines against SARS-CoV-2 from nucleic acid-based vaccine platforms, Arevalo et al developed a nucleoside-modified messenger RNA (mRNA)–lipid nanoparticle vaccine encoding hemagglutinin antigens from all 20 known influenza A virus subtypes and influenza B virus lineages. In mice and ferrets, this multivalent vaccine elicited high levels of cross-reactive and subtype-specific antibodies that reacted to all 20 encoded antigens. Vaccination protected mice and ferrets challenged with matched and mismatched viral strains, and this protection was at least partially dependent on antibodies. Studies in humans are underway.[92]

Meanwhile, the 2023–2024 US flu season is almost over with the CDC estimating that there have been at least 1.2 million illnesses, 12,000 hospitalizations, and 740 deaths from flu this season. Unfortunately, so far, flu vaccination coverage is lower among children and adults this year compared to the same time last year despite strong evidence that flu vaccination last season substantially reduced the risk of serious outcomes.[93] Regardless of how this flu season evolves, we know the next influenza season begins in less than 7 months and a lethal new influenza strain emerging in China is only a transpolar flight away …

★★★★★★★★

I still look up in wonder when I hear the call of Canada geese overhead. I think I always will. But some component of the awe I feel now includes comprehension of the critical role that migratory water birds play as the reservoir of the amazing and terrifying influenza virus.

HISTORIC PERSPECTIVE: INFLUENZA AND THE PUBLIC HEALTH MOVEMENT

Influenza struck North America in late 1918 and created an epidemic memorialized for its high mortality rate and seeming predilection for healthy young adults. The North American outbreak was part of the global pandemic that affected the entire world, killing 21 million worldwide and more than half a million in the United States. Some of its reach can be attributed to the troop movements associated with the First World War. The effectiveness of the public health movement rallied in opposition to the epidemic also owes a great debt to the infrastructure attached to the war; this produced the framework – especially the tight links between the government and public health – upon which modern US public health still rests. This historic perspective will examine responses to influenza across the United States and demonstrate its resilience in current public health architecture.

The fall of 1918 saw the American public health service hard at work promoting worker welfare in areas essential to the war effort, including health care of military personnel, an aggressive campaign against venereal disease, and improved working conditions and health promotion for industrial workers participating in manufacturing. Those efforts might have distracted the Surgeon General and the rest of the public health infrastructure from the early flu reports surfacing across the Northeast in the spring and summer. But by October, which saw the deaths of 4500 in Philadelphia and 2300 in Chicago in a single week, the effort to combat the flu was in full swing. That meant coordinating reports from all over the country on mortality rates, mass public education, and the appointment of state influenza directors to distribute doctors and nurses to the most severely affected areas. The volunteer medical corps was also raided to provide additional physicians and nurses to join the influenza combat ranks. Their salaries became part of the government payroll during the epidemic, and they were deemed vital to the nation's health. These efforts were fueled by a one million dollar appropriation by Congress. Tremendous power was also granted to the Attorney General including the right to restrict fundamental Constitutional rights, like the freedom of assembly. The Attorney General exercised this right on October 5, 1918 to close all areas of public assembly. His order was carried out by local public health departments, and across the country, schools, theaters, churches and restaurants closed. Anti-spitting laws originally designed to curb tuberculosis were enforced, and in many areas, new laws were written to order the wearing of masks in public.

These prevention efforts proved insignificant in light of the vast number of new and critically ill influenza cases. The public health service responded by appointing new officers specifically to address the epidemic, creating a network of emergency hospitals, hiring thousands of physicians to staff these new facilities and beginning vaccine trials. When the number of new cases finally began to decline at the end of November, the public health service found itself in a new role: no longer devoted to prevention and treatment, it turned its attention to damage assessment. A team of interviewers began conducting door-to-door surveys across the nation, and their findings were analyzed by a PHS statistician. It was these findings that, despite the relatively small sample, showed the most vulnerable population to have been previously healthy 20–40 year olds and the baseline mortality rate to have been at least 55,000.[94] All these efforts reflected the need for a stronger federal public health authority, since the PHS was left scrambling at the beginning of the epidemic to hire staff and establish the necessary infrastructure to educate about the disease, disseminate information about how it was transmitted, reduce transmission rates, treat the sick, and assess national and regional morbidity and mortality. Most of the PHS's success was due to local and regional efforts, and it is both by examining those and dividing the effort by race that it becomes clear that this was not yet a truly national public health service.

The American Red Cross was perhaps the most effective of the groups mobilized in the fight against influenza, and it worked with the PHS to provide treatment and propagate information about the means of transmission. Its standing was bolstered by its links to the government, which included reporting directly to Congress and its status as the official organization designated to respond to disasters and carry out the US government's responsibilities under the Geneva Convention. The ARC operated through a network of regional and local offices, and these expanded considerably during the course of the Firest World War. President Wilson organized a board to control the Red Cross when the United States entered the war, and that board expanded the organization substantially, recruiting at least 8 million female volunteers as well as reorganizing to include 14 regional divisions with 12,700 staff and 20 million members. Part of the ARC's mandate included hiring nurses, as well as recruiting female volunteers. It is worth noting that black women consistently faced rejection, both as nursing candidates and as volunteers. This racial divide would limit the opportunities for black women to serve overseas, as well as have significant repercussions for public health efforts, including those mobilized against influenza. The very African American women who were refused the chance to serve overseas were assigned to care for servicemen on military bases afflicted by the flu; other women also rejected as unsuitable, such as married women, joined their ranks. The white nurses who had previously held the gates of their profession closed against black women and kept their numbers restricted to those who were unmarried, found they no longer had sufficient personnel to justify these decisions. Although it would take many more decades to end racial segregation in the ARC and the medical profession, the work of African American women in the influenza epidemic initiated a slow shift in nursing demographics. Even in the midst of the epidemic, however, white officials were reluctant to permit African American nurses to care for white civilian patients.[95] Ironically, racial segregation might have benefited African Americans when it came to influenza, since this is one of the factors to which their lower mortality rate during the epidemic has been attributed. Other factors include the poor conditions in African American neighborhoods that might have increased the number of cases in the spring influenza season and thus provided immunity during the deadlier fall outbreak, and inaccurate reporting of African American flu mortality.[96] The lower morbidity and mortality rate among African Americans did nothing to erase racial medical theories that defined African Americans as biologically inferior and more prone to sickness, and it reinforced the idea that black and white people were constitutionally different in their responses to disease.[97] The long-term effects of this racialized medical thinking would be experienced at least through the end of the Tuskeegee Syphilis study in 1972.

The ARC effort was nationally organized, but it was locally run. Regional and local offices were responsible for a significant effort to combat the flu, including provision of approximately $2 million in supplies and equipment to hospitals, transportation of health care workers, supplies, and bodies, creation of institutions to care for patients and to feed and house those left homeless and orphaned by the disease, and recruitment of nurses and other volunteers to serve alongside PHS personnel.[98] As Moser Jones argues, however, the success of the ARC's efforts showed high regional variation that demonstrated the weaknesses inherent in a system dependent upon coordinating even a quasi-governmental organization with the governmental wing responsible for public health and the importance of cooperation on the ground among all acting agencies.[95] She contends that the regional variation in response efficacy reflected not just a disconnect between what the federal government and the ARC central authority deemed "the right way to respond" but also the centrality of a culture that valued volunteerism at the community level as an important aspect of citizenship.[99]

The nation might have valued volunteerism, but the federal government viewed the inconsistent regional cooperation with central authority to be a significant weakness in the public health infrastructure. Federal efforts to promote public health had begun as early as 1798, when Congress passed a law authorizing the establishment of hospitals to care for sick and disabled seamen. It continued in 1871 when Congress created the position of Surgeon General, originally intended to head the Marine Health Service, and became more institutionally bound when Congress passed the National Quarantine Act in 1878, transferring the power of quarantine from states to the Marine Health Service, and when a federally funded lab was established on Staten Island to study communicable diseases in 1887. Eventually the three areas of federal responsibility for public health would be handled by the National Institutes of Health (established in 1930), the Centers for Disease Control (established in 1946), and the Federal Emergency Management Agency (established in 1979).[100] It was the influenza epidemic that prompted the first articulation of the need for a federally controlled and funded public health infrastructure that was resilient to regional variation. It took 60 years to fully realize that initial goal which has since expanded. FEMA and the CDC have the federal power to quarantine, first granted during the 1918 influenza epidemic but not used since, though states and cities have exercised their right to quarantine as recently as the Ebola outbreak of 2014.[101]

References

(1) Magner LM. (2005) *A History of Medicine.* Second edition. New York, NY. Informa Healthcare. p.496–497.

(2) Magner. 2005. p.502, 516.

(3) Levine AI. (1992) *Viruses.* New York, NY. Scientific American Library. Distributed by W.H. Freeman and Company. Chapter 1.

(4) Fernandez MO, Thomas RJ, Garton NJ et al. Assessing the airborne survival of bacteria in populations of aerosol droplets with a novel technology. *J R Soc Interface* 2019; 16(150): 20180779 doi: 10.1098/rsif.2018.0779.

(5) Paules C, Subbarao K. Influenza. *Lancet* 2017; 390(10095): 697–708.

(6) Taubenberger JK, Morens DM. The pathology of influenza virus infections. *Annu Rev Pathol* 2008; 3:499–522.

(7) Kash JC, Taubenberger JK. The role of viral, host and secondary bacterial factors in influenza pathogenesis. *Amer J Pathol* 2015; 185:1528–1536.

(8) Hsu AC-Y. Influenza virus: a master tactician in innate immune evasion and novel therapeutic interventions. *Front Immunol* 2018; 9:1–11. Article 743.

(9) WHO | Influenza (Seasonal), March 2014. Available at: www.who.int/mediacentre/factsheets/fs211/en/. Accessed 7/7/2016.

(10) Leung NHL, Cuilling X, Ip DKM, Cowling BJ. The fraction of influenza virus infections that are asymptomatic: a systematic review and meta-analysis. *Epidemiol* 2015; 26(6): 862–872.

(11) Lofgren E, Fefferman NH, Naumov YN et al. Influenza seasonality: underlying causes and modeling theories. *J Virol* 2007; 81(11): 5429–5436.

(12) Barry JM. (2004) *The Great Influenza: The Epic Story of the Deadliest Pandemic in History.* New York, NY. Viking Penguin. Chapters 14–19.

(13) Langford C. Did the 1918–19 influenza pandemic originate in China? *Population and Development Review* 2005; 31(3): 473–505.

(14) Humphries MO. Paths of infection: The First World War and the origins of the 1918 influenza pandemic. *War Hist* 2013; 21(1): 55–81.

(15) Barry. 2004. Chapters 22–25.

(16) Taubenberger JK, Morens DM. 1918 Influenza: the Mother of All Pandemics. *Emerg Infect Dis.* 2006; 12(1): 15–22.

(17) Tisoncik JR, Korth MJ, Simmons CP et al. Into the eye of the cytokine storm. *Microbio Mol Biol Rev* 2012; 76: 16–32.

(18) Liu Q, Zhou Y-H, Yang Z-Q. The cytokine storm of severe influenza and development of immunomodulatory therapy. *Cellular Molec Immunol* 2016; 13: 3–10.

(19) Morens DM, Taubenberger JK, Fauci AS. The persistent legacy of the 1918 influenza virus. *N Engl J Med* 2009; 361:225–229.

(20) Bell FC, Miller ML. Life Tables for the United States Social Security Area 1900–2100; *Actuarial Study* No. 116. Figure 2(a).

(21) Pfeiffer RJM. Ztschr. f. Hyg. *U. Infectionskrankh.*, 1893. P.357.

(22) Brooks H. The treatment of pneumonia. *Med Clin North Amer* 1922; 5: 993–1006.

(23) Nicolle C, LeBailly C. Recherches experimentale sur la grippe. *Annales de l'Institut Pasteur.* 1919; 33:395–402.

(24) Yamanouchi T. Skakami K, Iwashima S. The infecting agent in Influenza. *Lancet* 1919; 193: 971.

(25) Shope RE. Swine influenza, Experimental transmission and pathology. *J Exp Med* 1931; 54: 349–373.

(26) Smith W, Andrewes CH, Laidlaw PP. A virus obtained from influenza patients. *Lancet* 1933; 2:66–8.

(27) Francis T, Magill TP. The antibody response of human subjects vaccinated with the virus of human influenza. *J Exp Med* 1938; 68:147–60.

(28) Francis T, Salk JE, Pearson HE, Brown PN. Protective effect of vaccination against induced influenza A. *J Clin Invest.* 1945 Jul; 24(4):536–546.

(29) Kausche GA, Pfankuch E, Ruska H. Die Sichtbarmachung von pflanzlichem Virus im Übermikroskop. *Naturwissenschaften.* 1939; 27(18): 292–299.

(30) Luria SE, Delbruck M, Anderson, TF. Electron microscope studies of bacterial viruses. *J Bacteriol* 1943; 46: 57–76.

(31) Luria SE. Mutations of bacterial viruses affecting their host range. *Genetics* 1945; 30: 84–99.

(32) The Nobel Prize in Physiology or Medicine 1969. Nobel Media AB 2013, Available at: *Nobelprize.org.* Accessed October 12, 2016.

(33) Mosley VM, Wyckoff RWG. Electron micrography of the virus of influenza. *Nature* 1946; 3983: 263.

(34) Noda T. Native morphology of influenza virions. *Frontiers in Micro.* 2012; 2: 1–5.

(35) Laver WG, Valentine RC. Morphology of isolated hemagglutinin and neuraminidase subunits of influenza virus. *Virol* 1969; 38: 105–119.

(36) Bouvier NM, Palese. The biology of influenza viruses. *Vaccine* 2008;26(Suppl 4): D49–D53.

(37) Sakai T, Nishimura SI, Naito T, Saito M. Influenza A virus hemagglutinin and neuraminidase act as novel motile machinery. *Sci Rep* 2017; PMID 28344335.

(38) Hershey A, Chase M. Independent functions of viral protein and nucleic acid in growth of bacteriophage. *J Gen Physiol.* 1952; 36(1): 39–56.

(39) Mathews AP. Professor Albrecht Kossel. *Science.* 1927 Sep 30; 66(1709):293–293.

(40) Chargaff, E, Zamenhof S, Green C. Composition of human deoxypentose nucleic acid. *Nature* 1950; 165(4202): 756–7.

(41) Crick F, Watson JD. Molecular structure of nucleic acids: A structure for deoxyribose nucleic acid. *Nature* 1953; 171: 737–738.

(42) Pennazio S, Roggero P. Tobacco mosaic virus RNA as genetic determinant: genesis of a discovery. *Riv Biol.* 2000; 93(3): 431–55.

(43) McCauley JW, Mahy BWJ. Structure and function of the influenza virus genome. *Biochem J* 1983; 211: 281–294.

(44) Steinhauer DA, Holland JJ. Rapid evolution of RNA viruses. *Ann Rev Microbiol* 1987; 41: 409–433.

(45) Drake JW. Rates of spontaneous mutation among RNA viruses. *Proc Nat Acad Sci* 1993; 90(9): 4171–4175.

(46) Burnet FM, Lind PE. A genetic approach to variation in influenza viruses: recombination of characters in influenza virus strains used in mixed infections. *J Gen Microbiol* 1951; 5(1): 67–82.

(47) Matrosovich M, Stech J, Klenk HD. Influenza receptors, polymerase and host range. *Rev Sci Tech.* 2009 Apr; 28(1): 203–17.

(48) Hinshaw VS, Webster RG, Turner B. The perpetuation of orthomyxoviruses and paramyxoviruses in Canadian waterfowl. *Can J Microbiol* 1980 May; 26(5): 622–9.

(49) Webster RG, Bean WJ, Gorman OT et al. Evolution and ecology of influenza A viruses. *Microbiol. Rev.* 1992; 56: 152–179.

(50) Webster RG, Wright SM, Castrucci MR et al. Influenza – a model of an emerging virus disease. *Intervirology* 1993; 35: 16–25.

(51) Scholtissek C, Rohde W, Von Hoyningen V, Rott R. On the origin of the human influenza subtypes H2N2 and H3N2. *Virology* 1978; 87: 13–20.

(52) Lindstrom SE, Cox NJ, Klimov A. Genetic analysis of human H2N2 and early H3N2 influenza viruses, 1957–1972: evidence for genetic divergence and multiple reassortment events. *Virology* 2004; 328: 101–19.

(53) CDC Novel H1N1 Flu | The 2009 H1N1 Pandemic: Summary Available at: www.cdc.gov/h1n1flu/cdcresponse.htm

(54) Osterholm MT, Kelley NS, Sommer A, Belongia EA. Efficacy and effectiveness of influenza vaccines: a systematic review and meta-analysis. *Lancet Infectious Dis.* 2012; 12(1): 36–44.

(55) Sanger F, Nicklen S, Coulson AR. DNA sequencing with chain-terminating inhibitors. *Proceedings of the National Academy of Sciences USA,* 1977; 74(12): 5463–5467.

(56) Mullis KF, Faloona F, Scharf S et al. Specific enzymatic amplification of DNA in vitro: The polymerase chain reaction. *Cold Spring Harb. Symp Quant Biol* 1986; 51: 263–273.

(57) Taubenberger JK, Reid AH, Krafft AE et al. Initial genetic characterization of the 1918 "Spanish" influenza virus. *Science* 1997; 275: 1793–1796.

(58) Taubenberger JK, Morens DM. 1918 Influenza: the mother of all pandemics. *Emerg Infect Dis* 2006; 12(1): 15–22.

(59) Taubenberger JK et al. Molecular virology: Was the 1918 pandemic caused by a bird flu? Was the 1918 flu avian in origin? *Nature* 2006; 440(7988): E9-E10.

(60) Heather HM, Chain B. The sequence of sequencers: the history of sequencing DNA. *Genomics* 2016; 107: 1–8.

(61) Ho S. The molecular clock and estimating species divergence. *Nature Education* 2008; 1(1): 168–169.

(62) Worobey M, Han G-Z, Rambaut A. Genesis and pathogenesis of the 1918 pandemic H1N1 influenza A virus. *Proc Nat Acad Sci* 2014; 111(22): 8107–8112.

(63) Uyeki TM, Bernstein HH, Bradley JS, et al. Clinical Practice Guidelines by the Infectious Diseases Society of America: 2018 Update on Diagnosis, Treatment, Chemoprophylaxis, and Institutional Outbreak Management of Seasonal Influenza. *Clin Infect Dis* 2019; 68:e1.

(64) Centers for Disease Control and Prevention: Seasonal Influenza (Flu): Information for Health Professionals. Available at: www.cdc.gov/flu/professionals/index.htm

(65) Liu Q, Zhou Y-H, Yang Z-Q. The cytokine storm of severe influenza and development of immunomodulatory therapy. *Cellular Molec Immunol* 2016; 13: 3–10.

(66) Hui DS, Lee N., Chan PK, Beigel JH. The role of adjuvant immunomodulatory agents for treatment of severe influenza. *Antiviral Res* 2018; 150: 202–216.

(67) Boere, G.C. & Stroud, D.A. 2006. The flyway concept: what it is and what it isn't. In *Waterbirds around the world*. Eds. G.C. Boere, C.A. Galbraith & D.A. Stroud. The Stationery Office, Edinburgh, UK. pp. 40–47.

(68) Hagemeijer W, Mundkur T. Migratory flyways in Europe, Africa and Asia and the spread of HPAI H5N1. Wetlands International. Report of the UNEP/CMS Scientific Taskforce on Avian Influenza and Wild Birds. Accessed Sept. 23, 2016.

(69) Chan PKS. Outbreak of avian influenza A(H5N1) virus infection in Hong Kong in 1997. *Clinical Infectious Diseases* 2002; 34(Suppl 2):S58–64.

(70) Kile JC, Ren R, Liu L et al. Update: Increase in Human Infections with Novel Asian Lineage Avian Influenza A(H7N9) Viruses During the Fifth Epidemic – China, October 1, 2016–August 7, 2017. *MMWR* 2017; 66(35):928–932.

(71) WHO. Avian Influenza Weekly Update Number 692. June 7, 2019.

(72) WHO: Influenza at the human-animal interface. Summary and assessment, 20 December to 16 January 2017. Available at: www.who.int/influenza/human_anima l_interface/en/

(73) Dusek RJ, Hallgrímsson GT, Ip, HS et al. North Atlantic migratory bird flyways provide routes for intercontinental movement of avian influenza viruses. *PLoS ONE*, 2014; v. 9, p. e92075, doi: 10 .1371/journal.pone.0092075. Accessed October 2, 2016.

(74) USDA–Animal and Plant Inspection Service. Veterinary Services. 2016 HPA1 Preparedness and Response Plan, January 11, 2016. Available at: www.aphis.usda. gov/animal_health/downloads/animal_diseases/ai/hpai-preparedness-and-respo nse-plan-2016.pdf. Accessed October 1, 2016.

(75) Charostad J, Rezaei Zadeh Rukerd M, Mahmoudvand S et al. A comprehensive review of highly pathogenic avian influenza (HPAI) H5N1: An imminent threat at doorstep. *Travel Medicine and Infectious Disease* 2023; 55:102638. https://doi. org/10.1016/j.tmaid.2023.102638

(76) One-on-one with Dr. Margaret Chan. Harvard Business School Journal: Stories. March 1, 2006.

(77) McKenna M. Big pharma has the flu. Available at: www.wired.com/story/flu-vacc ine-big-pharma/

(78) Neu KE, Henry Dunand CJ, Wilson PC. Heads, stalks and everything else: how can antibodies eradicate influenza as a human disease? *Curr Opin Immunol.* 2016 Oct; 42: 48–55.

(79) Joyce MG, Wheatley AK, Thomas PV et al. Vaccine-induced antibodies that neutralize group 1 and group 2 Influenza A viruses. *Cell* 2016; 166(3): 609–623.

(80) Sheikh QM, Gatherer D, Reche PA et al. Towards the knowledge-based design of universal influenza epitope ensemble vaccines. *Bioinformatics* 2016: btw399. Available at: doi: 10.1093/ bioinformatics/btw399. Accessed October 12, 2016.

(81) Wenqian H, Tan GS, Mullarkey CE et al. Epitope specificity plays a critical role in regulating antibody-dependent cell-mediated cytotoxicity against Influenza A virus. *Proc Nat Acad Sci* 2016. doi: 10.1073/pnas.1609316113.

(82) Protecting Humanity from Future Health Crises: Report of the High-level United Nations Panel on the Global Response to Health Crises. p.7

(83) Du Y, Xin L, Shi Y, Sun R et al. Genome-wide identification of interferon-sensitive mutations enables influenza vaccine design. *Science* 2018; 359(6373): 290–296.

(84) Deng L, Mohan T, Chang TZ, Wang B-A et al. Double-layered protein nanoparticles induce broad protection against divergent influenza A viruses. *Nature Comm* 2018; 9: 359–371.

(85) Ping J, Lopes TJS, Nidom CA… Neumann G, Kawaoka Y. Development of high-yield influenza A virus vaccine viruses. *Nature Comm* 2015; 6: 8148.

(86) Dormitzer PR, Suphaphipat P, Gibson D et al. Synthetic generation of influenza vaccine viruses for rapid response to pandemics. *Sci Transl Med* 2013; 5(185): 185r68.

(87) Dunkle LM, Izikson R, Patrirca P. Efficacy of recombinant influenza vaccine in adults 50 years of age or older. *N Engl J Med* 2017; 376: 2427–2436.

(88) Esparza J. *Confronting Emerging Viral Threats: From HIV/AIDS to Zika.* Penn State Berks Science Colloquium. April 1, 2016.

(89) Shattuck Flu Map. Available at: YouTube/GatesFoundation/Institute of Disease Modeling

(90) Bill & Melinda Gates Foundation. Ending the Pandemic Threat: A Grand Challenge for Universal Influenza Vaccine Development. Available at: https://gcgh.grandchallenges.org/challenge/ending-pandemic-threat-grand-challenge-universal influenza-vaccine-development

(91) Eiden J, Fierro C, Schwartz H et al. Intranasal M2SR (M2-Deficient Single Replication) H3N2 influenza vaccine provides enhanced mucosal and serum antibodies in adults. *J Infect Dis.* 2022 Dec 28; 227(1):103–112. doi: 10.1093/infdis/jiac433.

(92) Arevalo CP, Bolton MJ, Le Sage V et al. A multivalent nucleoside-modified mRNA vaccine against all known influenza virus subtypes. *Science* 2022; 378: 899–904. doi:10.1126/science.abm0271

(93) Lewis NM, Zhu Y, Peltan ID et al. Vaccine Effectiveness Against Influenza A–Associated Hospitalization, Organ Failure, and Death: United States, 2022–2023, *Clinical Infectious Diseases*, 2023: ciad677, https://doi.org/10.1093/cid/ciad677

(94) Gernhart G. A forgotten enemy: PHS's fight against the 1918 influenza epidemic. *Public Heath Rep* Nov–Dec, 1999; 114(6): 559–561.

(95) Moser Jones M. The American red cross and local response to the 1918 influenza pandemic: A four city case study. *Public Health Reports* 2010; 125: 92–104.

(96) Northington Gamble V. There wasn't a lot of comforts in those days: African Americans, public health, and the 1918 Influenza epidemic. *Public Health Rep* 2010; 125: Suppl 3:114–122.

(97) Northington Gamble, 120.

(98) Jones, 93.

(99) Jones, 102.

(100) www.fema.gov/about-agency; www.hhs.gov/about/historical-highlights/index.html

(101) Drazen JM, Kanapathapillai R, Campion EW et al. Ebola and Quarantine. *N Engl J Med* 2014; 371: 2029–2030. www.cdc.gov/quarantine/aboutlawsregulationsquar antineisolation.html

Bibliography

Gina Kolata. *The Story of the Great Influenza Pandemic of 1918 and the Search for the Virus That Caused It.* Farrar, Straus and Giroux. New York. 1999.

JN Hays. *The Burdens of Disease: Epidemics and Human Response in Western History.* Rutgers University Press. Piscataway, NJ. 2009.

John M Barry. *The Great Influenza: The Epic Story of the Deadliest Pandemic in History.* Viking. New York. 2004.

Michael BA Oldstone. *Viruses, Plagues & History.* Oxford University Press. New York. 2010.

Michael Greger. *Bird Flu: A Virus of Our Own Hatching.* Lantern Books. New York. 2006.

5

POLIO

The Plague of Summer

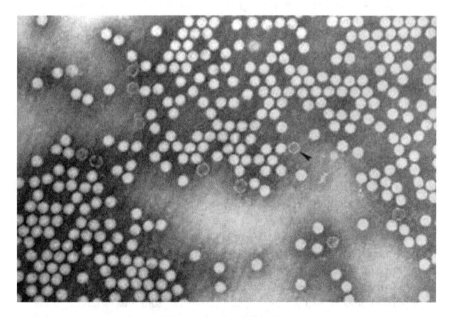

FIGURE 5.1 Electron micrograph of polio virus.

Source: cdc.gov

DOI: 10.4324/9781003427667-5

A POLIO STORY

Our family has its own polio story. I was only 5 so I don't remember the details myself but it is part of family lore so I have heard it many, many times. Every time anyone mentioned polio, my mother told this story – and she always started the same way:

It was the October after Brian was born – Rae-Ellen was 5, Sally was 3 and the baby was 2 months. Rae-Ellen was always the healthy one, never sick and never tired. But early in the fall of first grade, she came home from school and fell asleep in the big armchair in the living room. When I went to wake her for dinner, her cheeks were bright red and she was very hot – burning up with fever as her grandmother used to say. Her temperature was 104 degrees, almost as high as my little brother Sam's had been, back when he was so sick with mastoiditis and had to have surgery. She said her throat hurt and she wouldn't eat anything. I gave her a baby aspirin and a cool sponge bath and then moved her into the bedroom downstairs, hoping her sister would not get sick too. In the night, she woke up crying and I found her shivering so hard her teeth were chattering. I gave her more aspirin, wrapped her up in a quilt and rocked her in the old chair we used to have by her crib when she was a baby. I couldn't remember the last time I had held her in my arms – with the new baby and Sally, Rae-Ellen was my big girl. I held her tight and finally the shivering stopped – she was still glowing with fever but she was asleep so I slid her back into bed.

In the morning, she seemed a little better – she even drank a little apple juice. Her dad didn't think we needed to call the doctor and he left for work. I was racing around trying to clean up the kitchen and feed the baby with Sally coloring at her little table when I heard Rae-Ellen crying. I could see right away she was worse, with spasms of shaking that racked her whole body before subsiding, only to start again. I tried to get her to take more aspirin but she wouldn't even try to swallow. She said her throat hurt and her ears and her neck. I remember that moment so well – my heart just stopped because I knew neck pain was a sign of polio. We had had a few polio cases in our neighborhood that summer and a little girl from our street was still in the hospital with it. My women's group at the church had a special meeting in July to go over the signs of polio and I remembered that neck pain was an important one. A new member who had moved to Edmonton from the states brought something called "The Polio Pledge" which we were all supposed to sign – with Brian born in August, I hadn't gotten around to signing it but it was still thumbtacked to the bulletin board in the kitchen and sure enough, neck pain was right at the top of the list of things to watch for. I went straight to the phone and called the doctor's office.

It was late afternoon before Dr. Fraser arrived and by then, I was a wreck from worry. We had only been living in Edmonton for a year and I didn't know him well but I tried to be calm, hanging up his coat and offering tea as I pointed the way to the bedroom. He headed straight down the hall, looking back over his shoulder to ask what was going on. As soon as I said, "She says her neck hurts," I saw him stiffen, just for a moment.

"What about her legs? Is she able to walk alright?" he asked. And I was so glad I could say that she had just walked to the bathroom by herself.

He carried his black bag into the bedroom and right away, I liked the way he was so cheerful and gentle with Rae-Ellen who at that moment was glowing like a light bulb.

"Well – what have we here? A pretty girl like you shouldn't be sick. Can you tell me what's bothering you?"

She looked very small in the bed but she spoke right up, just like she always did. "My throat hurts. And my neck and my ears."

"Can I take a look? I will need you to help me – can you do that?" Rae-Ellen gave a little nod and he took out a small flashlight and a tongue depressor that smelled like peppermint.

"Now you hold this special stick and open your mouth up wide – as wide you can. If you can open wide enough, I'll let you keep that special stick."

She did her best, opening her mouth and sticking her tongue out when he asked.

"Great job! Now you keep holding that stick while I look in your ears."

He used an instrument with a light to look in her ears and then felt her neck – I could see Rae-Ellen wince as he moved his fingers along her jaw. Then he asked her to lift up her head and look at her belly button – and she did with no problem.

"Let's see how strong you are – can you push my hands away?" He put his palms against the soles of her feet and I could see both legs straighten.

"Do you know something? You are a very brave little girl – can I have that stick back for a minute?" He took out his pen and drew a little face on one end of the stick, a little girl with big eyes and long straight hair. "There you go – a little portrait for a very good girl."

He was turning away when Rae-Ellen asked, "What is this stick for?"

The doctor looked surprised. "It's called a tongue depressor – I use it to push the tongue out of the way so I can see the back of the throat."

There was a pause. "You mean if someone doesn't open up their mouth you use this stick?"

"That's right – but you did such a good job by yourself that I could see perfectly without the stick. Now I'm going to talk to your mum for a few minutes and then I'll be back."

Out in the hall, I was rigid with fear but he said right away, "I know you're worried about polio but you don't need to be – there is nothing that suggests it. She has a bad strep throat and her neck is sore because all her lymph nodes are swollen and tender. I'm going to give her a shot of penicillin and she should start to feel better by tomorrow. If she doesn't, call the office and I'll come back out."

I was so relieved I just burst into tears. "She'll be okay?"

He patted my arm, "She's going to be fine. Thank goodness the polio season is pretty much over for this year."

And she was better by the next day and back to school by two days after that. That should have been the end of it but all that long, cold winter, it seemed like she would have a "bad throat," as my mother called it, every few weeks. By the time spring finally came, I felt like I knew the doctor well and Rae-Ellen really liked him. Whenever he came to the house or we went to his office, she brought her special stick along. She even asked me to help her write a letter thanking him for taking care of her. But the bad throats kept coming back and eventually, he told us she needed to have her tonsils out. The operation was scheduled for July.

It was 1953 – the year of the biggest polio epidemic in Edmonton's history. Starting in May, our city newspaper – *The Edmonton Journal* – reported the number of new polio cases on the front page every day. It said this epidemic was the worst medical emergency Alberta had ever faced. Right in the Polio Pledge it said that children were at special risk for paralyzing polio after tonsillectomy so Rae-Ellen's operation was cancelled. That summer was one of the hardest things I've ever experienced. It's impossible to describe the feelings of near panic and helplessness that I felt whenever any of our three had the slightest symptom. I knew polio could strike at any time, no matter how careful I was. One of our neighbor's children – a 7-year-old boy – came down with it in August and was in the special polio unit at the Royal Alexandra Hospital, paralyzed, on an iron lung. I had signed the Polio Pledge and I stuck with all the rules: all summer, I kept the children at home in the house or in our yard, away from other children and away from the community swimming pool where they usually took lessons – I never did learn to swim myself and I was determined that my children would learn – but not that summer. We didn't even go to church. Schools did not open until October when a heavy frost thankfully ended the epidemic. Rae-Ellen finally had her tonsils out in November and went right back to being the healthy one. But polio was never far from my mind until the vaccine came out in 1955 and all three of our children were vaccinated.

Polio: The Plague of Summer

So that's the story. I only remember a few details myself and none have anything to do with polio. I remember waking up in the big bed in the downstairs bedroom, all by myself. My grandmother – my mother's mother – had severe rheumatoid arthritis and had been in a wheelchair since she was in her twenties. She lived with us in the summer and fall and this was her bedroom on the main floor so she didn't have to deal with the stairs. She had a real hospital bed with a crank that you turned to raise and lower it and we loved playing with that, but I had never slept in the bed and had never been alone at night – as long as I could remember, my sister and I had shared a bedroom so I was scared. I do remember the doctor coming. Strangely, I don't remember the tongue depressor but I do remember the shot. Of course, I had had shots before but none like this. The doctor took two thin glass cylinders from his bag and slid them together, one inside the other. Then he attached a long thin needle. He told me this was a special shot with medicine that would make my throat better – the shot would hurt but only for a minute and then I would start to feel better. He broke open a small bottle and filled the glass cylinder with liquid. There was a strong smell of alcohol and then a terrible burning pain in my bum. My mum held my hand and I didn't cry. Afterwards, she put me on one of my grandmother's heating pads and I fell asleep – and when I woke up, I already felt better.

I cannot remember that doctor's face or writing him a letter. But I do remember how he made me feel special and that when I was sick, I knew he would make things right again. I am sure my experience with him is where my own interest in becoming a doctor began.

In his memoir about the 1953 polio epidemic in Edmonton, Alberta, Dr. Russell Taylor begins this way:

> It was as if this vibrant, optimistic city had been smitten by a medieval plague; it engendered the same fear and helplessness. Arbitrary and insidious, it struck all ages and conditions, sweeping its victims from buoyant health to paralysis and death within a week. Like war and like plague, it left its mark on three generations. To those on the ground that year, there was no apparent pattern. It seemed that once the disease touched down, the whole prairie lit up like an old-fashioned switchboard.[1]

Taylor was an internist who became director of an Isolation Ward turned Polio ICU at Edmonton's Royal Alexandra Hospital in response to the epidemic. Between June 1953 and March 1954, the unit admitted 415 patients with polio – 25% of them required a respirator and 43 died. At the beginning, the unit had only one iron lung and the shortage of respirators was a desperate problem throughout the epidemic. The memoir is a gripping record of how medically challenging and emotionally agonizing it was to care for these young, desperately ill patients.

The "Polio Pledge" was developed in 1952 by the National Foundation for Infantile Paralysis, founded by FDR in 1938 to support polio research and provide care for polio victims; the Foundation eventually became the March of Dimes. In 1952, the Pledge was mailed to 35 million homes in the United States and delivered to every American school child.

The link between tonsillectomy and polio was first reported in 1929 and by the 1950s, the association had been confirmed in surveys from three continents.[2,3] Analysis of extensive epidemiologic data revealed a potential causal relationship between removal of the tonsils and the onset of bulbar poliomyelitis – the most serious form, associated with paralysis of the respiratory muscles – within one month after surgery. It was theorized that if the throat was exposed to the polio virus in the early hours and days after surgery when the mucosal surface was still traumatized, the virus could pass directly into the central nervous system along exposed and traumatized nerve fibers. The summer pattern of polio infections was well known so the potential link with tonsillectomy led to recommendations to avoid elective tonsillectomy during the summer months and during polio outbreaks. This concern is essentially a thing of the past since the indications for tonsillectomy have resulted in a marked decrease in this procedure and polio vaccines have eliminated polio in North America. But 1952 was a different story: that was the year that the United States experienced the worst polio epidemic in the nation's history. Nearly 58,000 cases were reported and more than 21,000 people – mostly children and young adults – were left with some degree of paralysis.

There would be very few opportunities for my mother to tell her polio story today: at this point, almost no-one outside of physicians involved in global health has ever seen a case of acute poliomyelitis. Most North American medical schools would have little opportunity to demonstrate conditions related specifically to polio.[4] If the global polio eradication campaign is finally successful, it is tempting to think that polio will be completely relegated to the past. But the story of polio – a virus that traumatized the world for more than half a century – has much to teach us.

Polio: The Plague of Summer

This was how it began. Out of nowhere, young children were stricken with a strange disease that began with fever and ended with weakness and then, paralysis of the legs. A *New York Times* report from August 4, 1899 tells the story of an epidemic of infantile paralysis in Poughkeepsie, NY with half the victims under 3 years of age.[1] The treating physician was quoted as saying,

> The disease is such an uncommon one that very little is known about it. I find that among specialists of disease in children, the remote cause is a mystery. The general symptom is a weakness of the muscles of the legs. Some cases show rapid improvement while others seem to do no better (over time).… . there is a danger (of permanent paralysis) leaving the muscles of the leg drawn up like a club foot.

The last sentence of the report carries an important clue, not much attended at the time "… sufferers are found in families of rich and poor alike."[1]

The Disease: A Chronology of Discovery

Infantile paralysis – the original name for poliomyelitis – was not unknown: Egyptian carved stone images from between 1580 and 1345 BC show a man with the typical withered calf muscles of a polio survivor and there are scattered references to paralyzed children thought to be polio victims in the Middle Ages and throughout the Renaissance. The disease was given its first clinical description in 1789 by the British physician Michael Underwood who called it "debility of the lower extremities."[2] In 1840, it was recognized as a unique condition by Jakob Heine who suggested it might be a contagious disease.[3] The term poliomyelitis was coined by a German physician named Adolph Kussmaul in 1874, from the Greek *polio* for "grey" plus *myelos* for "marrow" because the pathology showed inflammation of the grey matter in the anterior columns of the spinal cord.[4]

The first modern polio outbreaks occurred along with the increase in population density in cities during the Industrial Revolution. By the mid-1800s, small outbreaks of acute infantile paralysis were being reported in Europe, distinguished by the young age of the victims and seasonal occurrence in the summer. But it was not until the end of the century that sporadic epidemics of the disease characterized by headache, fever, nausea and stiff neck with weakness of the extremities and permanent paralysis in a significant percentage of victims began to occur in North America.[5] The first well- recorded epidemic in the United States occurred in the summer of 1894 in Vermont. A young doctor named Christopher Caverly took care of all the victims and recorded the experience carefully. He described 123 recorded cases, 84 under 6 years of age, with permanent paralysis in 50 children and death in 18.[6]

This was one of many similar outbreaks in western Europe and North America reported at around this time, characterized by the same insidious onset, primarily in young children in the summer months and with the same serious residua of localized paralysis in up to half of symptomatic survivors. In 1907 and in 1911, after devastating polio epidemics in Sweden, Ivar Wickman published three important facts based on his careful observation of polio outbreaks in families in isolated rural communities. First, he confirmed the seasonal occurrence of the disease in late summer and early fall. More importantly, he reported that polio was spread directly from person to person and that there was subclinical infection, based on his observations that a new case in a family without polio often occurred after a visit from an asymptomatic individual whose family had an affected member. Finally, he identified the community school as the common source of the infections and deduced that apparently healthy children could carry the disease home, where family members developed varied clinical presentations. He was the first to recognize that polio could be present in completely asymptomatic people and identified the importance of these cases in the spread of the disease.[7] In addition, if infected individuals could be asymptomatic, the actual rates of paralytic disease and mortality were far lower than in original descriptions of the disease. Nonetheless, each summer brought terror to the hearts of parents all over the developed world.

In the United States at the turn of the twentieth century, medical research was in its infancy with only a small number of scientists, most trained in Europe, engaged in original investigation. In 1901, the Rockefeller Institute for Medical Research opened, modeled along the lines of the Pasteur Institute in Paris, supporting investigators so they could work independently. Simon Flexner, the first medical director of the Institute, dedicated himself to research in infectious diseases, specifically poliomyelitis. In 1908, Karl Landsteiner and Erwin Popper identified the causative agent for polio as a tiny filterable agent, invisible even with the strongest microscope – in other words, a virus (Figure 5.1).[8] In 1909 and again in 1913, Flexner and Paul Lewis published their research showing that this virus from human victims could be used to infect monkeys by swabbing the nasal mucosa and that the infection could be transmitted from one monkey to another, confirming that the disease was infectious and that the poliovirus was the infectious agent.[9] Led by Flexner and the Rockefeller Institute, this was the beginning of the intense American medical involvement with polio.

During the summer of 1911, three Rockefeller clinicians reported a classic clinical study of a polio outbreak in NYC, describing the natural history of the disease in 71 hospitalized children and 90 outpatient cases.[10] Their findings in families indicated that polio was highly contagious and confirmed that a significant number of those infected with the poliovirus had few if any symptoms. Their series emphasized that paralysis was not the presenting symptom of polio but instead followed an initial stage characterized by non-specific symptoms of fever, lethargy, muscle pain and headache. They reviewed multiple laboratory results trying to identify a defining diagnostic pattern, without success. Thirty-four cases were described in great detail including the history of the illness, the physical findings on presentation and the hospital course, day by day. These case descriptions illuminated the variety of presentations of infection with the poliovirus. The histories of 12 infants and children who died are described in heartrending detail as hour by hour, progressive paralysis of the intercostal muscles and the diaphragm led to respiratory failure and death.

After this exhaustive review, the authors concluded:

> At the present time there is no specific form of therapy by which the paralyses in acute poliomyelitis may be prevented, or by means of which resolution of the inflammatory process and, consequently, return of function may be hastened. The problem of treatment, therefore, consists in preventing the spread of the disease to other persons, in applying general symptomatic procedures, and in attempting the restoration of muscular efficiency and the prevention of deformities.[10]

That same year, Carl Kling and colleagues reported that polio virus was present in the throat and intestinal tissues of people who died from polio. Soon afterwards they isolated the polio virus from the intestines of patients suffering from acute polio, and importantly, from family members who did not display any symptoms, confirming that healthy carriers played an important role in spreading the disease.[11]

Unfortunately, this critically important finding did not gain much recognition at the time, at least among American researchers. Instead, led by Flexner, the Rockefeller researchers continued to investigate the disease using Rhesus monkeys infected by swabbing the nose. In this animal model, infection by way of the nasal mucosa was shown to lead to clinical paralytic poliomyelitis with pathologic findings in the brain and spinal cord that were indistinguishable from those seen in patients with the paralytic form of polio. On this basis, Flexner became convinced that the virus gained direct access to the brain and central nervous system in humans, solely by way of the cribriform plate above the nose.[11] Unfortunately, this incorrect focus on the polio virus as being "strictly neurotropic with entry to the body (only) by the nasal route" completely dominated polio research for the next 25 years so that well into the 1930s, there was very limited progress in understanding the true pathophysiology of the disease and therefore only limited progress in developing any approach to treatment or prevention.[12]

It was during this time that the germ theory of disease, first established in the 1890s, tragically intersected with the story of polio in the twentieth century. The culmination of the work of scientists dating back several centuries – recognition of how specific bacteria caused specific, distinct diseases – came simultaneously with understanding that ordinary actions including those of apparently healthy people were potential mechanisms for disease transmission. During the first part of the twentieth century, waterborne diseases like dysentery, cholera, and typhoid fever were the third leading cause of death in America. Major public health efforts then transformed the water supply using techniques of filtration and chlorination to purify the drinking water.[13] Jersey City, New Jersey, was the first city in the United States to chlorinate its water in 1908, followed that same year by Chicago. In those cities that had introduced chlorination and water disinfecting techniques, death rates from waterborne diseases plummeted and within 10 years, more than 1000 American cities were chlorinating the water supply. By 1923 the typhoid death rate had dropped by more than 90% from the level a decade before.[13] At the same time, municipal sanitation programs developed in the late nineteenth and early twentieth centuries and these were responsible for the design and construction of effective sewer systems.[14] Similar efforts improved sanitation and clean water access in the developed countries of Europe plus Australia and New Zealand.

In the United States, these public health efforts were combined with extensive advertising campaigns to educate the American public in domestic hygiene practices, designed to exclude dirt and disease from the home, with specific efforts to prevent illness from spreading. Industry responded with antibacterial soaps, special cleaning powders and disposable paper towels to help prevent the spread of germs on cloth towels in public restrooms. The country became obsessed with domestic and bodily cleanliness as markers of health and social responsibility. There were even posters exhorting mothers to keep their homes clean, specifically to protect their children from infantile paralysis. By the First World War, proper hygiene was represented as an obligation that citizens owed their society.[15]

Against this backdrop of immaculate cleanliness and dramatically improved public health, polio was an unexpected and devastating intruder. From the early 1900s onwards, small outbreaks occurred with increasing frequency all over North America including each of the Canadian provinces. Then, in the summer of 1916, there was a major polio epidemic in NY state. Beginning in June in Brooklyn, the disease ultimately spread throughout the state involving almost 30,000 symptomatic patients, 80% under the age of 5, before it ended. The New York Times covered the epidemic on its front page, reporting daily the number of new cases, their neighborhoods and the names of those who had died. The public reacted with panic and desperation:

> But this knowledge availed doctors little in the scourge summer of 1916. Local newspapers reported that by the first of July, 350 New York city children had been paralyzed by the disease and 75 of them had died... . one hundred thirteen new cases were counted on July 5, and 133 followed on the sixth. Terrorized New Yorkers began freelancing solutions ... (they) cabled and wrote the Department of Health with all manner of things they were certain were causing the plague.
>
> Tens of thousands of people decided to quit the city altogether. For families without the means to flee ... there was little to do but wait. In October ... the weather at last grew cool and New York City could begin to put the season of terror behind it. In the end, the doctors counted 27,000 cases of poliomyelitis around the country, 6,000 of them fatal. Nine thousand of the victims lived in the boroughs that made up New York City.[16]

By the time it was over, the 1916 epidemic in New York city was reported to have caused paralysis in 2% of all children under two years of age.[17]

Although it was reported to the American public as beginning in immigrant Italians from the slums of NYC, polio contradicted the usual rule that infectious diseases flourish in the poorest living conditions – good hygiene, the health mantra of the time, was no protection against this dreaded disease. The physicians who cared for children with polio recognized that it actually occurred in homes with the best living conditions and in areas with the lowest population density. Scientists were baffled by this disease which seemed to strike the young in the healthiest environments.

It was not until the 1950s that a definitive explanation emerged: an unintended consequence of the national obsession with cleanliness was decreased exposure to infectious viruses like the poliovirus early in life when maternal antibodies would minimize symptoms but allow natural antibodies to develop. As understanding of immunity increased, the increasing frequency of polio outbreaks beginning in the early 1900s was attributed to the increasingly sanitary home environments resulting in limited contact with the poliovirus early in infancy. This theory was confirmed when global antibody studies were carried out: in under-developed countries, most infants were found to have been exposed to the poliovirus very early in life without any symptoms of disease but with serologic evidence of immunity. By contrast, in industrialized countries, protective early immunizing infections were found to have occurred only in children living in crowded urban slums while in affluent areas, evidence of exposure to the poliovirus did not occur until later in life when the paralytic form of the disease was more likely.[18]

Back in the early 1900s, progress in understanding the disease and its spread remained slow. In her excellent book "Dirt and Disease: Polio Before FDR," Naomi Rogers quotes one participant at a national conference in Washington, DC in 1916, as saying "... polio is a disease the medical profession knows practically nothing about... . that we are groping in the dark (to understand).... . (we) are doing all we can to ascertain what is its cause and how it is disseminated."[19]

Polio and FDR

Then in August 1921, Franklin D. Roosevelt, former secretary of the navy and a recent candidate for vice president, came down with polio and was left with paralysis of both legs. FDR symbolized many of the characteristics of an individual at high risk of this infection. He had been tutored at home until high school and therefore had experienced none of the usual childhood diseases as a young child because of lack of exposure. Subsequently, while at boarding school and then at Harvard when most of his peers were disease-free, he had scarlet fever, measles, mumps and chronic sinus infections.[19] The week before he fell ill, he visited a Boy Scout camp where he was exposed to a large number of children in the age group now known to harbor the virus. He then engaged in a series of physically demanding activities which included extended running and swimming in ice cold water – histories of both excessive activity and "chilling" were reported in many cases of paralytic polio.[20] Although his age was not entirely typical, the age at polio diagnosis had been increasing and in 1921 when he fell ill, 30% of cases were in individuals over 10 years of age.

His diagnosis made polio front page news all over the country.

Roosevelt never walked again without assistance. He tried every available therapy, most notably swimming and exercising in natural hot springs in Warm Springs, Georgia and there is no doubt that his hard work there optimized his ultimate recovery. Despite his disability, Roosevelt campaigned for governor of NY state in 1928 and won. With the help of his family and staff, and the support of the press, he did his best to hide his inability to walk independently very skillfully, supporting himself with a cane on one side and the strong arm of his son or an aide on the other. With his powerful upper body for support, he used his shoulders to swing his legs – braced from the buttocks to the bottoms of

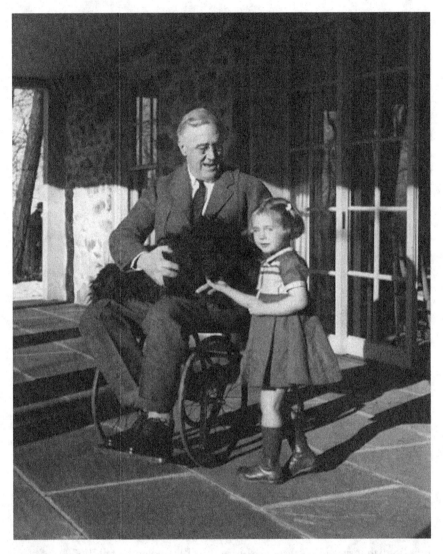

FIGURE 5.2 President Franklin D. Roosevelt in his wheelchair with his dog Nala and a young friend. This is a rare image revealing FDR's handicapped status.

Source: The National Archives. Franklin D. Roosevelt Library. 6/30/1941–6/30/1949. Archives.gov

his shoes – forward, shifting his weight from side to side, to simulate a normal walk. Eventually, he was able to use his right leg for support without a brace and to walk with a crutch and a cane but he always had to be helped to his feet. As shown in Figure 5.2, his disability was obvious to all who saw him despite all his efforts to disguise it.[21]

In 1929, the stock market crashed and the depression began. Many Americans blamed the Republican president, Herbert Hoover, so the field was wide open for an effective Democratic candidate like Roosevelt. Despite his significant handicap, Roosevelt campaigned hard and in 1932, he was elected President of the United States. This had very important ramifications for polio and for medical research. Simply by living his life in the public eye, FDR challenged the prevailing stigma against people with disabilities. More specifically, as President, he brought polio directly into the mainstream, with a fundraising plan to keep Warm Springs, Georgia going in the depths of the depression. He started by using a national advertising campaign to raise money. Local birthday balls were planned across the country to celebrate the president's birthday with one dollar from each ticket going to the Warm Springs endowment fund.[22] The response was amazing with more than 6000 parties held on the night of January 19, 1934; in the depths of the depression, Roosevelt received a check for over a million dollars! In subsequent years, with Warm Springs well taken care of, the plan shifted so that 70% of the income from the birthday balls would stay in local communities for care of polio victims. But with increasingly negative press from Republicans implying that the money raised was not being used appropriately, Roosevelt ended the fund-raising birthday balls and announced the founding of a nonpartisan "National Foundation for Infantile Paralysis" in 1938.[23]

Until that time, medical research was funded largely by individual researchers using their own income or in rare research institutes established by wealthy philanthropists including the Rockefeller Institute which had been researching polio without dramatic success since 1901. The National Foundation for Infantile Paralysis recruited Thomas Rivers from the Rockefeller to direct polio research and he outlined key basic priorities for conquering the disease, beginning with basic principles: understanding the pathology of polio, the portal of entry and the mode of human transmission – all still unknown despite decades of research. The Foundation established major virus laboratories at Yale, Johns Hopkins and the University of Michigan and the first coordinated research attack on polio began, funded entirely by public donations.[24]

The National Foundation for Infantile Paralysis successfully broadened its fundraising to include movie collection boxes and celebrity endorsements plus the collection of dimes mailed directly to the White House. Ultimately, this "March of Dimes" became the name for the entire organization. Even as the United States entered the Second World War after Pearl Harbor, the organization maintained its revenue stream to sustain ongoing research and fund the care of polio victims. In the early 1950s, the National Foundation for Infantile Paralysis, supported entirely by public donations, spent 10 times more on polio research than the tax-supported National Institutes of Health.[25]

The Disease: Epidemiology and Pathophysiology Defined

Over time and with the support of the Foundation, understanding of the clinical disease and its epidemiology progressed significantly. Originally, researchers who were unaware of clinical observations of the disease worked under the assumption that all cases of poliovirus infection resulted in paralysis, reflecting the prevailing hypothesis that the virus was neurotropic and passed directly into the nervous system from the nose. It was not until 1941 that research by Albert Sabin and his colleague Robert Ward, funded entirely by the National Foundation for Infantile Paralysis, definitively confirmed that the poliovirus enters the body through the mouth and subsequently the gastrointestinal tract. The primary site of virus multiplication was shown to be the mucosal lining of the mouth and the GI tract with drainage into the related lymphatic systems and then the blood. In most patients, there was brief transient viremia after which the patient recovered. In a very small subset, the virus entered the central nervous system, either directly through spinal axons or indirectly through the blood, and infected the anterior horn cells of the spinal column and/or motor neurons in the bulbar portion of the brainstem, resulting in the classic flaccid paralysis of poliomyelitis. Antibodies to the virus were present early after infection in lab animals and in patients.

By analyzing New York sewage at a time when paralytic polio was prevalent, Melnick found the poliovirus in "huge quantities."[26] Based on the case rate in the area from which the sewage came, he estimated a ratio of inapparent to paralytic infections of at least 100 to 1. During a polio epidemic in North Carolina, the same researchers found the number of age-specific sub-clinical infections per case to be 100–200:1.[27] These findings confirmed the earlier family observations of Wickman and family physicians caring for paralytic polio cases who recognized that a significant number of those infected with the poliovirus have few or no symptoms. Based on studies like these, the true epidemiology and clinical pattern of poliovirus infection emerged:[28]

- Humans were found to be the only known natural reservoir of poliovirus although chimpanzees and Old World monkeys could be experimentally infected.
- Poliovirus infection typically peaks in the summer months in temperate climates with no seasonal pattern in tropical climates.
- Polioviruses spread through the oral-fecal route, when viruses from infected feces are ingested, most often in contaminated water or food. The virus can also be transmitted directly from hand-to-mouth and from mouth-to-mouth.
- Poliovirus is highly infectious, with seroconversion rates among child contacts of nearly 100%, and greater than 90% among susceptible adults. Persons infected with poliovirus are most infectious from 7 to 10 days before and after the onset of symptoms, but poliovirus may be present in the stool for 3 to 6 weeks.

The response to poliovirus (PV) infection is highly variable with no symptoms at all in at least 90% of poliovirus infections; the ratio of inapparent to paralytic illness is at least 200:1. Infected persons without any symptoms still shed virus in their stools and are able to transmit the virus to others. In 4–8% of cases, infection spreads to the bloodstream, causing a range of minor, nonspecific symptoms, such as headache, sore throat, fever and vomiting; patients with this pattern are completely recovered within a week.

Non-paralytic aseptic meningitis with symptoms of stiffness of the neck and back and increased or abnormal neurologic sensation occurs in 1–2% of polio infections. Typically these symptoms will last from 2 to 10 days, followed by complete recovery. Finally, paralytic poliomyelitis, the most serious clinical outcome, occurs in approximately 0.5% of all poliovirus infections, when the virus invades the central nervous system (CNS), causing inflammation and destruction of motor neurons leading to muscle weakness and paralysis.[28]

The severity of paralytic polio depends largely on the site of motor neuron destruction, with highest morbidity and mortality resulting from respiratory or brain stem involvement. Weakness without sensory loss usually begins 1 to 10 days after initial symptoms and progresses for 2 to 3 days. Additional prodromal signs and symptoms can include changes in the reflexes and severe muscle aches and spasm in the limbs, neck or back. Even when the poliovirus reaches the CNS, the loss of motor skill may not noticeable if less than 20% of the motor neurons in any area are destroyed. When more than 20% of the neurons needed for movement are affected, partial or total paralysis will occur. The extent and pattern of paralysis is random but the lower extremities are affected with the greatest frequency. Generally, no further paralysis occurs after the temperature returns to normal. At no point do patients experience sensory losses or any changes in cognition. The illness progresses to flaccid paralysis with decreased deep tendon reflexes and reaches a plateau without change for days to weeks. Within 6 to 8 months, strength often begins to return. Many children and adults with paralytic poliomyelitis appear to recover completely and, in most, muscle function returns to some degree. Weakness or paralysis still present 12 –24 months after onset is usually permanent.[28]

Paralytic polio is classified into three types, depending on the level of involvement. *Spinal polio* is most common, accounting for ~80% of cases with manifest CNS involvement. It is characterized by asymmetric paralysis that most often involves the legs. *Bulbar polio* leads to weakness of muscles innervated by the cranial nerves and accounts for ~2% of cases. *Bulbospinal* polio, a combination of bulbar and spinal involvement, accounts for ~18% of cases. The overall death rate for paralytic polio is 2%–5% among children and up to 15%–30% for adults. Since bulbar polio can involve innervation of the muscles of respiration, the death rate is highest for bulbar and bulbospinal cases, as high as 75%.[28]

Treatment and Recovery

Until 1927, there was no effective treatment for what was often temporary paralysis of the muscles that control breathing. Researchers at the Harvard School of Public Health devised a negative pressure respirator called an iron lung that could maintain respiration artificially until a polio patient could breathe independently again. A pump alternately lowered and then raised the pressure inside a rectangular, airtight metal cylinder, passively pulling air in and out of the lungs. Inside the tank respirator, the patient lay on a bed that could slide in and out of the cylinder as needed. The iron lung was the first mechanical respirator, the very first method for temporary support of breathing. As muscle function recovered, patients could be weaned from the iron lung but there are many well-described cases of polio patients with persistent paralysis of the muscles of respiration who lived in iron lungs for decades. To this day, the iron lung is virtually pathognomonic of polio.[29]

In terms of residual paralysis, 10–40% of patients with paralytic polio reportedly recovered full muscle strength but 60–90% were left with variable paralysis, ranging from near total paralysis to isolated paralysis of individual muscles. Early muscle recovery reflected reduced inflammation of infected grey matter with improved function within weeks. Over time, remaining brainstem and spinal cord motor neurons developed new branches called axonal sprouts which could re-innervate orphaned muscle fibers, denervated by the acute infection, restoring the capacity to contract. Terminal sprouting could generate enlarged motor neuron units doing the work of multiple units: a single motor neuron that once controlled 200 muscle cells might control more than 800 cells. Finally, remaining muscle fibers with retained innervation hypertrophied and weaker muscles functioned at a higher than usual intensity, improving strength and function.[30] A critical factor in patients with paralytic polio was the preservation of normal sensation which typically allowed control of bowel, bladder and sexual function and made active participation in muscle recovery efforts possible.

Historically, the formal practice of medical rehabilitation – the process of promoting and facilitating recovery from physical damage or clinical disease – dates back to the end of the nineteenth century when the concept of motor re-education was first proposed.[31] Physiotherapy, one of the key components of medical rehabilitation, first appeared in the English language in 1900 where it was described as "the use of natural forces such as light, heat, air, water and exercise in the treatment of disease."[32] Gustav Zander, a Swedish physician, pioneered medico-mechanotherapy, the promotion of health and healing through the use of exercise machines that he designed in the late 1800s. In the early 1900s, two physicians trained by him established the Zander Room at the Massachusetts General Hospital, furnished with the earliest version of progressive resistance exercise equipment.[33] This progress in rehabilitation medicine was just in time for the influx of men injured in the First World War and young patients paralyzed by polio. In the early stages of recovery from paralytic polio, therapy evolved to focus on light stretching of paralyzed muscles to prevent contracture, positioning and support of weakened muscles and joints, and hot packs to reduce painful muscle spasms. As muscle strength returned and muscle spasms resolved, physical therapists used manual muscle testing to grade the specific strength of involved muscles. They then applied selective resistance to specific muscles to facilitate movement and increase strength. Patients were trained to perform repetitive muscle re-education exercises based on the response to daily physiotherapy sessions. They learned to substitute for a paralyzed muscle by using surrounding, stronger muscles to perform the same function, guided by the results of repeated muscle function evaluation. As strength improved, progressive resistance exercises were used, often with water submersion. Over time, there was an increased emphasis on function including self-care and mobility with specific focus on gait training using parallel bars and, when necessary, leg braces. Many of these techniques developed and evolved specifically as part of the effort to rehabilitate polio survivors, who included very young children.[31]

It is impossible to overstate the critical role that Franklin Roosevelt played in the development of physical rehabilitation for polio patients. From his first realization that he was paralyzed and that recovery was going to be a long, long process, he was absolutely determined to walk again. To that end, he pursued all potential avenues of treatment. At that time, physical rehabilitation medicine was in its infancy and there was no recognized approach to optimizing the recovery of polio patients so Roosevelt sought advice wherever he could find it. He had a physical therapist working with him daily from the early months of his recovery, stretching his muscles to prevent contractures and training him in what were eventually formalized as repetitive re-education exercises. He took daily baths in hot water mixed with salt, on the advice of his physician, Dr. Robert Lovett. Within two months, his upper body strength had recovered enough for him to sit upright – just barely – without support.[34] By one year after his acute illness, he could stand with full leg braces and some support and he was learning to walk with crutches after training at the Mass General Hospital in the Zander medico-mechanotherapy lab under Lovett's guidance, with the most skilled physiotherapy available. Lovett recommended swimming in salt water and lying in the sun, things he had noticed seemed to help some of his other post-polio patients: FDR lay in the sun and swam in the ocean.[35] Then in the fall of 1924, he heard about Warm Springs, Georgia where a young man paralyzed by polio was reported to have recovered the ability to walk after swimming in the highly mineralized water from a nearby natural hot spring. From his first day at Warm Springs, FDR was convinced of the power of the hot springs. The high mineral content enhanced buoyancy so he was able to stand and exercise for hours without the exhaustion associated with trying to support himself on land. That first visit was the beginning of a major association with Warm Springs. He returned many times and stayed for months, making slow but steady progress.[36]

Reports of his progress led to an influx of polio survivors from all over the world and Roosevelt welcomed them. He became actively involved with other patients, teaching them what he had learned about the benefits of aquatic exercise, testing and charting the strength of their muscle groups to measure progress, cheering them on.[37] In April 1926, he bought the property with the goal of developing a comprehensive rehabilitation center for polio survivors. He hired national experts in polio care and designed a program focused on functional goals supported by swimming and exercise in the mineralized waters, adaptation of orthotic devices, massage and recreational therapy. He even sought the endorsement of the American Orthopedic Association. By 1940, the Roosevelt Warm Springs Institute supported 400 residents who profited from not just the programs provided but also by living in a completely accessible community, the first of its kind for disabled individuals. By his personal fund-raising efforts and then by establishing the National Foundation of Infantile Paralysis (NFIP), Roosevelt insured the future of Warm Springs. The NFIP became actively involved in funding training and rehabilitation services while Warm Springs provided a model for successful physical rehabilitation and independent living that was applied to patients all over the world.

Despite his efforts to disguise his disability, Roosevelt's limitations were obvious to anyone who saw him. By living a public life with his disability simply part of who he was, FDR inspired people with disabilities of all kinds and helped to change the way individuals with physical handicaps were viewed. He became the champion for all people with disabilities and the de facto founder of physical medicine and rehabilitation as a recognized medical discipline.[38]

Early polio survivors – in fact individuals who were disabled from any cause early in the first decades of the 1900s – had remarkably limited resources since progress in disability support and access was essentially non-existent at the time. Looking back, I realize that my grandmother was the first disabled person I ever encountered, and she was very severely disabled. Her rheumatoid arthritis (RA) began in her late teens but this was before 1920 when the only treatment was aspirin for pain. It was not until 1929 that RA was identified as an autoimmune disease and there was still no specific treatment. By the time she was thirty, she already had multiple spontaneous joint fusions that severely limited her mobility. She was living on a farm outside a small town in Manitoba and had 4 young children. My mother remembered her cleaning the floor propped up on one crutch and using the other to propel the mop. I have no idea how she managed to produce three meals a day and clean house and care for her children with the pain and limitation that the disease imposed.

I remember her as so tiny, her back severely curved by kyphoscoliosis. Her fingers were frozen in a closed position and the joints in her feet, ankles and knees were fused so that she could not walk without crutches. Despite all her problems, Sally and I absolutely adored her. She always had time for us – I remember her playing checkers with me: I would set up the board and then she would nudge her pieces forward with the frozen knuckle of her right index finger. She taught us how to bake, propped up on her crutches in one corner of the kitchen and directing us through recipes for butter tarts and raisin pie. I realize now that she could not have dressed herself – buttons and zippers would have been impossible. Yet every day we would find her sitting in her massive, "one-size-fits-all" wheelchair looking so pretty, wearing a blouse and skirt with a matching sweater. My mother must have helped her to get up and dress but I remember none of that.

I never thought of this at the time, but she was very close to being a prisoner on one floor of the house since she could not go up or down stairs herself without much time and effort and my mother could not carry her. When she did go out, she was carried down the stairs in that huge, unwieldy chair by my father and my Uncle Sam. Amazingly, with no disabled access, she managed to travel by train across Canada, to live with each of her daughters and my Uncle Stan in succession. Her youngest son, my Uncle Sam, traveled with her and I can see now that she never could have managed without him since there was quite literally *no* wheelchair access to public transportation, schools, bathrooms or restaurants. These were the same problems faced by polio survivors at that time, struggling with braces and crutches and wheelchairs – or even worse, enormous iron lungs. The World Health Organization estimates that globally, there are more than 20 million people living with the sequelae of poliomyelitis. Reading the literature about polio survivors and how their leadership in the disability rights movement transformed the lives of millions of people is a true inspiration.

At Last: Progress in Polio Research

From 1938 forward, direction and support from the National Foundation for Infantile Paralysis resulted in dramatic progress in polio research after decades with limited results. At the Rockefeller Institute, Flexner's efforts to investigate the disease based on an animal model infected exclusively by way of the nasal mucosa were finally abandoned. There was important progress in polio research in 1931 when Australian researchers discovered there were two distinct serotypes of the polio virus while studying cross-immunity after experimental polio infection in monkeys. A third distinct type was identified subsequently in the United States. The three serotypes were named after the cases in which the type was first identified: type 1(Brunhilde); type 2(Lansing); type 3(Leon).[39,40] Type 1 is the serotype most often associated with paralyzing poliomyelitis.

Over the next decade, as both viral and immunologic research progressed, many different sub-strains of the poliomyelitis virus were identified and in the late 1940s, a major effort was made to classify these immunologically. The work of multiple laboratories (including those of Albert Sabin and Jonas Salk) ultimately concluded that all poliovirus strains can be classified into three major groups based on the three originally described serotypes, each with distinctly different antigenic constitutions. Each serotype has a slightly different capsid protein that defines cellular receptor specificity and virus antigenicity.[41,42] High antigenic variability characterizes strains but the variability was always confined to the limits of the three serotypes when subsequently tested against panels of neutralizing monoclonal antibodies. This proved to be critical information for future vaccine development.

The primary site of virus multiplication was confirmed to be the mucosal lining of the mouth and GI tract with drainage into the related lymphatic systems and then the blood.[43] In a very small subset, the virus was shown to enter the central nervous system, either directly through spinal axons or indirectly through the blood, and infect the anterior horn cells of the spinal column and/or motor neurons in the bulbar portion of the brainstem, resulting in the classic flaccid paralysis of poliomyelitis.[44] Importantly, regardless of the clinical picture, antibodies to the virus were shown to be present early after infection, first in lab animals and then in patients.[45]

Polio Prevention: Development of Polio Vaccines

Expanded understanding of the virus and the pathogenesis of the disease occurred against a background of increasingly frequent polio epidemics beginning in 1940. The average age at diagnosis had increased each decade with 50% of cases over 10 years of age by 1942. The risk of paralysis and death also increased significantly as age at infection increased.[5] The horrific nature of this disease that paralyzed children and the increasing number of victims led to enormous public pressure to find a solution. According to American historian William O' Neill, "Paralytic poliomyelitis was, if not the most serious, easily the most frightening public health problem of the postwar era."[46] Nearly 58,000 cases of polio were reported in the United States in 1952, with 3,145 people dying and 21,269 left with some degree of paralysis. There was a rising tide of panic in the country with Americans naming polio as their greatest fear after nuclear attack. In response to this and to the increasing base of scientific knowledge, scientists became completely engaged with developing a vaccine. Against this backdrop, the March of Dimes sustained its successful fundraising adding "poster children," polio survivors as models for what continued funding for care and research could achieve.

To this time, there had been only limited efforts at vaccine development since direct entry of the virus to the central nervous system was thought to preclude any role for circulating antibodies in blocking disease progression – and therefore any role for a vaccine. In addition, two disastrous vaccine attempts from the Rockefeller Institute in the mid-1930s had completely suppressed any enthusiasm for research in vaccine development.[47] The demonstration of viremia and of circulating antibodies early in polio virus infection were both critical factors for vaccine development, since vaccine-induced antibodies could potentially block the virus when it was circulating in the blood and prevent invasion of the central nervous system.[45]

Arising from the erroneous theory of direct CNS infection was a second incorrect doctrine bolstered by some failed experiments – that the polio virus could only grow in human nervous system tissue, a difficult process producing only a limited amount of virus. With recognition that the polio virus enters the body through the GI tract, the Harvard team of Enders, Weller and Robbins decided to attempt to cultivate it on non-neural tissue. Their 1949 report that the polio virus can be reliably grown on cultures of various embryonic tissues dramatically changed the potential for vaccine development. The team received the Nobel Prize for medicine or physiology for this discovery in 1954.[48] An accessible method to grow large amounts of polio virus galvanized vaccine development efforts and resulted in an historic rivalry between two young researchers, Jonas Salk and Albert Sabin, both funded by the National Foundation for Infantile Paralysis. This saga is described in detail in David Oshinsky's Pulitzer Prize-winning book.[49]

Salk had worked on development of a killed virus vaccine against influenza so he used this approach. His lab at the University of Pittsburgh developed a technique for isolating pure polio virus and he found the virus grew well in monkey kidney cultures, a more accessible approach than the use of embryonic tissues. He selected three poliovirus strains, one of each serotype, inactivated them with formaldehyde and then tested the most virulent Type 1 strain safely in monkeys. He then tested a killed virus vaccine containing all three virus serotypes in institutionalized children at two facilities, a rehabilitation facility for polio survivors, and a public institution for children with IQ scores below 50. (At that time, experiments on children in institutions were considered acceptable if they could theoretically benefit from the intervention.) In both settings, the vaccine proved safe with no illnesses reported and high antibody responses to all three types of polio virus persisting through months of follow-up.

In January 1953, Salk reported his killed virus vaccine results to the National Foundation's Committee on Immunization. There was discussion about a large field trial but no definitive plan emerged. Before Salk could even publish his work, news of the vaccine leaked into the lay press with a *Time* magazine article reporting "solid good news on the polio front."[50] Immediately, public demands for this vaccine accelerated in the context of the ongoing epidemic. Salk and the National Foundation were thrust into the awkward position of essentially denying Americans access to a vaccine developed by their own donations!

Salk's results were reported in the *Journal of the American Medical Association* and he and the National Foundation began immediate planning for a major polio vaccine trial.[51,52] There was a significant struggle over the design of the trial but ultimately, there were two study arms with injection of second graders with real vaccine and observed controls in the first and third grades in 127 counties, and inoculation of all first, second and third graders, half with vaccine and half with placebo, in 84 counties. Combined, the trial included almost 1.8 million schoolchildren from the United States, Canada and Finland in the largest public health experiment in history. Public attention was riveted on the vaccine trials which were extensively covered in the press. Two-thirds of all Americans(!) were reported to have donated money to the March of Dimes in 1954. The entire cost of the trial was supported by the March of Dimes which also undertook the training of all the trial personnel including 250,000 non-professional volunteers. Using March of Dimes dollars, a Vaccine Evaluation Center was opened at the University of Michigan. Despite negative commentaries from live virus vaccine advocates, the world's largest field trial began on April 26, 1954.

The trials ended in late spring of 1955, just before the beginning of the polio season. The results were announced at a press conference at the University of Michigan on April 12, 1955. The bottom line was clear: the vaccine was up to 80% effective in preventing paralytic poliomyelitis.[53] Edward R. Murrow, the father of broadcast news, announced the results from his show on location in the Vaccine Evaluation Center in Michigan that night, with Dr. Salk as his guest. When asked who owned the patent on the vaccine, Salk replied "Well, the people I would say. There is no patent. Could you patent the sun?" Salk was a hero. As David Oshinsky writes,

> Here, truly, was the people's vaccine, spearheaded by a charitable foun-
> dation, driven by the spirit of voluntarism, subsidized by millions of
> small contributions, aided by numerous scientists, tested by enthusiastic
> volunteers. Birthday balls, marching mothers, poster children – all had
> played a role. Developed in the public interest, this particular vaccine
> belonged to everybody.[54]

The Salk vaccine was not perfect. Three doses were required to develop complete immunity and antibody titers waned over time. In addition, a large number of monkeys had to be sacrificed during vaccine development, approximately 1500 animals for every 1 million inactivated vaccine doses. Shortly after the vaccine was licensed, failure to completely inactivate the vaccine virus at one of the production laboratories resulted in 260 cases of polio and 10 deaths. Despite these problems, the response to the Salk vaccine program was very dramatic as shown in Figure 5.3.

In 1954, there were 30,000 cases of polio in the United States, compared with less than 1000 cases in 1960. The vaccine program was not without problems but the dramatic results of the Salk vaccine were obvious.

Undeterred by the Salk vaccine's success, Albert Sabin continued research on a live virus vaccine at the Children's Hospital of Cincinnati. There were sound immunologic reasons to theoretically prefer a live virus vaccine, principally the fact that the antibody response was much more pronounced and long-lasting. While the Salk vaccine required three injections and subsequent boosters, a single oral dose of an attenuated live virus vaccine was projected to produce lifelong immunity. In addition, since those who ingested the oral vaccine would excrete the weakened virus in their stools, potentially infecting and immunizing many others in the population, the oral vaccine could theoretically eliminate susceptibility to the poliovirus completely. Finally, the oral, live attenuated virus vaccine produced local mucosal immunity via IgA induction in the gut, mimicking wild

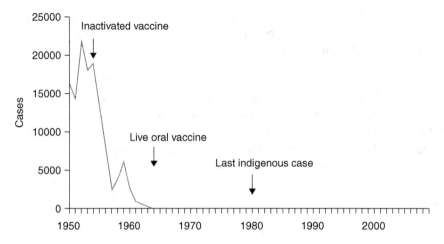

FIGURE 5.3 Poliomyelitis cases: United States 1950–2010.

Source: National Notifiable Disease Surveillance System, CDC. cdc.gov

polio virus infection. By contrast, the injected, killed virus vaccine produces serum antibodies against the poliovirus and prevents neurovirulence but does not induce intestinal mucosal immunity.[55]

Sabin carefully selected one strain of each poliovirus type that multiplied readily in the GI tract but demonstrated low neuro-virulence in monkeys and attenuated these by passing them through monkey tissue in rapid succession until a sufficiently weakened virus was produced – the same "passaging" technique used in developing the yellow fever vaccine. By 1954, he had developed three vaccines, one for each serotype, that did not produce paralysis when injected directly into the spinal column of monkeys. In the winter of 1955, he tested these vaccines in 30 adult prisoners who had no poliovirus antibodies. All 30 developed antibodies and none became ill.[56] However, proceeding with further live-virus testing, especially in children, was blocked over concerns about reversion of the live but attenuated virus back to a more virulent state coupled with loss of public interest in light of the successful Salk vaccine campaign.

With no public interest in a trial in the United Sates, Sabin established a relationship with the University of Leningrad in 1956 and with the approval of the US State Department, a mass immunization program using the oral attenuated virus vaccines began in Russia, with a plan to immunize every Russian under the age of twenty – 77 million individuals. Within a year, the first results were available with a dramatic decline in paralytic polio cases in Russia, verified by the World Health Organization. In 1960, the Soviets – and subsequently Sabin himself – presented the results of their national vaccination campaign, reporting very significant progress towards the eradication of polio.[57]

Back in the United States, the steep decline in polio cases in response to the Salk vaccine led to a major decrease in public interest and research support.

The National Foundation, now known as the March of Dimes, moved on to support research in birth defects and prematurity. With the success of the live-virus vaccines in Russia, Sabin conducted a new trial in the USA in which the three monovalent vaccines were each given orally as a single dose in 200,000 individuals, primarily young children. The results led to trial development of the Sabin vaccine in the United States in 1960.[58] Then, before that trial had even been completed, the American Medical Association voted that the Salk vaccine be replaced by the Sabin oral vaccine as soon as it became available. Despite Salk's efforts to defend it, 1961 was the last year in which his killed-virus vaccine was used exclusively in this era to prevent polio. After 1964, the oral polio vaccine was developed in a trivalent formulation and over the next three decades, this live-virus vaccine was the vaccine of choice.

However, a serious consequence of the oral polio vaccine was described as early as 1962: rare cases of vaccine-associated acute paralytic polio caused by rapid development of enhanced virulence of the attenuated virus strains in the vaccine.[59] Between 1961 and 1999, there were 1–2 cases of vaccine-associated paralytic polio (VAPP) per million primary immunizations with the oral polio vaccine.[60,61] From 1980 through 1999, 162 cases of paralytic polio were reported in the United States; 154 (95%) of these cases proved to be VAPP, with the remainder in persons who acquired wild-virus polio outside the United States. Some cases occurred in vaccine recipients and some in contacts of vaccine recipients. None of the vaccine recipients were known to be immunologically abnormal prior to vaccination. It became clear that the only way to eradicate polio completely in the United States was to eliminate live-virus immunizations by returning to the killed-virus vaccine and in 2000, the Salk killed-virus vaccine became the CDC's formal recommendation for immunization in the United States. With this change, all polio cases were eliminated in the United States.[62]

The polio experience is unique among American epidemics and within medical history: the pace and direction of scientific progress were dictated by the public, fueled by media reports of dying and paralyzed children, with the work of scientists funded almost entirely by public donations, unhampered by government regulations. There is no doubt that short-term development of the killed virus vaccine over long-term development of the live attenuated virus vaccine was driven by the intense public involvement. Until the mRNA vaccines developed for SARS-CoV-2, development of a vaccine was a much more complex and expensive undertaking and could take ten to fifteen years from concept to public availability.

The Poliovirus

The intense focus on discovering a polio vaccine occurred at the same time that understanding of viruses in general exploded, based on advances in imaging, genetics and molecular biology. With these techniques, understanding of the poliovirus began to develop although complete characterization required decades of research.

The virus was first visualized by electron microscopy in 1952 and was seen to be very small, only 30 nanometers in diameter, with striking icosahedral symmetry.[63] The genome is a single-stranded, positive-sense RNA, only 7500 nucleotides long. In 1981, the complete poliovirus genome was published simultaneously by two different groups.[64,65] That same year, Rancaniello and Baltimore successfully cloned the poliovirus and showed that the clone produced infectious polio when introduced into cultured mammalian cells. The technique used to create this clone has been applied to the study of many other viruses.[66] Using x-ray crystallography, the three-dimensional structure of the poliovirus was demonstrated in 1985, the first human virus to be resolved in this way.[67]

The poliovirus was shown to infect human cells by binding to a specific receptor on the cell surface – a glycoprotein in the immunoglubulin superfamily of proteins. Labelled CD155, it was identified in 1989 and its recognition finally made it clear why the virus causes disease in such a small number of species – this receptor is found only on the cells of humans, higher primates and Old World monkeys.[68] After the poliovirus binds to CD155, it is taken up by endocytosis and viral replication begins. Within 4 to 6 hours, up to 10,000 polio virions are released by cell lysis, the primary viremia of polio infection.[69]

The poliovirus genome has a very high mutation rate, among the fastest of all rapidly evolving RNA viruses, with both spontaneous point mutations and genetic recombination, just as we saw with the influenza virus.[70] Populations of polioviruses therefore always include multiple mutational variants but unlike influenza, the genomic and phenotypic variability occurs only within the bounds of the three well-defined serotypes. This means that immunity to any virus within a serotype will confer immunity for all mutations in that serotype. Albert Sabin exploited this known variability of the poliovirus genome in selecting the three serotypes to be attenuated in his vaccine, deliberately selecting mutants with the capacity to replicate efficiently in the human GI tract but not in the central nervous system.[71] His goal was to create a strong immune response in the gut with very limited neuro-virulence, characteristics which were critical in the success of his vaccine.

By classification, the poliovirus is an Enterovirus in the family Picornaviradae, which includes foot and mouth disease, the rhinoviruses, hepatitis A and the Coxsackie viruses. It is currently classified as part of a distinct cluster, (Human) Enterovirus C which consists of the three poliovirus serotypes and 11 Coxsackie A viruses.[72] The poliovirus is structurally similar to other human enteroviruses. The poliovirus is hardy: it can survive for 4–6 months in cold water and in feces for months at 4° C and for years at -20°. However, it is inactivated by pasteurization, formaldehyde, hydrochloric acid and chlorine – so there was actually little reason to worry about polio infection from swimming pools! It is resistant to lipid soluble agents like bile and proteolytic enzymes of intestine – hence its capacity to thrive in the GI tract.

Recent phylogenetic analysis suggests that the polio virus may have evolved from a C-cluster Coxsackie A virus ancestor through mutation resulting in replacement of the surface cellular receptor of the Coxsackie virus – intercellular adhesion molecule-1 – with CD155. C-cluster Coxsackie A viruses have the capacity to recombine with polio viruses to generate novel polio virus recombinants. Theoretically, this mechanism could contribute to the development of virulent vaccine-derived polio viruses.[73]

Global Polio: The Challenge

Polio is often considered to be an American disease because polio crippled an American President, because much of the critical research occurred here and because both vaccines were developed by American scientists. However, a parallel rise in disease outbreaks occurred in the first half of the twentieth century in developed countries all over the world including Canada, Europe (especially Denmark and Sweden), Australia and New Zealand. The introduction of the two effective polio vaccines quickly and dramatically reduced the incidence of polio in each of these first world settings. Compared with the immediately pre-vaccine years (1951–1955), the known global incidence of polio was reduced 700-fold by 1968. After the nation-wide trial of Sabin's oral polio vaccine in the USSR, the incidence there was also dramatically reduced.[57]

Belatedly, polio was also recognized as a major problem in developing countries, based on analysis of global statistics from the World Health Organization. Because the vast majority of individuals infected with polio have minimal if any acute phase symptoms, reports were based on "lameness surveys" that identified cases of acute flaccid paralysis with intact sensation.[74,75] Given the limitations of this case definition and problems with identification and reporting in resource-limited situations, the real incidence is far greater. From pre-vaccine reports, the global incidence of polio cases is estimated to have been at least 600,000 individuals annually.[5,76]

As the annual incidence of polio cases in the United States dropped exponentially following the introduction of the two polio vaccines, the wild poliovirus disappeared and has never been identified in the USA since the early 1970s.[50] This unexpected event raised the tantalizing possibility of global polio eradication. The poliovirus has a number of characteristics that theoretically make it a good candidate for eradication – humans are the only reservoir; although primates can be infected in a lab setting, there is no animal reservoir; there is an effective, inexpensive and easily administered oral vaccine; and previous mass vaccination campaigns to interrupt poliovirus transmission in Cuba and Brazil appeared to have been successful.[51] Beyond immunization, the attenuated poliovirus vaccine has another important advantage: children who take the oral vaccine excrete the weakened virus in their stools for up to 6 weeks, potentially infecting and immunizing multiple contacts in the population. Since the poliovirus needs a susceptible human population and a cycle of transmission for survival, mass vaccination could theoretically eliminate polio completely by exponentially enhancing the development of this herd immunity. The concept of herd immunity is based on the observation that if the number of pathogen-susceptible individuals is reduced to a sufficiently small number, then the pathogen will eventually die out.[77] It is estimated that 80–86% of individuals in a population must be immune to polio for the remaining susceptible individuals to be protected by herd immunity. Herd immunity has obvious theoretical advantages for disease eradication – but if routine immunization is stopped before eradication is achieved, the number of unvaccinated, susceptible individuals can rapidly exceed the capacity of herd immunity to protect them and new epidemics of disease can develop.

In 1988 – the Assembly of the World Health Organization (WHO) – informed by the known science of the poliovirus, inspired by Rotary International's 1985 pledge to completely eradicate polio, and undoubtedly influenced by their success in eradicating smallpox – established global eradication of polio by the year 2000 as a goal, giving birth to the Global Polio Eradication Initiative (GPEI). The Initiative is a public-private partnership of the World Health Organization, UNICEF, the Rotary Foundation, the US Centers for Disease Control and Prevention and the Bill and Melinda Gates Foundation.[78] The original GPEI plan was organized around three parallel strategies: to achieve high infant vaccination coverage with the oral polio vaccine (OPV); to conduct supplementary mass vaccination campaigns for children in polio-endemic countries and other countries with active wild polio virus(WPV) transmission, with "mop-up" vaccination campaigns in focal geographic areas around any confirmed polio cases; and to continue ongoing surveillance for acute flaccid paralysis and confirmation of poliovirus infection by testing stool samples plus environmental surveillance using sewage testing for polioviruses.

The GPEI made rapid early progress, with a reduction in the number of polio-endemic countries from 125 in 1988 to 10 in 2001, including polio-free certification in the Americas (1994), Western Pacific Region (2000), and Europe (2002). By 2001, 575 million children (almost one-tenth the world's population) had received the oral polio vaccine.[78] This required major public health education and immunization campaigns in countries all over the world and was not accomplished without adversity. Even with the express support of political leaders, polio workers had been kidnapped, beaten, and assassinated and still, pockets of disease persisted. The goal of eradication by 2000 was not achieved, and the Initiative struggled during the next decade due to increased recognition of disease caused by circulating vaccine-derived polio viruses(cVDPV) and major programmatic challenges including the lack of basic health infrastructure limiting vaccine distribution and delivery; the crippling effects of civil war and internal strife; physically isolated population pockets; and the oppositional stance taken by some marginalized communities against what was perceived as a dangerous external intervention.[78]

Polio caused by vaccine-derived polioviruses is the most important of these problems. Recognition that new polio virus mutations could develop from the

OPV and cause disease occurred early after the introduction of the OPV when cases of vaccine-associated paralytic polio (VAPP) were first reported. This rare adverse outcome of oral polio vaccination occurs in what is now estimated to be one per million vaccinations, in either vaccinees or their close contacts. The risk of VAPP is highest after the first OPV dose and decreases sharply after that. Mutation and replication are time-limited in immunologically competent individuals with excretion of the OPV strains for only 30 to 60 days so very rare, vaccine-associated paralytic polio events occur in this early time frame.

Early in 2000, a different form of vaccine-derived poliovirus was recognized, arising from infection with OPV-derived virus strains with significant nucleotide sequence divergence from the original vaccine strains, reflecting increased virulence as a result of prolonged replication and transmission. Since the usual rate of spontaneous nucleotide substitution – genetic drift – in polioviruses is approximately 1% per year, poliovirus isolates that differ from the original strains in the OPV by more than 1% are defined as vaccine-derived polioviruses (VDPVs) and when these are detected in community contacts of vaccinees, they are called circulating VDPVs, or cVDPVs.[79] In immunocompromised individuals, these can cause prolonged infection in the original recipient but this has only rarely been associated with clinical disease – in this circumstance, these are called immunodeficiency-associated VDPVs (iVDPVs). In the more common cVDPVs, recombination is very often observed as the mutated virus has been transmitted to multiple hosts with the opportunity to recombine with other human enteroviruses, especially coxsackie A viruses. Polio outbreaks caused by cVDPVs – recognized by the tragic appearance of cases of flaccid paralysis in a vaccinated region – are a critical public health threat and require the same emergent response as polio cases caused by wild polio viruses. Recognition of cVDPVs allowed identification of previous cVDPV outbreaks: retrospectively, cVDPV outbreaks were recognized to have occurred, including in Egypt between 1988 and 1993 and on the island of Hispaniola in 2000–2001. Since 2001, cVDPV outbreaks have been directly monitored by the WHO by stool testing cases of acute flaccid paralysis (AFP) and testing of environmental samples with approximately 90 identified cases/year; 86% of AFP cases due to cVDPV have been derived from strain 2 of the oral polio vaccine (OPV).[79]

Recent molecular genetic analysis of a dataset of 424 vaccine-derived polioviruses from poliomyelitis outbreaks used genome sequence comparisons to evaluate how the attenuated type 2 strain in the vaccine evolves into a virulent strain capable of producing acute paralysis. With phylogenetic mapping, the researchers showed that within 14 days after vaccination, important gate-keeper mutations have already occurred, followed within months by multiple recombination events, presumably with other intestinal viruses. As with the influenza virus, these results show once again the importance of mutation by genetic shift in establishing virulence in RNA viruses. Findings in a tissue culture model suggest that a relatively small number of early transition mutations followed by recombination can rapidly transform the attenuated vaccine strain into a virulent pathogen.[80]

With determined efforts at international, national and local levels, slow progress at eradication continued and by 2006, only four countries in the world (Nigeria, India, Pakistan and Afghanistan) were reported to have endemic poliomyelitis cases due to the wild poliovirus (WPV). A relatively small number of cases continued to occur in other countries, attributed to importation of the wild virus. Each year until 2010, approximately 1500–2000 cases of polio were reported, with 80% occurring in the 4 endemic countries. By 2012, India completed its first polio-free year and was declared polio-free. However, in two of the remaining countries – Pakistan, and Afghanistan – endemic WPV transmission has never been interrupted. Despite all efforts, case counts increased, and importation of the poliovirus from these countries continued to cause outbreaks in countries that had been polio-free. In response, the World Health Assembly declared global polio eradication "a programmatic emergency for global public health" in 2012 and in late April 2013, the WHO announced a $5.5 billion, 6-year cooperative plan (called the 2013–18 Polio Eradication and Endgame Strategic Plan) to eradicate polio from its last reservoirs. The plan called for mass immunization campaigns in the remaining endemic countries. It also dictated a planned switch to inactivated virus injections, to eliminate the risk of cVDPV outbreaks.[81]

The declaration of "polio eradication as a public health emergency" initiated new emergency operations in GPEI partner agencies, designed to complete eradication in the last three remaining polio-endemic countries. With these renewed efforts, the Southeast Asia Region was certified polio-free in 2014 and the proportion of the world population living in polio-free regions reached 80%. But cases of acute flaccid paralysis caused by vaccine-derived polioviruses increased, sometimes exceeding cases due to the wild poliovirus. In response, the 66th World Health Assembly endorsed the *Polio Eradication and Endgame Strategic Plan, 2013–2018*, aimed at complete poliovirus eradication by elimination of all paralytic polio due to infection with either wild PV or circulating vaccine-derived polioviruses (cVDPVs).[82] In September 2015, the Global Commission for the Certification of Poliomyelitis Eradication (GCC) announced that wild poliovirus type 2(WPV2) had been eradicated worldwide, after reviewing formal documentation submitted by Member States, global poliovirus laboratory network and surveillance systems. The last detected type 2 wild poliovirus dated all the way back to 1999, from Aligarh, India.[5]

Global eradication of polio will require cessation of all oral polio vaccines. This process began in 2016 with removal of the type 2 strain by means of a switch from trivalent OPV (containing all three serotypes) to bivalent OPV (containing only types 1 and 3) in OPV-using countries. This was accomplished by a coordinated global switch in 2016. At the same time, the inactivated, injected polio vaccine (IPV) was added in all routine immunization programs where the wild poliovirus had been eradicated, to maintain immunity levels to type 2 polio. A global stockpile of monovalent OPV type 2 (mOPV2) was maintained to enable a rapid response if vaccine-derived type 2 poliovirus emerged, following the switch. All wild type 2 poliovirus and all Sabin type 2 viruses remaining in essential research facilities were secured under appropriate biocontainment levels to minimize the risk of accidental re-introduction.[82]

Progress remained precarious. In 2016, four cases of acute paralysis due to wild polio virus type 1 occurred in Nigeria, where the terrorist organization Boko Haram has blocked vaccine efforts and surveillance. These were the first WPV cases in that country since 2014. Pakistan reported 20 WPV cases and Afghanistan 13 cases in 2016, compared with 54 in Pakistan and 20 in Afghanistan in 2015. Both countries are politically unstable and there are trust issues with vaccinators, associated with increasing numbers of inaccessible, susceptible children. One fifth of the paralytic polio cases in the world occur in one small district of Afghanistan where vaccinators have been unable to reach children consistently for the last 4 years.[83,84] In February 2022, a year and a half after the continent was declared indigenous wild poliovirus-free, the virus resurfaced in south-eastern Africa, in Malawi and Mozambique, where eight children were paralyzed by an amazingly persistent infectious threat. Efforts to eliminate all WPV continue.

Cases of vaccine-derived disease continue to emerge in areas where population vaccination levels were low. Polio vaccine protects children from vaccine-derived strains of the virus just as it protects them from regular polio – but at the same time, use of the live, attenuated vaccine introduces new polioviruses which can mutate and cause new polio outbreaks when are sufficiently large numbers of unimmunized individuals to allow circulation of the vaccine-derived viruses. In 2015–16, there were multiple cases of vaccine-derived poliomyelitis in the Lao People's Democratic Republic (Lao PDR, formerly Laos) after no cases there for many years. After an intensified vaccination effort, the GPEI declared the Lao PDR officially free of circulating-vaccine derived polio virus. But in 2017, there were nine cases in the Democratic Republic of the Congo and tragically, in mid-2017, multiple cases of acute flaccid paralysis due to vaccine-derived polio virus type 2 were reported in war-torn Syria. It was 18 years since the last cases of polio in Syria but immunization rates had plummeted during the civil war from over 80% in 2011, to just over 40% in 2017.[85] The WHO mounted a massive campaign aimed at vaccinating more than a quarter of a million children in eastern Syria beginning in the summer of 2017: the goal was to reach every child below 5 years of age with two doses of two different polio vaccines, spaced one to two weeks apart, a formidable challenge anywhere but especially in that chaotic, risk-filled situation. Despite the extreme risks associated with large-scale military movements, deficient health infrastructure and personnel insecurity in an active war zone, the World Health Organization, Gavi, UNICEF, and the GPEI reported that the polio outbreak in Syria had been completely interrupted by December of 2018, without international spread.[86]

Unfortunately, Syria was not the last of the new outbreaks. Since 2017, cases of AFP due to both WPV and cVDPV have increased. In 2018, WPV1 cases increased in both Afghanistan and Pakistan, a total of 33 cases in 2018 and 55 by August in 2019 compared with 22 in 2017, according to WHO reports. Disturbingly, environmental surveillance in this area documents clusters of persistent mutated genetic variant viruses in core reservoirs along the shared trans-national border area between these two countries. Cases due to cVDPV were documented in nine countries in 2018, a dramatic increase from all previous years. Indonesia and Papua New Guinea (PNG) reported a total of 27 AFP cases due to cVDPV1 after more than 10 polio-free years. Most disturbingly, seven African countries – Democratic Republic of the Congo, Kenya, Mozambique, Niger, Nigeria, Syria and Somalia – experienced polio outbreaks due to cVDPV2 between January 2017 and March of 2019, indicating inadequate population immunization against the type 2 strain before the 2016 global switch from trivalent to bivalent OPV. When the type 2 strain was eliminated from the OPV, the GPEI anticipated that some cases of paralytic polio due to cVDPV2 would appear and they thought they were prepared to address this situation with a monovalent OPV type 2 vaccine (mOPV2). However, the dramatic upsurge in type 2 outbreaks in Africa has almost depleted the stockpile of at a time when eliminating the type 2 strain from the OPV means an increasing number of children lack immunity to that strain. The inactivated Salk vaccine (IPV) is an obvious but sub-optimal option since it is more difficult to deliver – requiring a series of three shots – and does not induce mucosal immunity. Emergent supplemental immunization programs were initiated in every instance but continued case identification indicates that these responses have either been too little or too late.[87]

In response, the WHO adopted the *Polio Endgame Strategy 2019–2023*, an updated plan – with yet another deadline – for global polio eradication designed to address the dual challenge of wild polio virus eradication and elimination of circulating vaccine-derived polio viruses.[88] Key features include a schedule for phasing out the oral polio vaccine and thereby ultimately eliminating vaccine-derived cases. The WHO and UNICEF will develop Rapid Response Teams capable of responding immediately with emergent vaccination campaigns if / when polio outbreaks occur. A partnership is being established in the Eastern Mediterranean region to support the National Polio Eradication Initiatives in Afghanistan and Pakistan. Problems with vaccine delivery in this area are formidable with the border area between Afghanistan and Pakistan functioning as one block with the population and the virus moving easily from one country to another. Limited health infrastructure, inaccessibility, political upheaval, and in Afghanistan, ongoing conflict, make vaccination progress exceptionally difficult. There is active resistance directed by local leaders and an ongoing disinformation campaign. Polio vaccinators in Pakistan must have police escorts and even with this protection, attacks against immunization teams are on the rise. Nonetheless, 1.07 million children were vaccinated in Pakistan during the 2019 May Case Response Campaign and 1.4 million children were vaccinated at 408 Permanent Transit Points along the border with Afghanistan. Aggressive political and diplomatic efforts to re-establish the immunization program in southern

Afghanistan and to complete eradication in Pakistan are ongoing but after years of steady progress and more than 16 billion dollars, the GPEI is now facing its biggest challenge.

Before the GPEI began, poliomyelitis was endemic in 125 countries around the globe and more than 350,000 children per year were paralyzed for life. Between 2000 and 2017, the World Health Organization (WHO) estimated that its campaign had reduced the burden of the disease by 99%, preventing more than 13 million children from becoming infected and risking potentially debilitating paralysis. There has been dramatic progress towards polio eradication – but the final steps are proving just how formidable an opponent the poliovirus can be.

Post-Polio Syndrome

Post-polio syndrome (PPS) is a serious constellation of symptoms that can occur in polio survivors many years after recovery from their initial episode of paralytic poliomyelitis. The syndrome was first described in the 1960s and criteria for diagnosis were established in 1972: (1) prior paralytic poliomyelitis with evidence of motor neuron loss; (2) a period of partial or complete functional recovery after the acute illness, followed by an interval of at least 15 years of stable neuromuscular function; (3) slowly progressive, persistent new muscle weakness or decreased endurance, with or without generalized fatigue, muscle atrophy, or muscle and joint pain; (4) symptoms lasting at least a year; and (5) exclusion of other neuromuscular, medical and skeletal causes. Approximately half of all patients with paralytic polio go on to develop post-polio syndrome, with an average time to symptoms from the original polio episode of 35 years. Risk factors for development of PPS include more severe acute poliomyelitis paralysis, older age at acute polio attack, and greater physical activity in the intervening years.[89]

The etiology and pathogenesis of PPS are unknown but it has been hypothesized that the new muscle weakness of PPS is related to degeneration of individual nerve terminals in recovered motor units. These recovered units have been overextended for many years, compensating for missing units lost at the time of the acute illness. Progressive inability to maintain the increased work demands leads to symptoms of reduced muscle strength and eventually, atrophy. This explanation corresponds with the gradual but progressive symptoms and recognition that previously affected muscles are much more likely to be involved. Generalized weakness and disproportionate fatigue are also common. New symptoms can also include respiratory insufficiency, difficulty swallowing or speaking and loss of vocal strength in individuals who had bulbar involvement at the time of their acute episode.[89]

There are currently no effective pharmaceutical treatments that can stop the deterioration or reverse deficits. However, multiple studies have shown that non-fatiguing exercise with rest periods can significantly improve mild to moderate muscle weakness. Aquatic exercise programs designed to avoid muscle overuse improve flexibility, strength and cardiorespiratory function. Use of assistive devices can also improve specific muscle and joint symptoms. Most patients with respiratory insufficiency respond to non-invasive positive pressure ventilation and do not progress to permanent, fulltime ventilation. Finally, aerobic conditioning has been shown to improve cardiac function without causing adverse effects.[90]

Since the last cases of acute poliomyelitis in developed countries occurred before 1980, the number of new cases of post-polio syndrome in the United States is steadily declining.[91] However, the story with global polio is one of ongoing outbreaks with more than 20 million people living with the sequelae of poliomyelitis.[92] The world will continue to be challenged by the medical and rehabilitation needs of individuals with the sequelae of polio including post-polio syndrome for many years to come.

Looking Back :: Moving Forward

Early in the twentieth century, small outbreaks of infantile paralysis metamorphosed from contained pockets of disease in developed countries into large and progressively larger polio epidemics in NA and Europe. Many polio survivors were marked for life, living with the tragic residua of the disease in wheelchairs, leg braces and even primitive respirators. At its peak in the 1940s and 1950s, polio paralyzed or killed over half a million people – mostly young children – in the developed world every year.

In response, major research efforts identified the causative poliovirus, the epidemiology and (ultimately), the pathophysiology of the disease. Within half a century of the first major polio epidemic in the United States, American researchers developed two highly effective vaccines and the incidence of polio plummeted in the Global North. In addition, major societal events dramatically affected the course of the disease. When polio survivor Franklin Delano Roosevelt became President of the United States, he mobilized the American public to support research to prevent and treat the disease. With his leadership, nation-wide grassroots fund-raising campaigns emerged, campaigns so successful that they completely funded all the research which led to development of the two vaccines and established the practice of public philanthropy for scientific research. FDR played another important role in the polio story. Desperate to restore his own physical health, he focused attention on physical rehabilitation which emerged as an important medical subspecialty, initially working to restore function, improve strength and teach compensatory skills to newly paralyzed polio survivors. The emergence of rehabilitation therapy is a legacy of FDR and a legion of determined polio survivors. Finally, as disabled polio survivors struggled to re-enter society, they galvanized the rise of social and civil disability rights. In developed countries, the legacy of poliomyelitis remains in ongoing medical philanthropy, the practice of modern rehabilitation therapy and the disability rights movement. With these successes, two effective vaccines and dramatically decreased polio cases, the history of polio reads like a success story.

It was only after the development of the polio vaccines that the world belatedly realized that polio was a global disease. From lameness surveys designed to identify flaccid paralysis, the unrecognized global incidence of polio cases was estimated to have been at least 600,000 individuals annually. Inspired by the success of the smallpox eradication campaign, the WHO established the Global Polio Eradication Initiative(GPEI) dedicated to complete eradication of the poliovirus since 1988. Using the oral polio vaccine (OPV), this largest public health program in history made dramatic progress. More than 2.5 billion children have been vaccinated against polio, with a global decrease in the number of poliomyelitis cases by more than 99% and a reduction in the number of polio-endemic countries from 125 in 1988 to two – Pakistan and Afghanistan – by 2020. But despite sustained efforts in Pakistan and Afghanistan, there have been new wild poliovirus cases every year with a tragic upsurge since 2019.

At the same time, more cases of vaccine-associated paralytic poliomyelitis continue to be recognized due to spontaneous mutation of the attenuated virus strains in the OPV with consequent recurrence of neurovirulence and transmissibility. Endemic circulation of the type 2 poliovirus has been eliminated and it was removed from the oral polio vaccine in 2016. Vaccination campaigns then shifted to bivalent OPVs (bOPVs), conferring protection against serotypes 1 and 3 only. A consequence of this change was the emergence of circulating vaccine-derived poliovirus 2 (cVDPV2) as the predominant strain, capable of human-to-human transmission and neurovirulence, causing paralysis in patients. To overcome the threat of paralytic polio from cVDPV2, the Salk inactivated polio vaccine (IPV) was incorporated into immunization schedules in 2019 since it provides humoral immunity against all three poliovirus types and reduces the risk of paralytic poliomyelitis. In September of 2019, the Global Polio Eradication Initiative reported that it has successfully achieved the global goal of all 128 OPV-using countries incorporating at least one dose of IPV into their immunization activities.[93] And a new polio vaccine has been developed, a novel oral polio vaccine for serotype 2 (nOPV2) which was genetically engineered to be more resistant to mutation and revision to neurovirulence.[94] Based on the most recent report of the Global Advisory Committee on Vaccine Safety, nOPV2 shows an acceptable safety profile and appears more genetically stable than mOPV2 in field use.[95,96] The Strategic Advisory Group of Experts on Immunization (SAGE) recommended the transition to wider use of nOPV2 beginning in October 2021.

Eradication of polio will require complete elimination of the oral polio vaccine, a serious challenge. In May 2019, the WHO adopted the *Polio Endgame Strategy 2019–2023,* designed to address the dual challenge of wild poliovirus eradication and elimination of circulating vaccine-derived polioviruses.[88] In clinical use, nOPV2 shows an acceptable safety profile and appears more genetically stable than mOPV2 with growing evidence of its effectiveness in clinical settings. There is research into development of a new killed virus vaccine based on the three strains in the OPV.[93,94] Immediate intervention after outbreak detection with sufficient coverage and scope to shut down virus transmission is as essential as development of new, type-specific vaccines. The Endgame Strategy also includes changes in policy and approach to address ongoing challenges to vaccine delivery.

The poliovirus is a formidable and enduring enemy. The quintessential characteristic of RNA viruses – their capacity for rapid and continuous muta-tion – prevents continued use of the oral, attenuated virus vaccine that was such a critical part of the early success of the polio eradication effort. Each use of the bivalent OPV or the monovalent OPV2 seeds potentially new cVDPV outbreaks; this is especially true for the mOPV2 since there have been dramatic population decreases in strain-specific immunity since the type 2 strain was removed from the OPV.

The Global Polio Eradication Initiative is at a critical crossroads faced with the need to maintain high population immunity while transitioning away from the OPV in the context of increasing wild and vaccine-derived poliovirus outbreaks. Success will require a better vaccine with no risk of pathogenic virus introduction and induction of improved mucosal immunity. Clinical and environmental sur-veillance and emergent vaccine response to disease outbreaks must be sustained since the threat of new outbreaks – and of international spread – persists as long as WPVs and cVDPVs exist. And for complete eradication, an approach must be developed for the small population of immunodeficient individuals who chron-ically excrete the poliovirus and serve as a perpetual source. Research and devel-opment will continue to address these issues. But on the ground, deficient health infrastructure, spreading disinformation campaigns, violence against vaccination teams, and inaccessible populations isolated by geography or conflict, are for-midable ongoing challenges to achieving the polio eradication endgame. And with all the decades of scientific, medical and public health expertise brought to this challenge, the poliovirus remains an enduring and daunting adversary.

HISTORIC PERSPECTIVE: RACE AND CLASS IN THE TIME OF POLIO

The story of the development of the polio vaccine and its application to American school children, resulting in the virtual eradication of the virus in this country and then throughout North America, is accepted as perhaps the biggest public health success story of the twentieth cen-tury. In the parlance of public health, the microbe was isolated, the vector identified, an effective vaccine developed and administered, and people stopped dying: a win-win-win. The truth is, as you have been reading, far more complex. The first historical focus in this chapter will bring to light ways in which the efforts to control polio mirrored serious class and race-based prejudices dividing American culture. The second will concentrate on what happened to disabled polio patients after the vaccine proved effective, a long story that reminds us how little room people with disabilities are still given in our society.

It took a very long time for public health officials to accurately identify the means of transmission for the polio virus, and in the interim, many opportunities arose for existing socioeconomic biases to be mapped on to polio prevention. The dependence on an old, trusted, and problematic model for combating the spread of infectious diseases was part of the problem. This model, which was created in the United Kingdom and expanded in the United States by Lemuel Shattuck (1793–1859), said that the poor were the population most affected by epidemic diseases because of the poor sanitary conditions of their homes and neighborhoods. This was actually a smart observation and produced important changes in American cities, such as mandatory garbage removal, the development and improvement of urban sewage systems, and in some cases, the faster introduction of running water in poor areas. And while it did not occur immediately after Shattuck's recommendations were published in *Report of a General Plan for the Promotion of Public and Personal Health* (1850), local boards of health did increasingly take control over aspects of public hygiene such as the disposal of dead bodies, the management of contagious diseases in schools, the licensing and oversight of physicians, and public quarantine. Shattuck's report, written primarily about Boston but containing observations about other cities (London) and the cost of disease upon society, certainly became the bedrock upon which the US Public Health infrastructure would be founded. Beyond its institutional strength and ability to tie in with existing municipal systems, another asset was that big public health gains could be made without having to know the specific microorganism causing a disease or the way it was transmitted. By improving public hygiene, including ensuring safe public water sources, improving sewage removal, and controlling pests such as rats and flies, Lemuel Shattuck and his public health workers did dramatically reduce the rates of diseases such as cholera and typhus. But their motivation to do this work was not solely to improve the lives of the suffering poor. In fact, protecting the wealthy from infection by the poor, who they might encounter in their homes as staff, in lower level positions in their offices, and even in the street, was a significant motivator for Shattuck. Eugenics, which was gaining ground as a way to prevent the sick placing undue burdens on American society, was also part of these public health efforts. The campaign against tuberculosis, which gained momentum in the late nineteenth century, reflected the ways in which Shattuck's approach could encourage dangerous socioeconomic prejudices within American society.

A "Discussion on the Advisability of the Registration of Tuberculosis" recorded in *The Transactions of The College of Physicians in Philadelphia* from 1894 reveals some of the ways in which race, class, and eugenics could become intertwined in public health discussions.[97] This debate occurred between noted physicians of the time, and the subject was whether people with consumption (tuberculosis) should be reported to the Board of Health. It is noteworthy that the College agreed that they should not because it would be "adding hardship to the lives of these unfortunates, stamping them as the outcasts of society."[97] This realization gives credit to the men involved in the debate, and it demonstrates an awareness of the long-term consequences quarantine or the label of "carrier" or "patient" could place upon people. Dr. Owen Wister terms the registration of patients "criminals guilty of consumption" who could face mob violence if the press encouraged an uproar over a growing number of cases.[98,99] The tenor of the debate itself, however, is problematic. First, there was no agreement about how tuberculosis was transmitted. While Robert Koch had just discovered the tubercle bacillus, many still believed that it was genetically transmitted. Others believed that it was passed through sputum coughed up by sick patients, and some of those believed that the only way to prevent its passage was the careful management of sputum (both at home and, of course, in the streets) and the disinfecting of homes after a tuberculosis patient died. Noting the prevalence of tuberculosis cases in poor districts and even in specific residences, these physicians urged the board of health to take action only by "disinfection of rooms in which consumptives have lived and died."[97,99,100] The socioeconomic biases emerge throughout the document, beginning with the assertion that the debate over registering consumptives need only apply to the poor, since the wealthy could be counted on to have responsible physicians manage the disinfecting of their homes after their death. The eugenics aspect emerges in response to the claim that tuberculosis was hereditary. Dr. Da Costa, for example, insisted that no public health measure other than the absolute refusal to allow tuberculosis patients to marry would prove effective. Black people, who lived in the poorest area of the cities under investigation and were thus doubly in jeopardy of having tuberculosis, were described as even less capable of basic hygiene than the white poor, a group defined as lacking even the most basic capacity for personal or interpersonal care because of limited means and abilities ("the poor and careless"). To borrow Dr. Wister's phrase, labeling a group as infected with a contagious disease made them into criminals. And even in the discourse of these learned physicians, the poor and the non-white are suspect before they show the first symptom. It comes as little surprise, then, that during the polio epidemic, these very individuals were once again suspected of endangering public health.

As Naomi Rogers ably demonstrates, the 1916 New York City polio epidemic reflected the racist and anti-immigrant anxieties reflected in the tuberculosis debates. Despite strong epidemiological evidence that polio disproportionately affected American born, white children living in areas with good sanitation, public health efforts in New York focused on poor, immigrant neighborhoods, especially Italians, whose neighborhoods were plagued by filth.[97] Nancy Tomes also identifies the role of this kind of thinking in public health efforts to control polio. Flies became a focus of polio eradication efforts from the epidemics during the First World War well into the 1940s, with officials believing the insects originated in filthy, poor neighborhoods and carried the disease to the upper-middle class neighborhoods where it thrived. Underneath this fear of insects also lay anxiety about black and immigrant servants who worked in the predominantly white, wealthier suburban homes where polio struck hard.[99] The tendency to close public swimming pools and playgrounds, where children of different classes and races could mix, served two masters. First, the obvious epidemiological approach to controlling contagious diseases with poorly understood modes of transmission is to limit contact among vulnerable people. By closing public places such as swimming pools and movie theaters, where children from different backgrounds might mingle, the hope was that poor, immigrant children from areas with poor sanitation could not infect wealthier, native-born children. More traditional quarantine methods, in which houses with active polio cases were required to identify themselves with window placards, were also used throughout the earlier twentieth century and, though they would certainly have resulted in the isolation of members of those households, they were less racially and socioeconomically divisive, since the majority of affected homes were in white, wealthier suburbs.

Naomi Rogers once again provides an important corrective to our understanding of the racially motivated public health efforts directed toward polio.[100] While it was predominantly understood to be a white disease through the 1930s, this reflected prevailing racial bias that claimed black people could not contract polio and came at a very high price for African American victims of the disease. A combination of factors made African American polio patients disappear from polio narrative that dominated the first three decades of the twentieth century. First, the South, where the majority of African Americans lived, did have a lower incidence of polio outbreaks than the Midwest and the Northeast. But that does not explain why black people were excluded from public health and patient records in areas that were affected by epidemics. One of the reasons was the continued predominance of racial medicine, which contended that people of different races had different susceptibilities to different diseases, contended that African Americans could not contract polio. Second, African American communities were primarily served by black physicians, and white medical schools did not admit them. Thus, they lacked access to the same level of education as those physicians serving white neighborhoods. African

Americans were also socioeconomically disadvantaged, and thus less able to seek treatment until the disease advanced. Morbidity and mortality statistics were not as aggressively reported from these communities, and polio cases easily dropped through the cracks.

Finally, most of the treatment centers for polio patients, including the one in Warm Springs, Georgia that was founded by President Roosevelt, only accepted white patients. Beginning in the 1930s, civil rights activists and African American physicians began to counter the narrative that polio did not affect African Americans, and though the predominant treatment centers continued to rely on the "susceptibility narrative" of racial medicine, the increasing visibility of African American polio victims became hard to ignore, especially as FDR faced his third presidential election and hoped for an unprecedented level of black support. This oversight was partially remedied finally in 1939 when the Tuskeegee Institute received a grant from the March of Dimes to open a center for treating black children with polio. It opened in 1941, promising to train African American physicians to treat polio and other orthopedic diseases as well as treat all affected children. In fact, with only 36 beds and minimal outpatient facilities, the center was insufficient to treat even a fraction of non-white polio patients. The Center did, however, become an important part of national efforts to correct the racialized approach to polio. John Chenault, the African American orthopedic surgeon chosen to head the center, countered the prevailing epidemiological studies, that demonstrated how rare the disease was in African American communities. In his own study focusing on epidemics in the South, he showed that African American cases had been significantly underreported due to medical oversight and lack of resources.[101] The 1940s was a decade of conflicting racial accounts about polio, with the old "racial susceptibility" argument still holding sway in a great deal of popular reporting on the disease and in the medical community. Separate medical facilities for people of different races remained the hallmark of American medicine through the 1960s, especially in the South, but increasingly the efforts to eradicate polio attempted to bridge this divide. The March of Dimes responded to Chenault's efforts and the increasing visibility of black polio victims resulting from civil rights efforts by attempting to integrate black children into its polio advertising and fundraising efforts. Rita Reed became the first African American poster child for the March of Dimes in 1947. Amazingly, by the time Salk's vaccine was introduced in public schools, black and white children received it equally and black medical professionals were an integral part of the trials. In the South, however, 1954 was the year Brown v Board of Education ended school segregation, and black children received their vaccines on the lawns outside white schools because they were not yet permitted inside them.

HISTORIC PERSPECTIVE: PHYSICAL DISABILITY BEFORE POLIO

The story of the polio vaccine is one of scientific triumph. Without question, the administration of Salk's vaccine to children through the public school system eradicated the virus in the United States and Canada. What it could not do, however, is bring back full mobility to those who had already been affected by the virus. Polio survivors were caught in an impossible landscape, in which the physical marks of their illness often defined their existence. Before polio, children born with physical disabilities or degenerative diseases such as cerebral palsy were frequently sent to institutions or kept at home. Public schools were not required to accommodate wheelchairs or any other forms of mobility assistance, and thus a standard education often fell beyond the reach of polio victims. For those who spent their childhoods in institutions, access to academic curriculum was often limited or non-existent. Patients with disabilities were not expected to require educations, since they were not expected to work, marry, or have families of their own. Physical disability, as defined before the mid-twentieth century, was a life sentence to a very limited life indeed. Some of this reflects the eugenics theory discussed in the previous section. The general treatment of people with physical disabilities before the 1940s–50s reflected eugenic thinking, which contended that anyone born with a disease or disability should be prevented from reproducing-either through isolation or sometimes forced sterilization – to protect the nation from having to support their "defective" offspring. The 1927 Supreme Court decision in *Buck v Bell* to uphold a 1924 Virginia law permitting the sterilization of those found to be "feeble-minded" or epileptic demonstrates the strength of eugenic thinking in the first half of the twentieth century.[102] Virginia was far from the first state to pass an involuntary sterilization law. That honor goes to Indiana, which did so in 1907, and thirty more states followed suit. The states that did not pass involuntary sterilization laws frequently proposed and debated them, demonstrating the prevalence of eugenic thinking in this country. In fact, Oliver Wendell Holmes' pronouncement that "three generations of imbeciles are enough" allowing the forced sterilization of anyone deemed to fit the very loose category of "feeble minded" still stands, though the state laws it upheld were finally repealed, with some still in place as late as the 1970s. Throughout its use, involuntary sterilization affected at least 70,000 people in this country, with reported numbers thought to be low because of the prevalence of sterilization within institutions that operated outside the law. Women were disproportionately the victims of forced sterilization, as were racial minorities and the poor. While those deemed to be mentally ill were the most common victims of this, the "feeble minded" were a close second.[103]

Forced sterilization of people with physical disabilities was rare, but their institutionalization was encouraged and accepted by the time the polio epidemic reached its height in the United States in 1952.

Polio changed the way America understood physical disability because the campaign to end it was so extensive, thanks to the March of Dimes, and because the virus was so prevalent that nearly everyone knew someone affected by it. Those affected in the final rounds of epidemics that occurred before Salk's vaccine came into effect had the numbers and visibility to produce a shift in American thinking about physical disability, much as the images of children in braces produced a shift in American charitable giving to end the disease. But it was not an easy transition to bring about, as Daniel Wilson demonstrates. Three primary challenges faced the families of polio survivors and the patients themselves as they returned home from rehabilitation facilities and tried to re-enter their lives. First, they were among the first people with physical disabilities other than war veterans to have lives to return to from the time before their disabilities. Men stricken with polio wanted to return to their jobs, if those were still available, or find some other means of making a living so they could help support their families and preserve their identities. Women afflicted by the virus hoped to marry and become parents or, if they were already wives and mothers, return to those roles. Adolescents and children, both male and female, wished to return to school and play with their friends. But decades still existed before the Americans with Disabilities Act (1990) would make accessibility a requirement for public facilities, and there were no legal requirements prohibiting hiring discrimination for those with disabilities. Schools and office buildings were a labyrinth of staircases, heavy doors, and narrow doorways that made wheelchairs incredibly difficult and crutches a daily challenge. Physical education requirements, the centrality of athletics in school social activities, and negotiating dating as polio patients entered high school were additional challenges.[104] The will and family support required to reintegrate those left disabled by this virus into the worlds they left behind were as exceptional as they were novel. Previous generations of polio survivors, like those born with physical disabilities or who suffered injuries at work or in the military, had largely lived quiet lives at home or, in extreme cases, in institutions. Polio survivors paved a new road for the physically disabled, living and working in "normal society."

The second challenge they faced in entering public life was acceptance. Not everyone agreed that people afflicted with the marks of the virus should be working or going to school, though the March of Dimes campaigns consistently featured children in braces or on crutches enjoying childhood activities. Larry McKenzie, for example, was the 1951 March of Dimes poster boy, and he was featured studying at the kitchen table on his family's farm and sharing a toasted marsh-mallow with a friend, all while wearing elaborate braces to support his arms.[105] Some families found themselves and their disabled children ostracized long after the possible threat of contagion had passed, as though the bad luck that had affected the family was itself contagious. Everyone affected by the disease faced the social stigma surrounding "cripples," the term applied to anyone with a physical disability. As Wilson puts it, "Because negative attitudes about individuals with disabilities were widespread in society, every encounter outside one's intimate circle risked rejection."[106] That rejection included stares, chas-tisement for being out in public at all, and even public declarations thanking god for protecting the viewer from winding up affected as the survivor had been.[106] Those who could hide their braces under shirtsleeves or pant legs were happy to do so, but those in wheelchairs or requiring respirators were stuck being immediately visible as a "polio," the term applied to physically disabled survivors.[107] The most horrible cases of discrimination occurred in schools based in commu-nities that reinforced existing stereotypes about handicapped people. Many schools allowed polio survivors back into their classes as soon as they were able to return though they did nothing to help them nego-tiate the physical obstacles posed by the buildings themselves; others did not. Some segregated students with disabilities of any kind from regular classes, placing those with physical, cognitive, and mental disabilities in the same room with a single teacher. Others required students with disabilities to receive tutoring at home, either through teachers sent by the district (often resulting in a very haphazard educa-tion) or through speakerphone. Some districts simply refused to allow polio survivors to come back. The parents of a polio survivor in rural southern Wisconsin were told by their daughter's school superintendent that it was not convenient to rearrange classes to accommodate her, especially since it was a waste of time to educate crippled children and it would be depressing for other children to see her. After two years of activism by members of her community and agreeing that she would not ask for any accommodations of any kind, she was allowed to return to high school. She was greeted by her homeroom teacher apologizing to the other students for having to see her every day. She persevered, navigating her wheelchair through a building that could not accom-modate it and graduating without ever having been inside one of the bathrooms, since the doorways were too narrow for her to enter.[108]

The fact that polio survivors were expected to fit into their surroundings, work hard, and hide their disabilities was a mixed blessing. Certainly, these individuals went on to live remarkable lives, often earning top grades in school and embarking upon university education and respected professions. But the cost of fitting in was very high. It took several decades of trying to be accepted as "normal" before survivors began to look for other people like them or even identify themselves as handicapped, because their fear of rejection was understandably very high. By choosing to fit in as much as possible, they also overstressed their bodies. The extremely hard work they put in during their rehabilitation to walk, use their legs and arms without visible braces, and even to breathe on their own would later show up as post-polio syndrome, when their overworked neural pathways began to degenerate.

The final challenge they faced was one they shared with other disabled individuals: making the world accept them on their own terms. It is not surprising that this took a very long time. While it is true that the majority of polio survivors were part of the Baby Boom generation that is renowned for breaking away from the conservative ethos of previous generations, forming a movement to gain disability rights required something other than bravery and a belief in the fundamental importance of justice. It meant publicly acknowledging that you were physically different and thus deserved accommodation to allow you to live your life to the fullest possible potential. It meant coming out of the shadows, wearing braces or using wheelchairs in public, and talking about what polio cost you. In short, it meant rejecting the Puritan work ethic instilled in so many survivors during rehabilitation, where they were told their ultimate goal was to seem normal, and that they could only accomplish it by working as hard as possible. Any failure to achieve physical therapy goals was interpreted as a failure of the patient's will, and thus patients were held responsible for their own recovery. The positive side of this is that it inspired patients to believe they could get better, sometimes in the face of extraordinary odds. But the negative side was omnipresent: few polio survivors with paralysis regained complete use of their bodies, and they were blamed for that. Choosing to publicly claim the identity of a disabled person meant rejecting this dictum, which so many had adopted as children or teenagers and not been able to question. It also meant accepting your body as it was – not as it had been born, as was the case for other civil rights movements and even many people with congenital disabilities, but as it had been transformed by a virus. The plethora of polio survivor narratives now available through the internet demonstrates the challenges these people encountered as they struggled to return to their lives, find meaningful work, marry, and have families. The narratives show the extraordinary strength of these individuals and, at the same time, make you see them as people whose bodies were hijacked by a virus but whose hearts, minds and souls remained inextricably their own.[109]

Notes

1 Taylor, Russell F. Polio '53: A Memorial for Russell Frederick Taylor. The University of Alberta Press. Edmonton, Alberta. 1990.
2 Aycock WL, Luther EH. The occurrence of poliomyelitis following tonsillectomy. N Engl J Med 1929; 200:164-167.
3 Maxcy KF. Tonsillectomy and poliomyelitis. Amer J Pub Health 1954; 44:1065-1067.
4 Groce NE, Banks LM, Stein MA. Surviving polio in a post-polio world. Soc Sci Med 2014; 107:171-178.

References

1. Puzzling Child Disease. Epidemic of Infantile Paralysis Baffles Physicians of Poughkeepsie – Believed to be Contagious. *Special to the New York Times.* Published: August 4, 1899. Copyright @ The New York Times.
2. Underwood M. Debility of the lower extremities in children. In: *Treatise on Diseases in Children.* London: J Matthews. 1789.
3. Heine, J. *Beobachtungen ilber Lahmungszustande der unteren Extremitaten und deren Behandlung.* F. H. K6hler, Stuttgart, 1840.
4. Batten FE. Acute poliomyelitis. The Lumleian Lectures for 1916 delivered before the Royal College of Physicians. *Brain* 1916; 39: 115-211.
5. Nathanson N, Kew OM. From emergence to eradication: the epidemiology of poliomyelitis deconstructed. *Amer J Epidemiol* 2010; 172:1213-1229.
6. Caverly CS. *Infantile paralysis in Vermont. 1894-1922. A Memorial to Christopher S. Caverly.* Vermont State Department of Publications, Burlington, VT. State Department of Public Health. 1924.
7. Eggers HJ. Milestones in early poliomyelitis research (1840 to 1949). *J Virol* 1999;73(6):4533-4535.
8. Landsteiner K, Popper E. Mikroscopische praparate von einem menschlichen und zwei affentuckermarker. *Wein kiln Wschr* 1930; 21:
9. Flexner S, Lewis PA. The transmission of acute poliomyelitis to monkeys. *JAMA* 1909; 53:1639-1640.
10. Peabody FW, Draper G, Dochez AR. *A Clinical Study of Acute Poliomyelitis.* Monographs of the Rockefeller Institute for Medical Research, 1912, no. 4.
11. Flexner S, Amoss HL. Experiments on the nasal route of infection in poliomyelitis. *J Exp Med* 1920; 31: 123-134.
12. Eggers HJ. Milestones in early poliomyelitis research (1840 to 1949). *J Virol* 1999;73(6):4533-4535.
13. CDC: History of Drinking Water Treatment. Available at: www.cdc.gov/healthywater/drinking/history.htm
14. Benidickson J. *The Culture of Flushing: A Social and Legal History of Sewage.* UBC Press. Vancouver. 2011.
15. Hygiene - Hygiene and Public Health, 1700–1945. <a href="http://science.jrank.org/pages/9722/Hygiene-Hygiene-Public-Health-1700–1945.html">Hygiene - Hygiene and Public Health, 1700–1945</a>
16. Kluger J. *Splendid Solution: Jonas Salk and the Conquest of Polio.* The Berkley Publishing Group. Penguin Group(USA) Inc. New York, NY. 2006. pp.15-17.
17. Wyatt HV. Ending polio immunization: stars and gutters. *Vaccine* 2000; 18:781-784.

18. Paul JR, Melnick JL, Riordan JT. Comparative neutralizing antibody patterns to Lansing (type 2) poliomyelitis virus in different populations. *Am J Hyg* 1952; 56:232–251.

19. Tobin, James. *The Man He Became: How FDR Defied Polio to Win the Presidency.* Simon & Schuster, Inc. 2013. pp. 38.

20. Tobin. pg. 40–43.

21. Tobin. pg. 27–72.

22. Oshinsky David M. *Polio. An American Story.* Oxford University Press, Inc. New York, NY. 2005. pp. 48–50.

23. Oshinsky. pg. 53.

24. Oshinsky. Pg. 58–59.

25. Spencer WA. Poliomyelitis: a review of current concepts. *Phys Ther Rev* 1953; 33:373–374.

26. Melnick JL. Poliovirus in urban sewage in epidemic and non-epidemic times. *Am. J. Hyg* 1947; 45:240–253.

27. Melnick JL, Ledinko N. Development of neutralizing antibodies against the three types of poliomyeoitis virus during an epidemic period. The ratio of inapparent infection to clinical poliomyelitis. *Am J Hyg* 1953; 58:207–222.

28. Murray PR, Rosenthal KS, Pfaller MA. In *Medical Microbiology, Eighth Edition*, pp 462–464. Elsevier, Inc. Philadelphia, PA. 2016.

29. Laurie G. "Ventilator users, home care, and independent living: a historical perspective." In Gilgoff, Irene S. *Breath of Life: The Role of the Ventilator in Managing Life-Threatening Illnesses.* 2002. Lanham, Maryland: Scarecrow Press, Inc. pp.161–201.

30. Carroll RL. Rate and amount of improvement in muscle strength following poliomyelitis. *Physiother Rev* 1942; 22:243–257.

31. Conti AA. Western medical rehabilitation through time: a historical and epistemological review. *Sci World J* 2014; 2014:1–5.

32. Sullivan M, Jampel A. The rich and remarkable history of physical therapy at MGH. *Caring Headlines* 2011; Oct 20: 4–7.

33. Neumann DA. Polio: its impact on the people of the United States and the emerging profession of physical therapy. *J Orthop Sports Phys Ther* 2004; 34:479–492.

34. Tobin. pg. 102–111.

35. Tobin. pg. 142–148.

36. Tobin. pg. 201–213.

37. Tobin. pg. 214–226.

38. Verville RE, Ditunno JF. Franklin Delano Roosevelt, polio and the Warm Springs experiment: its impact on Physical Medicine and Rehabilitation. *PM&R* 2013; 5:3–8.

39. Burnet FM, MacNamara J. Immunological differences between strains of poliomyelitic virus. *Br J Exp Path* 1931; Apr;12(2): 57–61.

40. Paul JR. *A history of poliomyelitis.* New Haven, CT: Yale University Press, 1971.

41. Wilson DJ. *Living with Polio: The Epidemic and Its Survivors.* Chicago: University of Chicago Press. 2007. p. 181.

42. Minor PD, Ferguson M, Evans DMA et al. Antigenic structure of polioviruses of serotypes 1,2 and 3. *J Gen Virol* 1986; 67: 1283–1291.

43. Trask JD, Paul JR, Vignec AJ. I. Poliomyelitic virus in human stools. *J Exp Med* 1940 May 31; 71(6): 751–763.

44. Sabin AB, Ward R. The natural history of human poliomyelitis: distribution of virus in nervous and non-nervous tissue. *J Exp Med* 1941; 73: 771–793.

45. Morgan IM, Howe HA, Bodian D. The role of antibody in experimental poliomyelitis: production of intracerebral immunity in monkeys by vaccination. *Am J Hyg.* 1947 May; 45(3): 379–89.
46. O'Neill WL. *American High: The Years of Confidence, 1945–1960.* New York: Simon and Schuster. 1989. pg.136.
47. Kluger J. Chapter In *Splendid Solution: Jonas Salk and the Conquest of Polio.* New York NY: The Berkley Publishing Group, published by the Penguin Group (USA) Inc. 2006.
48. Enders JF, Weller TH, Robbins FC. Cultivation of the Lansing strain of polio virus in cultures of various embryonic tissues. *Science* 1949; 109: 85–87.
49. Oshinsky. pg.150–268.
50. Oshinsky. pg. 167.
51. Salk JE. Studies in human subjects on active immunization against poliomyelitis. I. A preliminary report of experiments in progress. *JAMA* 1953; 151(13): 1081–98.
52. Salk, JE. Recent studies on immunization against poliomyelitis. *Pedatrics* 1953; 12: 471–475.
53. Salk JE. Considerations in the preparation and use of poliomyelitis virus vaccine. *JAMA* 1955; 158(14): 1239–1248.
54. Oshinsky. pg. 211.
55. Hird TR, Grassly NC. Systematic review of mucosal immunity induced by oral and inactivated poliovirus vaccines against virus shedding following oral poliovirus challenge. *PLoS Pathogens* 2012; 8: 1–9. E1002599.
56. Sabin AB. Oral poliovirus vaccine: History of its development and use and current challenge to eliminate poliomyelitis from the world. *J Inf Dis* 1985; 151(3): 420–436.
57. Sabin AB. Poliomyelitis incidence in the Soviet Union in 1960. *JAMA* 1961; 176: 231–232.
58. Sabin AB, Michaels RH, Spigland I, et al. Community-wide use of oral poliovirus vaccine. Effectiveness of the Cincinnati program. *Am J Dis Child* 1961; 101: 546–567.
59. Henderson DA, Witte JJ, Morris L et al. Paralytic disease associated with oral polio vaccines. *JAMA* 1964; 190(1): 41–48.
60. Schonberger LB, McGowan JE, Gregg MB. Vaccine-associated poliomyelitis in the United States: 1961–1972. *Am J Epidemiol* 1976; 104: 202–211.
61. Nkowane BM, Wassilak SG, Orenstein WA et al. Vaccine-associated paralytic poliomyelitis in the United States, 1973 through 1984. *JAMA* 1987; 257(10): 135–1340.
62. Alexander LN, Seward JF, Santibanez TA et al. Vaccine policy changes and epidemiology of poliomyelitis in the United States. *JAMA* 2004; 292(14): 1696–1701.
63. Reagan RL, Brueckner AL. Morphologic observations by electron microscopy of the Lansing strain of poliomyelitis virus after propagation in the Swiss albino mouse. *Tex Rep Biol Med* 1952; 10: 425–428.
64. Racaniello VR, Baltimore D. Molecular cloning of poliovirus cDNA and determination of the complete nucleotide sequence of the viral genome. *Proc Nat Acad Sci* 1981; 78: 4887–4891.
65. Kitamura N, Semler BL, Rothberg PG et al. Primary structure, gene organization and polypeptide expression of poliovirus RNA. *Nature* 1981; 291: 547–553.
66. Racaniello VR, Baltimore D. Cloned poliovirus complementary DNA is infectious in mammalian cells. *Science* 1981; 214: 916–919.
67. Hogle JM, Chow M, Filman DJ. Three-dimensional structure of poliovirus at 2.9 A resolution. *Science* 1985; 229: 1358–1365.

68. Mendelsohn C, Wimmer E, Racaniello VR. Cellular receptor for polio-virus: molecular cloning, nucleotide sequence and expression of a new member of the immunoglobulin superfamily. *Cell* 1989; 56: 855–865.

69. Racaniello VR. One hundred years of poliovirus pathogenesis. *Virol* 2006; 344: 9–16.

70. Kew OM, Nottay BK. Molecular epidemiology of polioviruses. *Rev Inf Dis* 1984; 6(Suppl 2): S499–S504.

71. Crainic R, Kew O. Evolution and polymorphism of poliovirus genomes. *Biologicals* 1993; 21: 379–384.

72. Carstens EB, Ball LA. Ratification vote on taxonomic proposals to the International Committee on Taxonomy of Viruses. *Arch Virol* 2009; 154(7): 1181–1188.

73. Jiang P, Faase JAJ, Toyoda H et al. Evidence for emergence of diverse polioviruses from C-cluster Coxsackie A viruses and implications for global poliovirus eradica-tion. *Proc Nat Acad Sci* 2007; 104: 9457–9462.

74. Cockburn WC, Drozdov SG. Poliomyelitis in the world. *Bull Wld Hlth Org* 1970; 42: 405–417.

75. Bernier RH. Some observations on poliomyelitis lameness surveys. *Rev Inf Dis* 1984; 6(Suppl 2): S371–S375.

76. Assaad F, Ljunges-Esteves K. World overview of poliomyelitis: regional patterns and trends. *Rev Inf Dis* 1984; 6(Suppl 2):S302–S307.

77. Fine P, Eames K, Heymann DL. "Herd immunity": a rough guide. *Clin Inf Dis* 2011; 52: 911–916.

78. Mast EE, Cochi SL. For the Record: A History of Polio Eradication Efforts. Available at: wwwnc.cdc.gov/travel/.../for-the-record-a-history-of-polio-eradicat ion-efforts

79. Kew OM, Wright PF, Agol VI et al. Circulating vaccine-derived polioviruses: current state of knowledge. *Bull WHO* 2004; 82: 16–23.

80. Stern A, Yeh MT, Zinger T et al. The evolutionary pathway to virulence of an RNA virus. *Cell* 2017; 169: 35–46.

81. Global Polio Eradication Initiative. Polio eradication and endgame strategic plan, 2013–2018. Geneva: World Health Organization; 2013 [cited 2016 Sep. 25]. Available at: www.polioeradication.org/resourcelibrary/strategyandwork.aspx

82. Snider CJ, Diop OM, Burns CC, Tangermann RH, Wassilak SG. Surveillance systems to track progress toward polio eradication – worldwide, 2014–2015. *MMWR* 2016 Apr 8; 65(13):346–51.

83. Soucheray S. Last steps in polio eradication prove challenging. *Center for Infectious Disease Research & Policy News.* Sept. 27, 2016.

84. Poliomyelitis. Report by the Secretariat. World Health Organization. *Seventieth World Health Assembly.* Document A70/14. 24 April 2017.

85. Beaubien J. Mutant strains of polio vaccine now cause more paralysis than wild polio. NPR News. *Infectious Disease.* June 28, 2017.

86. WHO. Syrian Arab Republic. Polio outbreak in Syria successfully stopped. Available at: www.emro.who.int/syria-nes/polio-outbreak-successfully-stopped.html

87. Greene SA, Ahmed J, Datta SD et al. Progress toward polio eradication – world-wide. January 2017 – March 2019. *MMWR* 2019; 68: 458–462. Available at: http://dx.doi.org/10.15585/mmwr.mm6820a3

88. World Health Organization. Polio: Statement of the Twenty-first IHR Emergency Committee. Regarding the International Spread of Poliovirus. 29 May 2019 Geneva. Available at: www.who.int/news-room/detail/29-05-2019-statement-of-the-twe nty-first-ihr-emergency-committee

89. Gawne AC. Halstead LS. Post-polio syndrome: historical perspective, epidemiology and clinical presentation. *Neuro Rehab* 1997; 8: 73–81.

90. Jubelt B, Agre JC. Characteristics and management of post-polio syndrome. *JAMA* 2000; 284: 412–414.

91. Becker LC. Polio survivors in the U.S., 1915–2000: age distribution data. Report to the Board of Directors of Post-Polio International. October, 2006.

92. Groce NE, Banks LM, Stein MA. Surviving polio in a post-polio world. *Soc Sci Med* 2014; 107: 171–178.

93. Polio Global Eradication Initiative. 2019. Inactivated polio vaccine now introduced worldwide. https://polioeradication.org/news-post/inactivated-polio-vaccine-now-introduced-worldwide/

94. Macklin GR, Peak C, Eisenhawer M et al. Enabling accelerated vaccine roll-out for Public Health Emergencies of International Concern (PHEICs): novel oral polio vaccine type 2 (nOPV2) experience. *Vaccine* 2023; 41(Suppl 1): A122–A127. doi: 10.1016/j.vaccine.2022.02.050. Epub 2022 Mar 17.

95. Van Damme P, De Coster I, Bandyopadhyay AS et al. The safety and immunogenicity of two novel live attenuated monovalent (serotype 2) oral poliovirus vaccines in healthy adults: a double-blind, single-center phase 1 study. *Lancet* 2019; 394: 148–158.

96. Shin W-J, Gbormittah F, Chang H et al. Development of thermostable lyophilized Sabin inactivated poliovirus vaccine. *mBio* 2018; (6): 9:e02287-18. Available at: https://doi.org/10.1128/mBio.02287-18

97. "A Discussion on the Advisability of the Registration of Tuberculosis," Special Meeting held January 12, 1984 in *The Transactions of the College of Physicians of Philadelphia*, third series, volume 16, 1894.

98. Rogers N. *Dirt and Disease: Polio Before FDR*. New Brunswick, NJ: Rutgers University Press. 1996, p.30–71.

99. Tomes N. *The Gospel of Germs: Men, Women, and the Microbe in American Life.* Cambridge, MA: Harvard University Press. 1998, p.246–247.

100. Rogers N. "Race and the Politics of Polio: Warm Springs, Tuskegee, and the March of Dimes," *American Journal of Public Health* 2007 May 97(5): 784–5.

101. John Chenault's speech at the ground-breaking ceremony for the Tuskegee Center in January 1940, "Infantile Paralysis Center Launched at Tuskegee," Birmingham (Alabama) News, January 12, 1940. He also published an article detailing his findings in *the Journal for the National Medical Association* in 1951.

102. For a scathing indictment of *Buck v Bell*, see Adam Cohen, *Imbeciles: The Supreme Court, American Eugenics, and the Sterilization of Carrie Buck*. NY: Penguin. 2017.

103. Kaelber L. "Eugenics: Compulsory Sterilization in 50 American States," presented to the Social Science History Association, 2012, www.uvm.edu/~lkaelber/eugenics/

104. Wilson, p. 169.

105. Wilson, 172–173.

106. Wilson, 178.

107. Wilson, 179.

108. Fairchild AL. "The Polio Narratives: Dialogues with FDR, "*Bull Hist Med* 75(3): 488–534.

109. Wilson, 181.

Suggested Reading

David M Oshinsky. *Polio. An American Story.* Oxford University Press. New York. 2005.

James Tobin. *The Man He Became: How FDR Defied Polio to Win the Presidency.* Simon & Schuster, Inc. New York. 2013.

Jane S Smith. *Patenting the Sun. Polio and the Salk Vaccine.* William Morrow and Company, Inc. New York. 1990.

Jeffrey Kluger. *Splendid Solution: Jonas Salk and the Conquest of Polio.* Berkley Publishing Group. Penguin Group(USA). New York. 2006.

Naomi Rogers. *Dirt and Disease: Polio before FDR.* Rutgers University Press. New Brunswick, NJ. 1990.

Tony Gould. *A Summer Plague. Polio and its Survivors.* Yale University Press. New Haven, London. 1995.

William L O'Neill. *American High: The Years of Confidence, 1945–1960.* Simon and Schuster. New York. 1986.

6

HIV AND AIDS

The Never-Ending Story

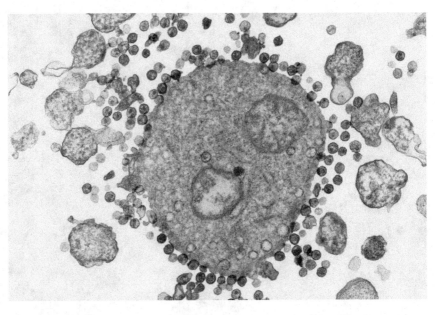

FIGURE 6.1 HIV virions budding and releasing from an infected cell.

Source: NIAID, NIH.

DOI: 10.4324/9781003427667-6

BLOOD IN THE OR

I have always loved the operating room. I'm a pediatric cardiologist, not a surgeon, but most of my critically ill patients were babies with heart defects for
whom surgery was the only effective treatment. Congenital heart defects occur
because of the complex process of cardiac development that begins in the early
weeks of pregnancy. An error in development at any stage can result in a defect
in the heart's structure – and in some newborns, these defects are fatal without
emergent correction. When I started in pediatric cardiology, congenital heart
surgery was just out of its infancy and pediatric cardiovascular surgeons were
beginning to attempt complete repairs in newborn infants with critical structural defects. In those days, the field was still new and very small so cardiologists
and cardiovascular surgeons worked together very closely. Cardiologists made
the baby's diagnosis using cardiac catheterization, a technique that involves
threading a tiny catheter from the blood vessels in the leg up into the heart
and then injecting radio-opaque dye to visualize the anatomy in detail. Once
the diagnosis was established, cardiologists met with the surgeon to plan the
surgical approach. My teachers – pioneers in the field of pediatric cardiology –
always went to the operating room with their patients and so did I.

I am talking here about open heart surgery – and when the heart is the
size of a golf ball as it is in a newborn – this means some of the most technic-
ally challenging procedures imaginable. Open heart surgery is exactly that –
opening the heart to perform surgery – and this means that the heart must
stop beating and the body's circulation supported for the surgeon to work.
This is accomplished with a cardiac bypass machine which oxygenates venous
blood, simulating the way the lungs function in life, and then routes it through
a tiny catheter – smaller than a drinking straw in a newborn – into the aorta, the
great vessel that carries blood to the body. A roller pump drives the oxygenated
blood through the aorta, to the heart muscle itself and to the entire body.

The heart revealed is a thing of great beauty, lying just under the breast-
bone, pumping continuously from the first weeks of pregnancy to the end
of life. It has always been a magical moment for me to see the anatomy that
I had worked to diagnose revealed, and to watch the intricate steps involved
in cardiac repair. My respect for the courage and skill of pediatric cardiovascular surgeons still verges on reverence. When the repair has been completed
and the heart begins to pump again, I am filled with awe. After all these years,
open heart surgery in a newborn still feels like a miracle.

But open heart surgery does expose the operating team to an enormous
amount of blood. Every step involves blood – venous blood flowing, arterial
blood pumping, random blood splashing – and sharp objects: saws, needles,
scalpels, retractors. There is obvious, ongoing risk of trauma to the hands,
evading protective gloves, of blood spurting onto the face, into the eyes.
Many times, I remember seeing a surgeon's forehead dotted with blood

above his mask. Blood exposure was always an issue but it suddenly became a major risk after the AIDS epidemic began. Our knowledge about AIDS in medical practice followed the epidemiologic pattern as it was uncovered by reports in the literature. At first, it was a strange new disease that attacked the immune system of young gay men causing unusual infections and malignancies – a problem for specialists in infectious disease and oncology. But less than a year after the very first cases, AIDS was reported to be caused by a transmissible agent carried in the blood – and suddenly it became a problem for all health care providers and especially for surgeons. Because the agent had not been identified there was no way to test for its presence and AIDS cases occurring after blood transfusions showed the agent was present in the blood supply. Open heart operations using cardiopulmonary bypass represent the largest routine exposure to blood in clinical medicine so cardiac surgical teams were thought to be at the greatest risk of accidental infection with the unknown agent that caused AIDS. Cardiac surgeons are among the bravest people I know, routinely facing the challenge of literally stopping the heart to repair it – but I have never seen fear like that I saw in the faces of my colleagues during those terrible early years of the AIDS pandemic. Early in the epidemic, an anonymous survey of cardiac surgeons suggested that almost 30% would not operate on a person with AIDS because of fear of infection.[a]

The dilemma of the contaminated blood supply continued until 1985, long after the human immunodeficiency virus had been identified, because of the conflicting priorities of the key groups involved: the public health community led by the CDC were convinced of an impending disaster involving potentially many thousands of recipients infected by contaminated transfusions of blood and blood products while the blood-banking community was concerned about fear of AIDS compromising their critical supply of donors. Without a definitive test, potential solutions were suggested and rejected while doctors struggled to deal with terrified patients and families as well as their own fears. During this time, many adults donated their own blood in advance of an operation, a complicated effort that involved going to a blood bank weeks before surgery when up to three units of blood could be taken and stored. Obviously, this was not an option for children or in an emergency situation so the process of directed donations arose in response to concerns about blood safety raised by the AIDS epidemic. A directed donation occurred when a patient's family and friends donated blood to be used only for that specific patient. Directed donations were extremely common before open heart surgery in the children I cared for in the early 1980s.

By 1985, an effective HIV screening test had been developed and within 6 months, the blood supply was declared safe – but not until more than 12,000 people in the United States had received contaminated transfusions of blood or blood products. By that time, the health care industry had a much greater understanding of the risk of infection related to multiple procedures including simple routine tasks like blood drawing. In terms of surgery, the procedures that exposed surgeons and their assistants to infection from contaminated blood had been found to primarily involve passing devices between operators with the highest risk associated with suture needles followed by scalpel blades and glass syringes. In a study of 234 observed surgeries, an astonishing 50% were reported to involve glove perforation with contamination of a co-worker's hand.[b] A 1992 glove study showed 51% contamination of the hands with single gloves versus 7% with double gloves – this report led to implementation of double gloving as a routine universal precaution along with masks with shields that protect the eyes.[c] Between 1985 and 2013, the CDC reported there were 58 confirmed and 150 possible cases of occupationally acquired HIV infection among American health care workers. Nurses were the largest affected group, with 41% of confirmed cases; there were no confirmed cases in surgeons.[d]

Pediatric cardiology progressed enormously during my time in the field – we almost always make the diagnosis of even the most complex congenital heart defects with ultrasound now, and surgical procedures that were revolutionary in the early days have become almost routine. Often, non-surgical, catheter-based procedures have replaced or augmented surgical approaches. And infection of the blood supply with HIV has been replaced by the risk of exposure to other serious viral pathogens like the hepatitis C virus.[e] The risk for health care workers of HIV infection due to exposure to contaminated blood has all but disappeared, but this history remains an important part of the story of AIDS.

[a] Condit, D and Frater, RWM. Human Immunodeficiency Virus and the cardiac surgeon: A survey of attitudes. *Ann Thorac Surg* 1989, 47: 182–186.
[b] Palmer JD and Rickett JW. The mechanisms and risks of surgical glove perforation. *J Hosp Infect* 1992, 22: 279–286.
[c] Quebbeman EJ et al. Double gloving: Protecting surgeons from blood contamination in the operating room. *Arch of Surg* 1992, 127: 213–217.
[d] CDC. Guidelines for prevention of surgical site infection. *Inf Control Hosp Epidemiol.* 1992: 20(4): 247.
[e] CDC. Notes from the field: Occupationally acquired HIV infection among health care workers – United States, 1985–2013. *MMWR* 2015, 65(53): 1245–1246.
[f] Centers for Disease Control and Prevention. Recommendations for health care workers potentially exposed to Hepatitis C. April 2018. www.cdc.gov/hepatitis/pdfs/testing-followup-exposed-hc-personnel.pdf. Accessed August 14, 2018.

HIV and AIDS: The Never-Ending Story

At first, it seemed like an American disease. In June 1981, the Centers for Disease Control and Prevention (CDC) in Atlanta reported in their *Morbidity and Mortality Weekly Report (MMWR)* that between October 1980 and May 1981, five young men in Los Angeles, all active homosexuals, were treated for biopsy-confirmed *Pneumocystis carinii* pneumonia (PCP). Three of these patients had evidence of depressed immune function and two died. *MMWR* is a weekly summary for the United States of important, time-sensitive public health information. In the comments accompanying this small case series, the editors noted that historically, *Pneumocystis* – a yeast-like fungus – infects only patients with severely compromised immune systems so its occurrence in these previously healthy individuals raised the possibility of immune dysfunction secondary to some predisposing common exposure. That all of the patients were homosexuals suggested an association with some aspect of homosexual lifestyle or a disease acquired through homosexual contact.[1]

From this first report, the CDC became the coordinator for emerging information on this new disease and *MMWR* the major information source as the knowledge base grew and evolved. Only four weeks after that first release, *MMWR* reported that over the last two and a half years, Kaposi's sarcoma (KS) had been diagnosed in 26 young homosexual men, 20 in New York City and 6 in California. Until that time, KS was known as a rare skin cancer that presented as circumscribed dark purple lesions and that only occurred in elderly men of Mediterranean descent – characteristics not shared by any of these young men. Notably, six of these KS patients had also developed *Pneumocystis* pneumonia. In contrast to the usual KS course where mean survival time was 8–13 years, eight patients died within two years of diagnosis.[2] By September, there was a second series of 8 patients with atypical KS. Again, all were young homosexual men and survival time was short: half of the patients were dead within 20 months of diagnosis. The authors reported the historic association of KS with an immune-compromised state in a subset of cases in Africa but no immune testing was performed in either of these two groups.[3]

The epidemiology of this new disease unrolled rapidly with critical new reports almost every month. By the end of 1981 – only six months after the first report – outbreaks of bizarre opportunistic infections and of unusual malignancies in young homosexuals had been reported from major cities all over the United States. By this time, these disparate cases were found to be linked by definite evidence of immune dysfunction focused on the cellular immune response of lymphocytes, the white blood cells that determine the body's response to infectious microorganisms and other foreign substances. The characteristic pattern was moderate to severe reduction in lymphocyte counts; low counts of helper/inducer T4+ lymphocytes – now called CD4 cells – and correspondingly, a low T4+ to T8+ lymphocyte ratio (T-8+ lymphocytes are suppressor/ cytotoxic lymphocytes, now called CD8 cells); and anergy (no lymphocyte response to antigen stimulation).

And then in December 1981, opportunistic infections associated with cellular immune dysfunction were reported for the first time in *heterosexual* men and women who were intravenous drug users (IDUs).[4] The combined evidence indicated a new disease caused by a transmissible agent that attacked the immune system in specific, vulnerable populations. Most concerning was the exponential increase in cases and the expanding base of susceptible populations – by the end of 1981 in the United States, there were 270 reported cases of this severe, new, acquired immune deficiency among gay men and 121 of these individuals had already died.[5]

****

Media coverage played a critical role in the evolution of the AIDS story. In the beginning, coverage of the new disease outbreak was very limited. Reports described a "new and mysterious illness" in gay men with little additional information. Quantitative content analysis of press coverage of HIV/AIDS in Australia, USA, France and Britain during the 1980s and 1990s revealed a common pattern with coverage focused almost exclusively on homosexuals.[6]

It is not a coincidence that AIDS emerged in the early 1980s when after centuries of persecution, the gay liberation movement was in full swing in the United States. For a minority of young homosexual men, liberation meant an extravagantly active sex life with multiple sexual partners in places like public bathhouses. In spite of gay pride parades and stories of "coming out," the longstanding stigma of homosexuality persisted with overt homophobia through the 1980s, even in New York City and San Francisco, both sophisticated metropolitan centers with flourishing gay sub-cultures – and both among the first cities to report cases of the new illness. From the beginning, news coverage of the disease was dominated by the initial CDC reports of "gay pneumonia," alluded to in 83% of stories in 1981.[6] The labels "gay plague" and Gay-Related Immune Disease (GRID) first appeared in 1981, establishing the public view of the illness as exclusively a contagious disease of homosexuals.[7]

On July 3, 1981, the same day this information was published in MMWR, the New York Times reported "Rare Cancer Seen in 41 Homosexuals," describing the outbreak of Kaposi's Sarcoma, "a rare and often rapidly fatal form of cancer," diagnosed in homosexual men. The article – one of the first in a lay publication to address the new outbreak – explained that the diagnoses had been made mostly in New York City and San Francisco, and that the CDC was alerting other doctors who treat "large numbers of homosexual men" of the problem.[8] Beginning with the headline, the article clearly suggested that this cancer was a homosexual problem, just like the unusual infections and the immune system dysfunction.

****

Early in 1982, a small case series described immunologic findings in 15 healthy homosexual men and two men with KS. Both KS patients and 7 of the 15 healthy gay volunteers had low T4+/T8+ lymphocyte ratios – the same pattern seen in individuals with opportunistic infections and KS. High cytomegalovirus (CMV) antibody titers – evidence of previous CMV infection – were found in 14 of the

15 men and half of the group reported exposure to inhaled nitrites. A history of CMV infection and of amyl nitrite use had been noted in prior reports of both opportunistic infections and KS, and the authors of this report suggested the combination might be the cause of the immune dysfunction. It would be many months before this immunologic pattern was instead recognized as a pre-clinical stage of the new infectious disease.[9]

Within months, a series of critical reports raised new concerns about spread of the epidemic. First, the CDC reported that between June 1981 and May 1982, a total of 355 cases of Kaposi's sarcoma and/or serious opportunistic infection had occurred in previously healthy people between 15 and 60 years of age. Sixteen percent of the group were heterosexual and, of these, the majority had a history of IV drug use. Similarities between the homosexual and heterosexual cases in age range, fatality rates, and geographic and temporal distribution strongly suggested that the cases were all part of the same disease outbreak.[10]

A critical report from the CDC in May 1982 described cases of persistent, generalized lymphadenopathy (lymph node enlargement) in homosexual males, reported by physicians from several major cities. In a subset of 8 of these men seen at medical centers in Atlanta, New York City and San Francisco, immunologic evaluation demonstrated immune dysfunction with abnormal T-lymphocyte helper-to-suppressor ratios, the same pattern described in individuals with overt opportunistic infections and KS. Approximately 70% of these patients also had some constitutional symptoms including fatigue, fever, night sweats and weight loss. Was this lymphadenopathy and immune dysfunction combination an early expression of infection with the same transmissible agent attacking homosexual men and IV drug users?[11]

Only a month later, the CDC reported the now familiar disease pattern of opportunistic infections in 34 Haitians (33 male) living in the United States; most had immigrated within the last 2 years. Age range was similar to other reported groups, but only a small minority were homosexuals or IV drug users. When immunologic studies were performed, there was evidence of severe immune dysfunction. For the entire group, the mortality rate on short-term follow-up was nearly 50%. The similarity of the disease pattern and immunologic picture to that described in American homosexual males and IV drug users, suggested an as yet unidentified common cause.[12]

Only a week later, the CDC reported three cases of opportunistic *pneumocystis carinii* pneumonia (PCP) in individuals with hemophilia but with no other underlying disease. All three were heterosexual males who had received repeated injections of factor VIII concentrate to stop uncontrolled bleeding. To treat clotting factor deficiencies like those found in hemophiliacs, pooled concentrates of the missing factor from hundreds of donors are needed. None of these three patients had a history of homosexual contact or intravenous drug abuse but two patients who were specifically tested had evidence of cellular immune deficiency and all had lymphopenia. The CDC editors of the report wrote,

The clinical and immunologic features of these three patients are strikingly similar to those recently observed among ... homosexual males, heterosexuals who abuse IV drugs, and Haitians who recently entered the United States. Although the cause of the severe immune dysfunction is unknown, the occurrence among the three hemophiliac cases suggests the *possible transmission of an agent through blood products.*[13]

By December 1982, the CDC reported that all three of the original hemophilia patients had died, and there were four more cases among hemophiliacs receiving frequent clotting factor transfusions; two were children under 10 years of age. All had the now familiar pattern of cellular immune dysfunction.[14] A national survey of hemophilia treatment centers revealed that 30% of all hemophiliacs had abnormal immunologic tests.[15]

With these cases, the evidence seemed clear that a dangerous new agent transmitted through blood was attacking the immune system of healthy individuals in multiple different settings. At an urgent meeting convened in July 1982 to specifically address this risk in individuals with hemophilia, the CDC adopted the term "acquired immune deficiency syndrome" to describe the clinical and immunologic pattern in all these groups and the acronym AIDS was born.[15]

Another intriguing piece of the puzzle emerged in September with evaluation of immune function in 81 male homosexual volunteer research subjects in NYC: 50 were asymptomatic and 31 had one or more of the constellation of symptoms described in association with generalized lymphadenopathy. T-cell subsets were abnormal in both groups compared with those of a control group of healthy heterosexual males and the T4/T8 ratio decreased as the number of sexual partners increased. These results suggested that a large proportion of sexually active homosexual males in NYC could already have been infected by the agent which causes AIDS with significant but, to this time, asymptomatic immune dysfunction.[16] The findings were a chilling premonition of what was to come.

In the September 24 edition of *MMWR*, the CDC provided the following case definition of AIDS which included recognition of a pre-symptomatic state:

AIDS is an opportunistic infection at least moderately predictive of a defect in cell-mediated immunity, occurring in a person with no known cause for diminished resistance to that disease. Such diseases include Kaposi's Sarcoma, Pneumocystis carinii pneumonia, and other serious opportunistic infections ... this case definition may not include the full spectrum of AIDS manifestations, which may range from absence of symptoms despite laboratory evidence of immune deficiency to non-specific symptoms (e.g., fever, weight loss, generalized, persistent lymphadenopathy) to specific diseases that are insufficiently predictive of cellular immunodeficiency to be included in incidence monitoring (e.g., tuberculosis, oral candidiasis, herpes zoster) to malignant neoplasms that cause, as well as result

from, immunodeficiency. Absence of a reliable ... test for AIDS makes
th(is) working case definition the best currently available for incidence
monitoring.[17]

By December 1982, the potential number of "at risk" groups had increased even
further with the report of AIDS in a 20-month-old baby who had unexplained
cellular immunodeficiency and repeated opportunistic infections after multiple
blood and platelet transfusions for Rh incompatibility as a newborn. One of the
platelet transfusions the baby received was ultimately found to have come from a
homosexual man who was well when he donated blood but who died of AIDS-
related opportunistic infection 17 months later.[18,19] This case was a bombshell
suggesting not only transmission of the infectious AIDS agent in blood transfusions
but also a long incubation period for the infectious agent before symptoms appear.

Only a week later, a whole new risk group emerged when the CDC reported
four cases of AIDS in babies less than 2 years of age. None had ever received
blood or blood products but three had mothers from groups at risk for AIDS and
the mother of the last child had AIDS. In addition, the cases of six young children
who died with opportunistic infections and unusual cellular immunodeficiencies
were also under investigation as were those of another 12 children with similar
immunodeficiencies but without life-threatening opportunistic infections.[20]
Clinical features in these infants included growth failure, oral candidiasis (fungal
infection), enlarged liver and spleen, generalized lymphadenopathy and chronic
pneumonitis without a demonstrable infection. Seven of the nine mothers for
whom information was available were intravenous drug abusers.

The pattern of immune dysfunction described in these infant AIDS cases closely
resembled that seen in adults with AIDS. One mother had already died with AIDS
and the others came from groups at risk for AIDS. Taken together, these cases
suggested the infectious agent had been transmitted from mothers with AIDS or
a pre-AIDS high-risk state to their children before birth or during delivery. Since
most of the mothers were well, the series supported the important, emerging concept of a long incubation period for the AIDS agent before symptoms appear.

By the end of 1982, the CDC reported a total of 788 AIDS cases, 95% from
one of four identified risk groups – homosexual men, heterosexual IV drug users,
Haitians and hemophiliacs – the "4H club," as it was called with predictable
stigmatizing results.[21] Although receipt of blood products, in general, did not
make the list of specified risk situations, the hemophiliac cases and the baby who
developed AIDS after a platelet transfusion from a man who subsequently died
of AIDS were considered important, confirmatory evidence that the AIDS agent
was blood-borne and could be transmitted by transfusion of blood and blood
products. Official meetings were initiated with the blood services community
to address this issue. Transmission from mother-to-child was not considered a
confirmed risk group at that time.

★★★★★★★★

The disease pattern changed dramatically in the first week of 1983 with a resulting major shift in the scientific and public response when the CDC reported AIDS in two women who had developed cellular immunodeficiency with no other risk factors except long-term sexual relationships with partners who had AIDS. AIDS had been diagnosed in an additional 41 previously healthy women who were in no other identified risk category: four of these women had steady sexual partners who were IV drug abusers.[22,23] It was suddenly and alarmingly clear that the unidentified AIDS agent could be transmitted by heterosexual sex.

And then there were the children. After the original report at the end of 1982, two more series reported AIDS cases in infants and young children.[24,25] All were small at birth and had severe growth failure with lymphadenopathy, hepato-splenomegaly (enlarged liver and spleen), and recurrent infections with rare organisms, associated with profound cell-mediated immunodeficiency. In each case, at least one parent had AIDS or a recognized high-risk condition for AIDS. At the time of the report, 27% of the children had already died.

An additional risk factor was confirmed by a national case-control study which compared 50 male homosexuals with AIDS to 120 matched healthy male homosexual controls, all volunteer research subjects from clinics in NYC, San Francisco, Los Angeles or Atlanta. The two groups were interviewed and their responses to a wide array of personal and socio-demographic questions were recorded. The most significant finding was a striking difference in the number of sexual partners: the AIDS patients had a median of 68 partners in the last 12 months compared with 35 for controls. The number of sex partners correlated significantly with many other high-risk variables including meeting partners in bathhouses, previous history of syphilis, and use of nitrite inhalants.[26] Increased AIDS risk with multiple partners suggesting increased risk with increased exposure had emerged in other studies but it had never been clarified as specifically as it was here.

Looking forward just 18 months from that first report in July 1981, that small case series sounded the alarm on a new epidemic caused by an unidentified agent that decimated the immune system. The pathogen that caused AIDS was carried in body fluids and was transmitted sexually and through the blood. Multiple high-risk groups had been defined: homosexual males (especially those with multiple partners); heterosexual IV drug users; women whose sex partners had or were at high risk for AIDS, i.e., bisexual males or IV drug users; hemophiliacs who had received multiple clotting factor infusions; infants born to mothers who had or were at high risk for AIDS; and recipients of infected blood transfusions. (Haitian immigrants were also identified as a high-risk group and resolution of this putative etiology – described later in this chapter – would take several more years; unfortunately, the stigmatizing association of AIDS with Haitian heritage persisted for many years beyond that.) For all intents and purposes, AIDS was a uniformly fatal diagnosis: the reported mortality rate was at least 50%, but the death rate continued to rise with time from the original identifying illness – the average survival time after the diagnosis of AIDS was only between 9.5 and 22 months. Most worrisome was evidence of a prolonged asymptomatic but contagious carrier state that suggested the number of potentially infected patients far exceeded current reports. And the possibility that the virus had contaminated the blood supply indicated a large new group of individuals at high risk. AIDS was a rapidly expanding epidemic, without an identified cause and with no effective treatment.

★★★★★★★★★

To this time, the general public had primarily seen AIDS as a mystery disease of gay men and drug addicts chased by epidemiologists in relative obscurity. With spread to women, babies and healthy people receiving blood transfusions, AIDS was suddenly a focus for the mainstream media and a cause of mounting public concern. At that time, the field of medicine was enjoying a genuine sense of accomplishment. In addition to the dramatic progress made in the development of antibiotics for treatment of infectious diseases, the twentieth century had seen major advances in almost every other area of medicine including development of vaccines against diphtheria, whooping cough, tetanus, yellow fever and polio. Insulin therapy for diabetes was discovered, transforming this previously fatal disease. The heart-lung machine had been invented allowing routine open-heart surgery. CT scanning and magnetic resonance imaging provided amazingly detailed views of the human body in health and disease. Kidney, liver, lung and heart transplants were successfully performed. Against this backdrop, the emergence of an epidemic caused by a new, fatal virus was an unanticipated and unwelcome surprise. And a disease that was transmitted sexually and was especially common in promiscuous homosexuals was especially unwelcome at a time when the sexual revolution that began in the 1960s had only just started to make sex outside of traditional heterosexual, married relationships acceptable.

It is hard to describe the terror that arose when AIDS was shown to potentially infect the whole population. With no identified cause and no treatment, the specter of the disease hung over the American population, fueled by media reports of seemingly random infections. Part of the rising public concern about AIDS was related to increasing media coverage, exemplified by the continuous 24 hour news reporting launched by CNN in 1980, just as the epidemic was beginning.[27] A complete CNN news cycle consisted of the media reporting on some event, followed by reporting on public and other reactions to that report. News stories were presented as continuous news with constant updating, a major contrast with the previous day-by-day pace of the cycle of daily newspapers and scheduled TV news broadcasts. With spread to heterosexuals, even sporadic AIDS cases received intense, ongoing media coverage. The obvious limits of medical knowledge also fueled fear. When the epidemic began, even understanding of immune compromise was relatively limited, obtained primarily from experience with patients receiving drugs to suppress the body's natural immune response after organ transplant or as part of the reaction to cancer chemotherapy. AIDS appeared to be uniformly fatal, often in a very short time. Media coverage often fixated on stories that sensationalized the spread of the disease. "AIDS: Fatal, Incurable, and Spreading" read a typical headline from a cover of *People* magazine. The article began:

> In recent months doctors have reported alarming signs that acquired immune deficiency syndrome (AIDS), the terrible, incurable disease that has ravaged the homosexual community for four years, now poses a growing threat to heterosexuals … 500,000 to 1 million Americans are carrying the virus that produces AIDS. About 10% will develop the disease over five years, doctors say; meanwhile they may transmit the virus, which has a latency period of three to five years, to their sexual partners …[28]

At the time, *People* had a weekly circulation of 2.8 million subscribers so the potential impact of stories like this was substantial.

★★★★★★★

Discovery of the Human Immunodeficiency Virus

Two years into the epidemic, basic research lagged well behind the epidemiologic findings. This was not for lack of effort on the part of the CDC – as early as the fall of 1981 when there had been only a handful of reported cases, James Curran, Director of the newly created Task Force on Kaposi's Sarcoma and Opportunistic Infections at the CDC, met with a group of National Institutes of Health (NIH) researchers to describe what was known about this new disease and to outline what he felt were important research questions. There was no response. A year later he returned armed with specific information about the new, unidentified agent carried in body fluids and transmitted sexually and through the blood, that caused severe, fatal immunodeficiency focused on T-lymphocytes.[29] That combination of descriptors caught the attention of Robert Gallo, an established scientist at the NIH, who had spent the last 20 years studying retroviruses as a potential cause of malignancy in humans.

Remember, all viruses have a very simple structure with a core genome carrying genetic material, either RNA or DNA, inside a protein coat. In the vast majority of viruses, the genetic material is RNA. Reverse transcribing viruses or retroviruses are a special subset: they have an RNA genome but use a DNA intermediate to replicate. Retroviruses had been discovered in the early 1900s and subsequently been shown to be RNA viruses that induced cancer in birds and mammals, but it was not until the enzyme reverse transcriptase was identified in 1970 that the process by which retroviruses turned viral RNA strands into DNA was understood.[30,31]

Working with his own team of scientists, Gallo had identified a factor that promoted growth of T-cell lymphocytes. The first identified cytokine, this was originally called T-cell growth factor, but it is now known as Interleukin-2 or IL-2. Using IL-2, Gallo's team had isolated human T-cell leukemia virus (HTLV-1) in 1981 – the first identified human retrovirus. HTLV-1 was subsequently shown to be the cause of adult T-cell leukemia, a very common form of leukemia in Japan.[32] The retrovirus HTLV-1 attacks T-lymphocytes and is transmitted from one person to another through the blood, by sex and in utero from mother to child.

A virus that attacked the T-lymphocytes of the immune system and was transmitted by body fluids sounded like an HTLV-like retrovirus to Gallo and he immediately began to explore the idea that some version of his newly discovered virus might be the cause of AIDS. At the same time, Max Essex, a Harvard researcher, was exploring a potential role for feline leukemia virus, another retrovirus that attacks the immune system of cats. Searching for a retrovirus as the cause of AIDS proved to be a serendipitous first step that arose from conversation between these two scientists.[29]

Gallo's lab was well prepared for this investigation after their years of experience culturing and growing T-cells in the process of identifying HTLV-1 and subsequently an additional retrovirus, HTLV-2. By May 1982, the lab had begun trying to identify a retrovirus in the blood of AIDS patients. Meanwhile, Luc Montagnier, a French virologist at the Pasteur Institute was studying the lymph nodes of patients with AIDS. In January 1983, his lab identified reverse transcriptase enzyme activity in lymph node cells from a gay man with generalized lymphadenopathy.[33] At that time, retroviruses were the only entity known to use reverse transcriptase – and the only retroviruses known to attack humans were HTLV-1 and HTLV-2.

Montagnier's findings appeared to confirm Gallo's hypothesis that the AIDS agent was an HTLV-related virus and all his subsequent research focused on proving this. In the same issue of the journal *Science* where Montagnier's group reported their lymph node findings, the Gallo group reported they had isolated a virus from a patient with AIDS and "shown that it was related to the HTLV subgroup 1."[34] Despite Gallo's repeated assertions, however, he was never able to prove that an HTLV-related virus was the cause of AIDS.[35] Instead, in September 1983 at a meeting of retrovirologists, it was Montagnier who reported that his group had isolated a virus from 5 pre-AIDS patients and 3 patients with AIDS. He called the virus "LAV" for "lymphadenopathy-associated virus" and reported two more important findings: LAV showed a specific affinity for CD4 T-cells; and detailed analysis showed that it was not a variant of the HTLV group but rather, a member of the lentivirus family, a retrovirus subgroup.[36,37] By the time the Pasteur group published these findings in April 1984, they had also shown that T-lymphocytes were the receptor for LAV and had isolated LAV from the French blood bank supply.[38,39]

Over the next year, an increasingly acrimonious competition between Montagnier and Gallo – LAV vs HTLV-III – played out until ultimately, the two viruses were shown to be identical by nucleotide sequencing and they were both renamed the human immunodeficiency virus – HIV, shown in Figure 6.1.[40,41]

Along the way, the Gallo group made critical contributions. They discovered how to grow HIV continuously in permanent culture – this allowed development of an accurate and sensitive blood test to detect antibodies against HIV which could be used to confirm infection with the virus and screen donated blood. The ability to confirm infection definitively clarified the epidemiology of the illness and theoretically would allow the earliest possible introduction of treatment. While Luc Montagnier and his colleague, Francoise Barre-Sinoussi, won the Nobel Prize in Medicine in 2008 for their discovery of the virus that caused AIDS, exclusion of Robert Gallo is hard to understand given his many important contributions to knowledge of HIV and AIDS.[42]

★★★★★★★

The Virus

Discovery of the Human Immunodeficiency Virus proved to be only a small first step in understanding the complex immuno-pathophysiology of the virus and the acquired immune deficiency syndrome. From Montagnier's work, HIV was identified as a retrovirus, from the family Retroviridae – these are enveloped, icosahedral viruses which replicate by converting the RNA genome into a DNA intermediate using the enzyme reverse transcriptase; the DNA intermediate is then converted to double-stranded DNA.[43]

The new virus causing immune deficiency in humans was identified as a Lentivirus, a subgroup of the Retroviradae family which produces chronic and ultimately fatal disease in mammals after a long incubation period.[44] There are five serogroups based on the vertebrate hosts they infect. The main difference between lentiviruses and standard retroviruses is that lentiviruses are capable of infecting both non-dividing and actively dividing cell types, while standard retroviruses can only infect actively dividing cells. Lentiviruses are also known to have high mutation and recombination rates, major factors in the future struggle to identify effective treatment for HIV infection.

In 1986, a different lentivirus was isolated from West African patients with AIDS.[45] The genomic organization was found to be very similar to HIV and the two viruses subsequently became known as HIV-1 and HIV-2. HIV-1 is responsible for the majority of all human immunodeficiency virus infections but HIV-2 causes a significant minority of cases, primarily in West Africa. Infection with either HIV-1 or HIV-2 will progress to AIDS if untreated but the rate of progress is much slower with HIV-2. HIV-1 as the cause of an ongoing global pandemic is the focus of this chapter.

Negative-staining electron microscopy shows HIV-1 and HIV-2 to be small, roughly spherical viruses, approximately 120 nm in diameter. Both are encapsulated viruses which contain a conical capsid enclosing the RNA genome plus all the enzymes essential for formation of new viruses.[46] Nucleotide sequencing was accomplished by 1985 and since that time, increasingly sophisticated molecular genetic techniques including cryo-electron microscopy and tomography, and all-atom large-scale molecular dynamic simulations have revealed that HIV is a very complex virus.[47,48] The HIV envelope includes glycoproteins displayed on the surface of the virus as spikes which are used for host cell entry. The envelope spikes bind to the host target cell CD4+ receptor and a chemokine co-receptor, typically CXCR4 or CCR5; this process anchors HIV to the host cell. The viral and host membranes fuse, the viral capsid enters the cell, and the core genome dissolves, releasing the HIV RNA copies. Reverse transcriptase then converts the single-stranded RNA to double-stranded DNA, using cellular nucleotides as the building blocks for DNA synthesis. The HIV DNA complex migrates inside the host nucleus and integrates into the host DNA, forming the HIV/DNA provirus. *The HIV provirus remains part of the host DNA forever, perceived by the cell as normal host cellular DNA.* Cellular enzymes can then transcribe the proviral DNA into messenger and genomic RNA which is exported out of the nucleus into the cytoplasm and reassembled as mature HIV virions, ready to infect other cells.[49–52] Despite intensive study for more than two decades and increasingly detailed knowledge of the virus, complete understanding of the HIV infection process remains the goal of ongoing research.[53]

Like all lentiviruses, HIV populations have enormous genetic variation revealed by molecular phylogenetic studies. HIV is reported to have the highest recorded biological mutation rate currently known to science. Point mutations due to base substitutions occur very frequently, primarily because – as in all RNA viruses – the absence of proofreading makes the process of RNA synthesis error-prone. This results in a baseline spontaneous mutation rate of at least 1% per year. Within a single infected individual, the virus evolves extremely frequently and rapidly, resulting in multiple mutant versions of the virus.[54] As with the influenza virus, there is a second important mechanism for genetic variation: recombination – the exchange of entire gene sequences at unselected positions – occurs when a target cell is infected with different HIV subtypes. Recombination of HIV-1 subtypes is considered a driving force for its diversity worldwide, responsible for frequent and important genetic variation in the virus. Approximately 1 in 400 newly produced HIV viruses is a recombinant virus containing combined genetic material. Such a recombinant is called a unique recombinant form (URF). If an inter-subtype recombinant virus succeeds in being transmitted to many people, it becomes one of the circulating strains in the HIV epidemic and is classified as a "circulating recombinant form (CRF)"; at least 89 different CRFs have been identified.[55]

Genetic variability has resulted in multiple HIV-1 variants which are classified into four major phylogenetic groups: M, N, O and P. Group M is responsible for pandemic HIV-1 infection and is further subdivided into 10 recognized, genetically distinct subtypes, labelled A to K. The dominant HIV-1 subtype in the Americas, Western Europe and Australasia is subtype B and the majority of clinical research has been conducted in populations where subtype B predominates. Globally, nearly 50% of all people living with HIV have subtype C which is very common in high prevalence HIV/AIDS areas like Africa.[56] HIV-2 has the same high degree of genetic diversity as HIV-1 with at least 7 HIV-2 subtypes [57] To this time, there is no evidence that any HIV-1 or HIV-2 subtype is more infectious than others. Population mixing means geographical patterns in the distribution of subtypes are continually changing. So far, tests to diagnose HIV and monitor the level of virus in the body are sensitive to the full range of subtypes. The extensive and ongoing genetic heterogeneity of HIV-1 is a major reason for rapid development of drug resistance and for problems with vaccine development.

The chemokine receptor CCR5 is a key player in HIV infection due to its role as the co-receptor for virus entry into CD4+ lymphocytes. A rare, naturally occurring nucleotide deletion in the CCR5 gene has been found to be strongly associated with resistance to HIV infection despite frequent sexual exposure to the virus, as well as long-term control of HIV infection in a subset of HIV seropositive people. These individuals are called long-term non-progressors and have most often been shown to have a rare homozygous deletion of CCR5. This allele was found in 8% of white gay men enrolled in the Multicenter AIDS Cohort Study, but in no participants of African or Asian descent.[58] These "natural" immunities have prompted strategies aimed at achieving anti-HIV humoral responses through CCR5 targeting.[58,59] Specific patterns of the human leukocyte antigen (HLA) system have also been shown to delay the progression of HIV infection. It is likely that other, as yet undiscovered genetic correlates of race, ethnicity and gender that confer resistance or susceptibility will explain some of the variability in HIV infection and disease progression rates.[60]

A final, critical factor in HIV infectivity was first recognized almost twenty years ago – but also twenty years after the first AIDS cases appeared – when HIV-infected individuals were found to harbor hidden reservoirs of HIV-infected cells. These are sites that allow persistence of the virus in a latent, non-replicating state. The reservoir for HIV is primarily in a subset of long-lived CD4+ T-lymphocytes called resting memory cells that are widely distributed throughout the body, primarily in secondary lymph nodes that line the G-I tract but also in the spleen and in the brain. The reservoir is established within the first few days after HIV infection; after initiation of long-term antiviral treatment, there is a fairly rapid initial decline in the size of the reservoir, but subsequently, there is only a very slow decline over the lifetime of infected individuals. HIV reservoirs explain the near impossibility of complete HIV eradication to this time. Ongoing research is focused on developing methods to reverse latency and then rapidly eliminate the reactivated virus population.[61]

The Disease: HIV Infection and the Acquired Immune Deficiency Syndrome

Identifying the human immunodeficiency virus and understanding its unique characteristics dramatically clarified critical components in the pathophysiology of the disease and the course of the epidemic: first, HIV infection is difficult to acquire: it can only be contracted through direct mucous membrane or blood contact with the body fluids – genital fluids, blood or breast milk – of an infected person. HIV is very slow-acting: the extremely long incubation period of the virus is a critical factor in understanding the disease. And, HIV is inexorable: without treatment, the virus progressively destroys the immune system in almost every infected individual, eventually leading to overwhelming opportunistic infections caused by bacteria and fungi, and/or opportunistic neoplasms related to infection with oncoviruses.

HIV is transmitted primarily via unprotected sexual intercourse including vaginal, anal and (very rarely) oral sex; contaminated hypodermic needles in IV drug users; and from mother to child during pregnancy, delivery and/or breastfeeding; infection via contaminated blood products has almost completely disappeared. The principal targets of invading HIV are the cells of the immune system, particularly CD4+ T-cells, whose role is to clear foreign pathogens from the body. After entering a host cell, the virus begins a relentless process of replication during which the immune system of the host organism is progressively destroyed. The human immunodeficiency virus produces up to 10 billion new viral particles and destroys up to 2 billion CD4+ cells per day.[62]

There are three stages of HIV infection: acute infection, clinical latency and AIDS, the acquired immunodeficiency syndrome. Acute HIV infection is characterized by a non-specific flu-like illness with fever, sore throat, large tender lymph nodes and rash. Much less frequently, there are sores in the mouth and on the genitalia, and GI or neurologic symptoms. These initial symptoms are transient, lasting only one or two weeks. During this time, immune function is severely compromised and viral counts are extremely high. Due to their mild and nonspecific character, these symptoms are often not recognized as signs of HIV infection.[63]

The initial symptoms are then followed by a stage called clinical latencyasymptomatic HIV, or chronic HIV which lasts from 3 to over 20(!) years as shown in Figure 6.2. Recognition of the long duration of the incubation period was one of the most startling realizations of the early AIDS epidemic. The original AIDS cases with opportunistic infections presented acutely with overwhelming illness so the question of a significant incubation period for the unknown transmission agent did not arise. Recognition that homosexuals without symptoms already had abnormalities of immune function first introduced the idea of an AIDS prodrome.[9,16] But it was from the transfusion history of individuals with AIDS who were infected by receiving contaminated blood products that a specific date of infection could be identified and the existence of a prolonged incubation period was verified.[64] Ultimately, follow-up of cohorts of individuals at high risk for HIV infection established an average incubation period of approximately 10 years.[65,66] Older age at infection was identified as a significant factor accelerating disease progression based on studies of hemophiliacs.[67]

During this period of viral incubation and clinical latency, viral multiplication and CD4+ cell destruction continue while the individual remains asymptomatic – CD4 lymphocyte counts decline by an average of 50 to 75 cells/μl/year, as shown in Figure 6.2.[64] Historically, the WHO used absolute CD4 lymphocyte count to categorize disease progression:

Stage 0: The time between a negative HIV test followed in less than 180 days by a positive test.

Stage 1: Early disease; No AIDS defining conditions; CD4 count ≥ 500 cells/μl.

Stage 2: Mid-stage disease; No AIDS defining conditions; CD4 count 200 to 500 cells/μl.

Stage 3: Advanced disease: AIDS-defining condition or CD4 count 50–200 cells/μl = AIDS diagnosis per CDC 1993 revised definition. End-Stage: CD4 count <50cells/μl.

Since approximately 1999, assays that measure the number of circulating viral RNA copies in the blood – the viral load – have been used to monitor therapy. CD4 cell count and viral load together are used to estimate prognosis but viral load is the single most powerful predictor of progression from HIV infection to AIDS and of AIDS progression to a terminal stage, with or without treatment.[68,69] Successful treatment aims for a viral load "below the level of detection" (<50 copies/ml).

In the absence of specific treatment, 98% of those infected with HIV will develop full-blown AIDS by 10 years and die within 20 years post infection. During this entire time, testing for HIV-1 RNA can be measured in the plasma and tests for HIV are positive.[68] At the end of the latency stage, patients may experience symptoms like recurrent fever, weight loss, gastrointestinal symptoms like chronic diarrhea, and muscle pain. Between 50% and 70% of people develop a prodrome of generalized, unexplained, non-painful enlargement of more than one group of lymph nodes lasting 3 to 6 months, as recognized by epidemiologists in the first years of the AIDS epidemic.[16] The onset of symptoms – and therefore the shift in diagnosis from HIV infection to AIDS – reflects near-total destruction of the immune system.

AIDS is officially diagnosed when patients develop opportunistic infections or HIV-related malignancies that are normally prevented by the body's immune system – these are labelled AIDS-defining events. Development of AIDS is also defined in terms of immune compromise using a CD4⁺ T cell count below 200 cells per μL without clinical symptoms. Those patients who presented as the first AIDS cases in 1981 were in this late stage at the time they were first seen. Twenty percent of AIDS patients will develop progressive severe weight loss with chronic diarrhea called HIV wasting syndrome, the equivalent of the so-called "slim disease" seen in Africa. Opportunistic infections include a wide array of pathogens but especially pneumocystis and other severe fungal infections in North America and tuberculosis in Africa.[70] This brief statement in no way describes the severity of the symptoms or the degree of suffering associated with full-blown AIDS: pneumonia with pneumocystis is often so overwhelming that patients require respirator support and even with intensive care and aggressive antifungal treatment, acute mortality can still be as high as 40%.[69] Fungal infection of the mouth and esophagus is very common in late stage HIV(+) individuals; the infection is usually secondary to the yeast *Candida albicans* and can cause such severe pain and swallowing difficulty that hospitalization for hydration and pain control is necessary.[71] And alas, surviving one severe opportunistic infection does not prevent a new – and often ultimately fatal – infection in the near future.

Neurologic complications are also common with AIDS, with neurologic symptoms like seizures as the first sign of HIV infection in 10–20% of individuals, while ~60% of patients with advanced HIV disease have clinical evidence of neurologic dysfunction. Autopsy studies of patients with advanced HIV disease show pathologic abnormalities of the nervous system in 75–90% of cases.[72] In the early days of the epidemic in North America – and still in developing countries – opportunistic infections of the central nervous system including cryptococcal meningitis, toxoplasmosis, fulminant bacterial meningitis, neuro-tuberculosis and neurosyphilis caused significant neurologic morbidity and mortality in AIDS patients.

The time course of the CD4+ T cell count and RNA viral load from the time of HIV infection are graphed in Figure 6.2; during the very prolonged latency period lasting 3 to 20 years, the CD4+ T cell count (and therefore immune competence) progressively decreases and viral load (HIV RNA copies) increases but patients are primarily asymptomatic. AIDS-defining events only occur with critical lowering of the CD4+ lymphocyte count.

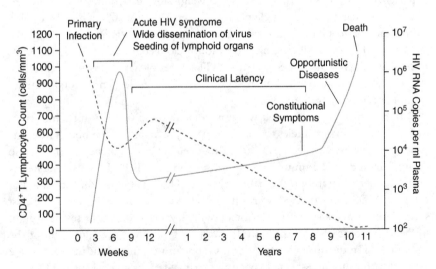

FIGURE 6.2 Timeline of CD4 T-cell and viral-load changes over time in untreated human immunodeficiency virus (HIV) infection.

Source: "The natural course of untreated HIV infection." Fauci AS et al. *Ann Intern Med* 1996; 124:654–663. niaid.nih.gov

People with HIV infection are also at increased risk for viral-induced malignancy (especially Kaposi's sarcoma), non-B cell lymphoma (especially primary central nervous system lymphoma), and invasive cervical cancer. Just as originally reported, Kaposi's sarcoma is the most common HIV-related cancer, occurring in 10–20% of untreated people with HIV infection, most often due to infection with the lymphotropic herpes virus, human herpes virus 8.[73] The second most common HIV-related cancer is lymphoma, with the increased risk related to multiple factors, including the transforming properties of the retrovirus itself, the immunosuppression that results from the disease, and opportunistic infections with lymphotrophic herpes viruses such as Epstein–Barr virus and – again – human herpes virus 8. The heterogeneity in the pathogenesis of lymphoma in HIV-infected patients is reflected in the variety of morphological subtypes. In the early years of the AIDS pandemic, lymphoma was the cause of death in nearly 16% of untreated individuals and was the initial sign of AIDS in 3–4%.[74] Cervical cancer is related to infection with the human papilloma virus (HPV) and is the most common AIDS-related malignancy in women.[75] These three malignancies are considered to be opportunistic neoplasms and are AIDS-defining cancers in HIV-infected patients.

Host genetics are significant co-factors in HIV infection and disease progression, potentially explaining differing rates of infection in different demographic, racial, ethnic and gender groups. As previously described, a minority of white HIV(+) individuals show very delayed progression from HIV infection to AIDS with stable CD4+ counts and low RNA virus loads for many years – perhaps indefinitely – due to a rare homozygous deletion of CCR5, the co-receptor for HIV entry into CD4+ lymphocytes. These individuals are also markedly resistant to HIV-1 infection.[58,59] Even heterozygotes for CCR5 have significantly less rapidly progressive disease. Of equal importance in determining rates of HIV infection and disease progression but much harder to measure and address are societal factors like poverty, racism, structural violence, homophobia, lack of knowledge and delayed/limited access to health care.

The immune response to foreign antigens is regulated by the human leukocyte antigen system (HLA) which is defined by major histocompatibility-complex genes. Another small subset of patients have specific HLA subtypes which are associated with HIV control.[60] By applying molecular and serologic techniques to HIV(+) individuals, HLA combination gene profiles were developed and analyzed statistically in a cohort of HIV(+) men and validated in a second unrelated cohort. In the validation cohort, specific profiles discriminated as much as a six-fold difference between groups in time to development of AIDS.[76] Patients with a high HLA score remained AIDS-free for a median of 10.7 years compared with those a low HLA score group who developed AIDS at a median of 5.2 years after seroconversion.[77]

Testing for HIV Infection

The ability to confirm HIV infection was a critical milestone in the AIDS epidemic. Individuals infected with HIV develop specific antibodies within 3–12 weeks of the initial infection and all the early tests focused on antibody detection. The first test – developed by the Gallo team – used blood and was known as an *enzyme-linked immunosorbent assay* or ELISA test. It was approved for use in 1985. This early test was designed to screen donated blood for possible infection. Although only 142 Americans were known to have contracted AIDS from blood transfusions at that time, public fear of contaminated blood was running high so blood donation centers began using the test in April 1985. By the end of July, only 3 months later, the US blood supply was declared free of HIV.[78]

This first-generation test was not designed for testing of individuals since it had a high false positive rate, not a problem for blood banks but definitely a major concern for frightened individuals. In addition, testing for HIV was associated with the very real threat of stigma and discrimination – being tested at all could be interpreted as a sign of belonging to one of the known high-risk groups which included homosexuals and IV drug users. With pressure to provide accurate testing for individual people, protocols were developed including retesting positive results with an additional procedure to improve accuracy before declaring test results positive. By March 1986, the US government had issued a recommendation that people in all "high-risk groups" seek periodic testing to determine if they were infected with the virus. Laws requiring specific informed consent for HIV testing were developed with mandatory before-and-after counseling and because of privacy concerns, HIV test results were excluded from lab and hospital system records.[79]

Since that time, a series of new testing methods has been developed, including the addition of a recombinant antigen. With each new generation of screening tests, the specificity has improved and the negative testing window post-infection has decreased. The most recent testing iteration was launched in 2015 and uses multiplex analysis to detect both HIV antibody and the selected HIV-1 antigen; the negative window has been reduced to 2 weeks. Independent testing reports 100% sensitivity and 99.5% specificity with this test. Rapid HIV assays for use in situations where results are needed immediately have also been developed using blood, serum or saliva. There are "at home" versions of these tests which have been shown to have 100% sensitivity and up to 96% specificity with results in as little as 30 minutes. In the window period between infection and the development of antibodies, accurate testing requires RNA tests which can detect the virus directly beginning about 10 days after infection. Positive results obtained by either antibody or PCR testing are confirmed by repeat testing. Over time, as public knowledge of HIV/AIDS increased, HIV testing became more accepted with screening results treated like other test results and included in lab and hospital records.[78]

Since 2006, the CDC has recommended routine, provider-initiated HIV screening for all adults with specific recommendations for adolescents and pregnant women.[79] Since 2007, WHO and UNAIDS guidance has also been given for provider-initiated HIV testing and counseling.[80,81] However, not everyone is following these recommendations. In 2014 when an estimated 1.1 million people in the USA were living with HIV, 15% were not diagnosed. Even more concerning, among Americans aged 13–24 with HIV infection, an estimated

44%(!) did not know their diagnosis. Thirty percent of new HIV infections were transmitted by people living with undiagnosed HIV infection.[82] Globally, the World Health Organization (WHO) estimated in 2016 that of 36.7 million people living with HIV, 30% did not know that they were infected with the virus.[83]

Prevention, Treatment and Treatment as Prevention: USA

By the mid-1980s, the AIDS epidemic in the United States had seen dramatic progress with description of the epidemiology of the disease, identification of the causative virus, understanding of the disease pathophysiology and development of a test to diagnose infection. But a diagnosis of AIDS was still, essentially, a death sentence with 16,301 known deaths by 1986. The development of effective methods for prevention and treatment was the dramatic story of the next decade …

Prevention

In the early years when there was no treatment, AIDS in the United States was exclusively associated with homosexuality, drug abuse, sexual transmission and death – AIDS patients were marginalized and ignored. Pictures of skeletal figures with disfiguring skin lesions fueled the prevalent public attitudes of fear, denial and discrimination. At least partially because knowledge was so limited, American health organizations at first declined to supply any information at all. Even health care workers at both the national and community levels were reluctant to care for patients with AIDS.

In this atmosphere, the first attempts at prevention arose from within the gay community where the forefront of early cases appeared. In 1982, Michael Callen and Richard Berkowitz, two gay men living with AIDS in New York City, published *How to Have Sex in an Epidemic*, which presented the concept that condoms could be used to protect against becoming infected and to prevent spreading the disease. That same year, the Sisters of Perpetual Indulgence, a gay activist group in San Francisco, self-published a pamphlet also promoting condom use to prevent infection – these were the first known descriptions of "safe sex" and a giant step forward in HIV prevention.[84] For many years, these two small books were the only available information about prevention of HIV infection.[85] Eventually, multiple HIV seroconversion studies showed that latex condoms are 90–95% effective when used consistently – validating the original, simple and clear "safe sex" message in these two pamphlets.[86]

In March 1983, the CDC issued its first recommendations for prevention:[87]

1. Sexual contact should be avoided with persons known or suspected to have AIDS. Members of high-risk groups should be aware that multiple sexual partners increase the probability of developing AIDS.

2. As a temporary measure, members of groups at increased risk for AIDS should refrain from donating plasma and/or blood. This recommendation includes all individuals belonging to such groups, even though many individuals are at little risk of AIDS. Centers collecting plasma and/or blood should inform potential donors of this recommendation. The Food and Drug Administration (FDA) is preparing new recommendations for manufacturers of plasma derivatives and for establishments collecting plasma or blood. This is an interim measure to protect recipients of blood products and blood until specific laboratory tests are available.

3. Studies should be conducted to evaluate screening procedures for their effectiveness in identifying and excluding plasma and blood with a high probability of transmitting AIDS. These procedures should include specific laboratory tests as well as careful histories and physical examinations.

4. Physicians should adhere strictly to medical indications for transfusions and autologous blood transfusions are encouraged.

5. Work should continue toward development of safer blood products for use by hemophilia patients. The National Hemophilia Foundation has made specific recommendations for management of patients with hemophilia.

In retrospect, these were extremely conservative recommendations given the gravity of the situation: since 1979, the number of patients diagnosed by the strict CDC definition had doubled every six months. Approximately 50 new cases of AIDS were being registered each week by the CDC and more than 2000 cases had been reported by the end of 1983. Despite this exponential increase, abstinence was the only recommendation for individuals "known or suspected to have AIDS" as was "awareness that multiple sexual partners increased the probability of developing AIDS"; there was no mention of condoms. Individuals from groups at increased risk for AIDS – not named – were asked to not donate blood and blood banks were tasked with communicating this message; but there was no recommendation for blood donation centers to question potential donors themselves. With no public education program, it was unclear how this information would reach the groups that needed it. Development of AIDS screening tests was recommended – who could disagree with that! – and doctors were asked to limit blood transfusions as much as possible; patients were encouraged to donate their own blood prior to surgical procedures with infusion of donated blood as needed. Hemophiliacs were referred to hematology recommendations developed specifically for them.[87] There was a strong sense of handwringing with no practical, evidence-based guidelines for prevention.

As described, the original test for HIV infection was released in 1985. Its limitations aside, the test was greeted enthusiastically by blood banks, health care providers and frightened individuals in high-risk groups. By March 1986, the CDC had issued a recommendation that people in all "high-risk groups seek periodic testing" to determine if they were infected with the virus. At that time, HIV testing required specific informed consent and test results were excluded from lab and hospital records.[78]

The first official public health response to the AIDS epidemic occurred in 1986 following years of silence during which federal funding for public health had been repeatedly cut, effectively limiting any potential response of agencies like the CDC or the NIH to the emerging threat. Open discrimination against people with AIDS was the common public attitude: they were routinely evicted from their homes, expelled from their classrooms and fired from their jobs. As the crisis unfolded, many doctors and nurses openly proclaimed they would not treat a patient with AIDS because of personal risk and the obligation to protect their own families. The response of the government and of elected officials encouraged this marginalization and discrimination against AIDS patients. President Reagan did not use the term AIDS in public until 1985, more than 4 years into the pandemic; by that time, there were more than 12,000 reported cases in the USA with 6,000 deaths and AIDS had spread to every populated continent on the planet. Even then, he questioned the safety of casual contact, specifically opposing allowing children with AIDS to continue in school, something already defined as safe by his own governmental medical experts.[88]

For years, Reagan prevented his Surgeon General, C. Everett Koop, from speaking out about AIDS. In 1986 when Koop was finally allowed to address the epidemic, his *Surgeon General's Report on Acquired Immune Deficiency Syndrome* used clear, candid language to review the ways the virus was transmitted and the disease symptoms. The report stated explicitly that AIDS could not be spread casually, reassuring the public that children attending schools with HIV(+) students were safe. It called for a nationwide education campaign with emphasis on early sex education in schools, increased use of condoms and voluntary HIV testing.[89] In 1988, Koop took the unprecedented action of mailing AIDS information directly to every US household, explicitly recommending the use of condoms as a highly effective defense against HIV infection. This report was a decisive advance, educating the public about how HIV is transmitted and the use of safe sex practices to prevent it. Surgeon General Koop helped redefine AIDS as a preventable disease and ultimately allowed the full integration of HIV(+) individuals into society.

Following Dr. Koop's lead, a national effort to educate the public about HIV and AIDS was launched in 1987 and the CDC created a comprehensive AIDS information resource, the CDC National AIDS Hotline and National AIDS Information Clearinghouse. Comprehensive school-based HIV education to inform and educate young people began in 1987, and funding for national, regional and community-based organizations began in 1988. The first research on effective behavior interventions to reduce transmission of HIV among sex partners started in the mid-1980s. Ultimately, selected behavioral interventions, including school-based programs, peer-to-peer interventions, strategies for parent-to-child communication and personalized risk-reduction strategies proved to be moderately effective in promoting behaviors that prevent HIV infection.[90]

Over time, public knowledge about AIDS increased and attitudes improved in response to advocacy of groups like ACTUP and celebrities like Elizabeth Taylor and Elizabeth Glazer who campaigned for acceptance and treatment.[88] Taylor founded *The Elizabeth Taylor Foundation*, to provide support services for people with HIV/AIDS and prevention education for populations most in need. In 1991, Magic Johnson, arguably the most famous basketball player in the world at the time, announced that he was HIV positive. His preseason bombshell made headlines worldwide. Phil Wilson, head of the Black AIDS Institute, was the AIDS coordinator for the city of Los Angeles at the time. He says Johnson's announcement shut down his switchboard. "It was the single most powerful event at the time to raise awareness about AIDS in black America." Kenny Smith, then of the rival Houston Rockets said, "Before then, people were ostracized, in my estimation, for having the disease. Magic was the person, because his name reached far beyond sports, to make HIV acceptable, more a disease than a mark of shame." Johnson went on to establish the *Magic Johnson Foundation*, dedicated to AIDS-related research and outreach.[91] He has remained very involved in AIDS activism, especially education about the risk for heterosexuals and African-Americans, launching the "I Stand with Magic" partnership to promote HIV testing and sustained treatment adherence for HIV positive individuals at a meeting of the National Minority AIDS Council in 2006.[92] Twenty-five years after the announcement that he was HIV positive, Rolling Stone wrote,

> … some moments truly transcend sports and shake the world. Great plays or broken records might resonate with fans, but there are usually only a handful of situations that can define a decade. We like to think that athletes do things that can change the world, but very few do. Earvin "Magic" Johnson's November 7th, 1991 announcement that he was HIV positive was one of those moments.[93]

Celebrity activists like Taylor and Johnson highlighted injustice and prejudice against people with HIV/AIDS, demanded increased government resources to fight the disease, established private foundations to support research and treatment and accelerated the slow process of changing public attitudes about HIV/AIDS.

New HIV infections in the United States peaked at 150,000/year in the mid-1980s with a gradual subsequent decline. However, despite education and prevention efforts, there were 50,000 new cases every year from 1992 to 2015. Although the CDC still only mandates annual HIV testing for gay and bisexual men, they recommend screening for STDs and HIV every 3 to 6 months for individuals who have more than one partner or have had casual sex with people they don't know.

After observational studies suggested a potential benefit of male circumcision in preventing HIV infection, a randomized controlled trial was performed in heterosexual men in South Africa. After a mean follow-up of 18 months, the relative risk of HIV infection in the circumcised group was 0.40 – less than half – compared to the control group, an impressive 60% protection rate.[94,95] Results of male circumcision show equivocal benefits in preventing homosexual acquisition of HIV.[96] Since 2007, WHO/UNAIDS has recommended male circumcision as an efficacious intervention for HIV prevention in countries and regions with heterosexual epidemics, high HIV prevalence and low male circumcision prevalence. Since 2014, the CDC recommends circumcision in male patients and in newborn males as effective prevention against infection with HIV and other STDs.[97]

Treatment

In the early years, a diagnosis of AIDS was essentially a death sentence because patients presented very late in the course of the disease with overwhelming infections when the immune system had been essentially destroyed. The only available treatment was for the existing, often rampant, infections and most AIDS patients died within months of presentation. As the critical role of immune compromise was better understood, anti-viral agents were prescribed but at that time, these were few in number and experience in the context of a disease like AIDS was non-existent. Recognition that prophylactic antibiotics could reduce/ prevent *pneumocystis* pneumonia led to CDC guidelines but not until 1989 with a revision in 1992.[98,99]

Early clinical tests showed that a drug called Azido-thymidine or zoluvidine (AZT), which had been developed in the 1960s as an anti-cancer agent, slowed the progress of HIV in humans. At that time, the drug approval process in the USA was extremely slow and since AZT was not FDA-approved, access was restricted to patients enrolled in clinical trials. Outraged by federal regulations and policies that slowed the development, testing and distribution of drugs to treat HIV/AIDS, activists and community-based organizations were galvanized to take action. Their public demonstrations ultimately helped change the way clinicians, researchers, drug companies, and local, state and national governments addressed the HIV/AIDS epidemic and by extension, drugs to treat any disease.[100] (For more on this, see the Historic Perspective section at the end of this chapter.)

Meanwhile AZT had been shown to inhibit reverse transcriptase – the critical retrovirus enzyme – in a mouse retrovirus model and with its precise mode of action known, the drug could be studied in detail. A randomized clinical trial was begun and six months after initiation, only one member of the study group receiving AZT had died, compared to 19 deaths in the control group. The trial was halted and AZT was approved as treatment for HIV and AIDS in 1987 – six years after the first cases appeared.[101] Although its arrival was greeted with great optimism, resistance to AZT was found to develop rapidly. In 1990, the second drug for the treatment of AIDS, dideoxyinosine (ddI), was made available to people with AIDS, even though only preliminary tests had been completed and one year later, a third drug, dideoxycytidine (ddC), was authorized by the FDA for use in patients intolerant of AZT.[102,103]

AZT, ddl and ddC are all nucleoside analog reverse transcriptase inhibitors. After 1991, another new class of anti-HIV drugs, the non-nucleoside analog reverse transcriptase inhibitors, was developed – these are more quickly activated once inside the bloodstream. Next were protease inhibitors which prevent an already infected cell from producing more copies of HIV. Each of these drugs appeared to be partly efficacious, with great variation in response between individuals. Despite this proliferation of drug options, the standard antiviral therapy for HIV-infected individuals between 1986 and 1995 for the most part remained treatment with a single drug, followed by another when resistance developed. In 1992, the FDA approved the use of combination therapy with ddC and AZT for patients with advanced HIV infection and clinical or immunological deterioration, the first successful use of combination drug therapy for the treatment of AIDS.[104]

Increased appreciation of the capacity of HIV for rapid mutation associated with development of drug resistance led to the emergence of combination therapy as a primary treatment approach, with drugs from two or more classes used simultaneously. This switch to combination therapy had dramatic effects because in most cases, the virus remained sensitive to at least one of the drugs used. When nucleoside analog drugs, the non-nucleoside analog drugs, and the protease inhibitors were used together, the combination was referred to as "highly active anti-retroviral therapy" or HAART.[105] As shown in Figure 6.3, introduction of

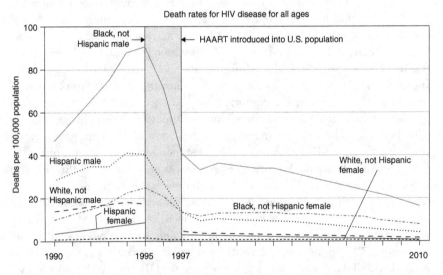

FIGURE 6.3 Death rate for HIV/AIDS for individuals of all ages by race/ethnicity and gender after introduction of highly active antiretroviral therapy (HAART). This dramatic change was the first decrease in mortality since the epidemic began in 1981.

Source: CDC/National Center for Health Statistics, United States, 2013. CDC.gov

HAART in 1995 led to a dramatic reduction in deaths from AIDS in the United States, the first decrease in mortality since the epidemic began

In addition to the decrease in death rates for all groups, this graph also reveals chronic disparities between Black and Hispanic individuals of either sex compared with Whites. These differences reflect ongoing structural barriers including not just race/ethnicity but also poverty, limited or difficult access to health care, lack of HIV education, fear and persistent stigma associated with homosexuality or drug use. Socio-economic barriers like these can result in delayed diagnosis and treatment initiation, and interruption and/or cessation of treatment, manifest as lower rates of linkage to care and viral suppression, and higher rates of death in race- and sex-defined, vulnerable populations.[105–107]

Over time, particular combinations of drugs were shown to have the most dramatic effects, reducing the amount of virus in the blood and increasing the number of CD4+ cells. By the end of 1996, the number of Americans dying from AIDS had declined 23% from the previous year, attributed primarily to the success of the new combination therapies. By the start of 1997, HAART – now cART/ART – combination therapy had become the standard of care for HIV-infected individuals with signs of significant immunosuppression. New drugs have been added to the ART armamentarium over time, with integrase strand transfer inhibitor (INSTI)-based regimens now recommended as part of initial therapy for most people with HIV.

★★★★★★★★

In all, the simultaneous treatment of people with HIV with different classes of antiviral drugs was the most significant scientific advance in the history of the AIDS pandemic. Now almost 20 years after its introduction, combination antiviral therapy has demonstrated impressive, sustained ability to control progressive disease in HIV-infected individuals. Along the way, treatment has evolved from the early "grueling regimens with high pill burden, inconvenient dosing, treatment-limiting toxicities, food and drug interactions, incomplete viral suppression and emergence of drug resistance to manageable one or two pill, once daily regimens that can be initiated in early HIV disease and continued with control of viral replication over an individual's lifetime."[104]

With the possible exception of two HIV(+) individuals who received stem cell transplants because of cancer, complete elimination, or "eradication," of HIV from an infected individual has never been achieved. Antiviral medications still allow full or partial resistance to develop with missed medication doses, irregular use, or incomplete doses, and cross-resistance is common so strict adherence to the prescribed drug regimen is necessary. Disparities in access to care persist in key affected populations. Nonetheless, the overall impact of combination antiretroviral therapy (cART or ART – the new acronyms for HAART) has been overwhelmingly positive.

Treatment as Prevention

With time and experience, the approach to initiation of anti-retroviral treatment – cART/ART – evolved. Measuring the viral load of circulating viral RNA copies in the blood was used to monitor therapy, and CD4 cell count and viral load together were shown to provide the most accurate prognosis of future outcomes. Successful treatment often led to a viral load "below the level of detection" (<50 copies/ml), indicating that the concentration of HIV in the blood was very low. Based on observations that rates of HIV transmission paralleled the viral load, the risk of infecting others was thought to potentially be very low in this situation.

Landmark research addressed this by investigating initiation of ART in healthy HIV(+) people with CD4 counts above 350 cells per cubic millimeter – the internationally recognized level below which ART initiation was recommended at that time. This was an international multi-center trial which included sites in the United States, Brazil, Thailand, India and multiple countries in Africa with two very important results: for HIV(-) partners, preventive ART significantly limited transmission of the virus by 96%. In the HIV(+) individual, early ART preserved CD4+ counts, delayed progression to AIDS and significantly decreased AIDS related outcomes.[108] Subsequently, a second large, multinational trial demonstrated a further reduction in morbidity and mortality among HIV(+) individuals who had normal CD4 counts, >500 cells/mm^3, and received ART immediately versus delayed initiation when CD4 counts fell below 350 cells/mm^3.[109,110] Finally, The PARTNER study of more than 1,000 mixed-status couples – one HIV(+), one HIV(-), 60% heterosexual, 40% homosexual – found *no* HIV transmissions with condomless sex when the viral load of the positive partner was very low, less than 200 copies/ml.[111]

This series of important studies has resulted in the current approach to use of ART – treatment as prevention (TasP): ART should begin as soon as HIV infection is confirmed, regardless of symptoms or timing, and for all AIDS patients, regardless of CD4 cell count or ongoing opportunistic infections.[112]

Incredibly, analysis of long-term multinational cohort studies now shows that HIV(+) individuals who started therapy after 2008 and had only a minimally depressed CD4+ count at the end of their first year on cART have a normal life expectancy.[113] There is still important work to be done since the survival benefits do not affect all HIV(+) individuals equally.[114] Long-term survival with HIV infection is dependent on early diagnosis, linkage to and retention in care, and adherence to treatment and these factors differ significantly by HIV transmission group. Specifically, life expectancies are lower in all periods for individuals with a history of injection drug use. Possible reasons for these differences include increased comorbidity with greater non-AIDS related mortality, as well as challenges with ART adherence, active drug use, hepatitis C co-infection, housing instability and lower socioeconomic status. Differences in life expectancy by race are also evident, with white individuals having higher life expectancies in all periods. These differences may be reflective of underlying discrepancies in socioeconomic conditions causing limited/difficult access to care and problems with adherence, absent or limited health insurance coverage, fear of drug side-effects and/or stigma and fear of social disclosure. The gap in life expectancy between white and non-white individuals has decreased substantially, from 23 years in 2000–02 to 8.5 years in 2006–07.[105–107] The disparity in observed life expectancy at age 20 narrowed for black versus white MSM from 33.0 vs. 52.3 years in 2012 to 50.9 vs 60.3 years in 2015.[106] Additional differences in life expectancies are associated with CD4 cell count at ART initiation – the lower the CD4 count even within the accepted range – the lower the life expectancy. Again, lower CD4 count at cART initiation can reflect delayed diagnosis and/or reduced access to care. These findings support the earliest possible identification of HIV infection and initiation of anti-retroviral therapy in all HIV positive individuals.[108–110,113] Even with recognized discrepancies in life expectancy, the results of early initiation of cART are truly amazing.[113,114]

Treatment as prevention (TasP) has the potential to radically change the global outcome of HIV infection, significantly reducing population levels of HIV transmission. However, its effectiveness relies on universal HIV testing and lifelong adherence to treatment since sustained viral suppression is the foundation for immune recovery, optimal health and prevention of resistance and transmission. Monitoring with viral load and CD4 cell count is recommended with treatment change based on these results in countries where these tests are available. HIV testing is widely available in the United States and AIDS programs actively advocate for universal testing with regular periodic testing for high-risk groups. Drug resistance is still an important cause of treatment failure regardless of the clinical setting. As HIV multiplies in the body, the virus mutates and new strains that develop while an individual is taking AR medications can be drug resistant. Drug-resistance testing is used to select an appropriate ART regimen. Careful medication adherence reduces the risk of drug resistance.

There have been other advances in preventing HIV infection in specific circumstances. Beginning in 2014, the CDC recommended prophylactic anti-retroviral treatment (PrEP) for individuals who are HIV negative but at high risk for HIV infection. Clinical trials in high risk groups show that daily use of a two-drug combination pill containing tenofovir and emtricitabine (called Truvada) substantially decreases the risk of infection and the viral load in those who do become infected. For example, among gay and bisexual men with detectable drug levels, PrEP reduced the risk of infection by as much as 92%.[115–117] In 2018, after a randomized trial showed similar positive results for PrEP in adolescents, the FDA approved Truvada for use in teenagers.

For people who need to prevent HIV after a single high-risk event of potential HIV exposure – such as unprotected sex, needle-sharing injection drug use, sexual assault or workplace accident – post-exposure prophylaxis, or PEP is recommended.[118] PEP should begin as soon as possible after exposure and must begin within 72 hours; treatment consists of a 28-day course of ART. If started within 72 hours after exposure and with 28-day adherence, PEP can reduce the risk of HIV infection by over 80%.

****

Evolving Epidemiology of HIV/AIDS in the United States: Implementation of Prevention and Treatment Advances

During the first four years of the epidemic, knowledge about AIDS increased dramatically as the epidemiology of the disease was described with identification of specific high-risk groups. As prevention and treatment regimens began to appear, the epidemiology of each high-risk group evolved independently, based on their unique demographics, their complex of social and economic determinants of health and the characteristics of the virus.

Sexual Transmission: Gay and Bisexual Men

Young homosexual men were the first group identified with AIDS and to this day, men who have sex with men (MSM) remain the group most frequently infected in North and South America and in Western and Central Europe. In 2016, the CDC reported that gay and bisexual men accounted for 67% of all HIV diagnoses and 82% of diagnoses among males in the United States.[119] MSM represent a much smaller proportion of new HIV diagnoses globally but even worldwide, this group continues to define a high-risk population.

As previously described, the first attempts at prevention arose from within the gay community in the United States with publication of information that condoms could be used as protection against becoming infected and spreading the epidemic. Multiple HIV seroconversion studies subsequently showed that latex condoms are 90–95% effective when used consistently.[84–86]

The story of the intense involvement of the American gay population in the early years of the epidemic is effectively told in many settings but perhaps nowhere better than in Randy Shilts' book *And the Band Played On*.[88,120] The work of gay advocacy groups and the involvement of committed celebrities were critical components in prevention efforts in the early years of the epidemic. However, until successful combination anti-retroviral therapy (HAART/cART/ART) was validated in 1995, HIV infection and AIDS cases continued to increase every year with MSM remaining the largest group of individuals in both categories. A peak of new AIDS diagnoses in 1993 was associated with expansion of the CDC surveillance case definition to include all HIV-infected individuals with severe immune-suppression (CD4+T-lymphocytes < 200/uL/ CD4+ T-lymphocyte percentage less than 14); or with pulmonary tuberculosis (TB), recurrent pneumonia or invasive cervical cancer.[121]

Between 1995 and 2005, there were consistent declines in AIDS incidence and deaths in all groups including MSM in response to the introduction of ART as shown in Figure 6.3.[122] By the end of 2000, the CDC reported there had been 774,467 people diagnosed with AIDS in the United States and 58% of these had died. There were more than 300,000 people living with AIDS, the highest ever reported, reflecting the large number being successfully treated with ART. Of these, 79% were men and 46% were infected through male-to-male sex.

In the early 1980s, most AIDS cases occurred among white males but cases among Blacks increased steadily and by the turn of the century, minority MSM emerged as the largest proportion of MSM with HIV/AIDS.[123] Socioeconomic factors like isolation due to the stigma of homosexuality and homophobia in some minorities and geographic areas, poverty and unemployment, and lack of access to health care were associated with high rates of HIV risk behaviors among minority MSM and served as barriers to accessing early HIV diagnosis and treatment.[124,125] With ongoing improvements in treatment of HIV positive individuals, AIDS deaths continued to decrease and the number of people living with AIDS continued to increase. Based on 2016–2020 statistics, gay and bisexual men remained the sub-population most affected by HIV in the United States, accounting for 71% of new HIV diagnoses: Black/African American MSM accounted for 26% of new HIV diagnoses and 39% of diagnoses among all MSM; Hispanic/Latino MSM made up 21% of new HIV diagnoses and 31% of diagnoses among all MSM.[126–129]

In theory, gay and bisexual men and their partners – both male and female – will be the groups to benefit most from initiation of combination ART as soon as HIV infection is confirmed.[107–110] The potential of ART to radically change the course of the HIV/AIDS pandemic relies on universal HIV testing and life-long adherence to treatment, both major challenges in the context of groups like young MSM and their partners who are among the most vulnerable to HIV infection. Innovative strategies are needed to increase the number of these at-risk individuals using safe sex methods and routinely testing for HIV infection.[130,131]

Annual new HIV infections in the United States have decreased by more than two-thirds since the height of the epidemic in the mid-1980s when there were more than 150,000 new infections every year. However, a 2016 study in 20 major US cities found that about 36% of black, gay and bisexual men were infected with HIV, compared to 22% of MSM overall.[131] A more effective approach to HIV prevention, diagnosis and treatment in MSM and their partners from every background is needed.

HIV/AIDS in Women

After the first cases of heterosexually acquired AIDS were reported at the end of 1981 in young women with sexual partners who had AIDS, the number of females with AIDS steadily increased. The CDC added "female sexual partners of males with AIDS" as a risk category for AIDS in 1983 reflecting understanding that receptive vaginal sex was a high-risk setting for HIV infection. The percentage of new AIDS cases attributed to heterosexual contact with HIV(+) individuals increased steadily from 13% in 1983 to 28% in 1988. From the beginning, HIV infection in women disproportionately affected racial/ethnic minority groups: in 1988, the cumulative incidence of AIDS attributable to heterosexual contact per million population was over 11 times greater for blacks and Hispanics than for whites.[132]

Over the next decade, AIDS cases in women continued to account for a significant proportion of all AIDS cases in the United States. By the end of 1990, AIDS cases among women accounted for 11% of all reported cases in adults, an increase of 29% in women, compared with 18% in men. Among all cases of AIDS in women, 85% occurred among women of childbearing age. Approximately one fourth of these women were only 20–29 years of age at the time of diagnosis; many were probably infected as teenagers. By 1993, AIDS was the leading cause of death for African American women aged 25–44 years.[133]

Over time, the number of new annual HIV diagnoses in women progressively declined. From latest CDC data, in 2020, 30,635 people aged 13 and older received an HIV diagnosis in the USA with adult and adolescent women accounting for 19% of new HIV diagnoses: 59% were African American; 20% white; and 16% Hispanic/Latina.[127–130,134–136] This increased risk among racial/ethnic minorities reflects a multitude of unequal socio-economic burdens including poverty, violent crime, social disorder, incarceration rates, and male-to-female sex ratios among US black adults.

Women urgently need more options for HIV prevention: currently available forms are limited and many women are unable to negotiate condom use with male sexual partners. Pre- and post-exposure prophylaxis are highly effective but problems with access, availability and daily pill compliance remain challenging. A vaginal ring which continuously releases the anti-HIV drug dapivirine has been found to be highly effective in preventing HIV infection.[137] Additional options for safe and effective prevention of HIV infection for women are under investigation.

Injection Drug Use (IDU)

In December 1981, just six months after the first AIDS reports in gay men, AIDS cases were reported for the first time in men and women who were intravenous drug users (IDUs).[4] By the end of 1985, 17% of all AIDS cases in the United States occurred in IDUs.[138] In this group, identified risk factors for HIV infection were shared syringes and other injection equipment, especially in communal settings like "shooting galleries"; the number of drug injections/month; and high-risk sexual behavior under the influence of drugs or in exchange for drugs. For women, the number of heterosexual partners who used drugs was also significantly associated with HIV infection.[139]

Prevention efforts have focused on these risk factors and from the beginning, these have been community-based, using mobile vans, storefronts and street corners to directly reach known at-risk populations and connect them to prevention programs, HIV testing, and care and treatment services. Needle and syringe programs that provide or exchange sterile equipment have been consistently shown to be highly effective at reducing new HIV infections, often also providing counseling, safer-sex education, HIV testing and referrals to drug treatment programs. The first comprehensive needle exchange programs were established in North America in 1988. Despite their proven success, there has never been consistent federal funding for needle/syringe supply programs so their distribution is inconsistent, based on state funding and community support.[140] Medication-assisted addiction treatment programs where drugs like methadone are substituted for opioids are effective treatment for drug dependence, eliminating risk behaviors associated with injection drug use and preventing HIV transmission. IDUs who do not enter addiction treatment programs are up to 6 times more likely to become infected with HIV. Again, funding is a critical deterrent to access to treatment for drug dependence.[141] HIV infection in IDUs is an ongoing problem: with the recent dramatic increase in opioid abuse in the United States, there have been community outbreaks of HIV infection related to injection of these drugs.[142]

Overall, the combination of education and intervention has significantly decreased the proportion of new HIV infections in IDUs in the United States. By 2020, people who inject drugs accounted for 7% of new HIV infections in the USA; another 3% combined homosexual behavior with drug injection.[127–130,143]

Transfusion of HIV-Contaminated Blood and Blood Products

Individuals with hemophilia who became infected with HIV were critical in understanding the pattern of HIV infection, providing the first suggestion that the then-theoretical agent that caused AIDS might be transmissible in blood products.[12] Testing of frozen stored plasma in a single-center series revealed that the first HIV infections in this group occurred as early as 1978.[144] Prospective follow-up of a cohort of 310 hemophiliacs with HIV seroconversion definitively confirmed the long incubation period between infection and the appearance of AIDS. The incidence rate of AIDS after HIV infection was found to be directly related to age, ranging from an average 8-year cumulative rate of 13% for individuals less than 17 years to 44% for those over 35.[144] Because of widespread prior contamination of blood factor concentrate, the HIV infection rate in the earliest years of the AIDS epidemic was higher among hemophiliacs than among any other group. From the late 1970s to the mid-1980s, about half of all people with hemophilia became infected with HIV after receiving contaminated blood products – among those with severe hemophilia who required repeated clotting factor infusions, an estimated 90% were infected with HIV. Ultimately, ~6000 American hemophiliacs and at least 8000 globally were infected with HIV by receiving contaminated clotting factor transfusions.

Despite suggestive guidance from the CDC, the plasma fractionation industry failed to initiate any approach to identifying infected blood donations so new infections continued until 1985 when the HIV screening test was validated.[145]

Universal screening of the blood supply dramatically reduced the risk of HIV transmission through clotting factor transfusions. Since 1987, specific inactivation methods have been used to effectively eliminate all viral contaminants in clotting factor products with no further transmissions of HIV through clotting factor products in the United States.

The history of HIV infection following transfusion with contaminated blood parallels the story in hemophiliacs. The first case was recognized in December 1982 when a 20-month-old baby was diagnosed with AIDS; as a newborn, he had received a platelet transfusion from a homosexual who was well when he donated blood but who subsequently died of AIDS.[18,19] Within months, there were multiple reports of transfusion-associated AIDS cases, many with confirmation that transfused blood components were from donors with AIDS.[146,147] At this early stage in the epidemic, it was these reports combined with the evidence from hemophiliacs that confirmed that the AIDS agent was blood-borne and could be transmitted by transfusion of blood and blood products. The CDC initiated official meetings with the blood services community to address this issue but despite these efforts and mounting concern on the part of many scientists and physicians, the blood donor industry was skeptical, reportedly because the number of AIDS cases was small compared to the enormous number of transfusions received, and concern that the volunteer donor supply would be interrupted if any screening procedures were put in place.[145] The CDC's 1983 official recommendations for the prevention of AIDS did include a specific recommendation that members of "high risk" groups should not donate blood but no surrogate screening procedures or direct questioning of donors about potential risk categories was recommended.[86] Spurred by news reports of AIDS from transfusions, blood donation before a planned procedure to be used for autologous transfusion, and directed donations from family members became very popular during this time period. Mathematical projections estimate that approximately 12,000 people in the United States acquired a transfusion-associated HIV infection between 1978 and 1984.[147,148] When the ELISA test for identification of HIV infection was adopted as the universal standard for screening donated blood in 1985, there was an immediate, precipitous decline in transfusion-associated HIV infection.[78] By 1995, less than one in half a million screened blood donations were estimated to be contaminated with HIV.[149]

Since then, the risk for transfusion-transmitted HIV infection has been almost eliminated, estimated conservatively to be one in 1.5 million. Very rarely, an individual donates blood during the window period after HIV infection and the donated blood tests positive. The last time this was reported in the United States was 2008.[150]

Babies with HIV/AIDS: Maternal-Infant Transmission of HIV

In 1982, the CDC first reported cases of AIDS in infants and young children whose mothers had AIDS included 6 young children who died with opportunistic infections and unusual cellular immune-deficiencies like those seen in adults with AIDS. The reports suggested the horrible possibility of transmission of the still unknown AIDS agent from mother to child, in utero or shortly after birth.[20] After the 1985 development of antibody testing, a more accurate picture of perinatally-acquired HIV infection emerged. In this time period, the incidence of HIV/AIDS in women was increasing exponentially with two major sources of infection: injected drug use and sex with partners infected with HIV. Eventually, it became clear that 15–40% of infants born to HIV-infected mothers become infected, either in utero, during labor and delivery and/or by breast-feeding.[151] Mothers with high viral counts and/or low CD4+ counts were found to have significantly higher rates of HIV infection in their babies.[152]

The natural history of vertically-acquired HIV infection in children is extraordinarily variable with a wide spectrum of age at symptom onset and clinical manifestations. In 15–20% of infected infants, severe immunodeficiency develops in the first year of life with failure to thrive and recurrent serious infections and/or encephalopathy, predicting early mortality. In a small subset – often those who are infected after birth by breast-feeding – the children can be completely well for several years before recurrent infections develop, reflecting immune compromise. Overall, without anti-viral treatment, median survival ranges from 75 to 90 months with only 70% of children surviving to 6 years of age.[153]

In the early days, diagnosing HIV infection in infants and children was challenging because antibodies cross the placenta so testing newborns was not an effective way to detect those who were infected. The only recommendation was that pregnant women in high-risk groups be offered counseling and voluntary HIV testing.[154] Using this voluntary system, a majority of HIV(+) pregnant women were not identified and the number of children with perinatally acquired HIV infection increased dramatically. In 1993, the CDC estimated that 14,920 HIV-infected infants had been born in the United States; 84% of these cases were African-American or Hispanic infants.[155]

With no effective treatment, management was limited to prophylactic gamma globulin injections and broad-spectrum antibiotic prophylaxis. Over time, *Pneumocystis carinii* pneumonia (PCP) – the same rare presentation seen in the original AIDS cases in young homosexual males – proved to be the most common opportunistic infection in American children with AIDS and in 1991, the first guidelines for PCP prophylaxis were published, based on age-associated CD4+ cell counts.[156] The guidelines had little impact on the dismal prognosis of these young children so they were revised, recommending specific PCP prophylaxis beginning at 4–6 weeks of age in all HIV-infected infants. At this time, AIDS was the seventh leading cause of death among children 1 to 4 years of age.[157]

From 1985 to 1999, AIDS cases among children declined 81% but with women accounting for 23% of AIDS cases in the USA (compared with 7% in 1985) and one-third of new HIV infections occurring among women, the problem of perinatal infection remained an ongoing challenge.[158] A major breakthrough occurred in 1994 when a three-part zidovudine (AZT) regimen given during pregnancy and labor to HIV-infected mothers and to their newborn infants reduced HIV transmission by almost 70%.[159] This was immediately recommended by the CDC and the US Public Health Service along with a repeat recommendation for voluntary HIV testing of all women during pregnancy.1[60–162] There was a steep and sustained decline in new HV/AIDS cases in infants and children in the United States from this point forward. Universal HIV testing is now recommended in all pregnancies and prenatal testing has increased dramatically. The combination of prenatal HIV testing, cART and avoidance of breastfeeding has dramatically decreased the incidence of new, perinatally acquired HIV cases in the United States every year since 1995. Perinatal HIV infections decreased 41% from 2015 to 2019, with only 84 cases of perinatal HIV infection in 2019.16[3]

HIV Infection/AIDS in the USA (2016–2020)

- At year-end 2019, an estimated 1.2 million people in the United States aged 13 and older were infected with HIV, including an estimated 13% who were unaware of their diagnosis.[127–130]
- Annual new HIV infections in the United States have decreased by more than two-thirds since the height of the epidemic in the mid-1980s when there were more than 150,000 new infections every year. From latest CDC data, 30,635 people aged 13 and older received an HIV diagnosis in 2020. About 65.9% received some HIV care and 56.8% were virally suppressed or undetectable.
- Gay and bisexual men (MSM) remain the sub-population most affected by HIV in the United States, accounting for 71% of new HIV diagnoses in 2020. Black/ African American MSM accounted for 26% (8,064) of new HIV diagnoses and 39% of diagnoses among all MSM; Hispanic/Latino MSM made up 21% (6,359) of new HIV diagnoses and 31% of diagnosis among all MSM.
- People who inject drugs accounted for 7% of new HIV infections in the USA in 2020.
- From 2016 to 2019, HIV diagnoses from heterosexual contact decreased 13% overall, constituting 22% of HIV diagnoses, 7% male and 15% female.
- Women accounted for 19% of the 36,801 new HIV diagnoses in the US in 2019; 86% were attributed to heterosexual sex and 14% to injection drug use.
- Teens and young adults continue to be at risk, with people aged 13 to 34 accounting for more than half (57%) of new diagnoses. People aged 25 to 34 represented 37% of those newly diagnosed. Among young people, gay and bisexual men and minorities have been particularly affected.
- In 2020, there were 18,489 deaths among adults and adolescents with diagnosed HIV infection in the United States. These deaths may be due to any cause, including COVID-19.
- As of 2020, about 700,000 people have died of HIV/AIDS in the United States since the beginning of the HIV/AIDS epidemic.[130]

****

Global HIV/AIDS

History of Global Spread

In 1982, the first recognized AIDS case from outside the United States was reported in France.[164] Early in the pandemic, European doctors had recognized and reported episodes of illness corresponding to the description of AIDS which had occurred before 1979 in Europeans and Africans.[165–168] By June 30, 1983, the WHO was aware of 153 European AIDS cases, predominantly from Belgium, France, West Germany, Switzerland, Britain and Denmark. The same risk groups as in American cases were identified in the majority of patients but a subset were Africans from sub-Saharan Africa and visitors to that area who had subsequently relocated to Europe.[169] The disease reports of the Africa-related cases matched the AIDS definition from the CDC but the epidemiologic profile did not match the profile defined by US cases – instead, cases occurred equally in men and women and there was no history of homosexuality, drug addiction or blood transfusions.[170,171] By November 1983, 22% of all European AIDS cases were among people originally from sub-Saharan Africa.[172] Based on personal experience, Chumeck et al. wrote: "We believe that AIDS is a new disease that is spreading in Central Africa."[173]

The African AIDS cases led Belgian researchers to begin investigating in Zaire (now the Democratic Republic of the Congo or DRC), the country of origin for many of these patients. Zaire was previously known as the Belgian Congo and Belgium still had strong connections with this part of Africa. In 1983, the US Agency for International Development (USAID) funded a limited investigation by American and Belgian investigators in Kinshasa, the capital of Zaire. Working with local physicians, the team identified 38 cases of AIDS in the main hospitals of Kinshasa, most already very ill. As with the small number of cases of African heritage seen in Europe, half the patients were women. On average, they had been symptomatic for 10 months with severe progressive weight loss during that time. There was no history of intravenous drug use or homosexuality in any case but as a group, the patients had multiple sex partners in the year before the illness began. Astonishingly, 26% of the patients died during the 3 weeks the research team was in Kinshasa.[174,175]

In this same time period, doctors in Uganda were confronted by a surge in cases of a severe wasting disease known locally as "slim disease," accompanied by a dramatic increase in opportunistic infections, especially tuberculosis. Females and males were equally affected and most patients were heterosexuals with a history of multiple sex partners. The doctors who described these patients recognized the similarity to the cases of acquired immunodeficiency syndrome seen in neighboring Zaire and subsequent testing confirmed that 80% of these cases were HIV positive.[176]

After the initial clinical recognition of the link between "slim disease" and AIDS, research was initiated to discover transmission patterns, risk factors, and the prevalence of HIV in Uganda. By 1990, HIV prevalence in pregnant women in Uganda's capital had peaked at over 30%. At around this time, the cases reported from Zaire/DRC and Uganda were recognized as just the very tip of the HIV/AIDS infection pyramid in Africa.

****

Origin of HIV

In reading about this time period, it is clear that after seeing their first patients with AIDS, physicians in Europe, Africa and the United States began to recall unusual, undiagnosed patients they had taken care of in the past whose case profiles resembled the devastated immune status seen with AIDS. When the first test for HIV became available in 1985, blood and tissue samples from some of these patients were tested and identified as HIV positive. In the United States, the earliest identified case was a 15-year-old boy who presented with disseminated chlamydial infection in 1968 and died of pneumonia in 1969; at autopsy he was found to have disseminated Kaposi's sarcoma and antibody testing for HIV was positive.[177] A Norwegian sailor with a history of visiting ports in Africa in the early 1960s developed the picture of clinical AIDS in 1966, followed by his wife and child. Subsequently, serum testing was positive for HIV in all three.[178] Recovery of HIV-1 sequences from a paraffin-preserved lymph node sample of a female from Kinshasa confirmed the presence of HIV infection there in 1960. Viral sequencing of a plasma sample from an African male from Kinshasa obtained in 1959, definitively confirmed the presence of HIV-1 and authenticated this case as the oldest proven human HIV-1 infection.[179]

Inevitably, identification of these cases led to a search for the origin of the human immunodeficiency virus with a focus on central, sub-Saharan Africa where the earliest known cases were identified. As early as the mid-1980s, a monkey or simian virus that very closely resembled HIV-2 was discovered to cause immunodeficiency in captive macaques. Subsequently, this simian immunodeficiency virus(SIV) was found in multiple primates in sub-Saharan Africa with the prevalence of naturally occurring infection ranging widely; in most species, the virus appeared to cause no detectable illness. Ultimately, phylogenetic studies show that SIV_{smm} – for "SIV sooty mangabey" – was confirmed as the monkey ancestor for HIV-2 with transfer to humans by skin or mucous membrane contact with blood, presumably related to bushmeat hunting. A simian virus that closely resembled HIV-1 was discovered in chimpanzees in 1990 in southeast Cameroon. Using noninvasive analysis of urine and fecal samples, scientists discovered that in monkeys, SIV_{cpz} (SIV chimpanzee) is spread primarily through sexual routes with animal migration carrying the infection from one community to another. Combined behavioral and virologic studies show that SIV_{cpz} infection is associated with an AIDS-like illness in chimpanzee colonies. As with SIV_{smm}, spread of SIV_{cpz} to humans is thought to have occurred via incidents related to hunting and slaughtering of chimpanzees as bushmeat.

Molecular phylogenetic studies like the ones we first encountered relative to the influenza virus can be used to analyze the genetic sequences of a cluster of similar viruses. The greater the similarity between the genetic sequences of two viruses, the greater the likelihood that they share a recent common ancestor; based on analyses like these, a family tree that shows the pattern of evolution of a virus can be created. From phylogenetic studies, the ancestral simian viruses to SIV_{cpz} and SIV_{smm} are thought to have evolved from primate lentiviruses that emerged in Africa sometime after the divergence between African and Asian Old World monkeys, within the last 10 million years.[180] Applying these same techniques to viruses from humans, a common ancestor of HIV-1, group M, the pandemic form of the virus, has been shown to have emerged in Kinshasa, the Democratic Republic of the Congo(DRC) – once Leopoldville, the Belgian Congo – in the 1920s.[181] Genetic sequencing of the two earliest human tissue samples from Kinshasa in 1959 and 1960 showed significant diversity indicating that by 1960, HIV had evolved enough that there were two distinct subtypes in circulation. Based on this rate of HIV mutation, phylogenetic analysis indicates the virus emerged as early as the turn of the century.[182] The viruses infecting monkeys and apes are thought to have crossed over into humans sporadically for a long time, most likely when humans were scratched or cut while hunting and butchering monkeys and chimps. That enabled the virus to adapt to humans. Those ancient infections never spread because human population density was so low in the jungle at that time. It was only when the virus traveled to Kinshasa at a time of explosive population growth that the HIV/AIDS epidemic started.

The cross-species transmission of SIV to humans likely occurred in Cameroon where the chimpanzees with SIV_{cpz} most closely resembling HIV group M were identified and the virus then travelled to Kinshasa in jungle hunters via the river system that linked the two countries for rubber and ivory transport. It is speculated that HIV was brought to the city by an infected individual who travelled from Cameroon by river down into the Democratic Republic of the Congo (DRC). This theory is wonderfully expounded by David Quammen in his book, *The Chimp and the River: How AIDS Emerged from an African Forest.*[183] On arrival in Kinshasa, the virus entered a large urban sexual network and spread quickly. Using the earliest archival HIV-1 sample from 1959 and molecular genetic analysis, researchers have created a phylo-geographic model demonstrating that HIV-1 spread from Kinshasa throughout the DRC and the Congo River basin as the population migrated over the next 30 to 40 years.[182] Historical transportation data from this period suggest that travel on railways and waterways is compatible with this migration path and therefore, transport of HIV-1 from Kinshasa to the other major population centers of the region. Based on this analysis, HIV group M had spread to all the major cities of the DRC by 1970. The development of the AIDS epidemic in Africa reflects the period of "massive demographic growth, urbanization and associated social change" that occurred in the region at that time.[184]

By linking phylogenetic tree shape to the demographic history of sampled populations, group M was shown to have undergone slow exponential growth between 1920 and 1960 followed by much faster exponential growth – almost 3 times faster – after 1960. This coincides with public health data that suggests that transmission rates of group M increased dramatically in this time period, as commerce and the sex trade expanded along with increased travel. Analysis of group M subtypes shows that the lineage ancestor of subtype B originated in Kinshasa in ~1944 before it was carried to North America. HIV-1 group M subtype B is the original virus identified by Montagnier and Gallo in 1982. Subtype B remains the dominant subtype in the United States from which it spread to become the most widely dispersed pattern all over the world. The same analytic techniques show that subtype C was carried from southern DRC mining regions to southern Africa where it is now the dominant group M subtype.[185]

The question of Haiti's involvement in the early AIDS epidemic in North America was also addressed by combining phylogenetic, molecular evolutionary, historic and epidemiologic data. Based on early reports of a high prevalence of AIDS in Haitian immigrants to the United States, there had always been speculation that the unknown originators of HIV were Haitian. Combining phylogenetic, molecular evolutionary, historic and epidemiologic data from the earliest known AIDS patients from Africa and the earliest Haitian AIDS patients, researchers showed that HIV-1, group M, subtype B moved from Africa to Haiti in ~1966, a time when Haitian professionals who had worked in what was the Belgian Congo in the 1960s returned home. Phylogenetic analysis and molecular clock techniques indicate that subtype B spread from there to the United States and Canada after a chance migration of the virus out of Haiti in 1969.[185] This is compatible with the average HIV incubation period of 10 years, with the first historic HIV infections in Americans occurring in ~1969 and the first clinical cases of AIDS appearing in the late 1970s.

The Pattern of Global Spread

With understanding of the origin and early spread of HIV-1, the development of the global pandemic of HIV/AIDS is more easily appreciated. After the first cases in Europe were infected by contact with HIV carriers from North America, spread was rapid – by the end of 1985, AIDS had been reported in 51 countries and on every continent except Antarctica.

Analysis of a large dataset of globally-representative HIV-1 group M subtype B strains using phylogeographic and statistical techniques mapped the global migration of this original virus subtype from the United States over the last 40 years.[186,187] Viral sequences from multiple countries revealed that the American continent and the Caribbean acted as the predominant source for outward spread of the epidemic. As documented by the original cases of AIDS, Western Europe was a region where subtype B infections were introduced early from

North America and multiple other geographic areas and spread mainly among regional populations. Early spread to Central and Eastern Europe was minimal and delayed until the end of the Cold War when travel between Western and Eastern European countries increased dramatically, accompanied by the arrival of HIV-1 in the east. In summary, HIV spread around the globe after the mid-1960s reflected both the pattern and volume of human mobility over this time period, with the predominant migration path from North America to Western Europe and then, beyond.[186,187]

As the pandemic evolved around the world, the disease pattern reflected the demographics and sexual/ social customs as well as multiple structural and societal determinants of health like poverty, health care access, socioeconomic status, education and homophobia in the involved regions. In Africa, after the original clinical cases in the 1970s, HIV/AIDS spread quietly but inexorably in heterosexual relationships from Eastern and Central Africa to Southern Africa through the 1980s until the early 1990s associated with multiple sexual partners. This was followed by a period of rapid exponential growth resulting in this area becoming the largest HIV/AIDS site in the world.[188,189] By 1995, the WHO estimated that of 20.1 million adults with HIV/AIDS worldwide, 12.9 million cases were in sub-Saharan Africa. Throughout Africa, tuberculosis was (and is) the infection that took greatest advantage of the compromised immune system in people with AIDS, not the rare opportunistic infections seen in North America and elsewhere in the developed world. To this day, tuberculosis remains the leading cause of death among African people living with HIV. In 2012, people with HIV infection accounted for 1.1 million (13%) of the estimated 8.7 million people who developed tuberculosis globally.

In industrialized countries like the United Kingdom and Western Europe, HIV appeared in the early 1980s among homosexual men and IV drug users and then spread to the heterosexual population, just as it did in the US.[186–189] Beginning in the late 1980s, the epidemic grew rapidly in South-East Asia where spread was predominantly in commercial sex workers and intravenous drug users. The epidemic is known to have been well-established in urban centers in India by the early 1990s although actual surveillance data is limited. In Japan, the largest proportion of early reported AIDS cases was in hemophiliacs who received HIV-infected blood products in the early to mid-1980s. Finally, in Eastern Europe and Central Asia, the pattern and magnitude of early HIV infection was not defined until after 1987 when the Soviet Union began to officially report HIV infections. After the fall of the Soviet Union in 1991, heroin and other injectable drugs became easily accessible to Russians. From the late 1990s onward, as trafficking routes into Russia further developed, HIV infection rates across the region began to rise steadily to currently 10–15% each year – a pace comparable to the infection rate in the United States in the early 1980s. There are currently at least 1.5 million people in Russia from a population of 140 million who have been diagnosed with HIV/AIDS. In 2014, the Russian Federal AIDS Center reported that intravenous drug use accounted for 58% of HIV infections with the rest from sexual transmission.[190] In 2017, the Russian Federation reportedly had the highest number of HIV-positive people of any country in Europe.

The Evolving Global Epidemiology of HIV Infection and AIDS: Implementation of Prevention and Treatment Advances

The first official responses to the global epidemic emerged in 1988, when the WHO launched the Special Program on AIDS, later called the Global Program on AIDS or GPA. Led by Jonathan Mann, the program demanded a human-rights-based response to the pandemic. Over the next decade, the GPA became the largest program in the history of the WHO, providing a basic international framework for HIV prevention. The GPA strongly supported individual behavior change with sex education in schools and explicit condom promotion and provision. Safe sex interventions directed at heterosexual populations were also extended to gay and bisexual men. By the early 1990s with GPA leadership, almost all developing countries had established their own, national HIV prevention programs with varying degrees of success reflecting the difficult political issues associated with a sexually transmitted disease in a wide variety of cultures.[191]

When successful anti-retroviral therapy appeared in 1995, global spread of the infection was still increasing: peak incidence of new HIV infections globally was in 1998 and by the end of 2002, AIDS was the leading cause of death worldwide among people aged 15–59.[192] By 2004, 15 million children worldwide had lost one or both parents to HIV/AIDS and AIDS-related deaths were still on the rise, peaking in 2005. In 1996, in response to the growing global pandemic, the United Nations established UNAIDS, the Joint United Nations Program on HIV/AIDS, to address the critical international need to focus aid and resources on treatment: for example, in 2000, there were more than 20 million people living with AIDS in sub-Saharan Africa, but only 8,000 were accessing drug treatment.

The 13th International AIDS Conference in 2000 marked a critical turning point, with UNAIDS raising global public consciousness about the spiraling AIDS mortality in Africa and the impossibly high cost of antiretroviral drugs. Under international pressure led by UNAIDS, generic producers made ART drugs available at much lower costs and pharmaceutical companies dropped their prices on brand-name products. This was followed by the Doha Declaration that certified that states could circumvent patent rights to access medicines deemed essential for public health.[192] In 2001, the Global Fund to Fight AIDS, Tuberculosis and Malaria was created under UN direction to fund country-owned initiatives against these diseases – since its creation, 60% of funds have gone to fund HIV/AIDS programs. In 2003, US President George Bush announced the President's Emergency Plan for AIDS Relief (PEPFAR); working in over 60 countries, PEPFAR has made major contributions to the global HIV/AIDS response, providing ART to millions of people. With these international funding sources, there has been dramatic progress with major gains in global initiation of antiretroviral therapy. By the end of 2005, a report released by the WHO and UNAIDS showed that the number of people on HIV antiretroviral treatment in developing countries had more than tripled since 2003 to 1.3 million.[193] Prevention and treatment efforts in different HIV transmission groups differ from one country to another, reflecting resources and the regional socio-political climate. As an example, global HIV infections caused by contaminated transfusions of blood and blood products varied widely between countries. After development of HIV testing in 1985, screening of the blood supply dramatically reduced the risk of HIV transmission through blood, blood product and clotting factor transfusions. Use of specific inactivation methods ultimately eliminated all viral contaminants in clotting factor products although the time for this to be accomplished varied between countries. Thousands of individuals were infected by transfusion of contaminated blood products with scandals involving government officials and the commercial blood supply widely reported in the United Kingdom and Japan.

Sexual Transmission of HIV

Gay and Bisexual Men (MSM); Female Partners of HIV(+) Men

While HIV infection in gay and bisexual men has never been a major transmission group in Africa or any other developing country, it remains a high-risk group in highly developed societies, especially in Western Europe, Latin America and South America. Globally, gay men and other men who have sex with men are 19 times more likely to be living with HIV than the general population.[193] Global prevention efforts have included homosexuals but specific prevention and treatment campaigns directed at MSM are seen much more commonly in areas where this pattern of transmission predominates. In 2007, the American Foundation for AIDS Research launched the MSM Initiative, a global program to support HIV prevention, treatment, and advocacy efforts for men who have sex with men. Early initiation of ART in HIV(+) individuals and effective use of pre- and post-exposure prophylaxis can radically change the global course of HIV infection and HIV transmission in this high-risk population.[108–118] As in the United States, strategies to increase the number of MSM testing for HIV and committing to treatment adherence are critically important.

Heterosexual transmission of HIV infection has always been much more important globally than in the United States, especially in sub-Saharan Africa. In 2017, HIV was the leading cause of death worldwide among women of reproductive age, and half of adults living with HIV worldwide were women.[193] HIV/AIDS is a major public health crisis for women, especially young women:[194] in South Africa for example, there are estimated to be 2300 HIV infections per week in adolescent girls, and girls in this age group are twice as likely as men to contract HIV. The global health impact of HIV/AIDS is particularly important in vulnerable female populations like adolescents and children, commercial sex workers, women who have suffered trauma, abuse, violence, substance abuse and serious mental illness, and women who have been trafficked for labor or sex work. HIV/AIDS is a critical factor in the global health of women who urgently need more options for HIV prevention – in 2017 alone, nearly 870,000 women and girls acquired HIV, according to UNAIDS.[193] Currently available forms of HIV prevention for women are limited, and many women are unable to negotiate condom use with male sexual partners. Pre- and post-exposure prophylaxis are highly effective but problems with access, availability and daily pill compliance remain challenging. Additional long-acting methods to prevent HIV infection in women are urgently needed.

Injection Drug Users (IDU)

Injection drug use has become a major and increasing cause of global HIV infection extending into Eastern Europe, Central Asia and the Far East. As of 2015, nearly 30% of global HIV infections were due to unsafe injection drug use. Implementation of effective treatment programs has varied widely between countries. For example, early in the global epidemic, Amsterdam had one of the world's highest rates of injection drug use – and one of the worst drug-associated HIV epidemics. In 1984, Amsterdam set up one of the first needle and syringe programs as concerns about the growing epidemic of HIV increased. This long-established needle exchange program is reported to have virtually eliminated IDU-transmitted HIV transmission there.[195] Rapid localized spread of HIV among IDUs was reported from multiple geographic centers extending from Western Europe to the Far East in the 1980s and 1990s. In most of these areas, the steep increasing incidence leveled off as specific intervention policies for IDUs and safe sex education practices were implemented. By contrast, the rate of HIV infection in Russia has still been rising, with intravenous drug use reportedly accounting for at least 58% of HIV infections. The Kremlin has refused to adopt the globally accepted, evidence-based strategy of drug substitution therapy that has significantly reduced the spread of the epidemic among drug users in other countries. Access to needle exchange programs in Russia is also very limited. Instead, the Russian government focuses on the criminalization of drug use and the stigmatization of key populations at risk.[190] In summary, injection drug use remains an important cause of global HIV infection with the introduction of education, treatment and prevention programs varying widely between countries.

Global Perinatal Infection

The global picture of perinatal HIV infection is best exemplified in sub-Saharan Africa, the epicenter of the global pandemic which has accounted for 65–70% of all new HIV infections since the first cases appeared there. From the outset, more than half of these new infections have been in women with a corresponding very high rate of perinatal transmission. Through the mid-1980s, accurate estimates of maternal and perinatal involvement were unavailable but by 1989, the WHO Global Program on AIDS reported there were 2.5 million women and half a million children infected with HIV-1 in sub-Saharan Africa alone.[196] With no virus-specific treatment, the number of infected women and infants skyrocketed. In 1991, perinatal AIDS was estimated to have increased global infant and child mortality by 30%.[197] By 1997, UNAIDS reported that the number of children less than 15 years of age infected with HIV since the start of the epidemic in the late 1970s had reached 3.8 million and 2.7 million of these children had already died.[198]

In 1994, the discovery that AZT treatment of the mother and baby at the time of delivery effectively blocked HIV infection in 70% of cases was a tremendous advance but one that was initially largely unavailable outside of industrialized countries.[156] Controversy arose about the ethics of prophylactic research trials to prevent maternal-fetal transmission of HIV in the less-developed world, centered around the need for placebo-controlled trials, the virtual impossibility of true informed consent, failure to provide an intervention of known efficacy and potential subject exploitation.[199–202] While this discussion was still ongoing, the CDC reported that a short course of oral AZT given late in pregnancy and during delivery with no infant dose had proven effective in reducing perinatal HIV transmission in a placebo-controlled study in Thailand.[203] Confirmation that there was an available, effective and relatively easy to implement intervention appeared to resolve the research trial controversy. Ultimately, subsequent studies showed that when HIV(+) mothers received combination anti-retroviral treatment and avoided breastfeeding, the rate of perinatal HIV transmission was reduced to less than 2%.[158] Breastfeeding as an infection route was addressed by considering the balance of factors – in a developing country, breastfeeding was almost always the better choice for nutrition and safety reasons and often the only choice because of economic and practical constraints.

Initially, efforts to extend the use of ART to resource-poor settings like sub-Saharan Africa were limited.[204] In 2000, with the major breakthrough in international access to ART, UNAIDS negotiated an Accelerating Access Initiative which was followed in 2001 by a United Nations Special Session Declaration that ART was essential to the fight on HIV/AIDS. The WHO followed by adding antiviral medications to their Essential Medicines List and developing a public health approach to treating individuals in resource-poor settings.[192] Over the next 15 years, multiple strategies were attempted in the effort to diagnose maternal HIV infection and prevent infant transmission by delivering antiretroviral therapy in resource-limited settings all over the world.[204–206] All these studies underscored the importance of offering ART interventions to pregnant women with HIV infection whenever and wherever they were identified – during pregnancy, during labor and delivery, or as an intervention with the newborn baby. Over the next decade, there was a progressive increase in ART use for prevention of HIV transmission from mother to child using a variety of protocols. Each program was theoretically efficacious for preventing transmission but implementation was fraught with problems because of the variability and complexity of the recommendations – and most importantly, because many iterations inexplicably left HIV(+) women without treatment after delivery.

The WHO followed the emerging evidence with serial recommendations for the prevention of peripartum mother-to-child transmission in developing countries with the first published guidelines on the use of ART for HIV infection among adults and adolescents in 2002, and on the use of ART to prevent mother-to-child HIV transmission in 2004.[207] The 2006 update of the guidelines introduced the concept of a public health approach, with simplified and harmonized ART regimens.[208] Then, in 2013, for the first time, WHO revised and combined all ART-related documents into consolidated guidelines recommending ART drugs for HIV treatment and prevention across all age groups and populations including pregnant women. These guidelines were updated in 2016 with augmented global guidance to reflect the strong science base supporting the benefit of early and sustained HIV treatment.[207-210] The 2016 WHO guidelines now call for "test and treat" strategies – initiating ART treatment in all people diagnosed with HIV as soon as possible after diagnosis, to decrease community viral load and reduce the rate of new HIV infections. While this "Treatment as Prevention (TasP)" approach will only be effective with scaling up of testing programs and ART adherence support, the recommendation that all pregnant and breastfeeding women living with HIV should initiate ART and remain on lifelong treatment regardless of clinical or CD4 stage of disease is a major breakthrough. For the first time, the ART strategy for pregnant women is fully aligned with the recommended first-line regimen for all non-pregnant adults. Providing ART to all pregnant and breastfeeding women living with HIV serves three synergistic purposes: it improves individual health outcomes for mothers; it prevents mother-to-child transmission of HIV; and it prevents transmission of HIV from the mother to an uninfected sexual partner. The TasP approach holds enormous promise for women, their babies and their families.

The proportion of pregnant women living with HIV receiving ART more than doubled in 21 of the 22 Global Plan priority countries, from 36% in 2009 to 80% in 2015. Perhaps more importantly, 93% of pregnant women receiving treatment were prescribed lifelong treatment, up significantly from 73% in 2014.[211] There is broad theoretical support for universal treatment and many countries are committed to adopting a "Treat All" policy. But there are ongoing problems in resource-limited settings that must be addressed for successful implementation of these goals. For example, a recent report from China documents prolonged delay in repeat HIV testing in infants born to HIV(+) women; in two-thirds of infants, testing was delayed until after 18 months of age and by that time, one third of the babies had died or were lost to follow-up.[212]

In 2016, there were 11.5 million women and girls living with HIV in eastern and southern Africa. On average, 76% of pregnant women living with HIV had access to antiretroviral medicines to prevent transmission of HIV to their babies. With optimized public health efforts, there is meaningful progress in preventing global mother-to-child transmission of HIV. There were 130,000 new HIV infections among children under five in 2022, dramatically declining from 310,000 in 2010 and representing a 58 per cent decline.[213]

HIV/AIDS Prevention and Treatment: Global Status

- By the end of 2022, more than 85.6 million people had been infected with HIV and 40.4 million people had died of AIDS, a figure that threatens to eclipse the cumulative tens of millions who died in the 1918–19 influenza pandemic, our gold standard for pandemic mortality.[213–216]
- Globally, UNAIDS statistics report that 39 million people – 0.7% of the world's population – were living with HIV at the end of 2018.[213]
- Prevalence varies widely from well below that level in countries like the United States to 3.2% of adults in the WHO African Region living with HIV in 2022. This accounts for two-thirds of the people living with HIV worldwide.
- Sub-Saharan Africa, which bears the heaviest burden of HIV/AIDS worldwide, accounts for 65% of all new HIV infections. Nearly 1 in every 25 adults is living with HIV and this accounts for more than two-thirds of the people living with HIV worldwide. Other regions most significantly affected by HIV/AIDS include Asia and the Pacific, Latin America and the Caribbean, and Eastern Europe and Central Asia.
- In the last several years, Russia has been the country with the largest number of new HIV cases and AIDS deaths. In January 2016, Russia reached its millionth case of HIV with currently at least 850,000 people living with HIV; a large number of these cases are undiagnosed.[215]
- Gains in treatment are largely responsible for a steep decline in AIDS-related deaths globally, from an estimated 2 million in 2005 to 1.5 million in 2010 and 630,000 in 2022.
- At the end of 2022, 76% of people living with HIV were accessing antiretroviral therapy, up from 24% in 2010. Globally, there were 1.2 million pregnant women with HIV in 2022, of which an estimated 82% received antiretroviral drugs to prevent mother-to-child transmission.
- At the end of 2022, there were 1.5 million children living with HIV globally, down from 2.5 million in 2010.

If even the current rate of progress can be sustained, there is potential to end the global HIV/AIDS pandemic by 2040. UNAIDS and the ONE Campaign reported that in 2013, a tipping point was reached in the fight against the disease when the number of people newly added to treatment that year was more than the number of people newly infected with HIV. If the number of people on treatment continues to increase and the number of new infections continues to decrease, we can theoretically end the HIV/AIDS epidemic in the next 15 years.

Looking Back :: Moving Forward

HIV infection is responsible for one of the most devastating human pandemics of all time but its story is also one of enormous scientific accomplishment. Against formidable odds, five years after recognition of the first cases in the USA, the epidemiology of the disease had been described, the causative virus had been identified, the pathophysiology of the disease was recognized and a test to diagnose infection had been developed. For those who lived through this time when thousands of people died tragically and horribly, this progress must have felt discouragingly irrelevant and interminably slow, since at that time, a diagnosis of AIDS was essentially a death sentence. It was not until 1996 – *15 years* after the first reported cases – that development of combined treatment with antiretroviral medications (ART) proved to be effective for treatment of AIDS and for control of HIV infection. The advent of effective ART dramatically changed the course of the pandemic, transforming HIV infection into a treatable chronic disease and saving millions of lives. This was followed by demonstration that if viral load is effectively suppressed in HIV(+) individuals, the virus is no longer transmissible. But HIV infection is still not curable. Future progress focuses on maximizing delivery of known, effective treatment and development of a definitive preventive and curative strategy.

Despite the enormous progress made since the first AIDS cases appeared, even antiretroviral therapy is still far from perfect. Treatment adherence is a powerful predictor of survival for individuals living with HIV infection, with an established required level for effective viral suppression of 95%. Despite development of new, potent antiretrovirals and once daily, single pill treatment regimens, average individual adherence to antiretroviral therapy is far below that, varying from 27–80% across different populations. In terms of treatment, 76% of people living with HIV were accessing antiretroviral therapy in 2022, up from 24% in 2010. Globally, there were 1.2 million pregnant women with HIV in 2022, of which an estimated 82% received ART to prevent mother-to-child transmission.[216] Even achieving the goals of "treatment as prevention" is an enormous challenge, requiring identification of all HIV-infected individuals, provision of effective, lifetime anti-HIV medication and viral suppression in treated individuals to undetectable levels. We are far from achieving any of these goals with an estimated 1.2 million people in the United States aged 13 and older with HIV infection, including 13% who are unaware of their diagnosis. This proportion is at least as large in other parts of the world. In response to statistics like these, scientific strategies to combat HIV/AIDS have developed in four major areas: virus eradication; new approaches to prevention and treatment; reduction of structural barriers to diagnosis and treatment; and vaccine development.

- The major biologic barrier to HIV eradication is latency, the persistence of integrated replication-competent HIV reservoirs in memory CD4+ T cells which emerge whenever antiretroviral treatment is stopped.[217] The most studied approach for eliminating latently-infected T cells is based on the "shock and kill" theory where a latency-reversing agent is used to flush out the reservoirs and then a cytolytic agent clears the latent viruses.[218–220] Research directed at every stage of this process is ongoing, from the development of biomarkers to quantify HIV persistence to engineering T cells to eliminate HIV-infected cells to enhancing the capacity of an individual's own immune system to clear HIV-infected cells. A 2023 study found the cancer drug venetoclax can kill hibernating HIV-infected cells and, crucially, delay the virus from re-emerging. A clinical trial based on these findings will launch in Denmark and Australia, to test whether venetoclax can be used as a potential pathway to develop a cure for HIV. Ruxolitinib, a Janus k inhibitors, has also been shown to significantly decay the reservoir in people living with HIV – further results of study of this methodology are pending.[218–220]

- Women urgently need more ways to prevent HIV infection. A new option is a vaginal ring which continuously releases the anti-HIV drug dapivirine. This was designed to be a discreet, long-acting HIV prevention option for women with the wearer replacing the product herself every four weeks. In an open-label study of women in southern and eastern Africa, the dapivirine vaginal ring (DPV-VR) reduced the risk of HIV infection by 39%, according to statistical modeling.[221] After two randomized controlled trials found that using the DPV-VR was well-tolerated and reduced the risk of HIV infection in women to 27%, the WHO recommended in 2021 that DPV-VR be offered as an additional prevention choice for women at risk of HIV infection as part of combination prevention approaches.[221]

- Since publication of the first edition of this book in 2020, effective, injectable, long-acting medications to treat HIV infection have been developed. Intramuscular cabotegravir (CAB) and rilpivirine (RPV) are long-acting antiretroviral therapies given every other month to people with HIV who have been shown to have virologic suppression with use of oral ART before initiating injectables. They have been shown to be as effective as daily oral ART in achieving and maintaining viral suppression.[222]

- With clear demonstration that ART significantly improves the health of HIV(+) individuals and dramatically reduces HIV transmission, social and behavioral research is focusing on known structural barriers to effective ART by increasing diagnosis rates, treatment initiation and viral suppression in at risk populations. UNAIDS established the "95-95-95" global targets, aiming to have 95% of HIV-infected people identified, 95% of those with HIV infection receiving antiretroviral treatment and 95% of those on treatment achieving undetectable viral levels. In 2022, Botswana, Eswatini, Rwanda, the United Republic of Tanzania, and Zimbabwe had already achieved the "95-95-95" targets. A further 16 other countries, eight of them in sub-Saharan Africa, the region which accounts for 65% of all people living with HIV, are close to doing so. Mathematical models show that universal

HIV testing followed by immediate antiretroviral therapy could theoretically eliminate viral transmissibility, effectively ending the 40 year-long global HIV/AIDS pandemic.[223]

- Two recent studies show the potential power of effective interventions directed at structural barriers to prevention and treatment: A community-based testing and treatment program in rural Kenya and Uganda used a public campaign to establish annual HIV testing linked to universal ART access and facilitated care for HIV(+) individuals. After two years, the 2020 goals were being achieved with 95.9% of HIV(+) individuals identified, 93.4% on ART and 89.5% of those virally suppressed.[224] A randomized trial compared standard ART initiation following weeks after HIV testing to same-day HIV testing and immediate ART initiation in eligible adults in Port-au-Prince, Haiti. In the standard group, ART was initiated a mean of 3 weeks after HIV testing. At 12 month follow-up, significantly more of the same day ART initiation group were retained in care and had appropriate viral suppression.[224]

- Efforts to develop a vaccine to prevent or modify HIV infection have been ongoing since the late 1980s, stymied primarily by the extravagant capacity of the virus for mutation which results in great genetic diversity, with multiple strains and subtypes prevalent in different parts of the world, and by the existence of replication-competent virus reservoirs. In 2000, the HIV Vaccine Trials Network (HVTN) was established linking a network of 25 clinical sites in the United States, Africa, Asia, South America, and the Caribbean dedicated to developing a preventive HIV vaccine by testing and evaluating candidate vaccines in all phases of clinical trials. To this time, results have been unsuccessful despite serial trials.

For example, on November 30, 2017, multiple international partners including the NIH and the Bill and Melinda Gates Foundation announced the HVTN 705/ HPX2008 study of an investigational HIV-1-preventive "mosaic" vaccine. Despite high hopes, this randomized trial ended in 2021 because it failed to protect participants from HIV infection.[225–227]

An ongoing complementary Phase 3 HIV vaccine study called Mosaico (HVTN 706/HPX3002) tested the safety and efficacy of a different investigational HIV vaccine among a different patient population (MSM men and transgender populations) in the Americas and Europe. The regimen was found to be safe but did not provide protection from HIV acquisition compared with placebo, ultimately leading Janssen to stop the phase 3 trial in January 2023.[225–227]

A novel preventative vaccine candidate which has been in development since 2004 has begun phase 1 clinical trial enrollment in the United States and South Africa.

Known as VIR-1388, the vaccine is designed to instruct the immune system to produce T cells that recognize HIV and signal an immune response to prevent the virus from establishing chronic infection using an attenuated cytomegalovirus to deliver the vaccine material. This safety trial is funded by NIAID with the Bill & Melinda Gates Foundation and Vir Biotechnology through the HVTN as study HVTN 142 and will enroll 95 HIV-negative participants, randomly assigned to one of four study arms: three arms will each receive a different dose of the vaccine, and one will receive a placebo. Initial results are expected in late 2024.[228]

★★★★★★★★★★

Extraordinary scientific achievements mark the current understanding of HIV/AIDS as it has evolved from a universally fatal global pandemic with no identified agent and no treatment, to a treatable chronic disease associated with a normal lifespan when treatment is initiated early and continually sustained. New approaches addressing all aspects of care hold the potential to end the current pandemic and prevent future infection. From the outset, the nature of the virus has characterized the disease: the secrets to any curative strategy and an effective vaccine lie in a complete understanding of the capacity of this unique virus to produce acute and persistent infection.

★★★★★★★★★★

I wanted to end this chapter on a purely positive note – after all, the progress made has been impressive and ending the HIV pandemic by virus eradication or complete global suppression seems almost within reach. But one Sunday just a few years ago, I was reading the obituaries in the *New York Times* when a headline leapt out at me: "Michael Friedman, Co-Creator of 'Bloody, Bloody Andrew Jackson' Dies at 41." The article confirmed what the headline already told me – the cause of death for this "versatile, cerebral and witty composer and lyricist" was complications of HIV/AIDS.

I cannot remember the last time I read an AIDS obituary like this, but I can easily remember a time when there were at least several every Sunday. Of course, in the early days – through the 1980s – no-one explicitly identified AIDS as the cause of death. The small type read something like "after a long illness," with only parents and siblings listed as survivors. "Donations in his memory to God's Love We Deliver." Or ACT UP. Or Bailey House. Or rarely, the Gay Men's Health Crisis. The number of talented young men who died of AIDS in those years was overwhelming. Right at that time, a friend told me about his "Triscuit Index" – based on his grandfather's advice, he had been following the status of the stock market by checking the price of Triscuits every year on his birthday. I had already been keeping a rough mental tally of AIDS obituaries in the Sunday Times and I began to think of it as the "AIDS Inventory" – a personal way to keep a handle on one small corner of the pandemic. Over the years, it proved to be a surprisingly accurate reflection of the evolution of the AIDS epidemic in NYC. In the early 1990s, the Inventory numbers peaked, reflecting the fact that at that time, AIDS was the leading cause of death for men in New York City between the ages of 25 and 44. As time passed, the men who died gradually became older. Sometimes they were survived by a life partner. And eventually, the cause of death was actually given as "complications of AIDS." After 1996 when anti-retroviral therapy became widely available, the numbers dwindled and then seemed to disappear.

I hadn't thought of the AIDS Inventory in many years but Michael Friedman's death notice brought that terrible time right back. The last line of his obituary reads, "His death stunned the theater community which had lost many artists to AIDS in the 1980s and '90s but fewer in recent years." In the days that followed, there was a memorial service and some details of Michael's illness emerged. He had reportedly been working very hard in the preceding 6 months, opening a new children's musical in Minnesota while simultaneously acting as the artistic director of Encores! Off-Center!, an annual summer program at New York City Center. Friends noticed he had lost weight and even the appearance of small purple lesions on his face but he was not tested for HIV until 9 weeks before he died when he presented with full-blown Pneumocystis pneumonia. Antiretroviral treatment was started imme-diately but despite all efforts, he died.

How did this happen? A gay man in NYC, the first identified high-risk AIDS group; a man who worked in the theater, the community that had suffered the greatest losses to AIDS in the early years of the epidemic; a man with many HIV positive friends on treatment – *this* man had not been tested for HIV for at least several years. Here I am writing about programs to increase HIV testing and treatment in the southern United States and in sub-Saharan Africa and right here in NYC, a gay man is not diagnosed with HIV until he presents with AIDS, just weeks before he dies. No matter where in the world we live, all the amazing treatment advances of the last 25 years are useless without proactive testing and early diagnosis.

Yes, there has been great progress – and yes, there is still more work to be done.

Historic Perspective: The Power of Activism

The federal public health network discussed in the section on influ-enza failed most profoundly when it was faced with HIV. The virus hit humans where we are least capable of changing and most constrained by prejudice: sex. The first group to be identified as victims of the dis-ease was gay men, to such an extent that it was originally identified as Gay Related Immune Deficiency (GRID) before the cases linked to IV drug use and blood transfusions rendered this label inaccurate and obsolete. Because this group of people was not granted equal rights as citizens by every member of the United States Congress, a view that was representative of the country at the time, funding AIDS research became a political football. In 1987, Senator Jesse Helms of North Carolina famously led his house of Congress in passing an amendment to an appropriations bill that prevented funding of AIDS education programs (that were proven to be highly effective) by the Centers for Disease Control because they might "promote, encourage, or condone homosexual activities."[229] Only two senators, Daniel Patrick Moynihan and Lowell Weicker, voted against this amendment, which essentially starved federal funding for AIDS prevention. Where the government failed, however, independent organizations succeeded. Due to the tireless efforts of the Gay Men's Health Crisis, Act Up, and other groups around the country, HIV/AIDS rates among gay men fell precipitously within five years. These organizations also provided care for those affected, funded research, and defended the civil rights of AIDS patients and their partners. In an era when being gay was still accepted as a rationale for discrimination, these individuals declared war on the federal government and its elected officials who refused to recognize their rights to privacy or the critical importance of a centralized education effort to prevent the spread of this terrible disease.

Gay Men's Health Crisis (GMHC) formed in 1981 in New York City in response to what was then considered "gay cancer." It was called that in response to the CDC warning about the sudden proliferation of the relatively rare cancer, Kaposi's sarcoma (KS), among gay men. CDC researchers and others would quickly notice the correlation between KS, pneumocystis carinii pneumonia, and other immune deficiencies among gay men and rename the disease GRID. Larry Kramer and about 80 other gay men met in his living room to discuss raising funds for research. Their efforts to inform gay men about HIV transmission and the critical importance of condom use over the next six years directly contributed to Jesse Helms' hateful amendment.[230] By 1982, GMHC opened the first AIDS hotline, a telephone that rang in a volunteer's New York City apartment and fielded over 100 calls the first night.[231] And in 1983, they funded the first AIDS discrimination lawsuit, which was brought by the Lambda Legal Defense and Education Fund.[231] New York's gay men had every reason to organize: they were in an epicenter of the AIDS epidemic, there was little accurate information about the disease available to the general public, and AIDS patients consistently faced discrimination by health care professionals. They met before the CDC declared the disease an epidemic (also in 1981) and over a year before AIDS research received any federal funds. In 1982, the CDC still was not sure women could get AIDS, though cases associated with blood transfusions and IV drug use would quickly change that misperception.[231] The men who founded the GMHC met because their lovers and friends were dying, and nobody seemed to care. Some were even openly happy, claiming the disease was divine vengeance against homosexuals. Gay people in New York City had already demonstrated the power of activism in the first wave of the gay rights movement beginning with the Stonewall Riots, and the gay activist network in New York City was strong, identifiable, and relatively wealthy. Using their existing network for fundraising and community support, GMHC produced educational material that would become the foundation for AIDS prevention, provided daily help to people with AIDS in New York City, created a vital legal bulwark against AIDS discrimination, and funded research into effective treatments. This is an extraordinary example of an identifiable community of people uniting to create a self-funded public health response based on education and awareness, and it is a model of how to create an effective community response to a public health threat. When GMHC began its work, condom use among gay men was very rare. Long before it was proven to be an effective deterrent to AIDS transmission (1988), condom use among gay men had increased to such an extent that in 1988 in New York City, more new cases were attributed to intravenous drug use than sex.[231] The fact that the majority (two thirds) of new cases were also among African American men points to the slow acceptance of homosexuality in the African American community and one of the areas in which the GMHC was least effective: bridging the racial gap in the gay rights movement.

The GMHC did three things exceptionally well: it produced educational material about HIV and its transmission and distributed it within the gay community, to health care workers, and to the general public; it raised enormous amounts of money to support people with AIDS and provided care for them, as well as legal defense when necessary; and it made AIDS part of popular culture through theater and film, as well as part of political culture by appearing before Congress, insisting on Constitutional protection for people with AIDS, and demanding funding for research and education. While President Reagan was still insisting against all evidence, in 1986, that there was no reason for the general public to worry about AIDS because it only affected gay men and drug users, Larry Kramer's "A Normal Heart" had been on stage for a year and "An Early Frost," a television film featuring a main character with AIDS, had already aired.[232,233] The importance of making AIDS and AIDS patients visible to the public cannot be overlooked, especially since gay activism was much harder to find outside of large cities. Ryan White, the teenage hemophiliac from Indiana who died of AIDS at 18 after facing extreme discrimination for his condition, has been credited with making AIDS patients "victims" rather than sinners who deserved their fate, but a great deal of credit for making AIDS victims visible and human also goes to Kramer and other writers, such as Paul Monette (*Borrowed Time: An AIDS Memoir*, 1988), who put them on stage and in readers' hands where their humanity could not be denied.

For all the incredible work GMHC did and continues to do, however, it could not prevent the epidemic spreading across the world. The version of the virus that reached North America was a direct import from Haiti, but it had its roots deep in sub-Saharan Africa. And in an increasingly global world, diseases travel faster than the human response to them. But it is worth remembering that a group of men who fit in a living room founded a movement that fundamentally changed their world – and ours – for the better. Activism matters. Because if Paul Monette wrote, "It will be recorded that the dead in the first decade of the calamity died of our indifference," he also declared, "Grief is a sword."[234]

References

1. Gottlieb MS, Schanker HM, Fan PT et al. *Pneumocystis* pneumonia – Los Angeles. *Morbid Mortal Weekly Rep* 1981; 30:250–252.
2. Friedman A, Laubenstein L, Marmor M et al. Kaposi's sarcoma and *Pneumocystis* pneumonia among homosexual men – New York City and California. *Morbid Mortal Weekly Rep* 1981; 30:305–308.
3. Hymes KB, Greene JB, Marcus A et al. Kaposi's sarcoma in homosexual men – a report of eight cases. *Lancet* 1981; 2:598–600.
4. Masur H, Michelis MA, Greene JB et al. An outbreak of community-acquired pneumocystis carinii pneumonia. Initial manifestation of cellular immune dysfunction. *N Engl J Med* 1981; 305:1431–1438.
5. AVERT website. History of HIV and AIDS: Timeline. Available at: www.avert.org. Downloaded September 30, 2017.
6. Cullen T. HIV/AIDS: 20 years of press coverage. *Australian Studies in Journalism* 2003; 12: 227.
7. Karpf A. *Doctoring the Media: The Reporting of Health and Medicine.* London. Routledge, 1988.
8. Altman L. *Rare Cancer Seen in 41 Homosexuals.* The New York Times. July 3, 1981. Downloaded August 14, 2017.
9. Goedert JJ, Neuland CY, Wallen WC et al. Amyl nitrite may alter lymphocytes in homosexual men. *Lancet* 1982; 1(8269):412–416.
10. Epidemiologic Notes and Reports. *Update on Kaposi's Sarcoma and Opportunistic Infections in Previously Healthy Persons – United States.* CDC Task Force on Kaposi's Sarcoma and Opportunistic Infections, Field Services Div, Epidemiology Program Office, CDC. *MMWR* 1982; 30:409–10.
11. Center for Disease Control and Prevention. Epidemiologic Notes and Reports. Persistent, Generalized Lymphadenopathy among Homosexual Males. *MMWR* May 21, 1982; 31(19):249–51

12. Centers for Disease Control and Prevention July 9, 1982. Opportunistic infections and Kaposi's sarcoma among Haitians in the United States. *MMWR* 1982; 31(26):353–354,360–361.

13. Centers for Disease Control and Prevention. Epidemiologic Notes and Reports. July 16, 1982. Pneumocystis carinii pneumonia among persons with hemophilia A. *MMWR* 1982; 31(27):365–367.

14. Centers for Disease Control and Prevention. Epidemiologic Notes and Reports. Dec. 10, 1982. Update on Acquired Immune Deficiency Syndrome (AIDS) among Patients with Hemophilia A. *MMWR* 1982; 31(48):644–646.

15. Leveton LB, Sox HC Jr, Stoto MA, editors. Institute of Medicine Committee to study HIV transmission through blood and blood products. *HIV and the Blood Supply: an Analysis of Crisis Decision-making. Chapter 3. History of the Controversy.* Washington(DC): National Academies Press (US); 1995. www.ncbi.nlm.nih.gov/books/NBK232419/

16. Kornfeld H, Vande Stouwe RA, Lange M, Reddy MM, Grieco MH. T-lymphocyte subpopulations in homosexual men. *N Engl J Med* 1982; 307:729–31.

17. Task Force for Acquired Immune Disorder. Centers for Disease Control and Prevention. Current Trends Update on Acquired Immune Deficiency Syndrome (AIDS) – United States. *MMWR* September 24, 1982; 31(37);507–508, 513–514.

18. Centers for Disease Control and Prevention. Epidemiologic Notes and Reports. Possible transfusion associated acquired immunodeficiency syndrome (AIDS) – California. *MMWR* 1982; 31:652–654.

19. Ammann AJ, Cowan MJ, Wara DW et al. Acquired immunodeficiency in an infant: possible transmission by means of blood products. *Lancet* 1983; 1:956–958.

20. Centers for Disease Control and Prevention. Epidemiologic Notes and Reports. Unexplained Immunodeficiency and Opportunistic Infections in Infants – New York, New Jersey, California. *Morbid Mortal Weekly Rev* 1982; 31(49):665–667.

21. Leveton LB, Sox HC Jr, Stoto MA, editors. Institute of Medicine Committee to study HIV transmission through blood and blood products. *HIV and the Blood Supply: an Analysis of Crisis Decision-making. Chapter 3. History of the Controversy.* Washington(DC): National Academies Press (US); 1995. www.ncbi.nlm.nih.gov/books/NBK232419/. Downloaded September 15, 2017.

22. Centers for Disease Control and Prevention. Epidemiologic Notes and Reports. Immunodeficiency among Female Sexual Partners of Males with Acquired Immune Deficiency Syndrome (AIDS). *Morbid Mortal Weekly Rev.* January 7, 1983; 31(52):697–698.

23. Harris C, Small CB, Klein RS, et al. Immunodeficiency in female sexual partners of men with the acquired immunodeficiency syndrome. *N Engl J Med* 1983; 308:1181–4.

24. Oleske J, Minnefor A, Cooper R et al. Immune deficiency syndrome in children. *JAMA* 1983; 249:2345–9.

25. Rubenstein A, Sicklick M, Gupta A et al. Acquired immunodeficiency with reversed T4/T8 ratios in infants born to promiscuous and drug-addicted mothers. *JAMA* 1983; 249:2350–6.

26. Jaffe HW, Choi K, Thomas PA et al. National case-control study of Kaposi's sarcoma and *Pneumocystis carinii* pneumonia in homosexual men: epidemiologic results. *Annals of Int Med* 1983; 99: 145–151.

27. CNN launches – Jun 01, 1980 – HISTORY.com. www.history.com/this-day-in-history/cnn-launches. Accessed Nov. 15, 2017.

28. Carlson P. AIDS: Fatal, Incurable, and Spreading. *People.* June 17, 1985 12:00 PM. Archive. Accessed Nov. 5, 2017.

29. Garrett L. *The Coming Plague. Newly Emerging Diseases in a World Out of Balance.* Penguin Books. New York, New York. 1995. From Chapter 11. Hatari: Vinidogodogo. pg. 316,317.

30. Baltimore D. Viral RNA-dependent DNA polymerase: RNA-dependent DNA polymerase in visions of RNA tumor viruses. *Nature* 1970; 226 (5252): 1209–1211.

31. Temin H. Viral RNA-dependent DNA Polymerase: RNA-dependent DNA Polymerase in Virions of Rous Sarcoma Virus. *Nature* 1970; 226 (5252): 1211–1213.

32. Poiesz BJ, Ruscetti FW, Reitz MS, Kalyanaraman VS, Gallo RC. Isolation of a new type C retrovirus (HTLV) in primary uncultured cells of a patient with Sezary T-cell leukemia. *Nature* 1981; 294:268–271.

33. Barre-Sinoussi F, Chermann JC, Rey F, Nugeyre MT, Chamaret S, Rozenbaum W, Montagnier L. Isolation of a T-lymphotrophic retrovirus from a patient at risk for acquired immune deficiency syndrome (AIDS). *Science* 1983; 220:868–871.

34. Gallo RC, Sarin PS, Gelmann EP et al. Isolation of human T-cell leukemia virus in acquired immune deficiency syndrome(AIDS). *Science* 1983; 220:865–867.

35. Broder S, Gallo RC. A pathogenic retrovirus (HTLV-III) linked to AIDS. *N Engl J Med* 1984; 311(20):1292–7.

36. Montagnier L, Chermann JC, Barre-Sinoussi C et al. *A new human T-lymphotropic retrovirus: characterization and possible role in lymphadenopathy and acquired immune deficiency syndromes.* New York: Cold Spring Harbor Laboratory; 1984.

37. Garrett. 1995. pg. 331.

38. Klatzmann D, Champagne E, Chamaret S et al. T-lymphocyte T4 molecule behaves as the receptor for human retrovirus LAV. *Nature* 1984 Dec 20-1985 Jan 2; 312(5996):767–8.

39. Vilmer E, Barre-Sinoussi C, Rouzioux C et al. Isolation of new lymphotrophic retrovirus from two siblings, one with hemophilia B, one with AIDS. *Lancet* 1984; 1: 753–757.

40. Wain-Hobson P, Sonigo P, Danos O. Nucleotide sequence of the AIDS virus, LAV. *Cell* 1985; 40:9–17.

41. Ratner L, Haseltine W, Patarca R et al. Complete nucleotide sequence of the AIDS virus, HTLV-III. *Nature* 1985; 313: 277–284.

42. Nobel Laureates in Physiology or Medicine. www.nobelprize.org/nobel_prizes/medicine/laureates/

43. Wong-Staal F, Ratner L, Shaw G et al. Molecular biology of human T-lymphotrophic retroviruses. *Cancer Res* 1985; 45(Suppl):4539s–4544s.

44. Montagnier L, Chermann JC, Barre-Sinoussi C et al. *A new human T-lymphotropic retrovirus: characterization and possible role in lymphadenopathy and acquired immune deficiency syndromes.* New York: Cold Spring Harbor Laboratory; 1984.

45. Clavel F, Guetard D, Brun-Vezinet F, et al. Isolation of a new human retrovirus from West African patients with AIDS. *Science* 1986; 233: 343–346.

46. Hockley DJ, Wood RD, Jacobs JP, Garrett AJ. Electron microscopy of Human Immunodeficiency Virus. *J Gen Virol* 1988; 69:2455–2469.

47. Wain-Hobson P, Sonigo P, Danos O. Nucleotide sequence of the AIDS virus, LAV. *Cell* 1985; 40:9–17.

48. Ratner L, Haseltine W, Patarca R et al. Complete nucleotide sequence of the AIDS virus, HTLV-III. *Nature* 1985; 313: 277–284.

49. Lu K, Heng X, Summers MF. Structural determinants and mechanism of HIV-1 genome packaging. *J Mol Biol* 2011; 410(4): 609–633.

50. Wilen CB, Tilton JC, Doms RW. *HIV: Cell binding and entry.* Cold Spring Harb Perspect Med 2012; 2:1–2.

51. Zhao G, Perilla JR, Yufenyuy EL et al. Mature HIV-1 capsid structure by cryo-electron microscopy and all-atom molecular dynamics. *Nature* 2013; 497: 643–646.

52. Earl LA, Lifson JD, Subramanain S. Catching HIV "in the act" with 3D electron microscopy. *Trends Microbiol* 2013; 21(8): 397–410.

53. Law KM, Satija N, Esposito AM, Chen BK. Cell-to-cell spread of HIV and viral pathogenesis. *Adv Virus Res* 2016; 95:43–85.

54. Iliffe J. *The African AIDS Epidemic. A History.* Ohio University Press. Athens, Ohio. James Currey Ltd. Oxford, UK. 2006. Chapter 2. Pg. 5.

55. McCutchan FE. Understanding the genetic diversity of HIV-1. *AIDS* 2000; 14(suppl 3):S31–S44.

56. Buonaguro L, Tornesello ML, Buonaguro FM. Human immunodeficiency virus type 1 subtype distribution in the worldwide epidemic: pathogenetic and therapeutic implications. *J Virol* 2007; 81(19): 10209–19219.

57. Reeves JD, Doms RW. Human immunodeficiency virus type 2. *J General Virology* 2002;83:1253–1265.

58. Liu R, Paxton WA, Choe S et al. Homozygous defect in HIV-1 co-receptor accounts for resistance of some multiply-exposed individuals to HIV-1 infection. *Cell* 1996; 86:367–377.

59. Huang Y, Paxton WA, Wolinsky SM et al. The role of a mutant CCR5 allele in HIV-1 transmission and disease progression. *Nature Medicine* 1996; 2:1240–1243.

60. Gonzalo-Gil E, Ikediobi U, Sutton RE. Mechanisms of viremic control and clinical characteristics of HIV+ elite/viremic controllers. *Yale J Biol Med* 2017; 90:245–259.

61. Churchill M, Deeks SG, Margolis DM et al. HIV reservoirs: what, where and how to target them. *Nature Rev Microbiol* 2016;14:

62. Iliffe J. 2006. Chapter 2. Pg. 8.

63. Vergis EN, Mellors JW. Natural history of HIV-1 infection. *Inf Dis Clinics NA* 2000; 14(4):809–825.

64. Groopman JE, Salahuddin SZ, Sarngadharan NG et al. Virologic studies in a case of transfusion-associated AIDS. *New Engl J Med* 1984; 311(22): 1419–1422.

65. Baccheti P, Moss AR. Incubation period of AIDS in San Francisco. *Nature* 1989; 338:251–253.

66. Brookmeyr R, Goedert JJ. Censoring an epidemic with an application to hemophilia-associated AIDS. *Biometrics* 1989; 45:325–335.

67. Goedert JJ, Kessler KM, Aledort LM et al. A prospective study of human immunodeficiency virus type 1 infection and the development of AIDS in subjects with hemophilia. *N Engl J Med* 1989; 312:1141–1148.

68. O'Brien WA, Hartigan PM, Martin D et al. Changes in plasma HIV-1 RNA and CD4+lymphocyte counts and the risk of progression to AIDS. *New Engl J Med* 1996; 334:426.

69. Mellors JW, Munoz A, Giorgi JV et al. Plasma viral load and CD4+ lymphocytes as prognostic markers in HIV-1 infection. *Ann Intern Med* 1997;126:946–954.

70. Fei MW, Kim EJ, Sant CA. Predicting mortality from HIV-associated Pneumocystis pneumonia at illness presentation: an observational cohort study. *Thorax* 2009; 64:1070–1076.

71. Klein RS, Harris CA, Small CB et al. Oral candidiasis in high-risk patients as the initial manifestation of the acquired immune deficiency syndrome. *New Engl J Med* 1984; 311:354–358.

72. Snider WD, Simpson DM, Nielsen S et al. Neurological complications of acquired immune deficiency syndrome: analysis of 50 patients. *Ann Neurol.* 1983 Oct;14(4):403–18.

73. Antman K, Chang Y. Kaposi's Sarcoma. *N Engl J Med* 2000; 342:1027–1038

74. Grogg KL, Miller RF, Dogan A. HIV infection and lymphoma. *J Clin Pathol* 2007; 60(12): 1365–1372.

75. Shiels MS, Engels EA. Evolving epidemiology of HIV-associated malignancies. *Curr Opin HIV AIDS* 2017; 12(1):6–11.

76. Kaslow RA, Carrington M, Apple R et al. Influence of combinations of human major histocompatibility complex genes on the course of HIV-1 infection. *Nat Med* 1996; 2: 405.

77. Saah AJ, Hoover DR, Weng S et al. Association of HLA profiles with early plasma viral load, CD4+ cell count and rate of progression to AIDS following acute HIV-1 infection. *AIDS* 1998; 12:2107–

78. Alexander TS. Human immunodeficiency virus diagnostic testing: 30 years of evolution. *Clin Vaccine Immunol* 2016; 23(4): 249–253.

79. Branson BM, Handsfield HH, Lampe MA et al. Revised recommendations for HIV testing of adults, adolescents and pregnant women in health-care settings. *MMWR Recommend Rep* 2006; 55(RR-17):1–17.

80. Guidance on provider-initiated HIV testing and counselling in health facilities. Joint UNAIDS and WHO statement. May, 2007. www.who.int/hiv

81. Centers for Disease Control and Prevention and Association of Public Health Laboratories. Laboratory testing for HIV infection. 2014. Available at: http://stacks.cdc.gov/view/cdc/23447. Downloaded Oct 25,2017.

82. Division of HIV/AIDS Prevention, National Center for HIV/AIDS, Viral Hepatitis, STD, and TB Prevention, Centers for Disease Control and Prevention. Available at: www.cdc.gov/hiv/statistics/overview/index.html. Downloaded 10/25/2017.

83. Global HIV and AIDS statistics | AVERT. Available at: www.avert.org

84. www.smithsonianmag.com/history/the-confusing-and-at-times-counterproduct ive-1980s-response-to-the-aids-epidemic-180948611/#MxHcOWSb8xqF5mEc.99

85. Merson MH, O'Malley J, Serwadda D, Apisuk C. The history and challenge of HIV prevention. *Lancet* 2008; 372: 475–488.

86. Pinkerton SD, Abramson PR. Effectiveness of condoms in preventing HIV transmission. *Social Science and Medicine* 1997; 44(9): 1303–1312.

87. MMWR. CDC Current Trends: Prevention of Acquired Immune Deficiency Syndrome (AIDS): Report of Inter-Agency Recommendations. *MMWR* 1983; 32:101–3.

88. Shilts R. *And the Band Played On*. St. Martin's Press. New York, NY. 1987. Pg. 55, 579.

89. Koop CE. Surgeon General's report on acquired immune deficiency syndrome. *Public Health Rep* 1987; 102(1):1–3.

90. CDC. *Compendium of HIV prevention interventions with evidence of effectiveness*. Atlanta, Georgia: US Department of Health and Human Services, CDC, March 1999.

91. Magic Johnson Foundation: MJF. www.Magicjohnson.org

92. Cavaretta J. *Magic Johnson Combats AIDS Misperceptions.* USA Today. 10/3/2006.

93. Diamond J. *Flashback: Magic Johnson Makes Earth-Shattering HIV Announcement.* Rolling Stone. 11/7/2016.

94. Auvert B, Taljaard D, Lagarde E et al. Randomized controlled intervention trial of male circumcision for reduction of HIV infection risk: The ANRS 1265 trial. *PLoS Med* 2007; 2(11): e298.

95. Siegfried N, Muller M, Volmink J, Deeks JJ, Egger M, Low N, Weiss H, Walker S, Williamson P. Male circumcision for prevention of heterosexual acquisition of HIV in men. *Cochrane Database of Syst Rev* 2009; 14:CD003362.

96. Wiysonge CS, Kongnyuy EJ, Shey M, Muula AS, Navti OB, Akl EA, Lo YR. Male circumcision for prevention of homosexual acquisition of HIV in men. *Cochrane Database Syst Rev* 2011; 14:CD007496.

97. U.S. Centers for Disease Control and Prevention (CDC). Recommendations for providers counseling male patients and parents regarding male circumcision and the prevention of HIV infection, STIs, and other health outcomes. A notice by the Centers for Disease Control and Prevention on 12/02/2014. [Docket No. CDC–2014–0012]. Fed Regist.2014; 79(231):71433. Available at: www.federalregis ter.gov/documents/2014/12/02/2014-27814/recommendations-for-providers-cou nseling-male-patients-and-parents-regarding-male-circumcision-

98. CDC. Guidelines for prophylaxis against *Pneumocystis carinii* pneumonia for persons infected with human immunodeficiency virus. *MMWR* 1989; 38(No. S-5):1–9.

99. Centers for Disease Control. Recommendations for prophylaxis against *Pneumocystis carinii* pneumonia for adults and adolescents infected with human immunodeficiency virus. *MMWR* 1992; 41(No. RR-4).

100. Epstein S. *Impure Science: AIDS, Activism, and the Politics of Knowledge.* University of California Press; December 9, 1996.

101. Fischl MA, Richman DD, Grieco MH et al. The efficacy of azidothymidine (AZT) in the treatment of patients with AIDS and AIDS-related complex. A double-blind, placebo-controlled trial. *N Engl J Med* 1987; 317(4):185–91.

102. Lambert JS, Seidlin M, Reichman RC et al. 2',3'-Dideoxyinosine (ddI) in Patients with the Acquired Immunodeficiency Syndrome or AIDS-Related Complex—A Phase I Trial. *N Engl J Med* 1990; 322:1333–

103. Skowron G, Bozzette SA, Lim L et al. Alternating and intermittent regimens of zidovudine and dideoxycytidine in patients with AIDS or AIDS-related complex. *Ann Intern Med* 1993; 118(5):321–30.

104. Tseng A, Seet J, Phillips EJ. The evolution of three decades of antiretroviral therapy: challenges, triumphs and the promise of the future. *Br J Clin Pharmacol* 2014; 79(2):182–194.

105. Losina E, Schackman BR, Sadownik SN et al. Racial and sex disparities in life expectancy losses among HIV-infected persons in the United States: impact of risk behavior, late initiation, and early discontinuation of antiretroviral therapy. *Clin Infect Dis* 2009; 49(10):1570–1578.

106. Althoff KN, Chandran A, Zhang J et al. Life-expectancy disparities among adults with HIV in the United States and Canada: the impact of a reduction in drug- and alcohol-related deaths using the lives saved simulation model. *American Journal of Epidemiology* 2019; 188(12): 2097–2109,

107. Govindasamy D, Ford N, Kranzer K. Risk factors, barriers and facilitators for linkage to antiretroviral therapy care: a systematic review. *AIDS* 2012; 26(16):2059–2067.

108. Cohen MS, Chen YQ, McCauley M et al. Prevention of HIV-1 infection with early antiretroviral therapy. *New England Journal of Medicine* 2011 Aug 11;365(6):493–505.

109. Lundgren JD, Babiker AG, Gordin F et al. The INSIGHT START Group. Initiation of antiretroviral therapy in early asymptomatic HIV infection. *N Engl J Med* 2015; 373(9):795–807.

110. TEMPRANO ANRS Study Group, Danel C, Moh R et al. A trial of early antiretrovirals and isoniazid preventive therapy in Africa. *N Engl J Med* 2015; 373(9):808–822.

111. Rodger AJ, Cambiano V, Bruun T et al. Sexual activity without condoms and risk of HIV transmission in serodifferent couples when the HIV-positive partner is using suppressive antiretroviral therapy. *JAMA* 2016; 316(2):171–181.

112. Panel on Antiretroviral Guidelines for Adults and Adolescents. *Guidelines for the use of antiretroviral agents in HIV-1-infected adults and adolescents. Department of Health and Human Services.* Available at: http://aidsinfo.nih.gov/contentfiles/lvguidelines/AdultandAdolescentGL.pdf (Accessed on October 10,2017).

113. The Antiretroviral Therapy Cohort Collaboration. Survival of HIV-positive patients starting antiretroviral therapy between 1996 and 2013: a collaborative analysis of cohort studies. *The Lancet HIV,* online publication 10 May 2017. Available at: http://dx.doi.org/10.1016/S2352-3018(17)30066-8

114. Katz IT and Maughan-Brown B. Improved life expectancy of people living with HIV: who is left behind? *The Lancet HIV, online publication* 10 May 2017. http://dx.doi.org/10.1016/S2352-3018(17)30086-3

115. Grant RM, Lama JR, Anderson PL et al. iPrEx Study Team. Preexposure chemoprophylaxis for HIV prevention in men who have sex with men. *N Engl J Med* 2010; 363(27):2587–99.

116. McCormack S, Dunn DT, Desai M et al. Pre-exposure prophylaxis to prevent the acquisition of HIV-1 infection (PROUD): effectiveness results from the pilot phase of a pragmatic open-label randomized trial. *Lancet* 2016; 387:53–60.

117. US Public Health Service. Pre-exposure prophylaxis for the prevention of HIV infection in the United States – 2014. A Clinical Practice Guideline. Division of HIV/AIDS Prevention, National Center for HIV/AIDS, Viral Hepatitis, STD, and TB Prevention, Centers for Disease Control and Prevention. www.cdc.gov/hiv/risk/prep/index.html. Downloaded October 29, 2017.

118. Sultan B, Benn P, Waters L. Current perspectives in HIV post-exposure prophylaxis. *HIV/AIDS–Research and Palliative Care* 2014:6 147–158. Available at: http://dx.doi.org/10.2147/HIV.S46585

119. CDC. HIV in the United States | Statistics Overview | Statistics Center | HIV. www.cdc.gov/hiv/statistics/overview/ataglance.html. Downloaded 10/31/2017.

120. Shilts R. *And the Band Played On.* St. Martin's Press. New York, NY.1987.

121. CDC. Impact of the Expanded AIDS Surveillance Case Definition on AIDS Case Reporting – United States, First Quarter, 1993. *MMWR* April 30, 1993; 42(16):308–310.

122. HIV and AIDS—United States, 1981—2000. *MMWR.* June 1, 2001; 50(21); 430–434.

123. CDC. HIV/AIDS among racial/ethnic minority men who have sex with men— United States, 1989–1998. *MMWR* 2000; 49:4–11.

124. HIV/AIDS Surveillance Report 2005 – Centers for Disease Control and Prevention. www.cdc.gov/hiv/pdf/statistics_2005_hiv_surveillance_report

125. Koblin BA, Mayer KH, Eshleman SH et al. Correlates of HIV acquisition in a cohort of Black men who have sex with men in the United States: HIV prevention trials network. *PLoS One* 2013;8(7): e70413.

126. CDC. Recommendations for HIV Prevention with Adults and Adolescents in the United States, 2016. www.cdc.gov/hiv/guidelines/recommendations/personswith hiv.html

127. CDC. Estimated HIV incidence and prevalence in the United States, 2010–2016. *HIV Surveill Suppl Rep* 2019; 24(1) www.cdc.gov/hiv/group/pregnant-people/ numbers.html

128. CDC's HIV Surveillance Report: Diagnoses of HIV Infection in the United States and Dependent Areas, 2017; vol. 29.

129. U.S. Statistics/ HIV.gov www.hiv.gov › hiv-basics › overview › data-and-trends › statistics

130. Hosek SG, Landowitz RJ, Kapoglannis B et al. Adolescent Trials Network for HIV/ AIDS Interventions. An HIV pre-exposure prophylaxis demonstration project and safety study for young MSM. *J Acquir Immune Defic Syndr* 2017; 74(1):21–29.

131. CDC. *HIV Surveillance Special Report, HIV infection risk, prevention, and testing behaviors among men who have sex with men*. National HIV Behavioral Surveillance, 20 U.S. Cities, 2014, No. 15; January 2016.

132. Holmes KK, Karon JM, Kreiss J. The increasing frequency of heterosexually acquired AIDS in the United States, 1983–88. *Am J Public Health* 1990; 80(7):858–63.

133. CDC. Current Trends in AIDS in Women – United States. *MMWR* 1990; 39(47):845–846.

134. Centers for Disease Control and Prevention, Division of HIV/AIDS Prevention, National Center for HIV/AIDS, Viral Hepatitis, STD, and TB Prevention. HIV in the United States: Diagnoses of HIV infection in the United States and dependent areas, 2015. www.cdc.gov/hiv/basics/statistics.html. Accessed November 6, 2017.

135. amfAR, The Foundation for AIDS Research. HIV and AIDS statistics – United States. June, 2019.

136. CDC. Diagnoses of HIV infection in the United States and dependent areas, 2017. *HIV Surveillance Report* 2018; 29.

137. Baetan J, Planee-Phillips T, Mgodi NM et al. High adherence and sustained impact on HIV-1 incidence: Final results of an open-label extension trial of the dapivirine vaginal ring. *10th IAS Conference on HIV Science* (IAS 2019). July 23, 2019

138. Changing epidemiology of HIV disease: cumulative reported U.S. adult and adolescent AIDS cases by risk group, through December 1985 and December 1995. Centers for Disease Control. HIV/AIDS Surveillance Report. December 1995.

139. Schoenbaum EE, Hartel D, Selwyn PA et al. Risk factors for human immunodeficiency virus infection in intravenous drug users. *N Engl J Med* 1989; 321(13):874–879.

140. Wodak A, Cooney A. Do needle syringe programs reduce HIV infection among injecting drug users: a comprehensive review of the international evidence. *Subst Use Misuse* 2006; 41:777–813.

141. Metzger D, Navaline H, Woody G. Drug abuse treatment as AIDS prevention. *Publ Health Reports* 1998; 113(Suppl): 97–106.

142. Conrad C, Bradley HM, Broz D et al. Community outbreak of HIV infection linked to injection drug use of Oxymorphone—Indiana, 2015. *MMWR* 2015; 64(16):443–444.

143. CDC. National Center for HIV/AIDS, Viral Hepatitis, STD and TB Prevention. Available at: www.cdc.gov/vitalsigns/hiv-drug-use/index.html

144. Eyester ME. Coping with the HIV epidemic 1982–2007: 25 year outcomes of the Hershey Hemophilia Cohort. *Hemophilia* 2008; 14:697–702.

145. Leveton LB, Sox HC Jr, Stoto MA, editors. Institute of Medicine (US) Committee to study HIV transmission through blood and blood products. *HIV and the Blood Supply: An Analysis of Crisis Decision-making. Chapter 3. History of the Controversy.* Washington(DC): National Academies Press (US); 1995. Available at: www.ncbi. nlm.nih.gov/books/NBK232419/

146. Curran JW, Lawrence DN, Jaffe H et al. Acquired immune deficiency syndrome (AIDS) associated with transfusions. *New Engl J Med* 1984; 310(2):69–75.

147. MMWR. Human Immunodeficiency Virus Infection in Transfusion Recipients and Their Family Members. *MMWR.* March 20, 1987; 36(10);137–40.

148. Selik RM, Ward JW, Buehler JW. Trends in transfusion-associated acquired immune deficiency syndrome in the United States, 1982–1991. *Transfusion* 1993; 33:890–893.

149. Lackritz EM, Satten GA, Aborle-Grasse J et al. Estimated risk of transmission of the human immunodeficiency virus by screened blood in the United States. *N Engl J Med* 1995; 333:1721–1725.

150. Zou S, Dorsey KA, Notari EP et al. Prevalence, incidence, and residual risk of human immunodeficiency virus and hepatitis C virus infections among United States blood donors since the introduction of nucleic acid testing. *Transfus* 2010; 50:1495–504.

151. Mofenson L. Epidemiology and determinants of vertical HIV transmission. *Semin Pediatr Infect Dis* 1994; 5:252–265.

152. Blanche S, Mayaux MJ, Rouzioux C et al. Relation of the course of HIV infection in children to the severity of disease in their mothers at delivery. *N Engl J Med* 1994; 330(5): 308–312.

153. Domachowske J. Pediatric human immunodeficiency virus infection. *Clin Microbiol Rev* 1996; 9:448–468.

154. CDC. Recommendations for assisting in the prevention of perinatal transmission of human T-lymphotropic virus typeIII/lymphadenopathy-associated virus and acquired immunodeficiency syndrome. *MMWR Morb Mortal Weekly Rep* 1985; 34(48):721–726.

155. Davis SF, Byers RH, Lindegren ML et al. Prevalence and incidence of vertically-acquired HIV infections in the United States. *JAMA* 1995; 274:952–955.

156. CDC. Guidelines for prophylaxis against *Pneumocystis carinii* pneumonia for children infected with human immunodeficiency virus. *MMWR Morb Mortal Weekly Rep* 1991; 40(RR 2):1–13.

157. Rogers MF. Epidemiology of HIV/AIDS in women and children in the USA. *Acta Paediatr Suppl* 1997; S-421:15–16.

158. CDC. Recommendations of the US Public Health Service Task Force on the use of zidovudine to reduce perinatal transmission of human immunodeficiency virus. *MMWR* 1994; 43 (no. RR-11).

159. Connor EM, Sperling RS, Gelber R et al. Reduction of maternal-infant transmission of human immunodeficiency virus type 1 with zidovudine treatment. *N Engl J Med* 1994; 331:1173–1180.

160. Shetty AK, Maldonado Y. Prevention of Perinatal HIV-1 Transmission in the United States. *AAP NeoReviews* 2001; 2(4).

161. Cooper ER, Charurat M, Mofenson LM, et al. Combination antiretroviral strategies for the treatment of pregnant HIV-1–infected women and prevention of perinatal HIV-1 transmission. *J Acquir Immune Defic Syndr* 2002; 29(5):484–494.

162. McKenna MT, Hu X. Recent trends in the incidence and morbidity associated with perinatal human immunodeficiency virus infection in the United States. *Am J Obstet Gynecol* 2007; 197(3)(suppl 1):S10–S16.

163. CDC. Diagnoses of HIV infection in the United States and dependent areas, 2019. *HIV Surveill Rep*, 2021; 32. www.cdc.gov/hiv/library/reports/hiv-surveillance.html

164. Rozenbaum W, Coulaid JP, Saimot AG et al. Multiple opportunistic infections in a male homosexual in France. *Lancet* 1982; 572–573.

165. Sterry W, Marmor M, Konrads A, Steigleder GK. Kaposi's sarcoma, aplastic pancytopenia, and multiple infections in a homosexual (Cologne,1976). *Lancet* 1983; i:924–5.

166. Bygbjerg IC. AIDS in a Danish surgeon (Zaire, 1976). *Lancet* 1983; i:925.

167. Vandepitte J, Verwilghen R, Zachee P. AIDS and cryptococcosis (Zaire,1977). *Lancet* 1983; i:925–6.

168. Dournon E, Penalba C, Saimot AG et al. AIDS in a Haitian couple in Paris. *Lancet* 1983; i:1040–1.

169. PHLS Communicable Disease Surveillance Centre. Acquired immune deficiency syndrome in Britain, August 1983. *Br Med J* 1983; 287:1205.

170. Ebbesen P, Biggar RJ, Melbye M. AIDS in Europe. *British Med J* 1983; 287:1324–136.

171. Clumeck N, Mascart-Lemone F, de Maubeuge A, Brenez D, Marcelis L. Acquired immune deficiency syndrome in black Africans. *Lancet* 1983; i:642.

172. Garrett. 1995. pg. 344.

173. Clumeck N, Sonnet J, Taelman H et al. Acquired immune deficiency in African patients. *New Engl J Med* 1984; 310:492–497.

174. Garrett. pg. 346–347.

175. Piot P, Quinn TC, Taelman H et al. Acquired immune deficiency syndrome in a heterosexual population in Zaire. *Lancet* 1984; 65–69.

176. Serwadda D, Sewankambo NK, Carswell JW et al. Slim disease: a new disease in Uganda and its association with HTLV-III infection. *Lancet* 1985; 2(8460):849–852.

177. Garry RF, Witte MH, Gottlieb AA et al. Documentation of an AIDS virus infection in the United States in 1968. *JAMA* 1988; 260(14):2085–2087.

178. Frøland SS, Jenum P, Lindboe CF et al. HIV-1 infection in a Norwegian family before 1970. *Lancet* 1988; 1(8598), 1344–1345.

179. Zhu T, Korber BT, Nahmias AJ et al. An African HIV-1 sequence from 1959 and implications for the origin of the epidemic. *Nature* 1998; 391: 594–597.

180. Sharp PM, Hahn BH. Origins of HIV and the AIDS pandemic. *Cold Spring Harbor Perspect Med* 2011; 1:a006841.

181. Worobey M, Gemmel M, Teuwen DE et al. Direct evidence of extensive diversity of HIV-1 in Kinshasa by 1960. *Nature* 2008; 455: 661–664.

182. Faria NR, Rambaut A, Suchard MA et al. The early spread and epidemic ignition of HIV-1 in human populations. *Science* 2014; 346(6205):56–61.

183. Quammen D. *The Chimp and the River: How AIDS Emerged from an African Forest.* David Quammen. New York: W.W. Norton & Company, 2015. Chapter 2.

184. Ihtte. 2006. Chapter 1. p. 2.

185. Gilbert MTP, Rambaut A, Wlasiuk G et al. The emergence of HIV/AIDS in the Americas and beyond. *PNAS* 2007; 104(47):18566–18570.

186. Magiorkinis G, Angelis K, Mamais I et al. The global spread of HIV-1 subtype B epidemic. *Infection Genetics Evolution* 2016; 46:169–179.

187. Cabello M, Romero H, Bello G. Multiple introductions and onward transmission of HIV-1 subtype B strains in North America and Europe. *Nat Sci Rep.* 2016; 6:33971.doi:10.1038/srep 33971.

188. Crocchiolo PR. AIDS epidemiology: the past ten years, the next ten years. *Arch Aid Res* 1991; 5(1–2):5–8.

189. Mertens TE, Low-Beer D. HIV and AIDS: where is the epidemic going? *Bull WHO* 1996; 74(2):121–129.

190. Hoskins R. Russia's Silent HIV Epidemic. *Foreign Policy*; November 22,2016.

191. Mann JM. The World Health Organization Global Strategy for the prevention and contrio of AIDS. *West J Med* 1987;147(6):732–734.

192. Witteveen, E, Schippers G. Needle and syringe exchange programs in Amsterdam. *Substance Use and Misuse* 2006; 41(6–7):835–6.

193. Ryder RW, Temmerman M. The effect of HIV-1 infection during pregnancy and the perinatal period on maternal and child health in Africa. *AIDS* 1911; 5 Suppl 1:S75–5.

194. Mandelbrot L, Henrion R. Human immunodeficiency virus and reproduction. *Ann NY Acad Sci* 1991;626:484–510.

195. WHO. United Nations AIDS. Report on the global HIV/AIDS epidemic – June 1998. data.unaids.org/pub/report/1998/19981125_global_epidemic_report_en.pdf

196. Wendland C. Research, therapy and bioethical hegemony: the controversy over perinatal AZT trials in Africa. *Africa Studies* 2008; 51:1–23.

197. Angell M. The ethics of clinical research in the third world. *N Engl J Med* 1997; 337:853–855.

198. Susser M. Editor's note: The prevention of perinatal HIV transmission in the less-developed world. *Amer J Public Health* 1998; 88(4):547–548.

199. Faden R, Kass N. Editorial: HIV research, ethics and the developing world. *Amer J Public Health* 1998; 88:548–550.

200. CDC. News Room: Press Release. Short-Course Regimen of AZT Proven Effective in Reducing Perinatal HIV Transmission. www.cdc.gov/media/pressrel/r980210.htm

201. Cohen MS, Levy JA, DeCock, Lange J. The spread, treatment, and prevention of HIV-1: evolution of a global pandemic. *J Clin Invest* 2008;118:1244–1254.

202. Creek TL, Sherma GG, Nkengasong J et al. Infant human immunodeficiency virus diagnosis in resource-limited settings: issues, technologies, and country experience. *Am J Obstet Gyneco* 2007; 197(3)(Suppl): S64–S71.

203. Guay LA, Musoke P, Fleming T, Bagenda D et al. Intrapartum and neonatal single-dose nevirapine compared with zidovudine for prevention of mother-to-child transmission of HIV-1 in Kampala, Uganda: HIVNET 012 randomised trial. *Lancet* 1999; 354(9181):795–802.

204. Lallemant M, Jourdain G, Le Coeur S et al. Single-dose perinatal Nevirapine plus standard Zidovudine to prevent mother-to-child transmission of HIV-1 in Thailand. *N Engl J Med* 2004; 351:217–228.

205. World Health Organization. Antiretroviral drugs and the prevention of mother-to-child transmission of HIV infection in resource-limited settings: expert consultation, Geneva, 5–6 February 2004: a summary of the main points from the meeting. Accessed Nov. 13, 2017.

206. World Health Organization. *Antiretroviral drugs and the prevention of mother-to-child transmission of HIV infection in resource-limited settings.* 2006. www.who.int/3by5/ arv_pmtct/en/

207. UNAIDS, President's Emergency Plan for AIDS Relief (PEPFAR) and Partners (2016) Start Free, Stay Free, AIDS Free: A super fast track framework for ending AIDS among children, adolescents and young women by 2020.

208. Zhao Y, Wang Y, Wang A et al. Median time to antiretroviral therapy initiation in a cohort of Chinese infants born with HIV. *JAMA Pediatr* 2017; Published online November 13, 2017. doi:10.1001/jamapediatrics.2017.3920.

209. WHO Consolidated guidelines on the use of antiretroviral drugs for treating and preventing HIV infection. 2016. www.unaids.org/sites/default/files/media_asset/ global-AIDS-update-2016_en.pdf

210. Global HIV & AIDS statistics — 2019 fact sheet. Available at: www.unaids.org › resources › fact-sheet

211. The Global HIV/AIDS Epidemic. The Henry J. Kaiser Family Foundation. www. kff.org/global-health-policy/fact-sheet/the-global-hivaids-epidemic/

212. European Center for Disease Prevention and Control(ECDC) and WHO Regional Office for Europe(WHO/Europe)(2016). Surveillance report: HIV/AIDS Surveillance in Europe 2015.

213. WHO. Global HIV/AIDS Update, 2022, Elimination of mother-to-child transmission. www.who.int/gho/hiv/epidemic_response/ART/en/; https://data.unicef. org/topic/hivaids/emtct/

214. At The Tipping Point – Tracking Global Commitments On AIDS. The ONE Campaign. www.one.org/us/policy/global-commitment-aids/

215. Gunthard HF, Saag MS, Benson CA et al. Antiretroviral drugs for treatment and prevention of HIV infection in adults: 2016 recommendations of the International Antiviral Society–USA Panel. *JAMA* 2016 July 12; 316(2): 191–210.

216. Deeks SG, Lewin SR, Ross AL et al. International AIDS Society global scientific strategy: towards an HIV cure 2016. *Nat Med* 2016;22(8):1–11.

217. Kristoff J, Palma ML, Garcia-Bates TM et al. Type 1-programmed dendritic cells drive antigen-specific latency reversal and immune elimination of persistent HIV-1. *EBioMedicine* 2019; 43:295–306.

218. Arandjelovic P, Kim Y, James P. Cooney JP et al. Venetoclax, alone and in combination with the BH3 mimetic S63845, depletes HIV-1 latently infected cells and delays rebound in humanized mice. *Cell Reports Medicine*, 2023; 101178 doi: 10.1016/j.xcrm.2023.101178

219. Reece MD et al. Ruxolitinib-mediated HIV-1 reservoir decay in A5336 phase 2a trial. *12th IAS Conference on HIV Science*, Brisbane, abstract TUPEB15, 2023.

220. Baetan J, Planee-Phillips T, Mgodi NM et al. High adherence and sustained impact on HIV-1 incidence: Final results of an open-label extension trial of the dapivirine vaginal ring. *10th IAS Conference on HIV Science (IAS 2019)*. July 23, 2019.

221. Ramgopal MN, Castagna A, Cazanave C et al. Efficacy, safety, and tolerability of switching to long-acting cabotegravir plus rilpivirine versus continuing

fixed-dose bictegravir, emtricitabine, and tenofovir alafenamide in virologically suppressed adults with HIV, 12-month results (SOLAR): a randomised, open-label, phase 3b, non-inferiority trial. *Lancet* 2023. Published: August 08,2023 doi: https://doi.org/10.1016/S2352-3018(23)00136-4

222. Granich RM, Gilks SF, Dye C et al. Universal HIV testing with immediate anti-retroviral therapy as a strategy for elimination of HIV transmission: a mathematical model. *Lancet* 2009; 373(9657):48–57.

223. Koenig S. Dorvil N, Devieux JG et al. Same-day HIV testing with initiation of anti-retroviral therapy versus standard care for persons living with HIV: A randomized unblinded trial. *PLoS Med* 2017; 14(7): e1002357. https://doi.org/10.1371/journal.pmed.1002357

224. Petersen M, Balzer L, Kwarsiima D et al. Association of implementation of uni-versal testing and treatment intervention with HIV diagnosis, receipt of antiviral therapy and viral suppression in East Africa. *JAMA* 2017;317(21):2196–2206.

225. Rerks-Ngarm S, Pitisuttithum P, Nitayaphan S et al. Vaccination with ALVAC and AIDSVAX to prevent HIV-1 infection in Thailand. *New Eng J Med* 2009; 361(23):2209–2220.

226. Fischer W, Perkins S, Theiler J et al. Polyvalent vaccines for optimal coverage of potential T-cell epitopes in global HIV-1 variants. *Nat Med.* 2007 Jan; 13(1): 100–6.

227. Gray GE, Laher F, Lazurus E, Cory L. Approaches to preventative and therapeutic HIV vaccines. *Curr Opin Virol.* 2016 Apr; 17:104–9.

228. Sept. 23, 2023. www.nih.gov/news-events/news-releases/clinical-trial-hiv-vacc ine-begins-united-states-south-africa

229. Edward Koch, "Senator Helms's Callousness toward AIDS Victims," *NYTimes.* November 7, 1987.

230. www.gmhc.org/about-us/about-us.

231. www.gmhc.org/about-us/gmhchivaids-timeline

232. Kramer L. *The Normal Heart.* Samual French Inc. NY,NY. 1985.

233. *An Early Frost.* Screenplay by Sherman Yellen. Directed by John Erman. NBC. 11/11/1985.

234. Monette P. *Borrowed Time: An AIDS Memoir* (NY: Harcourt Brace) 1988. https://books.google.com/books?id=lBD-AgAAQBAJ&printsec=frontcover&dq=Grie f+is+a+sword&hl=en&sa=X&ved=0ahUKEwjx8KPmw6bYAhXJSd8KHbQ6B NYQ6AEIOjAD#v=onepage&q&f=false

Suggested Reading

Avram Finkelstein. *After Silence.* University of California Press. Oakland, CA. 2018.

Elizabeth Glazer, Laura Palmer. *In the Absence of Angels.* G.P. Putnam & Sons. New York. 1991.

Gena Corea. *The Invisible Epidemic: The Story of Women and AIDS.* HarperCollins. New York. 1992.

John Iliffe. *The African AIDS Epidemic. A History.* Ohio University Press. Athens, OH. 2006.

Paul Farmer. *Infections and Inequalities: The Modern Plague.* With a new preface. University of California Press. Oakland, CA. 2001.

Paul Monette. *Borrowed Time: An AIDS Memoir*. Harcourt-Brace. New York. 1988.

Randall M Packard. *A History of Global Health: Interventions into the Lives of Other Peoples*. Johns Hopkins University Press. Baltimore, MD. 2016.

Randy Shilts. *And the Band Played On*. St. Martin's Press. New York. 1987.

Stephen Epstein. *Impure Science: AIDS, Activism and the Politics of Knowledge*. University of California Press. Berkeley. 1989.

7

OUT OF NOWHERE

West Nile Virus, SARS, Zika and Ebola

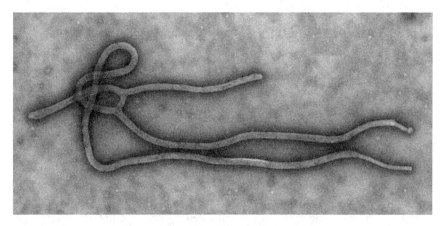

FIGURE 7.1 Electron micrograph of the Ebola virus.

Source: cdc.gov

DOI: 10.4324/9781003427667-7

A HOPEFUL EBOLA WARRIOR

At the end of September 2014, I retired as Professor of Pediatrics at the University of Rochester. October was my first month without full-time employment in the last 40 years, a simultaneously liberating and terrifying situation. One morning in that first week, I was drinking coffee and reading the *New York Times* at 10 o'clock in the morning – a previously unknown experience. The Ebola epidemic ravaging West Africa was front page news with 2400 deaths since the first reported case in the outbreak in December 2013 in Guinea. President Obama had just announced a major, military-led US response to the Ebola outbreak that "has reached epidemic proportions and now poses a potential threat to global security." Every channel was covering the epidemic 24/7, reporting that medical volunteers were desperately needed. All of a sudden, I realized this was something I could do, a way I could put all my years of medical experience to work. Online, the US Agency for International Development (USAID) had the following announcement:

MEDICAL VOLUNTEERS

If you are a qualified medical professional and want to volunteer to work in West Africa assisting those affected by the Ebola outbreak, please fill out the form embedded below to submit your contact information to USAID's Center for International Disaster Information.

I filled out the form the same day. According to the USAID website, all applications from experienced health sector workers would be reviewed and triaged to different agencies like the CDC, Project Hope and Medecin Sans Frontieres. Volunteers would be contacted within the next 2–4 weeks to arrange training and posting. I was tense but elated, ready to go. I reassured my anxious husband and was congratulated by my adventurous daughter. I began reading everything I could get my hands on about Ebola and identified the vaccinations I would need to enter West Africa. Every day, I checked the website for updates and my email for responses. Two weeks later, I received a very polite and extremely dismissive email reporting that because individuals over 59 years of age have a worse outcome if they contract Ebola, no volunteers in my age group were being accepted. I tried e-mailing and calling to no avail. My career as an Ebola fighter was over.

But my interest in Ebola was not. Initial recognition of this terrifying hemorrhagic fever occurred more than 40 years ago when simultaneous outbreaks occurred in two small villages in central Africa. From the outset, Ebola hemorrhagic fever was seen to have an extremely high fatality rate, more than 50% of all clinically apparent cases – one of the highest mortality rates of any known infectious disease. But previous outbreaks had occurred in localized small populations and the outbreaks had typically burned themselves out within months when the virus could find no new subjects to infect. The pandemic that began in Sierra Leone was different and galvanized scientists, ID specialists and public health practitioners – like me – all over the world.

Studying the Ebola pandemic as it evolved sparked the realization that epidemics caused by viruses have been increasing in frequency and ferocity over the last century. Terrifying disease outbreaks caused by new and re-emerging viral pathogens – like Ebola – have been occurring at closer and closer intervals. Often, the virus has jumped from an animal reservoir to infect humans and equally often, the virulence of the pathogen has been initially under-appreciated. Historians have identified recurrent themes that have marked almost every pandemic beginning with the plague in the thirteenth century: the sudden emergence of a previously unknown pathogen; the critical role of travel bringing a new contagion to a naïve population; the importance of poor general health and hygiene, overcrowding and lack of sanitation; and inadequate access to appropriate health care. But as with the Ebola pandemic of 2014–2015, our response to each new epidemic – the response of the medical establishment and the general public alike – almost always includes a sense that the outbreak sprang "out of nowhere!"

In fact, the most recent global epidemic challenges with Ebola and with West Nile virus, SARS and the Zika virus did expose new elements that have made us increasingly vulnerable to infectious threats: emerging viral pathogens; ever-increasing world population density with chaotic urbanization; rapid, frequent global travel and trade; and environmental change. Each epidemic originally seemed to emerge from nowhere to blast its way through the virology and epidemiology and disease characteristics that we thought we knew to create a terrifying narrative all its own. Each was originally a mysterious illness and as the narratives in this chapter will show, how quickly we responded by identifying and containing the pathogen was directly measured in lives lost or compromised. The stories are unique but identifying the critical connections between the power of new viral contagions and global inter-connectedness illuminates the terrifying capacity for deadly disease outbreaks in our current toxic environment. How rapidly we identify and how effectively we respond to viral disease outbreaks like these may well be critical factors in our survival as a species.

Out of Nowhere: West Nile Virus, Sars, Zika and Ebola

West Nile Virus

The dead birds came first. Near the end of June 1999, residents of northern Queens, one of New York (NYC) city's five boroughs, began to find bodies of dead birds, most often crows. From early July, officials at the Bronx Zoo received daily calls about dead birds and the zoo's chef pathologist, Dr. Tracey McNamara, became concerned about a potential pathogen that could infect the zoo's exotic bird collection. After a summer of "dead bird" calls, her concern was tragically realized in early September when two Chilean flamingoes, an Asian pheasant and a cormorant died suddenly over a three-day period. Autopsies of the dead birds revealed signs of brain inflammation and bleeding along with myocarditis, with no recognized pathogen. By this time, there had been many, many citizen reports of dead birds in Manhattan, Westchester and Connecticut. Dr. McNamara sent specimens from the zoo's cases to the National Veterinary Services Lab in Ames, Iowa and to the CDC in Atlanta, with initially no conclusive identification of the pathogen. Finally, she sent new specimens to the US Army Medical Research Institute of Infectious Diseases in Iowa where flavivirus-like particles were observed by electron microscopy.[1] These were forwarded to the CDC where West Nile virus was identified on September 21.[2] At the time, West Nile virus was a virus known to cause encephalitis but it had never previously been identified in North America nor ever reported to cause disease in birds.

Meanwhile, on August 23, an infectious disease specialist at Flushing Hospital in Queens contacted the NYC Health Department to report two elderly patients admitted with similar serious signs of encephalitis, an inflammation of the brain, with no identifiable cause. Over the next two weeks, seven new cases were admitted from the same area with similar alarming neurologic findings including signs of axonal neuropathy with flaccid paralysis like that seen with polio; three elderly patients died.[3] When an environmental investigation was performed, all the patients were found to have come from the same area in Queens and all were avid appreciators of the outdoors. Mosquito breeding sites were identified in the yards and/or neighborhoods of every patient. Urgent CDC evaluation of blood and spinal fluid samples using antibody testing originally led to identification of St. Louis encephalitis virus, a neurotropic virus known to cause encephalitis but never previously seen on the East Coast. Subsequently, DNA sequencing of viral isolates by polymerase chain reaction (PCR) analysis led to the identification of West Nile Virus as the cause of this cluster of encephalitis cases.[4] By September 28 when knowledge of the two parallel outbreaks converged, there had been countless avian WNV infections and deaths, and a total of 17 confirmed and 20 probable human cases of WNV encephalitis with four deaths reported from NYC and surrounding counties. A serious outbreak was underway.

The Disease and the Vector Identified

West Nile Virus was first isolated in 1937 from the blood of a febrile Ugandan woman during yellow fever surveillance screening.[5] That first patient's only symptom was fever but subsequent serologic studies with injection of her serum into mice led to isolation of a virus similar to two known flaviviruses shown to cause encephalitis – St. Louis encephalitis virus and Japanese B encephalitis – suggesting that this new virus might also be neurotropic.[6] The early pattern of clinical illness associated with WNV infection was defined in the 1950s when there were a series of outbreaks in the biogeographic region bordering the Mediterranean Sea. At that time, WNV fever was described as a generally mild flu-like illness with symptoms of fever, headache, myalgia, rash and vomiting. No fatalities or encephalitis cases were recorded in these early outbreaks.[7,8]

Studies in the 1940s demonstrated that WNV was carried by mosquitoes, suggesting vector-borne transmission. Detailed serologic and ecologic studies in humans and animals conducted by the US Naval Medical Research Unit with the Ministry of Public Health in Egypt in the early 1950s were the first to define the basic ecology and epidemiology of WNV infection.[9] The virus was found to be widely disseminated in the populations of the Nile Delta with clinical disease consistently described as a mild, flu-like illness with no cases of encephalitis and no fatalities. However, experimental infection of humans with terminal cancer (performed to induce a theoretically beneficial febrile reaction) did lead to several cases of encephalitis proving the WNV did have neurotropic properties. Viremia developed by 24 hours after infection and lasted up to 12 days, with the duration correlating with the severity of the illness. Besides mosquitoes, several additional hosts were also identified including camels, cows, donkeys, water buffalo, goats, horses, sheep and bats; horses often developed severe, symptomatic infections which could be fatal. Extensive studies of captured arthropods showed WNV only in mosquitoes, predominantly the *Culex* species. Multiple avian species including crows, herons and pigeons were found to be positive for WNV. On the basis of these studies, *Culex* mosquitoes were identified as host-vectors for WNV with birds as reservoir hosts. Humans and domestic quadrupeds were thought to be only incidentally infected. This was the first identification of the primary "bird-mosquito-bird" cycle of WNV shown in Figure 7.2.

In 1957, during a widespread outbreak of WNV in Israel, the first naturally occurring cases of encephalitis were reported in a group of elderly patients and over the next 20 years, rare cases of encephalitis were reported in a series of WNV outbreaks in Europe, Africa, Russia and India.[7,10]

Until the 1990s, large outbreaks of WNV were rare and the disease was consistently mild, but the epidemiology appeared to change with epidemics of increasing size and severity beginning with a large outbreak in Bucharest, Romania in 1996. The clinical spectrum was different with a reported preponderance of cases with central nervous system involvement – encephalitis or meningitis. In contrast to previous outbreaks which occurred where WNV disease was common and serologic evidence suggested widespread background infection, the Romanian population was largely serologically naïve to WNV and therefore highly susceptible to the infection.[11] This epidemic was followed by a series of widely disseminated, sporadic WNV outbreaks with significant CNS involvement and higher fatality rates in sub-Saharan Africa, the Middle East,

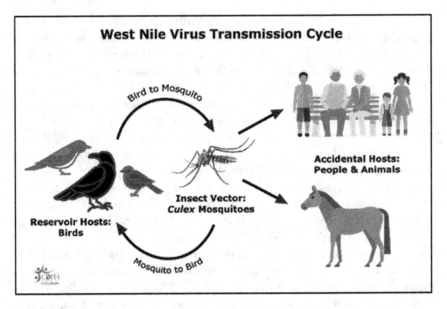

FIGURE 7.2 Reservoir bird cycle of the West Nile virus. Humans and animals are accidental hosts.

Source: www.cdc.gov.westnile

Europe, Southern Asia, India, China and the Far East, all thought to be spread by migrant birds originating in northern Africa.[12,13]

Until 1999, the western hemisphere was spared but that summer, multiple factors converged to bring the WNV to NYC. It is not known how the virus entered the United States – it could have been carried by infected humans or pets, by imported or migratory birds or by virus-infected mosquitoes.[14] However the virus traveled here, its arrival certainly reflected the importance of increased global connectivity in the spread of infections. The speed of spread and the extent of this new epidemic reflected the complete absence of immunity in both birds and humans in North America. The summer of 1999 was also the hottest and driest summer in a century and scientists believe the heat may have accelerated the breeding cycle of the Culex mosquito vectors and the replication rate of the virus during digestion.

In that first outbreak, active surveillance ultimately identified 62 patients, 59 of whom were hospitalized, all with laboratory evidence of recent WNV infection and clinical evidence of central nervous system involvement; 10% of patients had diffuse flaccid paralysis with findings compatible with an axonal polyneuropathy like that seen with polio. Extrapolating from this surveillance group, the attack rate of clinical WNV infection in the outbreak was reported to be at least 6.5 cases per million population. The overall case fatality rate was 12% but among patients with muscle weakness, it was much higher, reported to be 30%.[15] Even before the West Nile virus was confirmed as the cause, the outbreak provoked an extensive regional public health response with a telephone hotline to answer questions, and leaflets and messages on radio and television, warning the public to take precautions against mosquito bites. NYC distributed insect repellent at fire houses and for the first time, began to spray pesticides in areas where there was evidence of WNV activity, using aircraft in the outer boroughs and trucks in the streets of Manhattan.

The actual number of WNV infections in 1999 is impossible to determine but it is estimated to be many thousands since people with nervous system involvement are only a small fraction of cases. Birds were known as a reservoir for the virus – but this was the first reported WNV outbreak in which birds developed evidence of disease with many thousands of avian deaths primarily in crows and jays before the epidemic ended after fall frosts suppressed mosquito populations.

The Virus, the Reservoir and the Vector

After its original identification, serologic cross-reactivity studies identified WNV as a member of the *Flaviviradae* family in the genus *Flavivirus*, within the Japanese encephalitis serocomplex, along with the Japanese encephalitis virus and the St. Louis encephalitis virus.[2] WNV is often classified functionally as an arbovirus, a group of pathogens linked by mosquito or tick vectors as transmitters and shared seasonal incidence and geographic distribution determined by these transmitting vectors. While other viruses can cause encephalitis, only arboviruses have caused epidemics of viral encephalitis.[12]

WNV is a small, spherical single-stranded, positive-sense RNA virus with a lipid bilayer envelope. By cryo-electron microscopy – evaluation of ultra-thin frozen slices – it is seen to have icosahedral symmetry and a smooth surface with no visible projections or spikes.[16] The RNA genome encodes a single polyprotein which is cleaved into three structural proteins which form the capsid, membrane and envelope, and seven multi-functional, non-structural proteins which are important for viral synthesis and/or assembly, and modulate cell signaling and immune responses. The complex processes of viral attachment and cell entry remain the subject of ongoing investigation. Unlike other RNA viruses, WNV has a slow mutation rate with changes occurring almost exclusively by genetic drift.[13]

By phylogenetic analysis of published isolates, five distinct WNV genetic lineages have been identified with lineages 1 and 2 associated with disease outbreaks in humans. Lineage 1 has three clades: clade 1a includes isolates from Africa, Europe, the Middle East, Russia and the Americas; the strain identified in the 1999 NYC outbreak is part of this clade; clade 1b contains the Kunjin virus from Australia; clade 1c contains only isolates from India. Distribution of clade 1c is documented as far back as the early 1800s. Lineage 2 is found in isolates from sub-Saharan Africa, Madagascar and Russia. Lineages 3 and 4 have been isolated from potential vectors but have never been identified in association with human disease. By phylogeographic analysis, the most recent common ancestor of WNV 1a is thought to have originally emerged in Africa around 1921.[13,17]

In the 1999 NYC epidemic, genome sequencing of the virus from the brain of one of the two dead Chilean flamingoes and isolates from other bird species plus two human cases revealed identical genetic sequences, confirming that a single WNV strain caused the outbreak in both humans and birds. By phylogenetic analysis, the NYC WNV strain – termed NY99 – showed a very high degree of sequence similarity, greater than 99.8%, with a clade 1a Israeli virus isolated from a dead goose in 1998. Retrospectively, that same strain had previously been observed to be associated with disease in birds but this had never been reported in any WNV outbreak. Thus, the cause of the NY99 outbreak was originally thought to be a single WNV strain introduced from Israel.[7,14] Subsequent phylogeographic analysis indicates that that WNV strain from Israel and the NY99 strain plus several others now circulating in Europe actually originated from the same independent unknown location, probably in Africa. Of note, all these strains are associated with avian mortality, supporting the concept of their shared, common origin.[17]

Consistent with the original findings in Egypt in the 1950s, mosquitoes remain the natural vector for WNV transmission with at least 65 species identified as potential transmitters in the United States. Solely ornithophilic mosquitoes infect only birds and maintain the enzootic cycle between birds and mosquitoes but they do not infect humans. Mosquitoes who feed on both birds and humans are called bridge vectors because they carry the virus from the infected avian reservoir to incidental mammalian hosts – humans and domestic vertebrates. Mosquitoes from the *Culex* genus are the most important WNV bridge vectors in North America, Europe, Australia and South Africa with different *Culex* species dominating transmission in other areas.[13]

Among the hundreds of bird species shown to carry the WNV, passerine or "perching" birds are the primary reservoirs and infecting hosts because they develop high enough levels of viremia to efficiently infect mosquitoes. Certain birds – especially, crows, jays and robins – are called WNV amplifiers because they are favorite mosquito targets with high levels of viremia. Humans, horses and other domestic mammals can experience serious – even deadly disease – but they do not develop high enough serum virus levels to infect mosquitoes and are therefore known as dead-end hosts.[12,18] In North America, WNV infections occur in prime mosquito season, from July to September. When an infected mosquito bites a susceptible human host, components in the mosquito's saliva suppress the immune reaction at skin level. Infected cells then migrate to draining lymph nodes from which systemic viremia develops, carrying infection throughout the body and potentially to the central nervous system.[12]

The Disease, Updated

Over time, the contemporary clinical pattern of WNV infection has been clarified. As with polio and yellow fever, 75–80% of individuals infected with WNV are entirely asymptomatic. Approximately 25% develop a mild, self-limited, flu-like illness with some combination of fever, myalgias, headache, lymphadenopathy and truncal rash. A much lower percentage – less than 1% – experience the potentially devastating neuro-invasive manifestations with the likelihood of this kind of neurologic involvement increasing significantly with age. Symptoms of meningitis due to WNV are similar to those seen with other viral meningitides, namely fever, headache and photophobia with neck pain and stiffness. Signs of WNV encephalitis range from mild, transient confusion to severe encephalopathy with multiple kinetic symptoms, coma and death. Very rarely, acute, flaccid paralysis develops, secondary to anterior horn cell involvement; this dreaded pattern can result in quadriplegia and respiratory failure. The majority of patients with uncomplicated WNV fever and those with meningitis recover completely but the prognosis for those with encephalitis is variable, with more than a third reporting some residual symptoms at one year post infection. In the rare patients with acute flaccid paralysis, one third recover completely, one third have some improvement and one third have little or no improvement with time. Overall, among those individuals with clinical neurologic disease, the case fatality rate ranges from 4 to 13% and across outbreaks, is consistently highest among elderly patients over 70 years of age.[12,19]

While mosquito bites account for the vast majority of human WNV infections, the virus has also been transmitted by transfusion with infected blood and blood products and by heart, liver, lung and kidney transplant.[13] Blood donor screening with nucleic acid amplification-testing has dramatically decreased the risk for transfusion-related WNV infection in North America but every year, blood from several hundred asymptomatic donors tests positive for WNV and rare cases of post-transfusion disease occur.[20,21] Transplacental transmission can occur but is extremely rare with no definitive evidence of consequent fetal abnormalities. Peripartum transmission has also been reported. The risk of deadly, neuroinvasive disease is enhanced in WNV-infected patients receiving rituximab (Rituxan), a B-cell depleting monoclonal antibody used to treat hematologic malignancies.

Diagnosis, Treatment and Prevention

Because of its non-specific presentation, WNV fever can be difficult to diagnose. Even with clinical signs of meningitis or encephalitis, specific testing for WNV has been reported in less than half of cases so a high incidence of clinical suspicion is necessary.[22] If WNV infection is suspected, detection of IgM antibody in serum or spinal fluid by MAC-ELISA testing is the standard diagnostic test. Because only approximately 50% of the typical minimally symptomatic patients have ELISA testing at clinical presentation, testing of acute- and convalescent sera is often needed for definitive diagnosis of WNV fever. By contrast, 90% of patients with signs of involvement of the central nervous system are positive for IgM antibodies in spinal fluid within 8 days of symptom onset. In uncertain cases, nucleic-acid testing for virus-specific genetic material – the technique used to screen the donor blood supply – can be used.

Treatment of WNV infection remains supportive since none of a variety of theoretically-useful measures including anti-viral agents,

WNV-recombinant-humanized-monoclonal- antibody, and polyclonal gamma-globulin infusions have proven effective.[23]

Development of a safe and effective vaccine has been a major research focus. Approaches include vaccines containing cocktails of individual WNV proteins, chimeric vaccines which combine genes from more than one virus into a single vaccine and DNA vaccines, in which DNA that codes for a particular WNV protein is combined with bacterial DNA with the combined product injected directly into the skin of the vaccinee. Currently, there is no licensed WNV vaccine for people although several have been developed and shown real promise in Phase I and II trials. Unfortunately, with WNV's unpredictable outbreaks, Phase III trials may be very difficult to accomplish. In 2005, the US Department of Agriculture licensed a DNA vaccine to prevent equine WNV, and since then, at least four other types of WNV vaccines have been approved for use in horses.

There are barriers to developing a human vaccine against an unpredictable disease like WNV with varying outbreak size from year to year, including safety concerns and financial risk to manufacturers who carry a vaccine all the way to a phase 3 clinical trial but may not recoup their investment. Researchers had predicted prospects for a vaccine being developed were low unless WNV became an uncontrollable global epidemic.[24] Funded by the National Institute for Allergy and Infectious Disease (NIAID) HydroVax-001 is a new WNV vaccine based on a novel, hydrogen peroxide-based process that renders the virus inactive while still maintaining key immune-system triggering surface structures. In a Phase 1 clinical trial, the HydroVax-001 vaccine was found to be modestly immunogenic and well-tolerated at escalating dose levels.[25] Phase II trials are underway.

The other focus of prevention is directed at mosquito management with elimination of breeding sites and pesticides to reduce mosquito populations plus aggressive pesticide use during outbreaks. Public health programs recommend personal protection with protective clothing and insect repellant use against mosquitoes throughout the summer season, especially in high-risk individuals.

After NYC

The WNV already had an impressive global distribution with multiple viral strains identified throughout Africa, the Middle East, southern Europe, western Russia and Asia, and Australia when the NYC outbreak occurred but before the summer of 1999, no case of WNV disease had ever been reported in the Western Hemisphere. Astonishingly, from the original presentation in NYC, the virus spread across the entire continent to the Pacific Coast by 2003, to South America by 2005 and across Canada by 2009.[26,27]

Since 1999, there have been annual summer outbreaks of WNV disease in the United States of varying size and severity with peaks of activity in 2002–03, 2006, 2012 and 2021–22; each of these summer seasons were notably hot and dry. In 2002, a new WNV genotype, WN02, appeared, characterized by one amino acid substitution and 13 conserved nucleotide mutations. WN02 was found to be more efficiently transmitted by New World mosquitoes than the NY99 strain.[28] This genetic change coincided with large US outbreaks in 2002–2003 and may have contributed to the rapid spread of WNV across North America. A second new genotype termed SW/WN03, defined by two additional fixed amino acid substitutions was first observed in isolates collected in 2003. Since that time, WN02 and SW/WN03 genotypes have completely displaced the ancestor NY99 genotype in the United States.[29] High but stable WNV activity in the USA continued until the summer of 2012 when another large outbreak of WNV disease occurred with 2,873 reported neuro-invasive cases and 286 deaths. In the most recent large WNV outbreak – a 2021–2022 event in Arizona that resulted in close to 1,700 cases (two-thirds neuroinvasive) and 121 WNV-related deaths – a wetter-than-average summer monsoon season may have played a role, along with non-immune birds. Because the majority of WNV-infected individuals are asymptomatic, incidence tracking uses neuro-invasive disease cases where reporting is more complete. Based on this methodology, WNV is now endemic in the United States; yearly outbreaks have resulted in an estimated total of *4 to 5 million* human infections! Between 1999 and 2014, over 41,700 cases of West Nile disease – the proverbial tip of the iceberg – have been reported to the CDC, including 19,510 neuro-invasive cases and 1,861 deaths.[29,30]

Distribution of West Nile virus is determined by a complex of demographic, environmental and social factors. Increasing international travel and trade, rising population density and progressive urbanization have facilitated global spread. Higher temperatures and lower precipitation rates related to climate change have made transmission seasons longer and more intense.[31] Following its introduction to the United States in 1999, WNV has caused the three largest arboviral neuro-invasive disease outbreaks ever recorded with nearly 3000 cases each year in 2002, 2003 and 2012. Globally, there has been a continuous increase in WNV cases, most recently in Europe in the summer of 2018.[12,32] Now found on every continent except Antarctica, WNV is a major global health problem with – to this time – ongoing, unpredictable regional, national and international outbreaks, no standardized method of prevention and no effective therapy.

Looking Back :: Moving Forward

The introduction of West Nile virus (WNV) into North America in 1999 is a classic example of viral emergence in a new, naïve host environment. Subsequent dramatic dispersion across the continent reflects the impact the virus had on equally naïve bird reservoir populations, accompanied by an established, widely distributed mosquito vector. Understanding the spread of this virus is an important step towards effective prevention. Phylogenetic analysis of the complete genomes of avian isolates sampled across the United States between 2001 and 2012 reveals a star-like tree structure, indicative of explosive viral spread with minimal replacement of viral genotypes over time.[33]

Analysis of diffusion rates indicates that the spread of WNV occurred too quickly to be explained by simple contiguous spread, even with highly mobile avian reservoirs and mosquito vectors. The flyways of terrestrial birds including those that carry WNV are similar although distinct from those of waterfowl, like those that carry the influenza virus. There are three defined North American terrestrial bird flight paths – Western, Central and Eastern – within which individual birds use looped routes that allow them to maximize tail winds and access feeding sites. Recent avian phylogeographic studies suggest that the flight paths of terrestrial birds like those that carry WNV are important components in spread of the virus. This same approach identified optimal sites for WNV surveillance in New York, Illinois and Texas.[34] Targeted surveillance and vector migration analyses based on information like this represent important potential ways to predict the annual flow of WNV and implement focused interventions. Indeed, a recently released network model that includes WNV spreading by migratory birds using established flyways shows potential for prediction of virus spreading in simulation models.[35]

At least 75% of emerging and re-emerging diseases in the last half century are either zoonotic, vector-borne or – like WNV – both. Such diseases emphasize the importance of inter-relationships among humans, animals and the environment in the emergence and diffusion of disease in our increasingly connected world. The *One Health Initiative* is based on this concept – that human, animal and ecological health are inextricably linked.[36] No emerging disease narrative exemplifies this better than the arrival of WNV in New York city where a previously unknown virus established host reservoirs in local bird flocks from which mosquito vectors perpetuated the infection, incidentally infecting naïve human hosts and domestic farm animals and spreading rapidly throughout the entire Western Hemisphere. It was a veterinarian caring for exotic tropical birds who first identified the virus and crow deaths have subsequently been shown to be a sensitive sentinel surveillance system for WNV.[2,37] Direct collaboration between physicians, veterinarians and epidemiologists to address the animal and human interface behind zoonotic outbreaks is an important approach to creation of effective treatment and prevention strategies at local, national and international levels.

When WNV infection involves the central nervous system, morbidity and mortality are high so development of effective therapeutic options is of critical importance. Validation and standardization of prevention efforts are also a high priority. Effective surveillance systems to predict developing outbreaks are critical and lessons learned from experience with annual outbreaks in the United States and ongoing international research should facilitate development of such systems. Of equal importance is the implementation of sustainable vector management at local, national, and international levels coupled with aggressive execution of adult mosquito control programs as described in Chapter 3 on yellow fever. Finally, development of a safe, cost-effective vaccine to prevent WNV infection is a global priority.

Severe Acute Respiratory Syndrome – SARS

In November 2002, multiple inhabitants of the Chinese province of Guangdong on the coast of the South China Sea suddenly developed symptoms of a flu-like illness with headache, fever and dry cough. Over a period of approximately 5 days, a subset of these patients developed a worsening cough and shortness of breath. In these patients, chest x-rays showed signs of progressive air-space disease compatible with atypical pneumonia but lab work was remarkable only for a mild increase in total white cells with low lymphocyte and platelet counts. In some patients in this group, respiratory distress progressed rapidly to respiratory failure and death. The illness spread through six municipalities, apparently carried through direct contact with sick individuals. On February 11, 2003, the Chinese Ministry of Health notified the World Health Organization (WHO) that 305 cases of this acute respiratory illness of unknown etiology had occurred between November 16, 2002 and February 9, 2003.[38] The report stated that the disease was particularly noteworthy for transmission to health-care workers and household contacts; five deaths were reported in this group. Investigations had ruled out anthrax, pulmonary plague, leptospirosis and hemorrhagic fever. By the time of China's report, the outbreak had been in progress for at least two and a half months.

This new disease spread very rapidly. On February 26, an American businessman traveling from China developed respiratory distress while on a flight to Singapore. The plane landed emergently in Hanoi, Vietnam and the traveler was hospitalized at the Vietnam French Hospital. Doctors there suspected a possible atypical influenza virus and contacted the local office of the WHO for assistance. This is where fate intervened in the form of Dr. Carlo Urbani, a specialist in infectious diseases who provided that consultation.[39] Dr. Urbani had extensive experience in global medicine as a former president of Medecins sans Frontieres (MSF) and he immediately recognized the gravity of the illness and the potential for epidemic spread. He sent samples for emergent testing and created an isolation ward in the hospital to care for the growing number of cases that followed in the wake of the American traveler, half of whom were health care workers. The WHO responded with an emergency meeting with the Vietnamese Minister of Health and this led to city-wide infection control measures and an international appeal for assistance; experts from the CDC, WHO and MSF responded and with traditional disease control methods – isolation of sick individuals and quarantine of contacts – the Hanoi outbreak was brought under control. Tragically, Dr. Urbani himself became infected with the unknown pathogen and he died on March 18, 2003.[39]

Almost simultaneously, an outbreak of a similar respiratory illness was reported in Hong Kong. In this cluster, the index case was a nephrologist working in a hospital in southern China who traveled to Hong Kong on February 21. He originally stayed in a hotel but developed progressive respiratory distress and was subsequently hospitalized. Despite intensive support including ventilation, he died. Between February 22 and March 22, 10 additional patients with SARS were immediately identified in Hong Kong. Most had social or hospital care contact with the index patient but in at least one case, contact was at most very limited, confirming the highly contagious and infectious nature of this unknown disease pathogen.[40]

There was an important international connection with this Hong Kong outbreak: a couple from Canada stayed at the same hotel on the same floor and at the same time as the index case described above.[41] As far as could be determined, there had been no direct contact between them but on February 25, two days after returning to Toronto, the 78-year-old wife developed fever, anorexia and cough. Within five days, her cough worsened and she became progressively short of breath; she died at home 3 days later. Her 43-year-old son developed progressive symptoms beginning February 27 and despite intensive respiratory support, he died on March 13. It was at this point that the new Chinese respiratory illness was first considered as a possibility and four additional family members screened positive for possible or probable pulmonary compromise. Five additional contact cases were diagnosed, including the doctor who evaluated the index case in this outbreak and her husband, a man who was exposed to patient 2 in the hospital ED and a man from Vancouver who stayed in the same hotel implicated in the Hong Kong outbreak. In this cluster of 10 cases, four people died and one was still in Intensive Care being ventilated at the time of the report. Subsequent contact tracing identified an additional 100 individuals with probable or suspected Severe Acute Respiratory Syndrome or SARS – the newly defined acronym – with one additional death reported. In addition to the description of the epidemiology of the cases, the Canadian report described virologic studies in the Toronto cases which identified a new, previously unidentified coronavirus in 5 and human metapneumovirus in 4.[41]

With confirmation of a highly contagious, rapidly progressive, sometimes fatal viral pneumonia transmitted by direct contact, airborne droplets and fomites now reported in at least four countries, the WHO instituted worldwide surveillance on March 15, 2003 and issued a rare global travel alert about the outbreak as evidence mounted that this acute, atypical pneumonia was spreading by air travel along international routes.[42] The WHO named the mysterious illness after its symptoms: severe acute respiratory syndrome (SARS), and declared it "a worldwide health threat."[42] On March 21, 2013, the US Centers for Disease Control (CDC) provided an interim case definition.[43]

CDC INTERIM CASE DEFINITION FOR SEVERE ACUTE RESPIRATORY SYNDROME (SARS) SUSPECTED CASE

Respiratory illness of unknown etiology with onset after 2/1/2003 + the following criteria:

- Measured temperature >100.4 degrees F (38 degrees C).
- One or more clinical findings of respiratory illness (e.g., cough, shortness of breath, difficulty breathing, hypoxia or radiographic findings of pneumonia or acute respiratory distress syndrome).

- Travel within 10 days of symptom onset to an area with suspected or documented community transmission of SARS.

OR

- Close contact within 10 days of symptom onset with either a person with respiratory illness and travel to a SARS area, or a person under investigation for SARS.

By March 26, a total of 1,323 suspected and/or probable SARS cases including 49 deaths had been reported to the WHO from 14 different countries – a case-fatality ratio of ~4%. Chinese authorities reported an updated total of 792 suspected/probable cases and 31 deaths in Guangdong province between November 16, 2002 and February 28, 2003.

The Virus

On March 28, the CDC reported that a novel, previously unrecognized coronavirus had been identified in clinical specimens from two patients from Thailand with suspected SARS. The isolate was identified initially as a coronavirus by electron microscopy, corroborated by results of immunostaining, indirect immunefluorescence antibody (IFA) assays, and reverse transcriptase-polymerase chain reaction (RT-PCR) with sequencing of a segment of the polymerase gene. IFA testing of sera and RT-PCR analysis of clinical specimens from six other SARS cases were positive for the new coronavirus. Sequence analysis indicted that this new agent was distinct from all other known coronaviruses.[44]

Other laboratories collaborating in the WHO-led investigation including the team from Canada had found similar results and had also isolated human metapneumovirus from some of the patients with suspected SARS.[41] At that time, information was insufficient to determine what roles these two viruses might play in the etiology of SARS. By April 16, the WHO announced that the new pathogen, a member of the coronavirus family never before seen in humans, was confirmed as the cause of SARS and would be designated as SARS-CoV.[44] The speed at which the virus was identified was the result of the close international collaboration of 13 laboratories from 10 countries. WHO and the network of laboratories dedicated their detection and characterization of the SARS virus to Dr. Carlo Urbani, the scientist who first alerted the world to the existence of SARS and who subsequently died from the disease.[39]

Coronaviruses belong to the subfamily Coronavirinae in the Coronaviradae family. They are enveloped spherical viruses with a positive-sense single-stranded RNA genome. The size of the genome is the largest for any RNA virus, ranging from 26 to 32 kilobases. The name "coronavirus" is derived from the Latin *corona*, meaning crown, and refers to the characteristic appearance of the virus

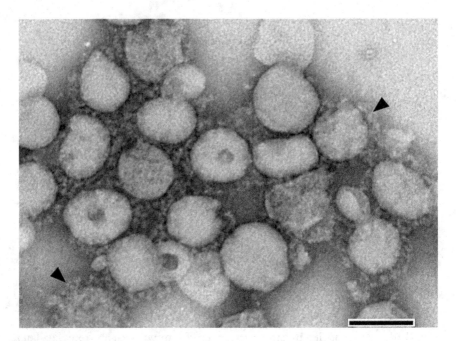

FIGURE 7.3 Transmission electron micrograph of original SARS Coronavirus. Arrows indicate surface spikes.

Source: cdc.gov

by electron microscopy which reveals a halo of spikes on the surface of the virus identified as S proteins, as shown in Figure 7.3.[45] These are the major antigenic determinants of coronaviruses, mediating receptor association and fusion of the viral and host cell membranes.

Coronaviruses are rapidly evolving viruses using the now familiar mechanisms of spontaneous point mutation and recombination to create ongoing genetic diversity. As a group, they cause respiratory and gastrointestinal disease in a wide variety of birds and mammals including cats, dogs, pigs, cows, chickens and ferrets. In humans, coronaviruses are responsible for 30–60% of common colds. Until SARS-CoV, no identified coronavirus was known to cause lower respiratory tract illness.

During the initial SARS outbreak in China in 2002–2003, animals from a Guangdong live animal "wet market" were identified as the likely immediate source of infection since all the early cases had a history of animal contact in this location. SARS-CoV was isolated from a majority of Himalayan palm civets in the market and subsequent culling of palm civets dramatically reduced the number of other infected animals in the marketplace. However, while the majority of civets in the market showed evidence of SARS-CoV infection, civets on farms and in the wild were free of the infection indicating that the market animals were only intermediate hosts for a virus that had first crossed species to infect them in the market setting, and then jumped to infect humans with whom the civets had direct contact

Bats had already been recognized as the natural reservoirs for a large variety of diverse viruses, including more coronaviruses than any other species. In 2005, two independent research groups reported almost simultaneously the discovery of novel coronaviruses related but not identical to SARS-CoV in horseshoe bats in China. After years of investigation, a live SARS-like CoV very closely resembling human SARS-CoV was isolated from bat fecal samples and was neutralized by convalescent SARS patient sera, providing convincing evidence that Chinese horseshoe bats are the ancestral origin of SARS-CoV.[46] While direct transmission of bat coronaviruses to humans is rare, human activity increasingly allows overlap with intermediate hosts like the civet that can mediate interspecies transmission.

Over the next 4 months, humans carried the SARS virus to 30 countries and areas of the world but it became deeply embedded in just six. In affected areas, approximately 20% of all cases were in health care workers. Ultimately, 8439 people were infected and 812 died from SARS in the 2002–2003 outbreak.[47] There were 4 cases of confirmed SARS in Guangdong province in the winter of 2003–2004 – all patients recovered. Since 2004, there has never been another identified case of SARS.

Looking Back :: Moving Forward

SARS presented emergent requirements to the global health system and despite concurrent outbreaks in multiple locations, these were met by a remarkable international collaboration coordinated by the WHO and the CDC. In the 5 months following the first cases of SARS in China, the epidemiology of this previously unknown disease was described and a novel causative organism identified.[48,49] Using a secure Internet site, laboratories shared information about the virus and the disease in real time. SARS-CoV was shown to be accurately diagnosed using enzyme-linked immunoassays (EIA) or reverse transcriptase polymerase chain reaction (RT-PCR) tests, performed on respiratory secretions or blood. Classic disease control measures – active surveillance, early diagnosis, infection control with isolation, contact tracing with quarantine, and international reporting – were aggressively implemented in multiple sites and proved effective. While a wide variety of antiviral and anti-inflammatory measures were attempted, there were no conclusive benefits so aggressive supportive care with prevention of viral spread was the recommended – and successful – approach.[50]

On July 5, 2003, the World Health Organization removed Taiwan, China, from the list of areas with recent local transmission of SARS, the last area to be cleared. Based on country surveillance reports, the chain of SARS-CoV transmission had been broken, everywhere in the world.[51] There have been no identified cases of SARS since 2004.

The SARS pandemic showed us how quickly a previously unknown virus can emerge from an animal reservoir and spread in our increasingly populous, highly mobile and interconnected world. This outbreak also emphasized the consequences of delayed and inaccurate reporting of a new disease outbreak – in the 3 months after the first cases appeared in China, the virus was able to establish a major outbreak there and initiate global spread. There was extreme under-reporting of the number of cases, the severity of the illness and its spread within China and this initially minimized the importance of the outbreak and therefore, the global response. Chinese authorities continued to cover up the extent of the outbreak for months before a brave whistleblowing physician, 72-year-old Jiang Yanyong, exposed the crisis through Western media, galvanizing the global response that ended the SARS pandemic. More recently Jiang, now 88, has had his contacts with the outside world cut off and movements restricted after he asked the authorities to reassess the 1989 Tiananmen pro-democracy movement. He is now under de facto house arrest.

The SARS pandemic foreshadowed many aspects of the COVID-19 pandemic to follow, including the speed with which a previously unknown virus can emerge and spread in our highly mobile and interconnected world. It also showed how concerted international cooperation and disease containment measures can allow health experts to effectively eliminate international spread of a highly contagious and virulent new disease – a model for the potential public health reaction to future new disease outbreaks. To that time, there had never been a better demonstration of the power of global collaboration.

ZIKA Virus

The discovery of the Zika virus, like the West Nile virus, was an incidental finding: while taking samples as part of routine yellow fever surveillance in the tropical forests of Uganda in 1947, scientists isolated a new virus from captive sentinel rhesus monkeys. Named Zika virus (ZIKV) for the Ugandan forest in which it was first identified, the virus was also recovered from an *Aedes africanus* mosquito on a tree platform in that same forest, suggesting vector-borne transmission.[51] In 1952, serological surveys in Uganda and Nigeria in Central Africa showed Zika antibodies in 75% of a sample population suggesting widespread unrecognized infection. The first definitive evidence that the virus could cause clinical illness in humans appeared in 1954 when a 10-year-old Nigerian girl with fever and rash showed a post-symptom rise in antibodies against ZIKV.

Over the next 40 years, the Zika virus was repeatedly detected in mosquitoes and monkeys used for yellow fever research in a narrow band of countries stretching across equatorial Africa. During that same time period, ZIKV migrated to Asia along with infected humans and mosquitos, with occasional cases of mild human illness detected along the way. The geographical distribution expanded to include India, Pakistan, Indonesia and Malaysia where seroprevalence studies indicated widespread population exposure but reports of overt disease remained mild and rare. During this time, the close resemblance between ZIKV, dengue and chikungunya in clinical disease symptoms and in viral characteristics was observed and confirmed.[52]

In 2007, the pattern changed abruptly when the Zika virus caused a large outbreak on the tiny Pacific island of Yap, located in the Philippine Sea, due north of Papua New Guinea.[53] Given the island's isolated location in the open ocean and the complete absence of monkeys, the virus is thought to have been carried to this naïve population by an infected person or an accidentally imported mosquito. Based on house-to-house surveys, 73% of Yap's 7391 citizens were infected with the Zika virus during this outbreak. Although there were no deaths, hospitalizations or severe complications reported, the dramatic size and rapid spread of the outbreak were remarkable, attributed to a combination of lack of population immunity and misidentification/under-reporting of cases in previous outbreaks.[53]

By this time, we thought we had a reasonable knowledge base about the Zika virus and ZIKV infection with 80% of those infected being completely asymptomatic. The vast majority of those with symptoms had a very mild illness characterized by low grade fever and headache associated with a non-specific itchy rash and mild, generalized body aches. The rash began on the face and spread throughout the body. There was conjunctivitis (inflamed red eyes) in approximately 60% of cases. In the absence of complications, recovery occurred in 4 to 7 days.[54] The primary mode of transmission was via the bite of Aedes mosquitoes – especially *A. aegypticus* and *A. aldopictus* – encountered previously by us as the agents for transmission of yellow fever. Infection with Zika virus was generally suspected based on symptoms and recent history of travel to an area with active Zika virus transmission.

Specific, accurate diagnosis of Zika virus infection is difficult because antibody response to related flaviviruses like dengue is cross-reactive, and antibody detection of ZIKV is nonspecific in populations previously exposed to any of the four dengue viruses or West Nile virus, and/or vaccinated against yellow fever virus. Laboratory evidence of a confirmed recent Zika virus infection is therefore quite complicated, requiring either detection of Zika virus or Zika virus RNA or antigen in any body fluid or tissue specimen; or a positive or equivocal Zika virus or Dengue virus IgM test on serum with a positive titer for Zika virus (≥10) from plaque reduction neutralization testing (PRNT) and a negative PRNT titer for dengue virus. The definitive diagnosis of ZIKV infections has increasingly depended on detection by nucleic acid tests. Similar to other flavivirus infections, Zika virus IgM antibodies can remain in the body for months after infection, making it difficult to use serologic tests to determine the timing of infection. A completely dependable, accurate and responsive diagnostic test for rapid confirmation of ZIKV diagnosis in the field has yet to be developed.[54]

The Virus

The Zika virus (ZIKV) is a member of the Flaviviridae virus family and the genus Flavivirus, and is thus directly related to the dengue, yellow fever, Japanese encephalitis, and West Nile viruses.[55] Like other members of the genus, Zika virus is enveloped and icosahedral and has a non-segmented, single-stranded, 10 kilobase positive-sense RNA genome, first sequenced in 2007. The RNA genome encodes seven nonstructural proteins and three structural proteins including the flavivirus envelope glycoprotein which initiates viral entry by endocytosis after binding to the endosomal membrane of the host cell.

In 2012, genetic researchers constructed phylogenetic trees using Zika virus strains collected in Africa (Uganda, Nigeria and Senegal), and Asia (Cambodia, Malaysia and Thailand). Two geographically distinct lineages were identified – Asian and African – with multiple strains within each lineage.[56]

★★★★★★★★

After the island-wide outbreak on Yap, there were sporadic cases of Zika virus infection reported from several countries in south-east Asia between 2010 and 2013. In 2013, the story changed again when there was a huge outbreak of ZIKV disease involving more than 28,000 people in French Polynesia. Serologic testing showed 66% of the population had been infected. French Polynesia is located in the middle of the South Pacific Ocean more than 5000 miles across the open sea from Yap Island but near-identical nucleotide sequencing indicates that the viral strain causing the outbreak was of Asian origin and originated from Yap Island. Given the distance between the two sites, the virus could only have been imported by an infected person.[57]

It was during this large outbreak that ZIKV disease was first observed to be associated with Guillain-Barre Syndrome (GBS), a rare, serious autoimmune disease of the nervous system in which an individual's immune system attacks the myelin sheaths of peripheral nerves. The condition often develops a few days or weeks after a viral infection with rapid onset of neurological symptoms which can progress from a tingling sensation in the extremities to paralysis of the muscles that control breathing. Patients respond to treatment with immunoglobulins or to plasma exchange but the mortality rate is 5%. During the Zika epidemic in French Polynesia, the incidence of GBS was estimated to be 20 fold higher than its basal island incidence.[58] Ninety-eight percent of patients with GBS were shown to have antibodies against ZIKV, compared with only 55% of antibody-negative individuals, strongly supporting a causative association.[59,60] These findings of neurovirulence suggested further viral evolution.

Meanwhile, in east central South America, Brazil was enjoying a time of relative infectious disease tranquility following the successful anti-mosquito campaigns of the last century. With yellow fever apparently vanquished, those programs had been largely dismantled. The infectious disease threat response shifted from building basic public health infrastructure and capacities for prevention as the first line of defense, to the use of surveillance to pick up early signals of an outbreak and then mounting an organized, emergency response. It was in this setting that doctors in northeastern Brazil first began seeing patients with a new, characteristic disease pattern in the summer of 2014. Almost all had the same signs and symptoms: fever, bloodshot eyes, headache and a flat, pink, itchy rash. Dengue was very common in this area and the symptoms were similar but serological tests excluded dengue as well as chikungunya. Although patients were not severely ill, their numbers were alarming and after investigation, authorities confirmed that this previously unknown disease was an ongoing outbreak of Zika fever, proven by RT-PCR performed by researchers from Brazil's Federal University of Bahia in May 2015. Zika had never previously been seen in South America. Local authorities linked the outbreak to the recent increased flow of foreign visitors prompted by a series of sporting events, coupled with the large population of the mosquito vectors, *Aedes aegypticus* and *Aedes albopictus*, that inhabit the region.[6]

At first, doctors and epidemiologists were reassured by this information as Zika was thought to cause only mild symptoms in a minority of infected individuals. But within weeks, there was a spike in cases of Guillain-Barre Syndrome as seen in the ZIKV outbreak in French Polynesia.

And Then – Out of Nowhere

Then, late in the summer of 2015, doctors began to report large numbers of newborns with microcephaly in northeastern Brazil associated with a maternal history of rash suggesting possible infection during the pregnancy.[61] Microcephaly is an exceedingly rare anomaly caused by underdevelopment of the brain; the baseline incidence is ~ 2–7 cases per 10,000 newborns. Microcephalic babies almost always have profoundly delayed development as well as other neurologic problems like seizures, vision abnormalities and deafness. It has been reported after maternal exposure to teratogenic compounds and to maternal gestational infection with viruses including cytomegalovirus, rubella and herpes, or toxoplasmosis.[62]

Case numbers accumulated rapidly and by November 2015, the Brazilian Government declared a national public health emergency.[63] A suspected association between maternal ZIKV infection and congenital microcephaly in their offspring then emerged from a retrospective analysis of the Zika disease outbreak in French Polynesia: serological and surveillance data found the baseline prevalence of microcephaly in the islands was 2 cases per 10,000 neonates compared with 95 cases per 10,000 women infected with Zika in the first trimester during the outbreak.[64]

Between November of 2015 and June of 2016, 7830(!) suspected cases of microcephaly were reported to the Brazilian Ministry of Health. From this group, 1500 infants were medically investigated with a strong association established between maternal history of rash during pregnancy and subsequent microcephaly. Infants with definite or highly probable ZIKV infection had severe intracranial calcifications and other major neuroimaging abnormalities including cortical malformations, ventriculomegaly, cerebellar hypoplasia, and abnormal hypodensity of the white matter. Many definite or probable cases of ZIKV syndrome were found to have normal head circumferences despite specific neuroimaging findings and lab evidence of ZIKV infection. Over time, a congenital Zika syndrome (CZS) was characterized with distinctive brain development abnormalities including some combination of microcephaly, intracranial calcifications, retinal manifestations, and defects of the extremities including congenital contractures and hypertonia.[65]

The striking increase in congenital microcephaly and other neurological abnormalities in northeast Brazil was so concerning that the WHO declared the Zika epidemic to be a Public Health Emergency of International Concern on February 1, 2016, the very rarely used designation that was put into effect late in the 2014–2015 Ebola epidemic.[66] But the potential spread of the Zika virus across the Americas and the possibility that a mosquito bite during pregnancy could cause such devastating neurologic damage in a developing fetus was so concerning that the declaration was felt to be justified. Over the next year, epidemiologic, pathologic and biologic evidence accumulated supporting a strong association between prenatal ZIKV infection and congenital microcephaly with associated severe brain anomalies and ultimately, it was concluded that this was a direct causal relationship.[67-71] *Birth defects resulting from a virus transmitted by a mosquito bite had never previously been reported.*

In response to confirmation of vertical transmission of ZIKV infection during pregnancy, countries including Brazil, Colombia, El Salvador and Jamaica advised their populations to postpone planned pregnancies, to control mosquitoes by reducing mosquito-breeding grounds; and to prevent mosquito bites in at-risk individuals, especially pregnant women. Mosquito transmission was still considered the primary mode of infection but human sexual transmission by vaginal, anal, or oral sex, and the sharing of sex toys was subsequently confirmed. Zika was found to be transmitted sexually even if the infected person was entirely asymptomatic at the time.[72] In response, the US Centers for Disease Control developed specific recommendations to prevent maternal ZIKV infection including: avoidance of travel to areas where ZIKV infection had been reported by women who were or planned to become pregnant; specific mosquito bite prevention efforts by pregnant women and their male and female partners who lived in or traveled to ZIKV-active areas; use of sexual protection for the length of pregnancy; testing for ZIKV infection in the first and second trimesters of pregnancy for women who live in ZIKV-active areas; and delayed attempts to conceive for eight weeks for women and 6 months for men after travel to ZIKV-affected areas.

****

As it turned out, we knew relatively little about the Zika virus at the outset of the outbreak in Brazil, given its low profile and what we thought was minimal pathogenicity. The sudden and enormous number of ZIKV cases and the recognition of severe associated fetal complications led to intense efforts to understand the dynamics of the epidemic and the pathophysiology of the infection.

Two hypotheses dominated investigation of the mechanisms responsible for the dramatic emergence of Zika virus as an epidemic pathogen with serious associated effects: the chance introduction of a virus with under-appreciated neurotropic characteristics into a large, immunologically naïve population with abundant *Aedes aegypti* mosquito vectors; or spontaneous genetic evolution enhancing human infection. Either or both mechanisms could theoretically result in enough severe ZIKV infection outcomes for definitive recognition of a previously unrecognized outcome.[73]

Comparative genomic and phylogenetic analyses identified several amino acid substitutions that may have contributed to increased ZIKV transmission and pathogenicity. Specifically, a spontaneous amino acid substitution in one of the virus's non-structural proteins has been identified in all clinical isolates from the Americas after 2013 but not from Cambodia back in 2010. The mutation increases ZIKV acquisition by mosquitoes from an infected mammalian host — and increased viral prevalence in mosquito vectors could have contributed to the rapid spread in the recent pandemic.[74]

Using molecular mapping and next generation sequencing, an international group of researchers explored spread of the Zika virus in the Americas. With a mobile genomics laboratory, they generated ZIKV genomes including one sequence from the earliest confirmed case of ZIKV infection in Brazil. Analysis of these viral genomes combined with ecological and epidemiologic data showed introduction of ZIKV into Brazil in February 2014, more than 12 months prior to the first report of clinical Zika infection in May 2015. The projected date of origin coincides with a documented increase in air travel to Brazil from ZIKV endemic areas, specifically the Pacific Islands including French Polynesia. This is critical information because it indicates the virus was circulating in human and mosquito populations causing subclinical and unrecognized disease and the now-identified serious neurologic complications for more than a year before it was recognized.[75] As with Ebola and HIV, delayed identification of an outbreak allows for exponential epidemic spread. With ZIKV, this was accelerated by the complete absence of immunity to ZIKV in the enormous, immunologically naïve population of Brazil.[76]

Another international study examined ZIKV genomes from clinical and mosquito samples from 10 countries and territories. Their phylogenetic analysis showed rapid expansion of the outbreak after the original introduction into Brazil with multiple subsequent introductions of ZIKV strains into Puerto Rico, Honduras, Columbia, other Caribbean islands and then the continental United States. Again, ZIKV was found to have circulated undetected for many months in every location before the first locally transmitted cases were recognized.[77]

Using phylogenetic trees from human and mosquito-derived genomes in Miami, researchers found evidence that Zika was introduced into Florida on multiple occasions, several months before it was detected. Their analyses suggested that ZIKV entered the United States from Caribbean countries, which are linked to Miami by extensive air- and cruise-ship travel. The presence of *Aedes Aegypti* mosquitoes coincident with large numbers of people arriving from high-incidence Zika areas supported successful introduction of the virus resulting in reported sporadic cases but the transmission rate was below the threshold level needed to establish an ongoing epidemic.[78]

Appropriately, the most intense contemporary focus of ZIKV research has been around the consequences of vertically-transmitted infection during pregnancy. A retrospective analysis of clinical and postmortem findings in nine infants with definite intrauterine ZIKV infection confirmed the strong predilection of the virus for fetal central nervous system cells, corroborating experimental in vitro and in vivo studies of neural specificity with ZIKV infection during pregnancy.[79]

One genetic mutation in the region coding for the ZIKV envelope protein is rare in African isolates but is consistently identified in all isolates from recent outbreaks. A recombinant ZIKV clone which contained this motif was highly pathogenic and lethal in a mouse model; by contrast, a recombinant clone in which this motif was deleted or mutated was highly attenuated and non-lethal with very limited replication in the brain of infected animals. These findings suggest that specific genetic changes in the ZIKV envelope protein are an important factor in ZIKV virulence and neuro-invasion.[80]

The absence of reported microcephaly in outbreaks before 2013 led researchers to search for a mutation that made the virus more virulent to the fetal brain. Chinese scientists investigated the *in vivo* neurovirulence of three contemporary ZIKV strains (VEN/2016) isolated in 2015–2016 and compared these to their Asian ancestral strain isolated in Cambodia in 2010 (CAM/2010) in one-day-old neonatal mice, comparable to human fetuses in the third trimester. Upon intracerebral injection, all three contemporary strains led to profound neuro-logical signs followed by 100% mortality, compared with death in only 17% of the CAM/2010 injected animals. Using an established mouse embryonic micro-cephaly model, the researchers then compared the effects of the contemporary and ancestral strains. Both viruses predominantly targeted neural progenitor cells but the VEN/2016 strain was much more virulent, causing a more significant microcephaly phenotype in the embryonic mouse brain. Based on these prelim-inary findings, the researchers compared the genome sequencing in the contem-porary ZIKV strains, using the ancestral strain as a reference. Phylogenetic analysis revealed that the contemporary strains had accumulated multiple nucleotide substitutions. In particular, a single serine to asparagine substitution in the viral polyprotein substantially increased ZIKV infectivity in both human and mice neural progenitor cells and led to more significant microcephaly in the mouse fetus and higher mortality in neonatal mice. Evolutionary analysis indicated that the S139N substitution arose before the 2013 outbreak in French Polynesia when microcephaly was first reported. The substitution has been stably maintained during subsequent spread to the Americas. This adaptation makes ZIKV more virulent to human neural progenitor cells, and could have contributed to the increased incidence of microcephaly in recent ZIKV pandemics. While this work has not been universally accepted, it strongly suggests a spontaneous ZIKV genetic mutation may underlie the development of microcephaly during first trimester maternal ZIKV infection.[81]

Researchers in Brazil identified a striking difference in the incidence of microcephaly at different times and locations in the ongoing epidemic. During the first massive wave of ZIKV infection in northeast Brazil in the spring and summer of 2105, the peak monthly occurrence of microcephaly was very markedly elevated at 49.9 cases per 10,000 livebirths. The second wave of Zika virus infection was much smaller but involved all regions of Brazil from September 2015 to September 2016 and the occurrence of microcephaly was much lower with estimated monthly peaks ranging from 3.2 to 15 cases per 10,000 livebirths. The explanation for these differences is unknown but could include the intensity of the Zika virus outbreak, and the success of public health efforts to protect pregnant women from ZIKV infection.[82]

Information is accumulating about the incidence of birth defects in pregnant American women with lab evidence of Zika infection. Among 442 completed pregnancies in the USA through 2016, 6% of all fetuses or infants had evidence of Zika-associated birth defects, primarily microcephaly and other brain abnormalities. With definite first trimester Zika infection, the prevalence was higher: 11% had evidence of Zika-associated birth defects.[83] Of the 250 pregnant women in the USA who had confirmed Zika infection in 2016, 10% had a fetus or baby with Zika-related birth defects. This report is the first to provide analysis of a subgroup of pregnant women in the USA with clear, confirmed test results of Zika virus infection.[84] By December of 2017, there were 1297 confirmed cases of Zika infection during pregnancy in women in the USA. A report from the ZODIAC study, a long-term follow-up of children born with Zika-related microcephaly describes the health and developmental effects of congenital Zika virus infection in children with microcephaly through 2 years of age. At a mean age of 19 to 24 months, more than half have severe health and developmental problems in multiple areas including seizures, profound motor delay with spasticity and inability to sit independently, difficulties with sleeping and feeding, and hearing and vision problems.[85]

★★★★★★★

Epidemic Spread

Wide distribution of *Aedes aegypti*, the principal vector of the virus, and other *Aedes* species has greatly facilitated the spread of the disease. As we learned with yellow fever, *Aedes aegypti* is an invasive mosquito species that has adapted well to densely populated urban environments. In addition to mosquito transmission, male-to-female human sexual transmission has increasingly been demonstrated in the USA and elsewhere. The globalization of the Zika virus was made possible by the widespread presence in various parts of the world of *Aedes* vectors and increased human travel that facilitated geographic spread just as occurred with West Nile, Ebola, Dengue and Chikungunya. Its ultimate spread was difficult to predict but it was hoped to be restricted through vigorous preventive measures. On the recommendation of its Emergency Committee on Zika Virus and Observed Increase in Neurological Disorders and Neonatal Malformations, WHO issued a group of recommendations to contain the epidemic.[86]

After the explosive onset of the epidemic in Brazil, it spread regionally and then globally, beginning with the Caribbean Islands and Mexico, and then into the United States, especially Texas and Florida, then Europe, India, the Far East and Australia – essentially, all over the globe. According to the Pan American Health Organization/World Health Organization, 48 countries and territories in the Americas had confirmed transmission of Zika virus disease through mosquitoes since 2015 and five countries in the Americas had reported sexually transmitted Zika cases.[87] Overall, some 250,000 cases were confirmed, more than half from Brazil. There were 2,618 children born with confirmed congenital syndrome associated with Zika virus infection, again, most in Brazil. Extrapolating from reported cases, by 2016, more than 1.5 million people were estimated to be infected in Brazil alone.

Since 2016, when Zika was declared by the World Health Organization as a Public Health Emergency of International Concern, the virus became established in more than 80 countries, infected millions of people, and left many babies with the collection of birth defects known as congenital Zika syndrome. Travelers have been confirmed as important sentinels of Zika virus transmission throughout the pandemic.[88]

Then, almost as suddenly as it began, the number of new cases of Zika fever began to fall precipitously. On November 19, 2016, the WHO announced that the Zika virus was no longer a "Public Health Emergency of International Concern" but should be considered a dangerous mosquito-borne disease like malaria or yellow fever with long-term efforts needed to address the virus.[89]

Researchers who reconstructed the temporal spread of ZIKV in northeastern Brazil where the disease was first identified have shown the most likely explanation for the end of the epidemic. Using specimens sampled from before, during and after the outbreak, they showed that ZIKV seroprevalence (antibody prevalence in the population) increased *from 4.2% in 2013 to 17.4% in 2015, and to 63.3% by the end of 2016.* Based on modeling projections, ZIKV reached the critical community protective immunity threshold – herd immunity level – within a single year. These results predict restricted ZIKV spread in the area until new, susceptible individuals are added to the population. This is compatible with the complete absence of reported, new ZIKV cases in the area since 2016.[90] This projection for future ZIKV cases is also compatible with the results of stochastic spatial modeling of Zika transmission which also predicted the end of the current epidemic within 3 years with herd immunity delaying future large epidemics for a decade or more.[91]

Those predictions are being borne out in real-time as the number of new cases of Zika fever has continued to decrease dramatically in South America, Central America and the Caribbean since mid-2016. Per the Pan American Health Organization, since epidemiological week 44 of 2016, no additional countries or territories of the Americas have confirmed vector-borne transmission of Zika virus disease. Compared with more than 205,000 probable cases in 2016, Brazil had reported only 13,253 cases as of July 2017.[92]

In 2016, the United States recorded 224 probable or confirmed locally trans-mitted cases in Florida and Texas – in 2017, there was just one local transmis-sion in Texas. The dramatic epidemic that began in 2015 had almost vanished.[93] Given the high community protective immunity threshold – the protective herd immunity we described in the polio chapter – a new epidemic in the next decade is very unlikely. Zika virus is believed to have been maintained pri-marily in nature in a sylvatic cycle of transmission between non-human primates and forest-dwelling mosquitoes, just like yellow fever. This could allow future outbreaks to occur as susceptible population groups appear but there is no evi-dence this pattern has been established in the Americas to this time

Prevention

There is no treatment for primary Zika infection and none is needed given the minor symptoms it produces. However, in light of the major neurologic and con-genital complications, effective preventive measures are of critical importance. Aside from the personal protective efforts recommended by the CDC and the WHO, research strategies for prevention of a global pandemic have focused on vector control programs and effective vaccine development.[94]

Traditional vector control measures like insecticides and elimination of larval breeding sites are still recommended but one new approach previously described for yellow fever involves development of mosquitoes that are resistant to arbo-virus infection. The bacterial symbiont Wolbachia has been transferred from Drosophila into the mosquito *Aedes aegypti* where it blocks the transmission of arboviruses including Zika. Mosquitoes infected with Wolbachia are resistant to current circulating Zika virus isolates with reduced virus prevalence, intensity and disseminated infection.[95] A *Wolbachia*-infected *A. Aegypti* mosquito has been developed and has already been shown to spread through mosquito populations after large-scale release. *Wolbachia*-infected mosquitoes were released in two Rio de Janeiro neighborhoods in 2014, and in a suburb of Medellín in 2015. Researchers plan to survey the insects for viral infection and track the local incidence of disease in areas with and without *Wolbachia*-infected mosquitoes. Proving that Wolbachia infection of wild mosquitos limits human infections is critical before the method can find widespread use.[96] A field trial in Townsville, Australia has eliminated local arbovirus disease transmission over more than

2 year follow-up.[97] The World Mosquito Program is reportedly testing this approach in 12 countries.

As with yellow fever, another alternative is development of a genetically modified *A.aegypti* mosquito which expresses a repressible lethal gene. Male mosquitoes are mass-reared in insect nurseries (a fascinating concept!) where they are given tetracycline as a dietary additive – tetracycline suppresses the activation of the lethal gene. After release, these mosquitoes compete with wild males to mate with females. Offspring carry the lethal gene and do not survive to become adults because they have no access to tetracycline. Known as RIDL for Release of Insects carrying Dominant Lethal genes, this approach is undergoing field testing. A field release of RIDL mosquitoes in Bahia, Brazil, reportedly achieved a 95% reduction in local mosquito populations.[98]

The association of Zika virus infection with congenital microcephaly and Guillain-Barré syndrome has resulted in accelerated vaccine development efforts. Based on prior flavivirus vaccine development programs, multiple vaccine strategies have already advanced to the stage of clinical evaluation. These include nucleic acid (DNA and messenger RNA), whole-inactivated virus, live-attenuated or chimeric virus, and protein or virus-like particle vaccines. Within a year from the declaration by the World Health Organization of Zika virus as a Public Health Emergency of International Concern, multiple vaccine candidates entered clinical trials, with additional candidate vaccines in preclinical development.[99] One NIH vaccine candidate, the VRC's investigational DNA vaccine, was created on a platform initially developed for a West Nile virus vaccine. In only 4 months, this vaccine was in a phase 1 clinical trial and then advanced to a phase 2/2b trial in Texas, Puerto Rico, South and Central America.[100,101] This rapid progress in vaccine development demonstrates the global capacity to respond to pandemic threats when the need is great and emergency funding is made available. However, the dramatic fall in Zika cases has made it difficult to complete clinical vaccine trials.

Looking Back :: Moving Forward

The Zika virus is the latest infectious disease pathogen to demonstrate the combined limitations of medicine and science to respond to an emergent viral threat. After more than half a century as a covert cause of trivial disease, the enormous numbers of cases of ZIKV disease in this pandemic revealed serious and previously unrecognized neurologic complications of mutation when the virus was introduced into a large, immunologically unprotected population. Fortunately, collaborative global research has begun to increase our knowledge of Zika pathogenesis and transmission, exemplified by two 2018 research reports.

- A study of nonhuman primates infected with Asian/African ZIKV in early gestation showed fetal demise in 26% of the animals without clinical signs of infection. The results suggest that pregnancy loss due to asymptomatic

ZIKV infection may be a common but under-recognized adverse outcome of maternal ZIKV infection.[102]

- Cryo-electron microscopic single-particle reconstruction of the ZIKV at a resolution of 3.1 Å revealed heretofore unseen glycoprotein interactions and surface properties of the virus. Compared with other mosquito-borne flavivirus structures, the largest structural differences and sequence variations were seen to occur at the glycosylation loop associated with receptor binding, potential sites for drug development and vaccine design.[103]

At the same time, the extraordinarily high infection rate created powerful herd immunity, significantly limiting new ZIKA infections at the present time. The intense ongoing research focus on ZIKV disease outcomes and on disease prevention through vector control programs and facilitated vaccine development engendered by the global spread of this "new" pathogen will hopefully result in an improved capacity to respond when the next viral disease emergency strikes.

Ebola

In the summer of 1976, there were two separate, near simultaneous outbreaks of a terrible illness in central Africa. Members of two small isolated communities – Yambuku in Zaire's tropical rainforest in the northern frontier, and Nzara in the grasslands of southern Sudan – suddenly began developing fever, headache, joint and muscle pain, sore throat and intense weakness, followed by stomach pain, diarrhea, vomiting and rash. Many developed red eyes (due to conjunctival injection), hiccups and then signs of bleeding, from the nose, mouth and GI tract. The fatality rate was high with many deaths in both locations. Within days, family members and care providers began to fall ill with the same symptoms. Calls for help to Kinshasa, the capital of Zaire brought the medical director for the zone to Yambuku where he found a scene of near panic with multiple desperately ill villagers and members of the local Belgian missionary group, the only source of health care in the area. His report led the Minister of Health to place the whole Bumba Zone around Yambuku under strict isolation and urgently request help from the CDC to determine the cause of the outbreak. Reports of the similarly devastating outbreak in southern Sudan sent health workers to collect samples from patients there as well.[104]

Under the direction of the WHO, blood and tissue samples from both outbreaks were sent to high-security labs in multiple locations for analysis. In Belgium, preliminary tests excluded yellow fever and typhoid – both considered possibilities – but under the electron microscope, the blood samples were found to contain a previously unrecognized virus with a long, curled, wormlike shape.[105] At the CDC in the United Staes, the microbiology team confirmed that finding, reporting that the illnesses in both locations were caused by a new, previously unrecognized virus that resembled the Marburg virus, a known cause of hemorrhagic fever.[106] In response, the WHO issued two urgent bulletins describing the outbreaks of hemorrhagic fever in northern Zaire and south Sudan caused by a new virus, morphologically similar to Marburg virus but antigenically different.[107] The virus was named Ebola, after the Ebola River in Zaire near which the disease was first recognized.

On the ground in both locations, the number of new cases gradually decreased over approximately two months and then stopped. A full-scale epidemiologic survey of the outbreak in northern Zaire reported that there had been 318 cases of the new viral disease and 280 were fatal, an alarmingly high mortality rate of 88%.[108] Investigation of the Sudanese epidemic found 284 cases with 151 deaths, a mortality rate of 53%.[109] Secondary cases were relatively rare, occurring only in those who had extensive direct contact with confirmed patients so the virus was not thought to be highly transmissible. Despite investigations in both locations, the origin of the Ebola virus was not identified. The WHO report of the Zaire outbreak concludes with this prophetic description: "No more dramatic or potentially explosive epidemic of a new viral disease has occurred in the world in the past 30 years."[108]

Epidemiologic History

After that impressive and alarming start, there was a long, unexpected hiatus with no recorded Ebola outbreaks for almost 15 years. During the interval, biologic studies of the virus from the Sudan and Zaire epidemics showed the original outbreaks were caused by two different subtypes of the virus, subsequently called Ebola Zaire and Ebola Sudan.[110]

In 1990, there was a dramatic development when a terrifying disease struck monkeys imported from the Philippines to the United States for research, while they were in quarantine in Virginia. Symptoms were similar to the clinical picture of Ebola hemorrhagic fever with 100% fatality but despite extensive contact between caretakers and monkeys, no humans developed any signs of illness and only 4 handlers even showed antibody evidence of infection. The virus was subsequently found to have originated in captive macaques in the Philippines and was identified as a new Ebola virus, named Ebola Reston.[111] There have still been no human illnesses attributed to Ebola Reston but in 2008, the Reston virus was identified as the cause of an epidemic of hemorrhagic fever in pigs; again, animal caretakers had antibody evidence of infection but no humans developed disease.[112,113] This is important because it suggests that pigs – known to also be infected with EBOV Zaire – could potentially serve as the site for development of a new recombinant virus capable of infecting humans with an extremely high fatality disease.

In November 1994 after 15 years of apparent epidemiologic silence, Ebola virus (EBOV) re-emerged in Côte d'Ivoire, West Africa. During an outbreak of fatal viral hemorrhagic fever among western chimpanzees in the Taï National Park, a new EBOV subtype was isolated when a scientist performing necropsies on the infected chimps developed symptoms of Ebola virus disease and a new subtype was isolated from her blood. The virus was called Ebola Cote d'Ivoire.[114] In 2010, the virus was renamed Ebola Tai Forest in honor of the rain forest where the virus was detected. There has never been another identified case of human disease related to infection with Ebola Tai Forest.

The next epidemic was not reported until 1995 in the Democratic Republic of Congo (DRC – once Zaire), but between that outbreak and 2014, 24 additional localized outbreaks of Ebola hemorrhagic fever (EVD) occurred in 7 African countries including the DRC, Sudan, Gabon, Cote d'Ivoire, South Africa and Uganda. Major outbreaks occurred in the Congo in 1995 (EBOV Zaire; 315 cases, mortality rate 81%), Uganda in 2000 (EBOV Sudan; 425 cases, 53% mortality rate) and the Congo in 2002 and 2005 (EBOV Zaire; 143 and 264 cases; mortality rates, 89% and 71%).[115]

After a major outbreak of Ebola Zaire disease in the DRC in 2007, there were numerous reports of a mysterious illness in the Bundibugyo District of western Uganda at the end of the year. A novel EBOV virus species was identified in diagnostic samples submitted to the Centers for Disease Control and Prevention. This fifth Ebola subtype was called *Bundibugyo ebolavirus* (BEBOV) and in response to its detection, an international outbreak response found a large number of the confirmed patients reported having had direct contact with a single person who died of a severe hemorrhagic febrile illness consistent with EVD in November, 2007. Bleeding from any site was reported in 54% of patients with a confirmed diagnosis. As with all previous large EBOV outbreaks, there was a temporal lag of approximately 3 months between the initial cases and the identification of Ebola virus as the cause of the outbreak, allowing for prolonged person-to-person transmission of the virus. Ultimately, there were 131 identified cases with a mortality rate of 32%.[116,117]

★★★★★★★★

During this period of increasingly frequent Ebola virus outbreak reports, the search for the source of the virus continued. Between 2002 and 2004, there were five documented human EBOV Zaire outbreaks in western central Africa, in Gabon and the DRC. Each human outbreak was accompanied by reports of gorilla and chimpanzee carcasses in neighboring forests.[118] In each outbreak, scientists found that the first human case had developed the illness after handling a distinct animal carcass: gorilla, chimpanzee or duiker (a small antelope that is known to eat carrion). The animal carcasses were located using global positioning satellite technology and evaluated by a combination of techniques. In total, the carcasses of ten gorillas, three chimpanzees and one duiker were confirmed to be infected by EBOV. Nucleotide sequencing of samples from all infected humans showed variation between epidemics but none between samples from the same outbreak, with eight EBOV Zaire strains identified in the 5 human outbreaks. In one case, serum from the index case for a human epidemic was positive for EBOV-specific IgG and virus sequences matched those detected in the bone marrow of the gorilla identified as the source of the outbreak. Nucleotide sequence variations distinct from those previously seen in humans were identified and matched those found in infected tissue from dead animals. Overall, this evidence suggests that these outbreaks were the result of multiple independent introductions of the Ebola virus into humans from infected great apes.[118] Subsequently, significant declines in the gorilla population in central Africa were reported with evaluation suggesting that in 2002 and 2003, EBOV Zaire killed about 5000 gorillas in this area. The lag in mortality onset between neighboring gorilla groups paralleled the Ebola disease cycle length, suggesting that group-to-group transmission had amplified gorilla die-offs.[119]

However, great apes and duikers cannot be the reservoir host for the Ebola virus since they are clearly, highly susceptible to EBOV infection and disease. Bats were long suspected to be the natural reservoir for the Ebola virus and in 2005, evidence of asymptomatic EBOV infection was detected in three species of fruit bat during evaluation of more than a thousand small vertebrates collected during Ebola outbreaks in humans and great apes between 2001 and 2003 in Gabon and the Republic of the Congo. Antibodies and nucleotide sequences specific for EBOV Zaire were detected in the liver and spleen of three fruit bat species in Gabon and the DRC (*Hypsignathus monstrosus*, *Epomops franquetti* and *Myonycteris torquata*). This finding has led to the working hypothesis that bats are the reservoir for this deadly virus with gorillas, chimpanzees and duikers as intermediate hosts.[120,121]

The Disease

In early outbreaks, the acute onset of the disease in isolated rain forest settings remote from medical and scientific facilities made acquisition of knowledge about the virus and the disease difficult. Over time, much has been learned: Ebola is contagious – i.e., it is transmittable from one infected individual or animal to another. The first human case in an outbreak of Ebola is usually acquired when blood, secretions or other body fluids of an infected animal enter a healthy person's body through the mucous membranes in the eyes, nose or mouth, or through an often very small break in the skin. This is most often associated with butchering an infected animal for food but can occur after handling an infected animal, eating food that infected animals have drooled or defecated on, or by touching surfaces covered in infected droppings and then touching the eyes, nose or mouth. Subsequent spread is direct, from person to person and the secondary transmission rate is reportedly low, averaging 1–4%. Surveys of surviving household members have shown that transmission requires extensive direct physical contact with an infected person in every case, especially with exposure to body fluids.[122] Those who touched the body of someone who had died especially if this involved traditional preparation for burial and those who were exposed during the late phase of the illness were at highest risk.[123] People can also become infected through contact with objects, such as needles or soiled clothing, contaminated with infected secretions (aka fomites). Health care workers – at risk for infection by both these methods – have frequently been infected in Ebola outbreaks with as many as half of some outbreak populations consisting of health care providers.[123] Once the virus makes direct contact with the blood or mucous membranes, it is highly infectious: an infinitesimally small amount of virus in direct contact with blood or mucous membranes can cause illness. Ebola virus is considered to be only moderately contagious because it is not spread through routine, social contact (such as shaking hands or sitting next to someone) and there is no evidence of transmission through intact skin or airborne spread through droplets with coughing or sneezing.[124] Over time, it has become clear that Ebola, like many other viral infections, presents with a spectrum of clinical manifestations, including minimally or even asymptomatic infection.[166] This means that a significant portion of Ebola transmission events may be undetected and that the mortality rate is likely considerably lower than that calculated for symptomatic patients.

The incubation period of Ebola virus disease (EVD) – previously known as Ebola hemorrhagic fever – ranges from 2 to 21 days but symptoms most commonly begin 8–10 days after contact with the virus. Illness onset is sudden, with fever, headache, joint and muscle pain, sore throat and intense weakness. This is followed by stomach pain, diarrhea, vomiting, rash and impaired kidney and liver function. Many patients develop red eyes due to conjunctival injection, hiccups and signs of internal and external bleeding. In 50–90% of cases, severe hemorrhage, multiple organ failure and shock develop, resulting in death. Survivors were previously not thought to be infectious but the virus persists in semen for many months post recovery and sexual transmission has been confirmed.[125]

The path from EBOV infection to clinical disease involves primarily a dramatically exaggerated immune response. Dendritic cells and macrophages, sentinels of the innate immune response, are involved early in the response to invasion. Activated dendritic cells carry the virus from the initial site of infection to lymph nodes, the spleen and the liver where intense replication takes place. Viral proteins inhibit immune responses, allowing relentless viral replication throughout the body. Extensive infection of monocytes and macrophages – the body's white cells that fight infection – leads to dramatic over-release of inflammatory and pro-inflammatory cytokines and chemokines, and this massive inflammatory response – similar to the cytokine storm seen with severe influenza – can result in impaired endothelial cell function and significant vascular leakage. There is massive cell death of T lymphocytes, eliminating a significant component of the adaptive immune response. In the worst cases, multifocal necrosis of hepatocytes (liver cells) leads to progressive liver failure; destruction of secondary lymphoid organs and other tissue damage results from direct cytopathic effects but also from the host response. Together, these events can lead to multi-organ failure, impairment of the vascular system, terminal shock and death.[126,127]

The characteristic hemorrhage seen with end-stage Ebola is the result of disseminated intravascular coagulation (DIC), a process in which the body's clotting system is inappropriately activated in response to specific triggers. With

Ebola virus infection, the trigger appears to be release of a transmembrane glycoprotein called tissue factor which is expressed by infected macrophages in response to inflammatory cytokines and vascular damage. Tissue factor initiates the clotting cascade and in response, small fibrin clots form in blood vessels all over the body. The clots can impede flow to vital organs, especially the liver, brain and kidneys leading to progressive organ damage. Because clotting factors are used up in the process of producing these clots, they are not available to prevent bleeding, leading to internal and external hemorrhage wherever vascular integrity is compromised. Even when overt bleeding does not occur, clotting times are prolonged and fibrin split products are often detected.[126,127]

Viral levels are dramatically higher from the beginning of the illness in patients who go on to die. High viral levels persist for up to seven days after death, explaining the high risk of infection associated with preparing bodies for burial.[128] It is the combination of direct viral effects and the excessive host response which drives the devastating pathophysiology of Ebola virus infection.

The Virus

Ebolaviruses are members of the family *Filoviridae*, which also includes the severe human pathogen Marburg virus (genus Marburgvirus) and the Lloviu virus (*Lloviu cuevavirus*; genus Cuevavirus). The *Filovaridae* family belongs to the order Mononegavirales, a group of viruses characterized by a linear, non-segmented, single-stranded negative RNA genome.[129] The morphology of the Ebola virus is unique among viruses: by electron microscopy, the virus appears as long filamentous strands about 14,000 nm long and 80 nm wide. The strands contain a tubular nucleo-capsid with surface spikes and on electron microscopy, they assume characteristic shapes including a shepherd's crook and the number six (Figure 7.1). The Ebola virus is a negative-sense single-strand RNA virus with a 19 kilobase genome, and like most other RNA viruses quickly generates mutations through error-prone replication. The RNA genome of the Ebola virus encodes seven viral proteins including a nucleoprotein, a glycoprotein, and a polymerase.[129]

There are 5 identified EBOV subtypes – Zaire, Sudan, Tai Forest, Bundibugyo and Reston – each named for the site where they were first identified. The Reston virus does not cause disease in humans. Significant outbreaks have been caused primarily by Ebola Zaire (aka ZEBOV) and Ebola Sudan (aka SEBOV). Nucleotide sequencing has shown significant variation in viral strains between epidemics but little or no variation between isolates from the same outbreak.[130]

Over the past 30 years, three basic methods for detecting infection and/ or disease with Ebola virus have been developed for use in clinical laboratory settings: serologic tests that detect host antibodies generated against the virus; antigen tests that detect viral proteins; and molecular tests that detect viral RNA sequences. In the early years, serologic tests were used to confirm the cause of disease outbreaks because antiviral antibodies persist for years following infection.

However, the variable onset of antibody responses during acute illness makes serology much less useful in the acute setting. Antigen detection and molecular tests are very effective for acute diagnosis as virus levels in the blood typically rise to high levels as soon as symptoms begin. No tests reliably detect Ebola virus prior to the onset of symptoms.

Accurate diagnosis of Ebola virus infection is a critical part of an effective outbreak response but establishing safe, rapid diagnostic testing in resource-poor environments has been challenging. Ultimately, real-time reverse transcriptase (RT-PCR) testing has become the standard for Ebola virus diagnosis. With RT-PCR, RNA molecules are converted into their complementary DNA sequences (cDNA) using reverse transcriptase enzymes, followed by amplification of the newly synthesized cDNA by standard PCR procedures. There are several standard, real-time RT-PCR tests approved for emergency use by the WHO and FDA, and four of these are commercially available as kits. Real-time RT-PCR diagnosis in an outbreak setting still requires field labs with substantial infrastructure and staff with expertise in molecular techniques.[128]

Treatment

There has been no specific treatment for EVD although experimental anti-viral medications were being tested during this outbreak. Outbreaks are managed by isolation of infected individuals, quarantine of contacts and barrier protection of health care workers. In the small, unsophisticated communities in which EVD typically develops, this requires active surveillance using several methods, including house-to-house search, review of hospital and dispensary records, interview of health care personnel, retrospective contact tracing, and direct follow-up of suspected cases, all carried out with sensitivity and tact. It is easy to appreciate how difficult this is to accomplish when outbreak management is most often attempted by teams of masked white foreigners in full-body protective suits descending upon frightened members of isolated African communities. In the usual situation, access to medical or scientific support is limited. Specific education to allow rapid identification and isolation of new cases and to halt the highly infectious traditional burial methods has been critical in arresting disease spread – again, this requires cooperation and trust between the community members and the outbreak support team.[131]

To avoid transmission of Ebola virus to care providers in hospital settings, great care needs to be taken to avoid contact with infected bodily fluids. This has proven very difficult to accomplish. Patients must be isolated, and strict barrier nursing techniques used, including masks, hoods with eye screens, double gloves, impermeable gowns and boots. Invasive procedures such as the placement of intravenous lines, handling of blood, secretions, catheters and suction devices are a particular risk and strict infection control is essential. Other infection control measures include proper use, disinfection, and disposal of instruments and equipment used in caring for patients. The bodies of those that have died of

Ebola virus infection remain highly infectious and must be promptly and safely buried or cremated.

In selected cases, infected Westerners and health care workers have been given antiviral agents like Zmapp, a combination of three anti-viral antibodies, and plasma transfusions from individuals who had recovered from Ebola and both measures seemed to possibly improve outcomes if given early in the course of the illness. There is ongoing investigation of several different therapeutic strategies that target specific viral structures and mechanisms of Ebola viruses, some of which have demonstrated promising results in animal studies. These include agents composed of interfering RNAs targeting specific proteins of Ebola viruses, hyperimmune globulin isolated from Ebola animal models, monoclonal antibodies, and morpholino oligomers, small molecules used to block viral gene expression. Limited reports indicated that simple provision of intravenous fluids and oxygen significantly improve patient outcomes.[132] The goals of therapeutic agents include prevention of disease development after exposure and moderation of EVD severity and duration.

2014: And Then, out of Nowhere ...

To this point, the Ebola virus had a well-established reputation as a guerilla pathogen in central Africa, emerging suddenly at random intervals in remote areas, infecting all those with extensive contact and causing severe disease which progressed rapidly to death within a few days in more than half of those infected, before disappearing almost as suddenly when no new potential victims remained. The mortality rate was formidable but in all the recorded epidemics between 1976 and 2013, there had been only a combined total of 2361 cases and in every outbreak, the disease burned itself out or was arrested by standard isolation techniques.

Then in December of 2013 a 2-year-old boy became suddenly and severely ill with fever, diarrhea and black stools (a sign of GI hemorrhage) in Meliandou, a small village in Guinea, West Africa. He died 2 days later followed by his grandmother, mother and sister. Because diarrhea was a prominent symptom, and because EVD had never occurred previously in West Africa, Ebola was not initially suspected as the cause, even as illness spread through the village. Some villagers sought help from a traditional healer in the next community and from there, the disease spread rapidly from one village to another without formal recognition as an Ebola outbreak for several months.[133] By March of 2014, almost 4 months later, cases of this severe illness were reported in neighboring Liberia and Sierra Leone, in people who had travelled from Guinea. The international medical aid group *Medecins sans Frontieres* (MSF) finally sent the first samples for confirmation of what turned out to be Ebola Zaire to labs in Hamburg and Lyon at that time. On May 25, scientists confirmed the first case of EVD in Sierra Leone. Epidemiologic investigation discovered a link between this case and the burial of a traditional healer who had treated EVD patients from Guinea.

Traditional burial involves preparation of the body by mourners and is associated with extremely high risk of infection. In this specific situation, there were 13 additional cases of Ebola, all women who attended the burial.

By this time, international aid was being provided by teams from the World Health Organization (WHO), Médecins Sans Frontières (MSF), and the CDC and initially, this appeared to curtail the outbreak in March and April 2014.[134,135] However, movement of untracked contacts across borders led to continued, uncontrolled spread and by June 2014, the situation had evolved into a public health crisis as the first documented multi-country Ebola epidemic. Ongoing transmission occurred in multiple districts in Guinea, Liberia, and Sierra Leone, including densely populated urban areas in these countries. Most previous Ebola outbreaks had occurred in remote areas in central Africa so chains of transmission were easier to track and break – familiarity with EVD and how it presents meant earlier recognition and therefore earlier implementation of isolation techniques. The current outbreak was different with large villages and urban areas as well as remote rural areas affected, vastly increasing opportunities for undiagnosed cases to interact with others and further spread the disease.

Intense fear ruled all three countries and mistrust of health care teams was prominent. As the outbreak progressed, overt community resistance began to emerge. Through June and July, containment efforts were increasingly hindered by local resistance and hostility toward doctors, flight of persons suspected to have the disease, involvement of multiple locations, and the cross-border movement of infected individuals. In some communities, aid workers were phys-ically threatened, and barriers were erected across roads preventing workers from reaching villages with suspected cases. Travel warnings for symptomatic persons leaving affected parts of Africa went unheeded. Case numbers from all three countries continued to increase and cases appeared in other parts of Africa where patients had traveled.

On August 8, 2014, the WHO officially declared the outbreak to be a Public Health Emergency of International Concern.[135] By this time, there had been 2000 known cases and more than half had died. Then in August, two American missionaries working with an international medical aid group, were infected.[136] Their emergency evacuation to the United States suddenly brought widespread international attention and then panic as health officials and the general public realized that this disease with its incredibly high mortality rate had the potential to spread around the world. By this time, more than 240 health care workers had developed EVD in Guinea, Liberia and Sierra Leone, and more than half of these individuals had died.[137] Shortages of personal protective equipment or its improper use, limited medical staff for large numbers of patients, and the compassion that caused medical staff to work in isolation wards far beyond the recommended number of hours, all contributed to the high rate of medical staff infection. In the early months of the epidemic, not even gloves or masks were available in some settings. Existing health care infrastructure was minimal – WHO estimates that, in these three hardest-hit countries, only one to two doctors were available to treat 100,000 people, and these doctors were heavily concentrated in urban areas. Before the outbreak, health indicators in West Africa were among the worst in the world, particularly in terms of maternal and child health. In this fragile context, the outbreak completely overwhelmed the existing health systems and this contributed to fear and mistrust of exhausted health care workers, closure of health facilities, and the deaths of health service staff.[137]

September 2014 – when I first became aware of the pandemic – saw the beginning of an international governmental response with the first official commitment from the USA of $500 million and 3000 troops deployed to the area to deliver supplies and build new treatment centers. Many other countries including China, France, the United Kingdom and Cuba sent nurses, doctors, infectious disease specialists, supplies and other forms of aid to augment existing relief efforts in West Africa. At that time, the United Nations described the severity of the outbreak as unparalleled. On September 30, 2014, an American who had travelled to the USA from Liberia was belatedly admitted to a Dallas hospital with a diagnosis of Ebola – he was the first case of Ebola diagnosed in the United States. Despite maximal care, albeit late in the course of the disease, this patient died and two of the nurses who cared for him were infected. Although they both survived, these cases created a public health crisis in the United States with widespread panic fueled by 24-hour media coverage.[138]

Through the fall of 2014, the epidemic continued to grow. Multiple health care workers were emergently transported back to their home countries with Ebola. On the ground in West Africa, medical teams struggled in protective gear that was so hot and confining they could only work 4-hour shifts – one nurse described literally pouring sweat out of her rubber boots at the end of her shift because it was so hot in her hazmat suit. Attempts were made by teams of international workers to identify and isolate all potential cases despite continuing bed and facility inadequacies. A new WHO report found that health workers were between 21 and 32 times more likely to be infected with Ebola than people in the general population – needless to say, this affected recruitment of additional health care workers.[139]

In early October, the UK announced that it would introduce temperature screening for passengers arriving at Gatwick and Heathrow airports from West Africa followed by a similar statement regarding JFK airport in the United States. On October 14, the WHO announced that the fatality rate from Ebola had reached 70%, with the total number of known cases at 6,353 and deaths at 4,447. Global panic was at its height.

On the ground in West Africa, efforts at public education gradually led to earlier identification of cases and cessation of the traditional burial techniques. Isolation of cases and quarantine of identified contacts gradually slowed the number of new cases with both Liberia and Sierra Leone reporting the lowest numbers in 6 months during the first week of January, 2015. By May 2015, Liberia was reportedly Ebola free with continually declining cases in Sierra Leone and Guinea. On May 9, 2015, WHO declared the end of the Ebola outbreak in Liberia and on

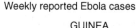

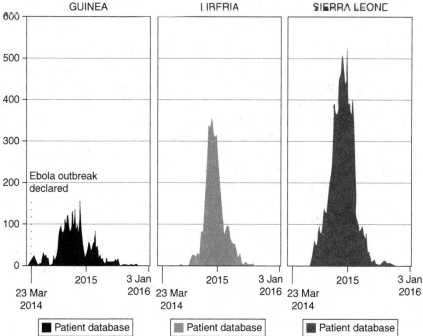

FIGURE 7.4 Ebola cases reported to the WHO from Guinea, Liberia and Sierra Leone, from March 23, 2014 to January 3, 2016.

Source: cdc.gov

November 7, 2015, WHO declared Sierra Leone free of Ebola virus transmission. On December 29, 2015, the WHO declared Guinea free of Ebola virus transmission. In toto, there were over 28,000 cases with more than 11,300 deaths in the 2014–2015 Ebola pandemic.[138,139] Figure 7.4 shows weekly Ebola case numbers in Guinea, Liberia and Sierra Leone from 2/2015 to 8/2015.[140]

Global Pandemic Averted

The Ebola virus was introduced into Nigeria on July 20, 2014 when an infected Liberian man arrived by air in Lagos, Africa's largest city with 21 million residents.[141] Lagos is an international travel hub with departures via every conceivable mode of transportation to cities throughout Africa and the world: spread of Ebola in Nigeria could have quickly turned a regional epidemic into a global catastrophe.

At the airport and in the hospital where he was admitted, the traveler came into direct contact with 72 people before he was diagnosed with Ebola. He infected 13 of these initial contacts with the virus, one of whom fled quarantine to travel by air to Port Harcourt, Nigeria's oil capital, further spreading the infection to doctors and others in that city. It looked as though a nightmare scenario – the exponential spread of Ebola in multiple urban centers – could become a reality.[141]

All the elements for a global epidemic were in place but prompt action by local and international public health teams prevented this from occurring. Unlike the three nations in West Africa where the Ebola epidemic was raging, Nigeria has a functioning public health infrastructure including an emergency operations center and incident management system established previously by the CDC and international partners as part of the global effort to eradicate polio. When the Ebola virus landed in Nigeria, the government had the critical systems already in place to detect people potentially infected with the virus and interrupt transmission before it could spread out of control.

Nigeria also had a team of epidemiologic disease detectives trained through the CDC's Field Epidemiology Training Program (FETP). Within hours after the initial patient's positive Ebola diagnosis, Nigeria's FETP trainees spread out across Lagos, looking for anyone who might have come in contact with the traveler – the process of contact tracing. CDC staff in Nigeria and from Atlanta became part of the incident management system providing a coordinated, urgent response. The teams identified 894 people at risk for Ebola and completed nearly 19,000 home visits to monitor these individuals for symptoms over the 21-day incubation period post exposure.

At the airports, more than 147,000 travelers were screened for fever that might indicate Ebola infection. Eventually, these efforts identified 19 additional people with Ebola across three generations of transmission in the two cities and ended the outbreak before it could spread further among Nigeria's population of about 180 million people, or beyond. The immediate, rapid response made possible by the existing infrastructure and trained epidemiologists in Nigeria is a model for how potential global pandemics can be contained and controlled.[1]

Identifying the Outbreak Source

The severe West African Ebola epidemic is thought to have stemmed from EVD in the 2-year-old index case in Meliandou, Guinea. Researchers explored the source of that original infection using wildlife surveys, interviews, and molecular analyses of bat and environmental samples, and showed that there had been no decline in larger wildlife like apes, gorillas and duikers in the Meliandou area before onset of the epidemic. Interviews with regional authorities, hunters, and women of the village revealed that primates are rare and difficult to hunt in southeastern Guinea. Most large game consumed in the region arrives smoked, from distant regions eliminating it as a source of the infection. If contaminated fresh bushmeat had been brought to the village by a hunter, the latter would likely be among the first cases, as observed in previous outbreaks in the Congo Basin. Instead, only children and women developed symptoms and died in the beginning of the 2013–2015 epidemic. Collectively, these findings suggested that larger wildlife did not serve as an intermediate amplifier leading to the infection of the index case in Guinea, by contrast with the majority of Central African Ebola outbreaks.[133]

As previously reported, bats are considered to be the natural reservoir of the Ebola virus. Children in Meliandou were known to regularly catch and play with small insect-eating bats in a large hollow tree very near the home of the index case. Researchers speculate that this 2-year-old child have been infected by playing near that tree which reportedly housed a very large colony of insectiv-orous free-tailed bats (*Mops condylurus*). Bats in this family are considered poten-tial sources for Ebola virus outbreaks, and experimental data have shown that this species can survive experimental infection.[142] Molecular analyses of bat and environmental samples identified 13 different bat species. Three of the species captured – *Eidolon helvum, Hypsignathus monstrosus,* and *Mops condylurus* – were previously reported as possible reservoirs for Ebola virus but no EBOV RNA was detected in any of the PCR-tested bat or environmental samples from Meliandou or the surrounding area. Attempts to demonstrate the presence of IgG antibodies against Ebola viruses were also inconclusive. The investigation suggested but did not prove that unlike the majority of previous outbreaks, infection of the index case in this epidemic most likely involved direct infection from a bat reservoir.[133]

Looking Back :: Moving Forward

This Ebola pandemic was unique: it was by far the largest Ebolavirus outbreak in history with more cases, survivors and deaths than all other outbreaks combined. It included cases in 10 countries with limited international spread and lasted for almost 2 and a half years. What happened? Analysis of the outbreak has iden-tified many critical factors, most important of which is delayed recognition of the cause of the disease as Ebola – EVD had never occurred previously in West Africa so awareness of its typical presentation was minimal. Formal disease sur-veillance systems, a critical factor in recognition and arrest of disease outbreaks, are limited in the affected West African countries. Once Ebola was recognized – a long 3 months after the index case – public health education campaigns were slow to begin and not optimally delivered. The primary countries affected by Ebola have some of the world's lowest literacy rates so messages and delivery needed to be tailored to address this. Health resources were already constrained when Ebola hit: Sierra Leone, Liberia and Guinea are among the poorest coun-tries in Africa with very fragile health systems so capacity to respond to a major health emergency was limited. The international community response was slow with the declaration of a Public Health Emergency of International Concern by the WHO delayed until *5 months* after the epidemic was recognized and *8 months* after it began – there is little doubt that the status of WHO has suffered in response to their handling of this epidemic. Finally, the outbreak emphasized the important role of increasing global interconnectedness associated with the acceleration of international travel and trade allowing greater opportunities for infectious diseases like Ebola to emerge and spread.[134,143-145]

This devastating Ebola pandemic led to immediate efforts to develop a vaccine to prevent and or/limit future outbreaks. A collaborative global effort coordinated by the WHO resulted in accelerated development of candidate vaccines funded by the US National Institutes of Health, the Wellcome Trust, the European Commission, the UK Medical Research Council and the Bill and Melinda Gates Foundation. After the attacks on the USA on September 11, 2001, several governments had invested in Ebola virus vaccine research because of concerns it could be used as a biological weapon.[146] Based on results from these studies, candidate vaccines were rapidly designed, developed and manufactured in the USA, Canada, Europe and Asia with trials initiated in these countries plus Africa and Australia. A total of 10 clinical studies were conducted in the USA, Europe and Africa in support of potential eventual registration of an Ebola vaccine. With a lethal pathogen like Ebola, licensure is approved on the basis of animal studies plus evidence of safety and a proven immune response.[147] Clinical trials used administration of the vaccine to healthy human subjects to evaluate the immune response and identify side effects in accelerated protocols. Viral-vectored vaccine candidates entered Phase I clinical trials including a recombinant replication-competent vesicular stomatitis virus (rVSV) model and a recombinant chimpanzee adenovirus serotype 3 (ChAd3), both encoding the EBOV glycoprotein. Both vectors were previously shown to be safe in human studies for other candidate vaccines. The rVSV-ZEBOV vaccine was studied in a phase 3 trial involving 11,841 people in Guinea at the end of the epidemic in 2015. Among the 5837 people who received the vaccine, no Ebola cases were recorded 10 days or more after vaccination. In comparison, there were 23 cases of EVD occurring 10 days or more after vaccination among those who did not receive the vaccine. The rVSV vaccine had no severe safety concerns and was shown to be 100% efficacious and 75% effective at the cluster level including herd immunity in unvaccinated cluster subjects.[148,149]

The rVSV vaccine was then chosen to be used on an expanded access basis in March of 2016 in response to a recurrent outbreak of EVD in Guinea. A ring vaccination strategy was used based on the technique developed and proven effective during the smallpox eradication campaign. This involved aggressive surveillance for EVD cases and contact tracing with vaccination of all contacts and people at risk. The rVSV trial, called *Ebola ca Suffit!*, showed the vaccine to be highly effective after a single dose when used in this setting. Over a 1-month period, 1510 individuals were vaccinated in four rings including 307 health care workers. No secondary cases of EVD developed among those vaccinated and there were no serious adverse events.[149-151]

The risk of human infection from pathogens like Ebola is ongoing, persistent and – to this point – unpredictable. Evidence from 40 years of previous Ebola outbreaks suggests that the classic disease response approach can be effective: early case detection and isolation based on community education and engagement;

comprehensive contact tracing and quarantine; supportive clinical care; and rigorous infection control including safe burial methods. To these we can now add the use of vaccine to halt outbreaks as soon as the first cases are identified. However, every effective response depends on early recognition of the first cases of a new disease outbreak – and this requires that existing health care inadequacies in countries like Guinea, Sierra Leone and Liberia be addressed. A robust national health service with an adequate health care infrastructure, an existing disease surveillance system and ongoing community health education programs are the minimum requirements for disease detection, the critical steps in controlling any potential epidemic infection. As the transport of Ebola to Nigeria showed, an existing public health system can swing into action and very effectively prevent disease spread.[141] Immediate development of national health services linked to continental and international programs is the critical first step in preserving the future of global health security. Achieving this transformation of health systems on a global basis will require sweeping reforms led by a re-invigorated and reorganized WHO backed by an enormous commitment of financial and human resources.[152,153]

On a more focused level, development of effective treatment methods was a very high priority. In September 2014, the World Health Organization launched a fast-track process to identify potential anti-Ebola drugs with four potential classes of products: immunomodulators, immunoglobulins, small inhibitory RNA and antivirals.[152] Three criteria were established for a drug to be acceptable as a candidate for clinical trials: available safety data in humans, evidence for in vivo efficacy against Ebola virus from preclinical studies, and sufficient drug supply.[153] Five potential drugs were identified: Favipiravir, an RNA polymerase inhibitor, originally developed and approved in Japan for the treatment of severe influenza; mAb114, a chimeric monoclonal antibody cocktail; Remdesivir, a novel nucleotide analog prodrug developed for treatment of filovirus infections that blocks replication; REGN3470-3471-3479, a co-formulated cocktail of three human monoclonal antibodies targeting the EBOV glycoprotein; and ZMapp, a triple monoclonal antibody cocktail, already tried in selected cases during the 2014–2015 epidemic that targets 3 Ebola glycoprotein epitopes.

The WHO concluded that large and complex trials in which treatments are randomized to a selected, homogeneous group of individuals – the usual standard for drug trials in a first world setting – are impractical/impossible in the field, given the typically fragile health care systems in countries with ongoing Ebola outbreaks. With the large number of patients presenting simultaneously, the very high mortality rate of the disease, and the impossibility of explaining a randomization process to very sick patients, it was concluded to be both ethically unacceptable and impractical to allocate patients from within the same family or village to receive or not receive an experimental drug.[152,153] The WHO therefore approved all five available experimental treatments for use at Ebola treatment centers using standardized protocols with each treatment chosen by clinicians on a case-by-case basis. The treatments would be used as long as informed consent was obtained from patients and protocols were followed, with close monitoring, standardized reporting of results and documentation of adverse events.

Update

There have been multiple new EVD outbreaks since the onset of the West African epidemic, all in the DRC. The first occurred between August and November of 2014 in the vicinity of Boende town in Equateur province, a dense rain forest area. The index case was a pregnant woman who butchered a monkey found dead in the jungle by her husband – the classic story for initiation of an Ebola outbreak. She developed symptoms on July 26 and died on August 7. After her death, a local doctor assisted by 3 health workers performed a postmortem cesarean section to separate the fetus from the mother before burial, per local custom. These 4 individuals all developed EVD and all died. Subsequently, 8 symptomatic individuals with suspected EVD were evaluated and cultured at the local health center for the province. All cultures were positive for Ebola Zaire; subsequent genomic sequencing revealed the virus was identical or closely related to the EBOV variant that caused the EVD outbreak in the DRC in 1995; it was unrelated to the variant associated with the epidemic in West Africa. Ultimately, there were 66 confirmed patients with most cases presenting in late August and early September. All cases and contacts were found to have arisen from contact with the index case. There were 8 infected health care workers and all died. Overall, the mortality rate was 74%. This outbreak, similar to many previous outbreaks in Central Africa proves that, unaddressed, Ebola remains a very serious, highly contagious virus. This outbreak burned out on its own and was declared over on November 14, 2014.[154]

On May 11, 2017, the WHO was notified that Ebolavirus Zaire had again been detected among a cluster of undiagnosed illnesses and deaths with hemorrhagic signs in Likati, a remote region of the DRC. Cases of the disease were reported in four health districts. This was DRC's eighth outbreak of EVD since the discovery of the virus in the country in 1976. An effective response to this latest EVD outbreak in Africa was achieved through the rapid identification of cases, immediate testing of blood samples due to strengthened national laboratory capacity, early announcement of the outbreak by the government, and rapid response activities by local and national health authorities with the support of international partners. Medical support by MSF and coordination support on the ground by the WHO Health Emergencies Program were critical; an Incident Management System with deployment of 50 experts was set up within 24 hours of the outbreak being announced. When the new EVD outbreak was announced in May of 2017, the rVSV vaccine was approved again for use but this did not prove necessary given the small size of the outbreak and the rapid control achieved.[155] The outbreak was officially declared over by the WHO on June 2, 2017, 42 days – or two complete infection cycles – after the last case. There were 8 identified cases with four deaths.[156] In April of 2019, a team of local epidemiologists, the WHO and MSF reported complete sequencing of the virus responsible for this outbreak, a novel variant of ZEBOV, genetically close to the Ebola virus Mayinga variant which was identified as the cause of one of the two original 1976 outbreaks in the DRC.[157] This outbreak shows again the effectiveness and power of traditional epidemiologic methods of disease control.

On May 8, 2018, local health officials reported a new outbreak with 21 patients showing signs of hemorrhagic fever and 17 deaths in Bikora, in the northwest part of the country, beginning in late April. Three days later, Ebola Zaire was confirmed by reverse transcription polymerase chain reaction (RT-PCR) testing and the WHO put the DRC and all its neighbors on high alert. Despite aggressive efforts at containment, EVD spread to Mbandaka, a major city in the DRC with a population of more than a million people. At that time, there had been 44 confirmed cases and 23 deaths. WHO officials were very concerned about a major urban outbreak since the Mbandaka cases were the first sign of urban spread in the DRC. They were also concerned about the spread of Ebola in Congo-Brazzaville and the Central African Republic, since they are both connected to the outbreak area through river systems. WHO and Doctors Without Borders initiated emergency vaccination based on contact tracing and by the end of June, 3,330 people had received the rVSV vaccine. New cases began to decrease and on 7/24/2018, the health ministry declared the outbreak over with 53 confirmed and possible cases of Ebola and 29 deaths. So – this outbreak lets us see the power of effective vaccination in preventing what could have been a major epidemic.

Only a week later on August 1, 2018, a new Ebola outbreak in DRC was reported in North Kivu Province in the easternmost part of the country; analysis of genetic sequencing showed that while the outbreak was new, in an area remote from Bikora, it was the same EBOV Zaire strain that caused the new outbreak, thousands of miles away.[158] Unfortunately, this outbreak was complicated from the outset by ongoing conflict with multiple armed groups in North Kivu Province, which shares a border with Uganda and Rwanda. For decades, eastern Congo has suffered from on-and-off war and it remains beset by ongoing conflicts over land and ethnicity. Since late 2014, approximately 1000 civilians have been killed by both local and state forces in the area around the city of Beni, where a number of health workers are currently based. Health workers in the region relied on the support of the United Nations peacekeeping force to allow them to work. The volatile security situation impacted the method of vaccination used by WHO to try and contain this epidemic – as with the previous outbreak, health workers were planning to use the ring vaccination method, which targets only those who have potentially been in contact with an infected individual. As of July 2019, more than 1700 people had been vaccinated using contact tracing. When security constraints made screening to identify and vaccinate contacts impossible, all available residents of any village where an EVD patient had been identified were vaccinated.[158] From the outset, sustained violence complicated all efforts at care delivery.[159]

Meanwhile, Congolese health officials began an experimental treatment trial in EVD patients in November 2018 with the monoclonal antibody cocktail mAb114, the antiviral Remdesivir, REGN3470-3471-3479 and ZMapp, all of which are infused intravenously. The four treatments were tested in units run by three medical charities: Doctors Without Borders, Alima and the International Medical Corps. Patients were assigned at random to get one of the treatments as part of the PALM trial, for Pamoja Tulinde Maisha, which means "Save Lives Together" in Swahili.[160] And in August 2019, the trial's cosponsors at the WHO and the National Institutes of Health announced that two of the experimental treatments, now known as Regeneron and mAb-114, dramatically boosted survival rates: among patients with low viral loads suggesting they had been infected only days before, only 6% of those who received Regeneron and only 11% of those who got the mAb-114 drug died. By contrast, 33% of those who received Remdesivir and 24% of those who got ZMapp died and these two drugs were eliminated from further use.[161] This clinical trial was carried out in the worst possible conditions but still, dramatic and important results were achieved. After further clinical trials, the WHO recommended these two monoclonal antibody treatments against Ebola, saying the use of such drugs combined with better care had revolutionized the treatment of a disease once seen as a near-certain killer.[162] The drugs – Regeneron's Inmazeb (REGN-EB3) and Ridgeback Bio's Ebanga (mAb114) – use synthetic monoclonal antibodies that mimic natural antibodies in fighting off infections. Dr. Janet Diaz, lead of the clinical management unit in WHO's Health Emergencies program, told journalists the drugs were currently available in Congo but more work was needed to improve affordability.

The DRC outbreak which began in 2018 was finally declared over by the World Health Organization (WHO) on June 25, 2020. Despite intensive international efforts including sustained attempts at contact identification and ring vaccination, despite discovery of effective treatment, conflict in the area continuously complicated efforts to treat infected patients and to identify contacts, with response teams facing daily challenges against a backdrop of sporadic violence from armed groups and mistrust in affected communities. There were more than 3470 confirmed cases and more than 2287 deaths.[163]

On September 20, 2022, the Ministry of Health confirmed another new outbreak of Ebola (Sudan virus) in Mubende District, in western Uganda, the sixth Ebola outbreak in Uganda. Five of the six have been caused by the species Sudan ebolavirus. The outbreak was declared over on January 11, 2023, with 142 confirmed cases (and 22 probable) and 55 confirmed deaths.

This last outbreak in an almost continuous series of outbreaks confirms that EBOV is endemic in central Africa, specifically in the DRC and Uganda. The incidence of EBOV outbreaks is escalating, a striking difference from the long period of what was thought to be epidemiologic silence after the first two reported outbreaks in 1976. However, earlier outbreaks that occurred in small, isolated villages could have burned out independently before ever being identified beyond the local level. At this time, important new risk factors combine to make the DRC particularly vulnerable to more and larger disease outbreaks:

- Over the last 60 years, there has been exponential population growth – from ~15 million in 1960 to more than 100 million in 2018. This population increase means people are living closer together in larger communities, and to jungle areas and the animals who inhabit them, both factors that facilitate disease spread.
- Since the 1960s, the Congolese have endured four decades of armed conflict with an ongoing civil war between government troops and rebels in Eastern Congo where current outbreaks have begun. The sustained levels of violence and conflict have caused massive infrastructural damage, population displacement and loss of life.
- Although the DRC is one of the richest countries on the planet with an estimated $24 trillion of natural resources, it has one of the highest levels of poverty in the world, ranking seventh among the world's poorest countries in 2023.
- In the past four decades, the political and economic collapse of the country has had a dramatic impact on the country's health care system. Hospitals and clinics lack personnel, equipment, medication and supplies. An estimated 70% of Congolese have little or no access to health care.
- Even basic infrastructure is deficient: in the DRC, only 1.8% of existing roads are tarred and less than 10% of the population has access to electricity.

In terms of risk factors for infectious disease outbreaks – high population density, urban overcrowding, war, poverty and deficient health care – the DRC has it all. Major efforts by international groups to improve health care infrastructure are ongoing but all the factors necessary for recurrent, disastrous pandemics persist.

Fortunately, the picture with specific regard to Ebola has also changed. For the last 40 years, the specter of the Ebola virus has hung over central Africa and haunted scientists, infectious disease specialists and public health experts all over the world. Until now, many believed that anyone infected with Ebola was "doomed to die alone among space-suited strangers and be buried without ceremony in a bleach-misted body bag."[164] But major scientific advances achieved on the ground in the last 5 years during the West African epidemic and the subsequent outbreaks in the eastern DRC and Uganda have resulted in an effective vaccine and powerful anti-viral treatments. As of February 20, 2020, the DRC, Burundi, Ghana and Zambia have licensed an Ebola vaccine, just 90 days after the WHO completed an accelerated pre-qualification process.[164] Licensing means that the manufacturer can stockpile and widely distribute this vaccine to African countries at risk of Ebola virus disease outbreaks. Disease prevention, deficient health infrastructure and delivery of care to distrustful infected individuals remain ongoing challenges but for the first time, there is major progress towards turning Ebola from a terrifying, highly fatal disease into one that is preventable and treatable. Pathways to access health care must be the next priority.

Out of Nowhere?

West Nile virus, SARS, Ebola and Zika are unique viruses but each led to a completely unanticipated, explosive global pandemic. Did they really come "out of nowhere"? Many of the characteristics associated with pandemics through history are readily identified, especially, the sudden emergence of a previously unknown/unrecognized disease and the critical role of travel bringing a new contagion to an immunologically naïve population. Only SARS was truly a previously unidentified pathogen while WNV, Ebola and Zika were all thought to have been well characterized. The importance of continuous viral evolution cannot be overemphasized, given the critical role it played with the WNV and Zika. For all four viruses, travel was important, introducing a new contagion to a location where the disease was unknown and the population had never previously been exposed. In fact, in today's highly interconnected world, rapid, frequent global travel played a critical role in the introduction and global spread of each of these viruses as did our exponentially increasing world population density and chaotic urbanization.

But perhaps most importantly, these pandemics emphasize the importance of the unique characteristics of viral pathogens in determining the frequency and gravity of disease outbreaks. WNV was known to be carried by mosquito vectors from avian reservoirs and was recognized in Africa, the Middle East, Eurasia and Australia for causing sporadic outbreaks of a generally mild disease but it was not until the virus reached NYC in 1999 that it was definitively shown to cause simultaneous deadly outbreaks in birds and serious neuro-invasive disease in people. We underestimated the power of spontaneous viral evolution leading to enhanced neurovirulence; and the incredible speed of disease transmission in an enormous, naïve population, replete with available reservoirs and carriers where global warming led to a longer period for disease transmission. That initial epidemic ended when cooler weather eliminated mosquitoes but astonishingly, the virus spread to infect millions of individuals and involve the entire Western Hemisphere over the next decade.

With SARS, a previously unidentified but very highly contagious virus caused a widely transmitted, rapidly progressive, sometimes fatal pneumonia that over a 6 month period affected more than 8000 individuals in thirty countries. Among its important lessons is the lethal capacity of viral pathogens that jump from animals to infect humans. And the SARS pandemic emphasized the power of international air travel in contemporary disease transmission – so powerful that the right pathogen can threaten the entire planet.

With Ebola, months of delay turned a theoretically containable local outbreak into a massive pandemic – and analysis of the delay identified the importance of high population density and poor existing health infrastructure as major risk factors for ongoing infectious disease spread.[165]

With both WNV and Zika, we underestimated the power of a minor virus we thought we knew, introduced by international air travel to countries replete with the necessary vector and an enormous, immunologically naive population – and we failed to identify the spontaneous development of enhanced neurovirulence with both viruses and the risk this posed for infected subjects and the developing fetus.

Analysis of these four pandemics does not support the "out of nowhere" concept but instead, highlights important themes in contemporary viral pandemic development: the critical roles of ongoing viral evolution and of emerging viruses that can cross over from other species to infect humans; the very high importance of global travel in disease introduction to new populations; the speed of disease spread in our crowded, increasingly connected world; and the importance of global scientific communication and collaboration. Critical evaluation of an outbreak focused on these characteristics could potentially interrupt disease spread.

There will be another viral pandemic – and the world may again feel that it came "out of nowhere." But the response to the WNV, SARS, Ebola and Zika epidemics will hopefully have left us better prepared to use intensive outbreak analysis of the virus itself plus international surveillance systems, continuous global pathogen-specific scientific investigation and communication, and immediate international collaboration to establish effective pandemic disease defenses.

References

1. Steinhauer J, Miller J. In New York outbreak, glimpse of gaps in biological defenses. Oct.11,1999. *Archives of the NY Times.*
2. Steele KE, Linn MJ, Schoepp RJ et al. Pathology of fatal West Nile Virus infections in native and exotic birds during the 1999 outbreak in New York City, New York. *Vet Pathol* 2000; 37:208–224.
3. Asnis DS, Conetta R, Teixeira AA et al.The West Nile Virus Outbreak of 1999 in New York: the Flushing hospital experience. *Clinical Infect Dis* 2000; 30:413–418.
4. MMWR. Outbreak of West Nile-like viral encephalitis – New York,1999. *MMWR* 1999; 48(38):845–849.
5. Smithburn KC, Hughes TP, Burke AW Paul JH. A neurotropic virus isolated from the blood of a native of Uganda. *Am. J. Trop. Med. Hyg* 1940; 20: 471–492.
6. Smithburn KC, Jacobs HR. Neutralization tests against neurotropic viruses with sera collected in central Africa. *J Immunol* 1942; 44:9–23.
7. Sejvar JJ. West Nile Virus: an historical overview. *Ochsner Journal* 2003; 5(3):6–10.
8. Marberg K, Goldblum M, Sterk VV et al. The natural history of West Nile fever. I. Clinical observations during an epidemic in Israel. *Am J Hyg* 1956; 64:259–269.1814.
9. Taylor RM, Work TH, Hurlbut HS, Rizk F. A study of the ecology of West Nile Virus in Egypt. *Am J Trop Med* 1956; 5:579–620.
10. Spigland, W. Jasinska-Klingberg, Hofshi E, Goldblum N. Clinical and laboratory observations in an outbreak of West Nile fever in Israel in 1957. *Harefuah* 1958; 54 (11): 275–280.

11. Tsai TF, Popovici F, Cernescu C et al. West Nile virus encephalitis in southeastern Romania. *Lancet* 1998; 352(9130): 767–771.

12. Petersen LR, Brault AC, Nasci RS. West Nile Virus: Review of the literature. *JAMA* 2013; 310(3):308–315.

13. Chancey C, Grinev A, Volkova E, Rios M. The global ecology and epidemiology of West Nile Virus. *Biomed Res Int* 2015; 4: 1–20. http://dx.doi.org/10.1135/2015/376230

14. Lanciotti RS, Roehrig JT, Deubel V et al. Origin of the West Nile virus responsible for an outbreak of encephalitis in the northeastern United States. *Science* 1999; 286:2333–2337.

15. Nash D, Mostashari F, Fine A et al. The outbreak of West Nile virus infection in the New York city area in 1999. *N Engl J Med* 2001; 344(24):1807–1814.

16. Brinton MA. The molecular biology of West Nile Virus: a new invader of the Western Hemisphere. *Annu Rev Microbiol* 2002; 56:371–402.

17. May FJ, Davis T, Tesh RB, Barrett ADT. Phylogeography of West Nile virus: from the cradle of evolution in Africa to Eurasia, Australia and the Americas. *J Virol* 2011; 85(6):2964–2974.

18. Robbins J. The ecology of disease. *NY Times Sunday review*. July 14, 2012.

19. Sejvar JJ, Leis AA, Stokic DS et al. Acute flaccid paralysis and West Nile virus infection. *Emerg Inf Dis* 2003; 9(7): 788–793.

20. Busch MP, Caglioti S, Robertson EF et al. Screening the blood supply for West Nile virus RNA by nucleic acid amplification testing. *N Engl J Med.* 2005 Aug 4; 353(5):460–7.

21. Centers for Disease Control and Prevention, National Center for Emerging and Zoonotic Infectious Diseases (NCEZID), Division of Vector-Borne Diseases (DVBD). West Nile Virus.

22. Weber IB, Lindsey NP, Bunko-Patterson AM et al. Completeness of West Nile virus testing in patients with meningitis and encephalitis during an outbreak in Arizona, USA. *Epidemiol Infect* 2011; 140(9): 1632–1636.

23. Acharya D, Bai F. An overview of current approaches toward the treatment and prevention of West Nile virus infection. *Methods Mol Biol* 2016; 1435:249–291.

24. Saxena V, Bolling BG, Wang T. West Nile virus. *Clin Lab Med* 2017; 37:243–252.

25. Woods CM, Sanchez AM, Swamy GK et al. An observer blinded, randomized, placebo-controlled, phase I dose escalation trial to evaluate the safety and immunogenicity of an inactivated West Nile virus Vaccine, HydroVax-001, in healthy adults. *Vaccine* 2019; 37(3):4222–4230

26. Lindsey NP, Staples JE, Lehman JA et al. Surveillance for human West Nile Virus disease. *MMWR Surveill Summ* 2010: 59(2):1–17.

27. Petersen LR, Hayes EB. West Nile virus in the Americas. *Med Clin North Am* 2008; 92(6):1307–1322.

28. Davis CT, Ebel GD, Lanciotti RS et al. Phylogenetic analysis of North American West Nile virus isolates, 2001–2004: evidence for the emergence of a dominant genotype. *Virology* 2005; 342: 252–265.

29. Grinev A, Chancey C, Volkova E et al. Genetic variability of West Nile virus in U.S. blood donors from the 2012 epidemic season. *PLoS Negl Trop Dis* 2016; 10(5):1–19.

30. Petersen LR, Carson PJ, Biggerstaff BJ et al. Estimated cumulative incidence of West Nile virus infection in US adults, 1999–2010. *Epidemiol Infect* 2012; 1–5.

31. Harrigan RJ, Thomassen HA, Buermann, Smith TB. A continental risk assessment of West Nile virus under climate change. *Glob Change Biol* 2014; 20(8): 2417–2425.

32. Burki T. Increase of West Nile virus cases in Europe for 2018. *Lancet Inf Dis* 2018; 392:1000.

33. Di Giallonardo F, Geoghegan JL, Docherty DE et al. Fluid spatial dynamics of West Nile virus in the United States: Rapid spread in a permissive host environment. *J Virol* 2015; 90(2):862–72.

34. Swetnam D, Widen SG, Wood TG et al. Terrestrial bird migration and West Nile virus circulation, United States. *Emerg Inf Dis* 2018; 24(12):2184–2194.

35. Moon SA, Cohnstaedt LW, McVey DS, Scoglio CM. A spatio-temporal individual-based network framework for West Nile virus in the USA: Spreading pattern of West Nile virus. *PLoS Comput Biol* 2019; 15(3): e1006875. https://doi.org/10.1371/journal.pcbi.1006875

36. Gyles C. One Medicine, One Health, One World. *Can Vet J* 2016; 57(4): 345–346.

37. Eidson M, Komar N, Sorhage F et al. Crow deaths as a sentinel surveillance system for West Nile virus in the northeastern United States, 1999. *Emerg Inf Dis* 2001; 7(4):615–620.

38. World Health Organization. Disease outbreak reported: acute respiratory syndrome in China-update 3. Available at www.who.int/csr/don/2003_2_20/en

39. Reilly B, Van Herp M, Sermand D et al. SARS and Carlo Urbani. *New Engl J Med* 2003;3 48(20):1951–1952.

40. Tsang KW, Ho PL, Ooi GC et al. A cluster of cases of severe acute respiratory syndrome in Hong Kong. *New Engl J Med* 2003; 348(20):1977–1985.

41. Poutanen SM, Low DE, Henry B et al. Identification of severe acute respiratory syndrome in Canada. *New Engl J Med* 2003; 348(20):1995–2005.

42. WHO. Disease outbreak news. Update 95 – SARS: Chronology of a serial killer. Available at: www.who.int/csr/don/2003_07_04/en/

43. CDC. Outbreak of Severe Acute Respiratory Syndrome---Worldwide, 2003. *MMWR*. March 21, 2003; 52(11):226–228.

44. CDC. Update: Outbreak of Severe Acute Respiratory Syndrome---Worldwide, 2003. *MMWR*. March 28, 2003: 52(12);241–248.

45. Li W, Wong S-K, Li F et al. Animal origins of the Severe Acute Respiratory Syndrome Coronavirus: Insight from ACE2-S-protein interactions. *J Virol* 2006; 80(9):4211–4219.

46. Hu B, Ge X, Wang L-F, Shi Z. Bat origin of human coronaviruses. *Virology J* 2015; 12:221–233.

47. World Health Organization. Summary of probable SARS cases with onset of illness from 1 November 2002 to 31 July 2003. www.who.int/csr/sars/country/table200 4_04_21/en/index.html

48. WHO Press Release 16 April 2003. Coronavirus never before seen in humans is the cause of SARS. Unprecedented collaboration identifies new pathogen in record time. Geneva, 16 April 2003.

49. Drosten C, Gunther S, Preiser W et al. Identification of a novel coronavirus in patients with Severe Acute Respiratory Syndrome. *New Engl J Med* 2003; 348(20): 1967–1976.

50. Wong GW, Hui DS. Severe acute respiratory syndrome (SARS): epidemiology, diagnosis and management. *Thorax*. 2003 Jul. 58(7):558–60.

51. WHO/ SARS outbreak contained worldwide – World Health Organization. www. who.int/mediacentre/news/releases/2003/pr56/en/

52. Dick GW, Kitchen SF, Haddow AJ. Zika virus. I. Isolation and serological specificity. *Trans R Soc Trop Med Hyg* 1952; 46(5):509–520.

53. Kindhauser MK, Allen T, Frank V et al. Zika: the origin and spread of a mosquito-borne virus. *Bull World Health Org* 2016; 94:675–686.

54. Duffy MR, Chen TH, Hancock WT et al. Zika virus outbreak on Yap Island, Federated States of Micronesia. *N Engl J Med* 2009; 360(24): 2536–2543.

55. Mo Y, Salada BMA, Tambyah PA. Zika virus – a review for clinicians. *Brit Med Bull* 2016; 119:25–36.

56. Kindhauser MK, Allen T, Frank V et al. Zika: the origin and spread of a mosquito-borne virus. *Bull World Health Org* 2016; 94:675–686.

57. Haddow AD, Schuh AJ, Yasuda CY et al. Genetic characterization of Zika virus strains: geographic expansion of the Asian lineage. *PLoS Negl Trop Dis* 2012; 6(2): e1477. Downloaded 12/16/2017.

58. ECDC Rapid Risk Assessment: Zika Virus Infection Outbreak, French Polynesia. European Centre for Disease Prevention and Control, Stockholm, Sweden. February 2014. http://ecdc.europe.eu/en/publications/Publications/Zika-virus-French-Polynesia-rapidrisk assessment.pdf

59. Oehler E, Watrin L, Larre P et al. Zika virus infection complicated by Guillain-Barre Syndrome – case report, French Polynesia, December, 2013. *Euro Surveill* 2014; 19: 20720.

60. Cao-Lormeau VM, Blake A, Mons S et al. Guillain-Barre Syndrome outbreak associated with Zika virus infection in French Polynesia. *Lancet* 2016; 387: 1531–1539.

61. Ai J-W, Zhang Y, Zhang W. Zika virus outbreak: a perfect storm. *Emerg Microbes Infect.* 2016 Mar; 5(3): e21. Published online 2016 Mar 9. doi: 10.1038/emi.2016.42

62. De Oliveira K, Cortez-Escalente J, De Oliveira WT et al. Increase in reported prevalence of microcephaly in infants born to women living in areas with confirmed Zika virus transmission during the first trimester of pregnancy – Brazil, 2015. *MMWR* 2016; 65:242–247.

63. Graham KA, Fox DJ, Talati A et al. Prevalence and clinical attributes of congenital microcephaly – New York, 2013–2015. *MMWR* 2017; 66(5):125–129.

64. Jaenisch T, Rosenberger KD, Brito C et al. Risk of microcephaly after Zika virus infection in Brazil, 2015 to 2016. *Bull WHO* 2017; 95:191–198. doi: http://dx.doi.org/10.2471/BLT.16.178608

65. Cauchemez S, Besnard M, Bompard P et al. Association between Zika virus and microcephaly in French Polynesia, 2013–15: a retrospective study. *Lancet* 2016; 387: 2125–32.

66. Franca GV, Schular-Faccini L, Oliveira WK et al. Congential Zika virus syndrome in Brazil: a case series of the first 1501 livebirths with complete investigation. *Lancet* 2016; 388(10047):891–897.

67. WHO. Zika Virus Epidemic. Public Health Emergency of International Concern. Feb 1, 2016. www.who.int/mediacentre/news/statements/2016/1st-emergency-committee-zika/en/

68. Rasmussen SA, Jamieson DJ, Honein MA et al. Zika virus and birth defects – reviewing the evidence for causality. *N Engl J Med* 2016; 374:1981–1987.

69. Souza BS, Sampaio GL, Pereira CS, Souza BS et al. Zika virus infection induces mitosis abnormalities and apoptotic cell death of human neural progenitor cells. *Sci Rep.* 2016; 6:39775. doi: 10.1038/srep39775.

70. Martines RB, Bhatnager J, de Oliveira Ramos AM et al. Pathology of congenital Zika syndrome in Brazil: a case series. *Lancet* 2016; 388(10047):898–904.

71. De Araujo TVB, de Alencar Ximenez RA, de Barros Miranda-D et al. Association between microcephaly, Zika virus infection and other risk factors in

Brazil: final report of a case-control study. *Lancet Infect Dis.* 2017 Dec 11. pii: S1473–3099(17)30727-2. doi: 10.1016/S1473-3099(17)30727-2. [Epub ahead of print]

72. Mlakar J, Korva M, Tul N et al. Zika virus associated with microcephaly. *N Engl J Med* 2016; 374(10):951–958.

73. Hastings AK, Fikrig E. Zika virus and sexual transmission: A new route of transmission for mosquito-borne Flaviviruses. *Yale J Biol Med.* 2017; 90(2):325–330.

74. Weaver SC. Emergence of epidemic Zika virus transmission and congenital Zika syndrome: are recently evolved traits to blame? *mBio* 2017; 8:e02063–16. https://doi.org/10.1128/mBio.02063-16

75. Liu Y, Liu J, Du S et al. Evolutionary enhancement of Zika virus infectivity in *Aedes aegypti* mosquitoes. *Nature* 2017; 545: 482–486.

76. Faria NR, da Silva Azevedo R de S, Moritz UG et al. Zika virus in the Americas: early epidemiologic and genetic findings. *Science* 2016; 352(6283):345–349.

77. Quick J, Grubaugh ND, Pullan ST et al. Multiplex PCR method for MinION and Illumina sequencing of Zika and other virus genomes directly from clinical samples in the field. *Nat Protoc* 2017; 12(6): 1261–1276.

78. Metsky HC, Matranga CB, Wohl S et al. Zika virus evolution and spread in the Americas. *Nature* 2017; 546(7658): 411–415.

79. Grubach ND, Ladner JT, Andersen KG. Genomic epidemiology reveals multiple introductions of Zika virus into the United States. *Nature* 2017; 546: 401–405.

80. Schwartz DA. Autopsy and postmortem studies are concordant: pathology of Zika virus infection is neurotropic in fetuses and infants with microcephaly following transplacental transmission. *Arch Path Lab Med* 2017; 141(1):68–72.

81. Annamalai AS, Pattnaik A, Sahoo BR et al. Zika virus encoding nonglycosylated envelope protein is attenuated and defective in neuroinvasion. *J Virol* 2017; 91(23):e01348–17.

82. Yuan L, Huang X-Y, Liu Z-Y et al. A single mutation in the prM protein of Zika virus contributes to fetal microcephaly. *Science* 2017; 358(6365):933–936.

83. De Oliveira WK, de Franca GVA, Carmo EH et al. Infection-related microcephaly after the 2015 and 2016 Zika virus outbreaks in Brazil: a surveillance-based analysis. *Lancet* 2017; 390(10097):861–870.

84. Honein MA, Dawson AL, Petersen EE et al. U.S. Zika Pregnancy Registry. Birth defects among fetuses and infants of US women with evidence of possible Zika virus infection during pregnancy. *JAMA* 2017; 317(1):59–68.

85. Reynolds MR, Jones AM, Petersen EE et al. Vital signs: Update on Zika virus–associated birth defects and evaluation of all U.S. Infants with congenital Zika virus exposure – U.S. Zika Pregnancy Registry, 2016; *MMWR* April 7, 2017; 66(13):366–373. www.cdc.gov/mmwr/volumes/66/wr/mm6613e1.htm

86. Satterfield-Nash A, Kotzky K, Allen J et al. Health and development at age 19–24 months of 19 children who were born with microcephaly and laboratory evidence of congenital Zika virus infection during the 2015 Zika virus outbreak – Brazil, 2017. *MMWR* December 15, 2017; 66(49):1347–1351. www.cdc.gov/media/releases/2017/p1214-congenital-zika-challenges.html

87. WHO statement on the 2nd meeting of IHR Emergency Committee on Zika virus and observed increase in neurological disorders and neonatal malformations. www.who.int/mediacentre/news/statements/2016/2nd-emergency-committee-zika/en/

88. Basu R, Tumbna E. Zika virus on a spending spree: what we now know that was unknown in the 1950s. *Virol J* 2016; 13: 165–174.

89. Leded K, Grobusch MP, Gautret P et al. Zika beyond the Americas: Travelers as sentinels of Zika virus transmission. A GeoSentinel analysis, 2012–2016. *PLoS ONE*; 12910: e0185689. https://doi.org/10.1371/journal.pone.0185689

90. Fifth meeting of the Emergency Committee under the International Health Regulations (2005) regarding microcephaly, other neurological disorders and Zika virus. www.who.int/emergencies/zika-virus/mediacentre/press-releases/en/

91. Netto EM, Moreira-Soto A, Pedroso C et al. High Zika virus seroprevalence in Salvador, northeastern Brazil limits the potential for further outbreaks. *mBio* 8:e01390–17. https://doi.org/10.1128/152

92. Ferguson NM, Cucunuba ZM, Dorigatti I et al. Countering the Zika epidemic in Latin America. *Science* 2016; 353(6297):353–354.

93. Pan American Health Organization / World Health Organization. Zika Epidemiological Update, 25 August 2017. Washington, D.C.: PAHO/WHO; 2017.

94. News Updates – Texas Department of State Health Services – Texas.gov. www.dshs.texas.gov/news/updates.shtm

95. Morens DM, Fauci AS. Pandemic Zika: a formidable challenge to medicine and public health. *J Inf Dis* 2017; 216 (suppl_10): S857 doi: 10.1093/infdis/jix383

96. Dutra HLC, Rocha MN, Stehling FB et al. Wolbachia blocks currently circulating Zika virus isolates in Brazilian *Aedes aegypti* mosquitoes. *Cell Host & Microbe* 2016; 19: 771–774.

97. Callaway E. Rio fights Zika with biggest release yet of bacteria-infected mosquitoes. *Nature* 2016; 539(7627):17–18. doi: 10.1038/nature.2016.20878

98. O'Neill SL, Ryan PA, Turley AP et al. Scaled deployment of Wolbachia to protect the community from Aedes transmitted arboviruses. *Gates Open Res* 2018; 2: 36–51.

99. Morabito KM, Graham BS. Zika virus vaccine development. *J Infectious Dis* 2017; 216 (suppl_10): S957–S963.

100. National Institute of Allergy and Infectious Diseases. NIH begins testing investigational Zika vaccine in humans. *Press release*. August 3, 2016. www.niaid.nih.gov/news-events/nih-begins-testing-investigational-zika-vaccine-humans

101. Morrison C. DNA vaccines against Zika virus speed into clinical trials. *Nat. Rev. Drug Discov* 2016; 15(8), 521–522.

102. Dudley DM, Rompay KK, O'Connor DH et al. Miscarriage and stillbirth following maternal Zika virus infection in nonhuman primates. *Nature Medicine* 2018; 24:1104–1107.

103. Sevvana M, Long F, Miller A et al. Refinement and analysis of the mature Zika virus cryo-EM Structure at 3.1 Angstrom resolution. *Cell Press/ Structure* 2018; 26: 1–9. https://doi.org/10.1016/j.str.2018.05.006

104. Garrett L. *The Coming Plague: Newly Emerging Diseases in a World Out of Balance.* Chapter 5. Yambuku. Pg.100–116.

105. Pattyn S, Jacob W, Van der Groen G et al. Isolation of Marburg-like virus from a case of haemorrhagic fever in Zaire. *Lancet* 1977; 1:573–574.

106. Johnson KM, Webb PA, Lange JV et al. Isolation and partial characterization of a new virus causing acute haemorrhagic fever in Zaire. *Lancet* 1977; 1:569–571.

107. Bowen ETW, Platt GS, Lloyd G et al. Viral haemorrhagic fever in southern Sudan and northern Zaire: preliminary studies on the aetiological agent. *Lancet* 1977; 1:571–573.

108. Ebola haemorrhagic fever in Zaire, 1976: report of an International Commission. *Bull WHO.* 1978; 56: 271–293.

109. Ebola haemorrhagic fever in Sudan, 1976: report of a WHO/International Study Team. *Bull WHO.* 1978; 56:247–70.
110. Richman DD, Cleveland PH, McCormick J et al. Antigenic analysis of strains of Ebola virus. Identification of two Ebola virus serotypes. *J Infect Dis* 1983; 147: 268–71.
111. WHO. Viral hemorrhagic fever in imported monkeys. *Weekly Epidem Record* 1992; 67(24):183–191.
112. Barrette RW, Metwally SA, Rowland JM et al. Discovery of swine as a host for the Reston ebolavirus. *Science* 2009; 325:204–206.
113. Kobinger GP, Leung A, Neufeld J, Richardson JS et al. Replication, pathogenicity, shedding, and transmission of Zaire ebolavirus in pigs. *J Infect Dis* 2011; 204(2): 200–208.
114. Formenty P, Hatz C, LeGuenno B et al. Human infection due to Ebola virus, subtype Côte d'Ivoire: clinical and biologic presentation. *J Infect Dis* 1999; 179 Suppl 1:S48–53.
115. Branch P. CDC. Outbreaks chronology: Ebola virus disease. https://stacks.cdc.gov/view/cdc/41088/cdc_41088_DS1.pdf
116. MacNeil A, Farnon EC, Wamala JF, Okware S, Cannon DL, Reed Z et al. Proportion of Deaths and Clinical Features in Bundibugyo Ebola Virus Infection, Uganda. *Emerg Infect Dis.* 2010; 16(12):1969–1972. https://dx.doi.org/10.3201/eid1612.100627
117. MacNeil A, Farnon EC, Morgan OW et al. Filovirus outbreak detection and surveillance: Lessons from Bundibugyo. *J Infect Dis,* 2011; 204, Suppl 3: S761–S767. https://doi.org/10.1093/infdis/jir294
118. Leroy EM, Rouquet P, Formenty P et al. Multiple Ebola virus transmission events and rapid decline of central African wildlife. *Science* 2004; 303:387–390.
119. Bermejo M, Rodriguez-Teijeiro JD, Illera G et al. Ebola outbreak killed 5000 gorillas. *Science* 2006; 314(5805):1564.
120. Leroy EM, Kumulungui B, Pourrut X et al. Fruit bats as reservoirs of Ebola virus. *Nature* 2005; 438:575–6.
121. Leendertz SA, Gogarten JF, Dux A et al. Assessing the evidence supporting fruit bats as the primary reservoirs for Ebola viruses. *EcoHealth* 2016; 13(1):18–25.
122. Dowell SF, Mukunu R, Ksiazek TG et al. Transmission of Ebola hemorrhagic fever: a study of risk factors in family members, Kikwit, Democratic Republic of the Congo, 1995. Commission de Lutte contre les Epidémies à Kikwit. *J Infect Dis* 1999 Feb; 179 Suppl 1:S87–91.
123. Khan AS, Tshioko FK, Heymann DL. The reemergence of Ebola hemorrhagic fever, Democratic Republic of the Congo, 1995. Commission de Lutte contre les Epidémies à Kikwit. *J Infect Dis.* 1999; 179 Suppl 1:S76–86.
124. Glynn JR, Bower H, Johnson S et al. Asymptomatic infection and unrecognized Ebola virus disease in Ebola-affected households in Sierra Leone: a cross-sectional study using a new non-invasive assay for antibodies to Ebola virus. *Lancet Infect Dis* 2017;7:645–653.
125. Christie A, Davies-Wayne GJ, Cordier-Lassalle T et al. Possible sexual transmission of Ebola virus – Liberia, 2015. Centers for Disease Control and Prevention (CDC). MMWR. *Morbidity and Mortality Weekly Report.* May 2015, 64(17):479–481.
126. Rivera A, Messaudi I. Pathophysiology of Ebola virus infection: current challenges and future hopes. *ACS Infect Dis.* 2015 May 8;1(5):186–97.

127. Dahlke C, Lunemann S, Kasonta R et al. Comprehensive characterization of cellular immune responses following Ebola virus infection. *J Infect Dis.* 2017; 215(2):287–292.

128. Towner JS, Rollin PE, Bausch DG et al. Rapid diagnosis of Ebola hemorrhagic fever by reverse transcription-PCR in an outbreak setting and assessment of patient viral load as a predictor of outcome. *J Virol* 2004; 78:4330–4341.

129. Holmes EC, Dudas G, Rambaut A, Andersen K. The evolution of Ebola virus: Insights from the 2013–2016 epidemic. *Nature.* 2016; 538(7624): 193–200.

130. Li ZJ, Tu WX, Wang XC et al. A practical community-based response strategy to interrupt Ebola transmission in Sierra Leone, 2014–2015. *Infect Dis Poverty* 2016; 5(1):74–84.

131. Weppelmann TA, Donewell B, Hague U et al. Determinants of patient survival during the 2014 Ebola Virus Disease outbreak in Bong County, Liberia. *Glob Health Res Policy* 2016; 1: 5–15.

132. Kilgore PE, Grabenstein JD, Salim AM, Rybak M. Treatment of Ebola virus disease. *Pharmacotherapy* 2015 Jan;35(1):43–53.

133. Saez AM, Weiss S, Nowak K et al. Investigating the zoonotic origin of the West African Ebola epidemic. *EMBO Molecular Medicine* 2015; 7(1): 17–23.

134. WHO Statement on the 1st meeting of the IHR Emergency Committee on the 2014 Ebola outbreak in West Africa. www.who.int/mediacentre/news/statements/2014/ebola-20140808/en/

135. WHO | Ebola outbreak 2014–2015 – World Health Organization Bulletin. www.who.int/csr/disease/ebola/en/

136. Cases of Ebola Diagnosed in the United States. www.cdc.gov/vhf/ebola/outbreaks/2014-west.../united-states-imported-case.ht

137. WHO. Health worker Ebola infections in Guinea, Liberia and Sierra Leone. Preliminary report. www.who.int/features/ebola/health-care-worker/en/

138. Dahl BA, Kinzer MH, Raghunathan PL et al. CDC's response to the 2014–2016 Ebola epidemic – Guinea, Liberia, and Sierra Leone. *MMWR Suppl* 2016; 65(Suppl-3):12–20. doi: http://dx.doi.org/10.15585/mmwr.su6503a3

139. WHO Ebola Situation Report. 20 May 2015. http://apps.who.int/ebola/en/ebola-situation-reports

140. Hersey S, Martel LD, Jambai S et al. Ebola virus disease – Sierra Leone and Guinea, August 2015. *MMWR* 2015; 64(35): 980–984. www.cdc.gov/mmwr

141. Shuaib F, Gunnala R, Musa EO et al. Ebola virus disease outbreak – Nigeria, July–September 2014. *MMWR* 2014; 63(39):867–872.

142. Olival KJ, Hayman DT. Filoviruses in bats: current knowledge and future directions. *Viruses* 2014; 6: 1759–1788

143. WHO Ebola Response team. After Ebola in West Africa – unpredictable risks, preventable epidemics. *New Engl J Med* 2016; 375(6):587–596.

144. Bell BP, Damon IK, Lernigan DB et al. Overview, control strategies and lessons learned in the CDC response to the 2014–2016 Ebola epidemic. *MMWR Suppl* 2016; 65(3):4–11.

145. Gostin LA, Friedman EA. A retrospective and prospective analysis of the West African Ebola virus disease epidemic: robust national health systems at the foundation and an empowered WHO at the apex. *Lancet* 2015; 385:1902–1909.

146. Marzi A, Feldmann H. Ebola virus vaccines: an overview of current approaches. *Expert Rev Vaccines.* 2014; 13: 521–531.

147. Milligan ID, Gibani MM, Sewell R, et al. Safety and immunogenicity of novel adenovirus type 26- and modified vaccinia ankara-vectored Ebola vaccines. *JAMA*. 2016; 315(15):1610–1623.
148. Osterholm M, Moore K, Ostrowsky J et al. Wellcome Trust-CIDRAP Ebola vaccine team B. The Ebola vaccine team B. *Lancet Infect Dis*. 2016; 16(1):e1–e9.
149. Henea-Restrepo AM, Longini IM, Egger M et al. Efficacy and effectiveness of an rVSV-vectored vaccine expressing Ebola surface glycoprotein: interim results from the Guinea ring vaccination cluster-randomised trial. *Lancet* 2015; 386:857–866.
150. Gsell P-S, Camacho A, Kucharski AJ et al. Ring vaccination with rVSV-ZEBOV under expanded access in response to an outbreak of Ebola virus disease in Guinea, 2016: an operational and vaccine safety report. *Lancet* 2017; 17:1276–1284.
151. Henao-Restrepo AM, Camacho A, Longini IM et al. Efficacy and effectiveness of an rVSV-vectored vaccine in preventing Ebola virus disease: final results from the Guinea ring vaccination, open-label, cluster-randomised trial (Ebola Ça Suffit!). *Lancet* 2017; 389(10068): 505–518.
152. World Health Organization. Categorization and prioritization of drugs for consideration for testing or use in patients infected with Ebola. Jan. 19, 2015. www.who.int/medicines/ebola-treatment/cat_prioritization_drugs_testing/en/
153. Ethical considerations for use of unregistered interventions for Ebola viral disease. Report of an advisory panel to WHO. http://apps.who.int/iris/bitstream/10665/130997/1/WHO_HIS_KER_GHE_14.1_eng.pdf?ua=1
154. Maganga GD, Kapetshi J, Berthet N et al. Ebola virus disease in the Democratic Republic of Congo. *New Engl J Med* 2014; 371(22):2083–2091.
155. Green A. Ebola outbreak in the DR Congo. *Lancet* 2017; 389:2092–2093.
156. WHO Bulletin. WHO declares an end to the Ebola outbreak in the Democratic Republic of the Congo. Brazzaville/Kinshasa, 2 July 2017. www.who.int/emergencies/ebola-DRC-2017/en/
157. Nsio J, Kapetshi J, Makiala S et al. 2017 outbreak of Ebola virus disease in northern Democratic Republic of Congo. *J Inf Dis* 2019.
158. Ebola situation reports – World Health Organization www.who.int/ebola/situation-reports/drc-2018/en/
159. WHO/ Ebola virus disease – Democratic Republic of the Congo. www.who.int/csr/don/24-august-2018-ebola-drc/en/
160. Clinical Trial of Investigational Ebola Treatments Begins in the Democratic Republic of the Congo. November 27, 2018 www.nih.gov/.../clinical-trial-investigational-ebola-treatments-begins-democratic-republic-congo
161. Kupferschmidt K. Finally, some good news about Ebola: Two new treatments dramatically lower the death rate in a trial. *Sci Mag*. August 12, 2019.
162. WHO recommends use of two antibody drugs against Ebola. *Reuters*. August 19, 2022, 8:26 AM EDT. www.reuters.com/business/healthcare-pharmaceuticals/who-recommends-use-two-antibody-drugs-against-ebola-2022-08-19/
163. Ebola health update – DRC, 2019 – World Health Organization www.who.int › emergencies › diseases › ebola › drc-2019
164. Kolata G. A Cure for Ebola? – *The New York Times*. August 12, 2019. www.nytimes.com › 2019/08/12 › health › ebola-outbreak-cure
165. Diallo MSK, Rabilloud M, Ayouba A et al. Prevalence of infection among asymptomatic and pauci-symptomatic contact persons exposed to Ebola virus in Guinea: a retrospective, cross-sectional observational study. *Lancet Inf Dis* 2019; Published February 11, 2019. doi: https://doi.org/10.1016/S1473-3099(18)30649-2

Suggested Reading

David Quammen. *Ebola: The Natural and Human History of a Deadly Virus.* W. W. Norton & Company. New York. 2014.

Debora Diniz. *Zika. From the Brazilian Backlands to Global Threat.* Diane G Whitty, Translator. Zed Books. London. 2017.

Dickson Despommier. *West Nile Story.* Robert J Demarest Illustrator. Apple Trees Productions Llc. New York. 2001.

Donald G. McNeil Jr. *Zika: The Emerging Epidemic.* W. W. Norton & Company. New York. 2016.

Laurie Garrett. *Ebola: Story of an Outbreak.* Hachette Books. New York. 2014.

Richard Preston. *Crisis in the Red Zone: The Story of the Deadliest Ebola Outbreak in History and of the Outbreaks to Come.* Random House. New York. 2019.

Thomas Abraham. *Twenty-First Century Plague: The Story of SARS.* Johns Hopkins University Press. Baltimore, MD. 2004.

8

AND NOW AS PROMISED

The SARS-CoV-2/COVID-19 Pandemic

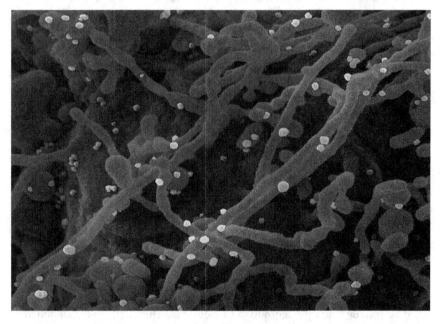

FIGURE 8.1 Scanning electron microscope image shows SARS–CoV–2 virions emerging from the surface of cells cultured in the lab.

Source: Photo courtesy of NIAID.US.gov

DOI: 10.4324/9781003427667-8

WE ARE ALL IN THIS TOGETHER: #wewantfreedomofspeech

Unlike all the other chapters in this book, this introductory essay is not a personal story. It is instead the story of a brave young Chinese physician named Li Wenliang, the nature of life in China's repressive and highly censored society, and the power of social media. In late December 2019, Doctor Li, a young ophthalmologist in Wuhan, China noticed that seven patients in his hospital quarantined with pneumonia had cultured positive for a virus resembling SARS-CoV. On December 30, 2019, he messaged his medical school alumni group on WeChat, a popular Chinese messaging app, telling them about the pneumonia patients and suggesting they consider wearing protective equipment at work to prevent infection. In China, memories of the 2003 SARS pandemic are powerful, as are memories of the Chinese government's delay in reporting the original outbreak that allowed global spread of the SARS virus. Li was among the first of a small group of doctors who tried to get the word out about the potential of a new SARS-like outbreak. Within hours, the message had gone viral with Li's name attached.[1]

On the same day in December that Li messaged his colleagues, the Wuhan Municipal Health Commission notified the World Health Association (WHO) about the cluster of cases and issued an emergency notice to the city's medical institutions, reporting that a series of patients from Wuhan, many of whom had contact with a local wet market, the Huanan Seafood and Wild Life Market, had a "pneumonia of unknown cause." However, the message also warned that "… no organizations or individuals were allowed to release any information to the public without authorization." Stunningly, while the global alarm had been officially raised, local communication measures in Wuhan were forbidden.

Li was called to a local police station on January 3, 2020 and reprimanded for "spreading rumors online" and acting illegally to "severely disrupt the social order" because of his message in the chat group. He was forced to sign a formal apology and agree to not discuss the disease further.[2] Frightened for himself and for his young family, he was grateful to be allowed to return home.[1] But in the days that followed, what had started as a local outbreak exploded, with dramatic daily increases in cases, including cases in health care providers indicating the new disease was already spreading from person to person. By January 7, a group of Chinese researchers definitively identified the cause of the atypical pneumonia as a coronavirus similar to the 2003 SARS-CoV. Still, no local measures were taken to provide information or to prevent the spread of infection.

It is dangerous to oppose the government of China. All communication channels are closely monitored and any hint of information that differs from the party line can result in arrest and imprisonment. As an example, you might remember that the original SARS outbreak began in November 2002 when multiple inhabitants of the Chinese province of Guangdong on the coast of the South China Sea developed a severe pneumonia. It was not until three long months later that the Chinese Ministry of Health notified the World Health Organization that 305 cases of this acute respiratory illness of unknown etiology had occurred between November 16, 2002 and February 9, 2003. Chinese doctors knew this was extreme under-reporting of the number of cases, the severity of the illness and its spread within China and that this misinformation deliberately minimized the importance of the outbreak and therefore, the global response. Chinese authorities continued to cover up the extent and severity of the disease for months before another whistleblowing doctor, Jiang Yanyong, exposed the crisis through Western media, galvanizing the global response that ended the SARS pandemic.[2] At the time, he was held in military custody for 45 days before international pressure led to his release. More recently Jiang, now 88, has had his contacts with the outside world cut off and movements restricted after he asked the authorities to reassess the 1989 Tiananmen pro-democracy movement. He is now under de facto house arrest. Yes, it is dangerous to oppose the government of China.[3]

Li returned to work but he himself was infected with the new coronavirus when he operated on a patient who did not know she was infected. On January 10, he started to feel sick, and his symptoms progressively worsened over the next 3 weeks. Hospitalized with fever and cough, too short of breath to speak, he decided to fight the government, going public online with details of how he had been silenced in the name of stability. He shared documents online and carried out interviews via text message, including photographs showing him wearing an oxygen mask and holding his ID badge to verify the authenticity of his posts.[4] His messages allowed reporters to follow the dangerous story of official suppression of the facts at a time when containment of the dangerous, new virus might have been most possible.[5]

Almost overnight, the 34-year-old doctor became a household name in China, identified by millions of people as the voice of truth in the escalating coronavirus crisis. His brave stance, and his illness, were particularly poignant because he was the father of a four-year-old and his wife was pregnant with their second child. As public anger about the cover-up spread, local authorities did eventually apologize to him and to the seven other physicians investigated for spreading rumors; the central government did finally acknowledge that the crisis had been mishandled in its early days. But the shift to implementation of aggressive local containment measures came too late for the thousands who had already been infected, including Li himself. On a social media post on January 30, he confirmed he was one of thousands of 2019-nCoV infected patients.

Late on Thursday, February 6, state-controlled media outlets reported that Li had died, triggering an enormous public outpouring of grief. Public assemblies are banned in China, and many overseas Chinese still fear ramifications from attending public events but messages and flowers were left outside the hospital where he died, and mourning ceremonies and vigils were held all over China and in many sites in North America. On social media, the news was met with a flood of posts expressing grief and anger. An hour after the announcement of Li's death, the trending topic "Wuhan government owes Dr. Li Wenliang an apology" appeared on the social platform Weibo before it was censored. The Chinese ambassador to Washington, Cui Tiankai, said on Twitter, a service the ruling party's internet censorship also blocks the public from seeing, "Really saddened by the death of Dr. Li Wenliang. He was a very devoted doctor. We are so grateful to him for what he has done in our joint efforts fighting against #2019nCoV." In a remarkable act of resistance, millions of Chinese posted: #WeWantFreedomOfSpeech. The government in Beijing responded by censoring every communication.[5]

The massive public response was an indication of how powerfully Li's story had resonated. In death, Dr. Li Wenliang was still the voice of truth, laying bare the facts of the Communist Party's efforts to suppress information about the outbreak and the reality that authorities prioritized maintaining the appearance of control over the health and safety of their people. With his words, Li made recognition of the divide between propaganda and reality, between suppression and truth, inescapable. While state TV broadcasts continued a steady stream of praise for the party's leadership, Chinese journalists with the help of online activists like Li exposed the government's systematic efforts to hide the disease outbreak. In a system designed to crush dissent, he dared to resist, dared to speak truth to power. While critically ill himself, he still exposed the true gravity of the 2019-nCoV outbreak, the incompetence of the government, and the need for aggressive defense. There is no greater hero.

And Now as Promised: The SARS-CoV-2/COVID-19 Pandemic

The First Six Months: December 2019–June 2020

On December 1, 2019 when the first reported case appeared in Wuhan, China, it might have seemed inconsequential, just one patient with a community-acquired pneumonia of unknown cause. But Wuhan in Hubei province is a major commerce and transportation hub with a population of more than 11 million people. On an average day, 30,000 people fly out of the city, and many more use bullet trains from three railway stations. Disease spread was inevitable. By December 31, there were 26 more hospitalized cases with a similar clinical picture and an unknown number who had not come to medical attention. By January 11, hospitalized cases had increased to 41 and review of the clinical features of this group revealed a history of fever, cough and fatigue that accelerated over several days to shortness of breath in predominantly middle-aged men.[6] In all patients, chest imaging was abnormal with x-ray findings of bilateral patchy pneumonia and/or CT scans showing distal, ground glass, lobular and subsegmental infiltrates. Within a week, more than half the group had severe breathing difficulty requiring some kind of respiratory support, one third needed ICU care and six had died.[6] Importantly, two-thirds of these patients had worked or shopped at a local fish and wild animal market, the Huanan Seafood Wholesale Market suggesting a possible origin for the virus. Of major concern is timing: if the first human illness appeared on December 1, infection must have occurred earlier, because of the incubation time – still undefined – between infection and symptoms. If so, the virus could have been spreading silently between people well before the cluster of cases was recognized in late December. On the same date, person-to-person transmission of the virus – already strongly suspected because of multiple cases of infection in hospital workers – was definitively confirmed by report of a cluster of five 2019-nCoV cases in a family who had travelled to Wuhan where only two family members visited a hospitalized relative.[7]

Against this alarming clinical backdrop, researchers with the China Center for Disease Control investigating the cause of infection in three of these adults with pneumonia of unknown etiology definitively identified a novel corona-virus (Figure 8.1) from broncho-alveolar lavage specimens just one week later, using whole-genome sequencing, direct polymerase chain reaction (PCR), and culture. Phylogenetic analysis showed that the previously unknown virus fell into the beta-coronavirus genus, which besides SARS-CoV and MERS-CoV, also includes a bat SARS-like coronavirus.[8,9] Based on the WHO temporary naming system, this new virus was called 2019-nCoV; as of 2/11/2020, it became SARS-CoV-2. The Huanan Market was closed on December 31 and the China Center for Disease Control reported on January 26 that of 585 collected samples, 33 tested positive for the virus. The 33 samples came from 22 stalls and a garbage vehicle in the market, most in the area where wild animals were traded.[10]

A focus on these dates in January is important because of the Chinese New Year festival which begins with the first new moon of the lunar calendar and ends on the first full moon, 15 days later; in 2020, the first day fell on January 25 and the festival lasted until February 8. This is the most important holiday of the year in China and involves travel for millions of people reuniting with their families. Travel by rail is the preferred mode of transportation with almost all Chinese people on holiday, and trains are densely packed with tightly confined families. I can think of no better environment for viral transmission.

On December 31, the Wuhan Municipal Health Commission announced the outbreak and alerted the World Health Organization (WHO) but in the two weeks that followed, local Wuhan health authorities remained the only official source in China for updates on the outbreak, reporting no new information despite the identification of the pathogen as a new coronavirus very similar to SARS-CoV by Chinese scientists on January 7. An expert team from the Chinese Ministry of Health visited Wuhan in early January, reporting that there was *no* person-to-person transmission and that the outbreak was well controlled, after the closing of the Huanan market: both statements were untrue. For a week, no new confirmed cases were announced and local health authorities continued to maintain there was "no obvious evidence for human to human transmission" and "no infection of healthcare workers" despite multiple reports to the contrary by medical professionals on social media; the outbreak was represented as "preventable and controllable."[1] At this critical turning point, the Chinese authorities put secrecy and order ahead of openly confronting the growing crisis and risking public alarm or political embarrassment – publicly portraying the outbreak as a well-managed situation, completely under control.

For the next two weeks, local health officials continued to assure the public that there were no new cases in Wuhan and no cases at all outside the city. This inaccurate portrayal of the outbreak allowed the virus to spread widely in Wuhan, to other cities in China and to the world. It was not until definite person-to-person transmission was finally confirmed with 2019-nCoV cases reported outside of China in Thailand and Japan, as well as in Chinese patients who had had no exposure to the Huanan market that the Minister of Health sent a second expert group to Wuhan on January 19.

This was accompanied by what was reported as a sudden jump in infections. Until January 17, only 41 cases of the virus had been reported. By January 20, that number had increased to 198. After the central government took over management on January 20, President Xi Jinping ordered "resolute efforts to curb the spread" of the coronavirus and explicitly stressed the need for the timely release of information – this was the first time Xi had publicly acknowledged the outbreak. Later that evening, a government-appointed respiratory expert, known for fighting SARS 17 years ago, declared on state TV that the new coronavirus was transmissible from person to person. Three days later, on January 23, authorities abruptly placed a complete lockdown on Wuhan, eliminating all forms of transportation and effectively sealing off the city. Other cities across Hubei Province rapidly instituted their own travel restrictions, putting much of the province of 59 million people in a de facto lockdown. By then, an estimated five million people had already left the city for the Lunar New Year holiday. And by January 24 when the information on the original 41 patients was published worldwide with the Wuhan lockdown in place, the number of confirmed 2019-nCoV infections in Wuhan had increased dramatically to 835 with 25 deaths.[11] Early suppression of knowledge about the outbreak squandered a critical window of opportunity when an informed Wuhan populace could have potentially changed its behavior to limit the virus's spread.

During the next two weeks, the epidemic grew exponentially with the number of cases doubling approximately every seven and a half days. The virus spread rapidly throughout and beyond China, exacerbated by Lunar New Year travel. By January 25, confirmed cases in mainland China stood at 2016 but there were already multiple cases in Thailand, Hong Kong, Macau, Australia, Malaysia, Singapore, France, Japan, South Korea, Taiwan, the United States, Vietnam, Nepal and Sweden; all cases outside of China were linked to travel to the Wuhan area or contact with travelers from Wuhan. While the Communist Party struggled to control spread of the virus throughout China, the majority of adjoining countries including Mongolia, Nepal, North Korea, Russia, Tajikistan and Vietnam, ordered immediate, partial closure of their borders with China and many international airlines reduced or suspended service to China.

The Virus

With explosive growth in cases in China, scientists there and around the world attempted to characterize the state of knowledge of the virus and the disease at that critical moment in time. Identification of the causative virus as a coronavirus provided important basic information very early in the epidemic[8,9] As a group, coronaviruses (CoV) are large, enveloped, positive-strand RNA viruses divided into four genera: alpha, beta, delta, and gamma; alpha and beta CoVs are known to infect humans. Four CoVs are endemic globally and cause 10–30% of mild upper respiratory tract infections in adults. However, as described in Chapter 7, two new well-known beta-CoVs – SARS-CoV and Middle East Respiratory Syndrome CoV (MERS-CoV) – have already caused epidemics of severe respiratory illness with high mortality just in the last 20 years. Coronaviruses are ecologically diverse with the greatest variety seen in bats, the suggested but unproven reservoir for these viruses.

The 2019-nCoV virus – officially now known as SARS-CoV-2 – is physically large among viruses, measuring 125 nanometers in diameter, and covered with spiky glycoprotein projections, critical for binding to host cell receptors as shown in Figure 8.2. Genetic analysis of samples from nine newly diagnosed patients in Hunan showed 99.98% sequence identity, indicating a very recent emergence of the virus in humans.[12] 2019-nCoV/SARS-CoV-2 is genetically distinct from SARS and MERS, although the spike protein of the new virus is similar to the SARS surface spike. When the 2019-nCoV sequence is compared to a library of viruses, the most closely related are two SARS-like bat viruses leading to the theory that this novel virus is also of bat origin with a currently unknown animal species potentially acting as an intermediate host between bats and humans.[12]

We know that the original SARS-CoV infects cells lining the respiratory tract using angiotensin converting enzyme 2 as a receptor; with the noted phylogenetic similarities between 2019-nCoV/SARS-CoV-2 and the original SARS-CoV on whole-genome sequencing studies, it was postulated and then shown that the novel coronavirus also uses the same host cell receptors in the nose and throat. An important CoV factor is their ability to expand their genetic diversity through ongoing mutation and recombination events. As with SARS, many scientists suspect that an unknown animal infected by bats with 2019-nCoV spread the virus to humans at the market in Wuhan where many of the early cases

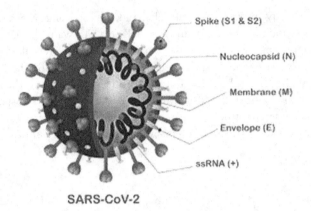

SARS-CoV-2

FIGURE 8.2 Computer rendering of the surface of SARS–CoV–2, the coronavirus strain that causes COVID–19.

Source: cdc.gov

were documented. With SARS, the intermediate host is thought to have been a palm civet. With SARS-CoV-2, the chief suspect has been the pangolin, a small ant-eating creature and the world's only scaled mammal; pangolins are prized in Asia as food and medicine. Pangolins were being sold in the now infamous seafood and wild animal market in Wuhan, linked to early cases of COVID19. The genome sequence of the novel coronavirus strain derived from pangolins was 89 per cent identical to that from infected people, China's official Xinhua news agency reported, suggesting that pangolins could potentially be the intermediate host between bats and humans.[13] Subsequently, analysis of genetic samples from the Huanan market which were uploaded to an international database suggested raccoon dogs could also have been the intermediate host.[14]

The Disease: Characteristics of Infection with SARS-CoV-2

Crucial findings with any new disease include the range of clinical severity, the extent of transmission and rates of infection – all remained unknown at this stage despite more than 71,000 cases of COVID-19 and 1600 deaths, as of February 17, 2020. At the time, the virus was thought to spread both directly – through physical transfer between people through contact with oral or nasal droplet secretions – and indirectly, through contact with droplets deposited on nearby surfaces when an infected person coughed or sneezed. On its own, SARS-CoV-2 was thought to be too big to stay suspended in the air for any significant length of time or to travel more than a few feet, so airborne transmission was not thought to be significant. However, as with SARS, aerosolized droplets generated during medical procedures were known to infect health care providers. Hand hygiene for both infected and uninfected individuals and personal protective barriers – gowns, gloves, masks and goggles – reduce droplet transmission. Estimates of the basic reproduction number or R_0 for the virus – the number of additional persons one case infects over the course of their illness in a non-immune population – ranged from 2.2 to 3.6 but there were estimates as high as 6.5.[15] (An R_0 of less than 1 indicates very low transmission potential; the higher the R_0, the greater the potential for sustained transmission. As an example, the R_0 for measles is 18!)

According to the WHO, most coronavirus cases reported to that date had a mild illness; in clinical series, 82% were mild, 15% severe and 3% critical.[16] Published details from three series of laboratory-confirmed, hospitalized cases in Wuhan, China gave us preliminary epidemiologic characteristics and transmission dynamics.[17–19] The median age of patients was 55–59 years with no cases in children below 15 years of age; in all early series, the preponderance of patients were male. Patients with earlier onset of symptoms were slightly younger, more likely to be male, and much more likely to report exposure to the Huanan Seafood Wholesale Market. In later cases, the majority of patients had no exposure to the market, supporting the increasingly important role of human-to-human transmission. The proportion of cases acquired in hospital by patients or hospital personnel increased over time, to 40% in one series. Based on exposure history and onset of symptoms, the mean incubation period was 5.2 days, with the 95th percentile of the distribution at 12.5 days. This preliminary estimate supported a 14-day medical observation/quarantine period for exposed persons. The most common clinical symptoms were fever, present in 80% of patients, followed by cough in 70%, shortness of breath in 30% and muscle ache in 10%. Bilateral pneumonia was present in 75% of these hospitalized patients on chest x-ray and/ or CT scan with multiple areas of consolidation and ground-glass opacifications. The median time from first symptom to shortness of breath was 5 days and to hospital admission was 7 days; ~60% of this hospitalized group developed acute respiratory distress syndrome (ARDS) at a median of 8 days after the first symptom. Mortality in severely ill patients ranged from 4–17%, predominantly in older patients, with deaths due to progressive respiratory and multi-organ failure. Overall, mortality was estimated at ~2%.

The outbreak of the 2019 novel coronavirus (SARS-CoV-2) is another example of the importance of infections at the animal-human interface, and the concerns that arise from the emergence of a newly identified organism as it spreads through human populations and across national and international borders. Yet another epidemic of human disease caused by a virus that is thought to live in bats underscores the perpetual challenge of emerging infectious diseases and the importance of ongoing, sustained global preparedness. Although it felt like a barn door exercise, China's decision to eliminate the zoonotic source of viruses like these by banning wild game markets in China will potentially be important for prevention of future zoonotic events.

Major questions remained: What was the course in non-hospitalized but sick patients and in patients with mild symptoms? What proportion of infected individuals had no symptoms at all? [Remember that with other viruses like polio, as many as 95% of infected individuals have no identifiable symptoms but are still contagious and infectious (Chapter 5)] What is the duration of viral replication and shedding in patients with varying degrees of illness severity? How long is viral survival on surfaces? What is the susceptibility, severity and infectivity in children? What is the true infection rate of the virus? Does transmission take place before the onset of symptoms as suggested by a single case report?[12] When are infected people most contagious? Right after they contract the virus? Only after symptoms begin? Or, do they become increasingly contagious over time? How long does the contagious stage last? Finally, what are virus-specific humoral and cellular immune responses in mild, moderate and severe cases of COVID-19? The answers to these questions were critically important for development of the most effective epidemic response.

Diagnosis

Identification and genetic analysis of 2019-nCoV allowed early development of three diagnostic techniques: isolation of the virus itself; positive RT-PCR assays; or identification of a genetic sequence that matches SARS-CoV-2. In practice, RT-PCR assays have been the method of choice. Beginning in January, the WHO published laboratory guidance for detection of the novel coronavirus including advice on biosafety, patient sampling, and pathogen detection and characterization. Within days of obtaining the sequence data, PCR assays were developed for clinical diagnostic use by multiple academic and public-sector groups, including the China Center for Disease Control.[20] These publicly available assays targeted areas of the genome for detection of sequences specific for 2019-nCoV/SARS-CoV-2.

Globally, the WHO established a network of specialized referral laboratories with expertise in the molecular detection of coronaviruses to serve as support for national labs performing diagnostic tests in their own countries. WHO also worked to ensure global test availability, sending 250,000 coronavirus tests to more than 70 laboratories around the world, as well as 500,000 masks, 350,000 pairs of gloves, 40,000 respirators, and nearly 18,000 isolation gowns to 24 countries. Early in the outbreak, only two labs in Africa – one in Senegal and one in South Africa – could test samples. The WHO goal was for 29 countries in Africa to have established diagnostic testing capacity.[15]

China appeared to be making major efforts to address rapid diagnosis.[21,22] A commercial nucleic acid reagent test kit and a sequencing system for the virus had been developed which could reportedly generate test results in 30 minutes. The complete kit was expected to speed up the diagnostic process and expand the supply capacity of virus detection products. Reports of diagnostic capacity in China varied widely and verification of these capabilities was unavailable.

By contrast with this organized plan, the situation on the ground in China appeared chaotic with reports of long lines of masked citizens awaiting testing.[22] From multiple online sources, test kits and labs were in short supply. As described further in the section on response to the outbreak, there had been major delays in diagnostic screening because of test kit/lab shortages and the overwhelming volume of individuals seeking care.

In the United States, the CDC also developed a laboratory test kit – the Real-Time Reverse Transcriptase RT-PCR Diagnostic Panel for 2019-nCoV/ SARS-CoV-2 testing. The test was intended for upper and lower respiratory specimens from individuals who met criteria for COVID-19 and had been FDA-approved for emergency use. However, within days of its release to pre-selected labs across the country, performance problems were identified and the test kits were recalled. In addition, at that time and going forward, the CDC guidelines allowed SARS-CoV-2 testing *only* in individuals who had been potentially exposed to the virus by travel to Wuhan, China or who had close contact with recent Chinese travelers. Testing could *only* be done with the CDC test kit and the tests had to be sent to the CDC which had a minimal turnaround time of 48 hours. This unfortunate approach definitively delayed identification of COVID-19 cases in the USA and led to a serious and prolonged misunderstanding of the status of the outbreak. The situation remained in place until February 28, 2020 and proved to be a major failure of the US public health response to the outbreak.[23]

Treatment

There were as yet no specific treatments for SARS-CoV-2 infection. Supportive care was being maximized for patients with severe lung involvement, including the use of lung bypass with heart-lung machines to rest the lungs and allow recovery when mechanical ventilation was no longer effective. In case series, doctors were trying a variety of anti-viral medications like the anti-influenza drug, oseltamivir (Tamiflu) as well as standard antibiotics when a patient's clinical condition deteriorated but no consistent results were available.[17–19]

There were reportedly 34 interventional studies in China recruiting subjects to investigate multiple aspects of care. As one example, a randomized, controlled trial to investigate the safety and efficacy of the investigational antiviral compound remdesivir was underway with the collaboration of the developer, Gilead Sciences, and the US Food and Drug Administration, the CDC, China's Center for Disease Control and Prevention, and the WHO.[24] Remdesivir is a nucleotide analogue prodrug initially developed as a treatment for Ebola and Marburg virus infections. In animal models, the drug had shown activity against other coronaviruses like SARS. A phase I study demonstrated the safety, tolerability and pharmacokinetics of remdesivir in healthy volunteers and a randomized, double-blind, placebo-controlled study to evaluate the efficacy and safety of remdesivir in hospitalized adult patients with mild and moderate 2019-nCoV infections began in China on February 3, 2020. Results were expected by April 2020. As of February 25, a parallel randomized, controlled trial of remdesivir began at the National Quarantine Unit at the University of Nebraska involving 13 people repatriated by the US State Department from the *Diamond Princess* cruise ship. The CDC reported that 11 people in the UNMC unit had confirmed SARS-CoV-2 infection and would participate in the trial.

Prevention/Vaccine Development

The WHO announced that the principal mode by which people are infected with SARS-CoV-2 was through exposure to respiratory droplets from the nose or mouth carrying infectious virus. For this reason, maintaining a distance of 6 feet between people was recommended. It was reportedly also possible for people to be infected through contact with contaminated surfaces or objects (fomites) so rigorous surface cleansing efforts and strict handwashing were recommended. There was a definitive statement that the virus was not airborne so masks were specifically not recommended.[25]

From the outset, development of effective vaccines was a priority.[26] On January 23, the Coalition for Epidemic Preparedness Innovations (CEPI) announced that it would give three companies a total of $12.5 million to develop SARS-CoV-2 vaccines. CEPI is a nonprofit organization formed in 2016 solely to support development of new vaccines against emerging infectious diseases.[27] Already available for potential evaluation in humans were three candidate vaccines for SARS-CoV and 5 for MERS-CoV. In response to CEPI's announcement, three different research proposals emerged, including one from the Vaccine Research Center at the U.S. National Institute of Allergy and Infectious Diseases (NIAID) working with the vaccine-maker Moderna. Based on the gene sequence of the virus reported by Chinese researchers, the company planned to utilize a messenger RNA platform developed after decades of research and previously shown to trigger an immune response in animals. Using this methodology, Moderna had already developed a vaccine for MERS-CoV but this had only been tested in animals. Incredibly, Moderna created a trial SARS-CoV-2 vaccine based on the mRNA platform just 42 days after the genetic sequence of the virus was described. The first batch had already been shipped to NIAID with phase I human testing planned as early as April 2020, evaluating safety and immune responses in small numbers of volunteers. In parallel to the human trials, researchers would test the vaccine's ability to protect an animal model intentionally exposed to the virus. Successful vaccines would then be tested in large human trials. The goal was a candidate vaccine ready for human tests in 16 weeks. This process can be accelerated in an active disease outbreak: if you recall, Ebola vaccine trials were initiated at the end of the 2014–2016 epidemic in West Africa with rapid validation of an effective vaccine used very effectively in subsequent Ebola outbreaks in the DRC.

In the United States, President Trump announced the creation of Operation Warp Speed on May 5, 2020, a public-private partnership to facilitate and accelerate the development, manufacturing and distribution of COVID-19 vaccines.[28] Funded at $10 billion initially from the CARES Act (Coronavirus Aid, Relief, and Economic Security), the program supported vaccine development by

Moderna and by AstraZeneca, Johnson & Johnson, Novavax, Merck and Sanofi/ GlaxoSmithKline. The goal was delivery of a vaccine for distribution by January 1, 2021.[28]

Epidemic Response: China

From December 2019, China was on the front line of a full-fledged war with SARS-CoV-2. According to the WHO, China had less than two physicians for every 10,000 residents, so response to this overwhelming epidemic was frenetic and desperate. By report, Hubei health care workers were exhausted and overwhelmed, with testing kits and personal protection items, such as face masks, hazmat suits, goggles and gloves, all in short supply. Hospitals and care providers without adequate protective gear and struggling with staff shortages were unable to respond to everyone seeking care.[29] In Wuhan, patients faced hours-long lines to receive any medical attention.[30]

Amid ongoing reports that people with symptoms of the virus were being denied admission to local hospitals in Wuhan because of limited beds and the requirement that all admissions had tested positive for the virus, the Chinese central government continued the lockdown on Wuhan and other cities in Hubei imposed on January 23, 2020, in an effort to quarantine the center of the outbreak.[31] All travel and transportation services connecting the city were blocked. In the following two weeks, all outdoor activities and gatherings were restricted, and public facilities were closed in most cities as well as in the countryside. The lockdown in Wuhan set the precedent for similar measures in other parts of China. Within hours, travel restrictions were also imposed on the nearby cities of Huanggang and Ezhou, and were eventually imposed on 15 other cities in Hubei, affecting a total of about 57 million people. As the days passed and COVID-19 numbers continued to increase, Hubei province enacted wartime measures, sealing off residential complexes and allowing only essential vehicles on the roads. Further restrictions followed: on February 2, 2020, Wenzhou, Zhejiang, implemented a seven-day lockdown in which only one person per household was allowed to exit the home, once every two days, and most highway exits were closed.

Subsequent lockdowns were introduced in other regions of China in response to localized outbreaks during the years that followed. Even if only a few COVID-19 cases were detected; neighborhoods and even entire cities were shut down for weeks to months at a time. Contract tracing apps were used by authorities to monitor people's movements to try to track the spread of the virus. Residents had to use the app to enter public places and were notified if they crossed paths with an infected person or traveled to a high-risk area, resulting in mandatory testing and/or isolation. The government carried out mass testing in places where COVID-19 had been reported. Even in places where there had been no new cases, residents often needed to have a recent negative COVID-19 test to be able to enter a business or public facility. Anyone who had been in contact with

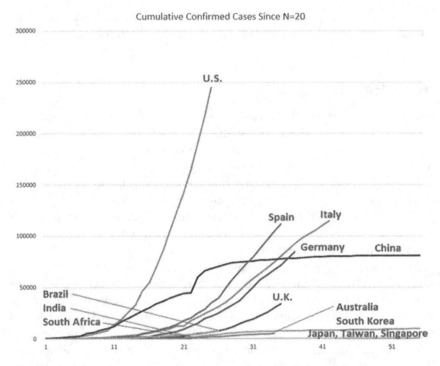

FIGURE 8.3 Total cases/country in the first 30 days after 500 confirmed cases. Note the abrupt flattening of the curve in China after lockdowns were imposed there in late January.

Source: Reprinted by permission from: *African J Reprod Health* 2020; 24(1): 14–21. doi:10.29063/ajrh2020/v24i1.2

an infected person was either put in government quarantine facilities or ordered to isolate. Even those who had only distant contact with a potentially infected person were made to isolate with isolation enforced by electronic seals attached to residents' doors. This combination of highly restrictive measures became known as China's Zero-COVID policy. Owing to these measures, the daily number of new cases in China plateaued and then decreased, as shown in Figure 8.3, while case numbers progressively increased in all other countries.

Epidemic Response: International

Led by the WHO, the international community were actively involved, beginning in the third week of January, 2020 when they convened an advisory Emergency Committee to review the situation in China. By their second meeting on January 30, person-to-person transmission had finally been definitively confirmed and there were increasing numbers of cases in China and in 20 other countries; the Committee concluded the outbreak had become a Public

Health Emergency of International Concern (PHEIC) on January 30, 2020. Following meeting in Beijing that week between China's President Xi Jinping and the WHO Director-General, China accepted the involvement of an international WHO-led collaborating team to work with Chinese counterparts on outbreak control. On February 5, WHO announced a $675 million 2019-nCoV/SARS-CoV-2 preparedness plan to provide international coordination and operational support, optimize readiness and response capacity, and accelerate research and innovation. The WHO organized a "Global Research and Innovation Forum" to mobilize international action in response to the 2019-nCoV emergency, on Feb. 11–12 in Geneva.[32] At the outset of the meeting, the WHO Director-General announced that the illness caused by 2019–nCoV now had an official name: COVID-19: the CO stands for corona, the VI for virus and the D for disease. In addition, the International Committee on Taxonomy of Viruses proposed a name for the novel coronavirus that causes COVID-19, SARS-CoV-2, formally recognizing this virus as a sister to the original SARS-CoV.[32]

Around the globe, nations developed their own initial responses to the epidemic. In the United States, President Trump announced the formation of the President's Coronavirus Task Force on January 29 and as of January 30, 2019-nCoV/SARS-CoV-2 was declared a public health emergency in the United States. The Department of Homeland Security issued instructions for quarantining U.S. citizens and permanent residents returning to the United States after stays in China, barring entry of other foreigners with recent travel to China and issuing a Level 3 advisory for travel to China. The State Department evacuated non-emergency US personnel and their family members and private US citizens from Wuhan beginning on February 11.[33]

Original responses by other countries were generally less aggressive but nearly all developed plans for dealing with the virus. The majority of adjoining countries including Mongolia, Nepal, North Korea, Russia, Tajikistan and Vietnam ordered partial closure of their borders with China. Hong Kong officials closed more than half the border crossing points to the mainland and shut down all high-speed rail and ferry service to China. In India, passengers coming from China were to be scanned at the airport and those who showed signs or symptoms of the virus quarantined. More than 20 countries including Canada, Singapore, Philippines, Uzbekisthan, Saudi Arabia, Indonesia and Thailand evacuated their own citizens. On February 7, the United Kingdom raised the risk to the public from low to moderate based on increasing person-to-person transmission and advised UK nationals to leave China where possible. On January 29, Russian president Vladimir Putin held a meeting on measures to counter the spread of coronavirus in Russia including requiring pool journalists to have their body temperature checked for signs of illness. On February 17, Russia temporarily suspended entry of Chinese citizens, banning them from traveling to Russia for employment, tourism or education. Taiwan banned all international cruise ships from docking and most international airlines reduced or suspended service to

China. International carriers, including British Airways, Air France, Lion Air and Lufthansa group announced they were canceling all flights to China.

Mid-February Assessment

While cases plateaued in China, the pandemic expanded rapidly all over the world. British researchers published a theoretical study predicting the spread of the virus over the next three months.[34] The researchers used international flight itineraries and mobile phone location data to plot the paths of almost 60,000 Wuhan residents who fled during the critical 2 weeks before the outbreak city was locked down. Their analysis estimated that 59,912 air passengers including 834 infected with 2019-nCoV flew from Wuhan to 382 cities outside of mainland China before the lockdown on January 23. The top 10 global destinations for Wuhan travelers were Thailand, Japan, Hong Kong, Taiwan, South Korea, the United States, Malaysia, Singapore, Vietnam and Australia but there were also multiple sites in Africa.

By February 14, the total number of cases in mainland China had exceeded 70,000 with more than 1500 fatalities officially reported by the Chinese National Health Commission from mainland China.[35,36] February14 turned out to be the peak of reported new cases in China and the beginning of a steady increase in cases reported from other countries, which had begun with confirmed cases in Japan, Thailand, and South Korea as early as January 20 (Figure 8.3). By far, the largest numbers of cases were in Asia. Outside China, 573 cases had been diagnosed in 26 other countries as of February 14 with three fatalities. There were reportedly only 15 cases in the United States and 9 in the United Kingdom, the latter all linked to the same individual, a British man who contracted the virus at a business conference meeting in Singapore from January 20–22.[37] More than 100 people took part in the conference, including at least one Chinese national from Hubei province – 12 cases of COVID-19 were linked to this meeting. The index British citizen was called a "super-spreader," a term coined during the SARS epidemic to describe someone who disproportionately infects a large number of people with a virus. The exact definition of a super-spreader varies from one outbreak to another, but this case demonstrated the potential for rapid and sustained person-to-person spread of SARS-CoV-2.

Another special cluster of COVID-19 cases outside of China was on the Diamond Princess cruise ship which had been quarantined in Yokohama, Japan since February 3.[38] The ship carried 3,700 passengers and crew and as of February 18, 542 passengers – a number which had been increasing every day – had tested positive for the virus, the largest known cluster of COVID-19 cases outside of China at that time. Concerned about exponential increases in new cases, the United States evacuated asymptomatic American passengers from the ship on February 16, to be quarantined for an additional 2 weeks in the United States. Among the hundreds of Americans evacuated from the ship, 14 tested positive for SARS-CoV-2 and had to be isolated on the flight home. Adding these patients to those already diagnosed meant there were theoretically 29 culture positive individuals in the United States at that time.

Emerging Epidemiologic, Virologic and Clinicopathologic Picture

A major epidemiologic review of more than 70,000 cases hospitalized with COVID-19 in China confirmed original findings: 87% of cases were 30–79 years of age with 3% over 80 years and only 2% less than 20 years of age.[39] There was a small male preponderance. Symptoms of fever and mild respiratory symptoms developed an average of 5–6 days after infection with a range from 1–14 days. Disease was mild in 81% with severe disease requiring at least some respiratory support in 14% and critical disease requiring intensive care in 5%. The median time from symptom onset to clinical recovery for mild cases was approximately 2 weeks compared with 3–6 weeks for patients with severe or critical disease. Overall, the case fatality rate was 2.3% but it increased dramatically with age, to 8% in patients aged 70–79 years and 14.8% in patients over 80 years. Among those with clinically critical disease, the mortality rate was 49%.

Information on viral dynamics in infected patients emerged from serial findings in 82 Sars-CoV-2-infected individuals.[40] Viral loads in throat swab and sputum samples peaked at ~5–6 days after symptom onset. Sputum samples generally showed higher viral loads than throat swab samples. Viral load was highest early after symptom onset but in a single patient who died, viral load was persistently very high. Stool samples from a small subset of pts were weakly positive.

A major series of more than 1000 patients correlated chest CT scan and RT-PCR results.[41] On initial evaluation, 59% of patients had positive RT-PCR results but 88% had positive chest CT scans. In patients with positive RT-PCR results, the sensitivity of chest CT in suggesting COVID-19 was 97%. Initial CT findings were consistent with COVID-19 prior or parallel to the initial positive RT-PCR results in 60–93% of cases. These findings suggested that chest CT might have been considered as a primary tool for diagnosis of COVID-19 infection in epidemic areas, when RT-PCR results were delayed.

February 14–28, 2020

After February 14, the number of new cases in China steadily decreased while the number in sites all over the world – 50 different countries as of 2/28 – steadily increased as shown in the preceding Figure 8.3. By February 28, there had been a total of 84,124 cases with 2862 deaths – almost 79,000 of those were in China and 2700 deaths had occurred in Hubei. But on that day, China reported 327 new cases while South Korea with a total of 2337 cases – the largest number outside of China – reported 511 new cases. Half of these were related to an outbreak that started in a church, reflecting increasing recognition of the importance of person-to-person spread in close quarters.[42]

There were new and increasing numbers of cases in northern Italy, in Iran and in Japan. And there were cases in three different countries in Africa. In response to this escalating situation, the still-cautious WHO raised the Outbreak Risk Assessment Level to "Very High," just below designation as a global pandemic.

In early March, COVID-19 literally exploded in multiple sites all over the world. From February 21– March 22, Italy went from the discovery of its first official COVID-19 case to a government lockdown of the whole territory including closure of all non-essential business activities. The country was hit by a tidal wave of cases with an incessant stream of deaths. In a foreshadowing of outbreaks all over the world, emergency and hospital services were completely overwhelmed and faced shortages of personal protective equipment (PPE), hospital beds, ventilators, and personnel. Military trucks were needed to transport bodies to crematoriums in nearby towns. Literally tons of medical equipment and teams of physicians from all over Europe and Asia arrived to help with the catastrophic situation.[43]

Global COVID-19 cases reached 100,000 on March 7 and on March 11 the COVID-19 epidemic was declared a pandemic by the WHO.[44] COVID-19 had rapidly transformed from being a severe problem primarily confined to China, to a global health emergency.

The pattern of the Italian outbreak proved prophetic in countries all over Europe with a similar sudden and explosive rise in cases, particularly in Spain and Great Britain.[45] In response to a severe lockdown, new cases peaked in Spain on March 16 at 8271 and the death toll surpassed that of mainland China on March 25. By March 13, when the number of new cases exceeded those in all of China, Europe was declared the epicenter of the pandemic with cases doubling every two to four days. By March 31, more than one-third of humanity was under some form of lockdown with increasingly dire predictions for future infections and deaths. One evaluation based on computer modeling estimated that in the absence of interventions, COVID-19 would have resulted in 7.0 billion infections and 40 million deaths globally in 2020. Mitigation strategies focusing on shielding the elderly and slowing but not interrupting transmission could reduce this burden by half, saving 20 million lives, but even in this scenario, health systems in all countries would be overwhelmed.[46]

Meanwhile, in the United States, an early effort by the administration – a February 2 limited travel ban preventing entry of foreign nationals with recent travel to China – was followed by a month of inaction with almost no testing and consistent downplaying of any threat by then President Trump. It was then revealed that the CDC had been denying testing for SARS-CoV-2 despite a diagnosis of pneumonia of unknown etiology if a patient did not meet the defined travel/exposure criteria for testing. In other words, testing was not being performed for the very clinical symptoms that defined the original outbreak! As of February 23, the CDC had tested only 479 persons from 43 states for COVID-19 – by comparison, South Korea had already tested more than 78,000 people.[22,47] In response to media reports of this situation, the CDC finally released expanded criteria for testing on February 28 2020 to include patients with a "severe acute lower respiratory illness" requiring hospitalization and without an "alternative explanatory diagnosis" and "no identified source of exposure."[48,49]

That announcement came as the CDC rushed to distribute new SARS-CoV-2 testing kits to state and local health departments amid concerns the virus had already spread beyond individuals known to have recently traveled to a country affected by outbreaks.[49] Initial rollout of test kits had been compromised by problems with the original tests but on 2/29, the FDA announced an "accelerated policy … to achieve more rapid testing capacity in the United States," allowing academic hospital labs capable of performing high-quality testing to develop and begin using their own tests to detect COVID-19. Before then, hospital labs weren't sent test kits by the CDC and the FDA required an extensive review process even if the hospitals had internally validated their tests. Under the new policy, the FDA review would still be required, but labs would be able to start using their own diagnostics once they were internally validated.[49]

Absence of testing did not mean absence of disease – in only the first 3 days after the CDC liberalized testing criteria and with still only a limited number of test sites, the first community-acquired cases were confirmed, Washington state reported the first death in the USA from COVID-19, the first health care worker to be infected with the disease, and most worrying, the first known outbreak in a long-term care facility.[50] Community transmission had clearly already been established and US cases were on the rise. On March 4, confirmed case numbers suddenly jumped from only a handful to more than 100. Only one week later, there were almost 1300 cases and 50 deaths. Trump announced new restrictions on foreign travelers from 26 European countries and declared a state of national emergency on March 13.[51]

Led by state governors, shelter-in-place efforts were urgently introduced and by April 7 roughly 95% of all Americans were under some form of lockdown. The shutdowns were described as aiming at "flattening the curve" – i.e., decreasing the rate of new infections. This was desirable for two reasons. First, it would prevent the health care system from being overwhelmed because the peak number of beds occupied at any one time would be lower. Second, it allowed time to improve clinical care strategies and capacity and to evaluate therapeutics. Despite these efforts, case numbers and deaths continued to increase. By April 25, the USA had more than 905,000 confirmed coronavirus cases and 52,000 deaths, a mortality rate of 5.7%. With more cases and deaths than any other country in the world, the USA was the new epicenter of the pandemic.[51]

A significant proportion of US COVID-19 cases occurred in New York City (NYC), where early infections were acquired not from Chinese contacts but from travelers from Europe. Case numbers grew exponentially: on March 20, with 5683 confirmed cases in NYC, the governor issued statewide shelter-in-place restrictions but by March 25 – only 5 days later – over 17,800 cases had been confirmed.[52] Major efforts to expand health care facilities included creation of a field hospital in Central Park and use of US Navy ships offshore in NY

Harbor. Severe shortages of PPE occurred here as they had all over the world. The city's infection rate was five times higher than the rest of the country with one-third of total confirmed US cases. Explosive growth in cases and deaths continued until April 12 when both categories began to gradually but steadily decrease, followed by a progressive withdrawal of shelter-in-place restrictions. By June 15, the US total confirmed case number was 2.1 million with 116,000 deaths, the highest national total in the world; there had been 215,000 cases and 21,000 deaths in NYC alone.[47]

A tragic feature of the COVID-19 pandemic first emerged in the USA: the critical involvement of nursing homes. At least 10,000 US deaths took place at senior care facilities – an estimated 27% of all deaths nationwide. In at least six states, nursing home fatalities accounted for half of all COVID-19 deaths.[53] Ultimately, investigation by the WHO revealed coronavirus fatalities in Europe and in Canada could similarly be traced to nursing homes.

Looking Back :: Moving Forward: The First Six Months (January 1–June 30, 2020)

There are three essential requirements for a global pandemic to occur: emergence of a new agent that infects humans; little or no population immunity to that agent; and easy pathogen transmission from one person to another: SARS-CoV-2 has them all. The demonstrated transmissibility and infectivity exemplify the power of this newly-emerged pathogen. Still, it was hard to believe the speed with which the pandemic evolved – the first rumors about a new coronavirus outbreak had emerged only months before. The current numbers were staggering but because the outbreak was evolving in real time, we couldn't yet see the total picture of those infected. This meant that calculation of things like the fatality rate was impossible – although we probably had a reasonable handle on the number of people who had died, we still did not know the number with mild or no symptoms who no one knew were infected. An enormous hidden population like this was alarming but a multitude of survivors who had minimal or no symptoms would mean a multitude of individuals with immunity – and herd immunity like this could theoretically have meant a dwindling population of susceptible people and even ultimately, the end of the outbreak.

Unfortunately, even if case identification was perfect, experts warned that as asymptomatic or very mild cases occurred and strict isolation efforts decreased, a new wave of cases would develop in international sites where only isolated cases primarily linked to contact with China were originally present. In China, the vast majority of confirmed cases had moderate to severe symptoms; by contrast, confirmed infections in other countries had milder symptomatology. Based on a combination of these statistics, epidemiologists estimated that only one in 19 people infected with the virus was being tested and that the true number of infected people was more than 800,000 as of February 11.[54] And experts were definitely right about global disease spread – as of February 28, there were reported cases in 50 countries with spiraling numbers in multiple locations including South Korea, Japan, Italy and Iran,

China's stringent quarantine efforts did limit disease spread as confirmed by the WHO with a massive effort in a compliant population.[55] The possibility of effective public health interventions on this scale in other countries – especially, the United States – was almost zero. As predicted, with ongoing exportation of pre-symptomatic cases, local spread was occurring with self-perpetuating outbreaks developing all over the world. It was still remotely possible that some combination of quarantine and travel bans and viral decrease in response to increasing herd immunity and rising temperatures would first halt the outbreak and then kill off the virus, and the world would never see SARS-CoV-2 again. After all, that's what happened with the original SARS in 2003. At that moment with the epidemic evolving all around us, it seemed much more likely that we were experiencing a true global pandemic, an expanding outbreak whose ultimate scope and duration were unknown. We were at a critical tipping point with the progressive increase in involved countries and independent self-sustaining person-to-person spread established in multiple sites around the globe, including many major population and transportation centers. To this time, the majority of cases had occurred in the global north in sites with well-developed health infrastructure – reports of cases in Africa and South America suggested a much more difficult situation for public health interventions in the future.

The Virus and the Disease

Early reports from China proved accurate in describing the basics of SARS-CoV-2 and the characteristics of COVID-19 but, with time, emerging research illustrated the extremely efficient spread of this virus. Reports of global superspreading events demonstrated significantly increased infectious risk associated with prolonged periods in crowded, indoor spaces. The importance of infection by asymptomatic or pre-symptomatic individuals was confirmed: the CDC estimated this pattern of spread to be responsible for at least 35% of infections. These combined findings led to the recommendations that the general public continue to maintain a physical distance of 6 feet and that the size of social gatherings be limited – both efforts to limit person-to-person droplet spread.

Original series from Wuhan accurately described a progressive respiratory illness. Subsequent reports during global spread revealed the important involvement of vascular injury and symptomatic hypercoagulation, with clots in as many as 30% of patients with severe COVID-19.[56,57]

Global outbreaks confirmed the dramatic increase with older age in disease severity and mortality in every setting, as shown for the US population in Figure 8.4.[58]

In China, the major disease co-morbidities aside from increasing age were related to pulmonary problems; by contrast, the most common comorbidities in

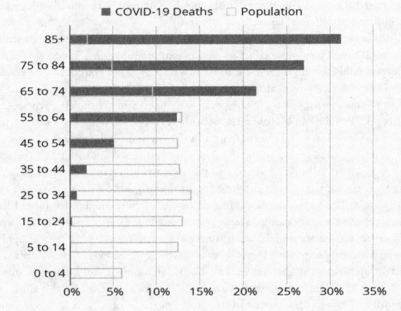

* COVID deaths as of Dec. 2, 2020; population estimates as of 2019
Sources: CDC, U.S. Census Bureau

 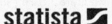

FIGURE 8.4 Distribution of COVID-19 deaths by age group in the USA.

Source: Created by Felix Richter. felix.richter@statista.com. Reprinted by permission from Statista.

subsequent sites were hypertension, obesity and diabetes. Modeling results from international data estimated that the average fatality rate ranged from 0.05% in Iceland to 1.3% in northern Italy. In individuals over 65, the fatality rate in the worst-case scenario was estimated to be ~3.2%. Many methodological issues complicated these calculations but the lower estimates were encouraging. Nonetheless, by June 15, 2020, at least 8 million cases of COVID-19 had been confirmed worldwide, with 435,000 deaths. [58]

New treatment options had emerged from active research protocols at sites all over the world, underway since the earliest days of the pandemic.

- A randomized trial of intravenous remdesivir in hospitalized adults showed those who received it had significantly faster recovery times than those who received placebo.[59] Mortality rates were also lower but results did not quite reach statistical significance.
- A triple combination of three anti-viral agents (interferon beta-1b, lopinavir–ritonavir, and ribavirin) in patients with mild-moderate COVID-19 disease

showed a significantly shorter median time to negative cultures for study patients.[60]

- Avifavir is a direct antiviral agent that disrupts coronavirus reproduction. The drug had been used in Japan since 2014 against severe forms of influenza and preliminary trials in COVID-19 patients have shown that it shortens recovery time.[61]
- In response to evidence of abnormal clotting, systemic anticoagulation (AC) showed early good results but further research was ongoing.[62]
- Low-dose steroid treatment with dexamethasone reduced deaths by one-third in ventilated patients and by one-fifth in patients requiring only oxygen.[63]

Results like these suggested that in the relative short term, a combination of agents would be defined to effectively address all COVID-19 presentations.

There had been impressive progress in vaccine development. Optimistic experts hoped that a viable vaccine against SARS-CoV-2 might even be ready by the end of 2020, with more than 150 potential vaccines under study.[64] For two candidate vaccines, phase II testing in humans had already begun and the beginning of large-scale, phase III testing of one of these based on messenger RNA technology was set for next month. Scientists at Oxford University had developed a vaccine from a weakened adenovirus combined with genes of the SARS-CoV-2 spike protein which triggered production of antibodies against the virus. A phase I/II clinical trial began in April in the UK to assess safety and efficacy in healthy volunteers and recruiting had begun for phase II/III trials.

The final trajectory of the SARS-CoV-2 pandemic was impossible to predict at that time. Despite signs of progress, the pandemic roared on with rising caseloads in Europe and multiple US states and dramatic increases in case numbers and deaths in South America and Africa. The highly politicized and flawed response to the pandemic in the USA and, to a lesser extent, in other countries emphasized that of all the knowledge that had emerged so far, perhaps recognition of the need for integration between science and policy, and the accurate communication of that information to the public was the most important revelation of all.

Evolution of a True Global Pandemic: July 1, 2020–December 31, 2023

The Disease: Epidemiology and Clinical Course

Over the summer of 2020, COVID-19 in China was reportedly effectively controlled but case numbers in Europe, the USA and other regions increased dramatically. As of August 11, 2020, 216 countries and regions from all six continents had reported more than 20 million cases of COVID-19, and more than 733,000 patients had died. High mortality occurred especially when health-care resources were overwhelmed. The United States remained the country with the largest number of confirmed cases and deaths. As cases and mortalities continued to increase, knowledge about the virus and the disease continued to emerge, as described below.

Prevalence of Asymptomatic/Mildly Symptomatic Infections

During the 2003 SARS-CoV pandemic, asymptomatic and clinically mild infections were rare and there were no reported instances of transmission before the onset of symptoms. This meant that disease spread could be – and was – contained by focusing on isolation of symptomatic individuals and quarantine of their contacts. The situation was strikingly different with SARS-CoV-2: within months of the first report of the disease, multiple reports suggested that SARS-CoV-2 was being transmitted from asymptomatic or pre-symptomatic individuals. When epidemiologic models were combined with serologic testing results, it was subsequently found that 40–45% of those infected with SARS-CoV-2 were asymptomatic.[65–67] In a decision analytic model of multiple scenarios of proportions of asymptomatic individuals with COVID-19 and infectious periods, transmission from asymptomatic individuals was again estimated to account for more than half of all infections.[68]

If a large proportion of infections resulted from virus transmission from asymptomatic individuals, new approaches to disease detection and prevention were clearly needed. This was critical information for efforts to contain the pandemic since effective control of spread meant population-based measures such as mask-wearing and strategic testing of people who are not ill would have to be added to hand hygiene and social distancing to slow the spread of COVID-19. Belated addition of these new measures was an unwelcome change and was met with considerable resistance in countries around the world. The transmission of SARS-CoV-2 induced by the large proportion of asymptomatic individuals remained a substantial challenge throughout the pandemic.[69]

Identification of Multisystem Inflammatory Syndrome in Children

From the outset of the disease outbreak in China and throughout global expansion, children were less frequently infected with SARS-CoV-2 and had less severe disease. According to the Centers for Disease Control, from March 2020 to June 2022 in the United States, there were 2.5 million cases of pediatric infection from SARS-COV-2 with a mortality rate of 0.05%, with deaths almost exclusively in children with identified, additional risk factors for COVID-19. However, in April 2020, a multisystem inflammatory syndrome associated with SARS-CoV-2 was observed among children in Europe and North America. The World Health Organization (WHO) named this syndrome Pediatric Multisystem Inflammatory Syndrome Temporarily associated with SARS-CoV-2 (PIMS-TS); the CDC used the term, Multisystem Inflammatory Syndrome in Children (MIS-C).[70–72] However named, the syndrome presented as an acute illness accompanied by a hyperinflammatory syndrome which could lead to shock and multiorgan failure.[73,74] The Centers for Disease Control and Prevention define MIS-C as a patient under 19 years of age with fever, evidence of inflammation, and clinically severe illness with involvement of multiple organ systems requiring hospitalization and no likely alternative diagnosis, along with recent SARS-CoV-2 infection or exposure to a confirmed or suspected COVID-19 case. The inflammatory picture can include rash, bilateral non-purulent conjunctivitis or mucocutaneous inflammation (oral/hands/feet) with hypotension or shock plus features of myocardial dysfunction, pericarditis, valvulitis, or coronary abnormalities (including ECHO findings or elevated Troponin/NT-pro-BNP), evidence of coagulopathy (by PT, PTT, elevated d-Dimers) and/or acute gastrointestinal problems (diarrhea, vomiting, or abdominal pain). Elevated markers of inflammation such as ESR, C-reactive protein, or procalcitonin are common and there is no other obvious microbial cause of inflammation, including bacterial sepsis, staphylococcal or streptococcal shock syndromes.

There is overlap of the clinical picture of MIS-C with Kawasaki Disease, also a pediatric multisystem inflammatory syndrome with a preponderance of male subjects, but children with MIS-C are significantly older and sicker, requiring ICU admission more frequently plus respiratory and circulatory support. Fortunately, MIS-C patients respond well to treatment with corticosteroids and intravenous gamma globulin and post-discharge sequelae are rare.[75]

As the COVID-19 pandemic evolved, the severity of MIS-C decreased with each subsequent SARS-CoV-2 variant.[76] As population immunity to SARS-CoV-2 increased, the incidence of MIS-C decreased dramatically and by early 2023, it had become a rare event.

Long Covid

Long COVID is a multisystem condition of mild to severe symptoms that follows acute SARS-CoV-2 infection. The World Health Organization defines long COVID as symptoms occurring 3 or more months after COVID-19 onset and lasting for at least 2 months.[77] Prevalence estimates vary but at least 65 million individuals around the world are said to have long COVID; prevalence is significantly lower for individuals who were not hospitalized with COVID and those who had been fully vaccinated. Long COVID is seen in people of all ages and acute phase disease severities, but the highest percentage of cases occur in females between 36 and 50 years of age.[78] A self-report symptom tracking study of more than 4000 individuals found rates of symptom persistence of 13.3% at 1 month after acute illness and 4.5% at 2 months.[79]

The symptoms and signs of long COVID involve every organ system with a wide variety of apparently overlapping pathologies. Apparent heart involvement is common with patient complaints of chest pain, palpitations and post-exertional fatigue. Central nervous system complaints like headache and brain fog are also common.[80] There is a significantly increased risk of a variety of cardiovascular problems in long-COVID patients, including heart failure, dysrhythmias and stroke, independent of the severity of initial COVID-19 presentation.[81]

Multiple causes of long COVID have been proposed including persisting reservoirs of SARS-CoV-2 in tissues; immune dysregulation; changes in the microbiota; autoimmune mechanisms and dysfunctional sympathetic/parasympathetic signaling. There is some consensus that long COVID is the result of a prolonged, low-grade inflammatory process. There is, as yet, no encompassing, evidence-based treatment for long COVID; individualized, symptom-specific management is recommended. An extended trial evaluating the use of metformin – a glucose-lowering drug used to treat people with type 2 diabetes – found that people with overweight or obesity who took metformin after testing positive for COVID were 41% less likely to develop long COVID in the following 10 months.[82] These promising results have yet to be evaluated in people without obesity.

Few people with long COVID demonstrate full recovery but the majority have decreasing symptoms over time. Ongoing research will hopefully begin to provide answers for this prevalent and troubling condition.[83]

The Virus: Emerging Information

Recognition of Airborne Transmission

Over time, it became clear that transmission occurred primarily by direct transmission from infected individuals rather than through fomites. Contact tracing studies in people with symptoms and case reports revealed a higher risk of direct transmission occurring in closed and crowded places and close-contact settings like weddings, bars and choir practices – all indoor settings characterized by loud vocalization and prolonged stays. Statistical analyses found that limitations on public gatherings and workplace closures were positively associated with lower levels of SARS-CoV-2 spread, corroborating the role of direct transmission in closed areas in facilitating the transmission of SARS-CoV-2. In response, the C.D.C. recommended that gatherings in the United States – including weddings, festivals, parades, concerts, sporting events and conferences – be limited to 50 people; at this time, there was no mention of masks.

By the fall of 2020, there was a major change in the description of the pattern of transmission of SARS-CoV-2 when scientists began to report overwhelming evidence that direct inhalation of airborne virus represented a major transmission route for the virus.[84] Previous research findings had shown that large droplets (larger than 100 μm) typically fell to the ground in seconds within 2 m of the source with potential infection only in individuals in that close range. Because of this limited travel range, physical distancing was thought to reduce exposure to the virus. By contrast, viruses in aerosols (smaller than 100 μm) could remain suspended in the air for seconds to hours, just like a cloud of smoke, and could travel away from their source and still be inhaled. Highly concentrated near an infected person, airborne viruses could infect people in close proximity but could also travel more than 2 m and accumulate in poorly ventilated indoor air, leading to the potential for superspreading events. Knowing that many individuals with COVID-19 have no symptoms means potential release of thousands of virus-laden aerosols with normal breathing and talking. Thus, virus transmission was shown to be far more likely to occur by inhaled aerosols than by droplet spray. This significant change in knowledge of virus transmission combined with the evidence of virus spread by asymptomatic individuals led to recommendations for mask-wearing beginning in the fall of 2020, plus recommendations for moving activities outdoors as much as possible and for improving indoor air using ventilation and filtration.[85]

Unfortunately, changing guidance for the public to include masking and avoidance of crowded indoor spaces was a difficult step for the WHO and for national public health organizations to take and for the public to accept, appearing as it did many months after an initial, apparently definitive, statement that masks were not necessary. Since the beginning of the pandemic, prevention efforts had focused on social distancing, handwashing and surface cleaning. It took the WHO until October 2020 to acknowledge that aerosols play a part in disease transmission in community settings and updated guidelines on mask use did not appear until December 2020.[86]

Even two years into the pandemic, there was confusion and ambiguity about the risks from airborne transmission and the benefits of mask wearing. This was especially true in the USA where then-President Trump stated publicly that he would not wear a mask. Governments around the world spent much of the pandemic focusing on hand washing and surface cleaning, ignoring the importance of ventilation and indoor masking. Changing messages undoubtedly contributed to resistance to masks and to other preventive efforts.

Virus Evolution: SARS-CoV-2 Variants of Concern over Time

Viral evolution is a constant so the emergence of new variants was anticipated and new mutations with a survival benefit like increased infectiousness or transmissibility would potentially become dominant. With SARS-CoV-2, the original Wuhan-Hu-1 reference genotype remained dominant globally until the fall of 2020, with disease pattern as previously described by reports from China plus inclusion of vascular and hypercoagulability findings.

Throughout the second half of 2020, SARS-CoV-2 cases ebbed and flowed, with waves peaking at different times in different countries and even in different regions in the same country. No new variant of concern (VOC) appeared until late summer of 2020 when the Alpha/B.1.1.7 strain appeared. Detected first in the United Kingdom, the Alpha variant spread rapidly and became the dominant strain globally into the fall of 2020. The survival advantage of the Alpha strain was increased transmissibility via enhanced binding to angiotensin-converting enzyme 2 (ACE2) receptor plus enhanced immune system evasion.[87,88] Symptoms of infection with the Alpha variant were similar to the original COVID-19 picture but with more complaints of muscle pain.

On October 5, 2020, a new variant was detected in India associated with a huge wave of SARS-CoV-2 infections. This emerging SARS-CoV-2 variant of concern – Delta/ B.1.6.17.2 – quickly displaced the Alpha variant and was associated with large increases in COVID-19 cases, first in India and then, globally. The Delta variant of concern had increased transmissibility, higher viral RNA loads in both unvaccinated and fully vaccinated individuals and decreased sensitivity to pre-existing host immune responses resulting in a massive wave of global infections.[89] Delta caused a slightly more severe form of illness with the addition of headache and anorexia to the original pattern, with somewhat higher hospitalization rates but no increase in mortality.[90] Delta and its descendants remained the dominant SARS-CoV-2 strain globally for more than a year until December of 2021.

Some variants caused important disease in the countries in which they emerged but did not become globally important. First documented in South Africa in May 2020, the Beta variant (B.1.351) had enhanced capacity to evade existing immune responses and was linked with increases in hospitalizations and deaths in South Africa. The Gamma variant (P.1) was first documented in Brazil in November 2020 and was estimated to be 1.7–2.4 times more transmissible than other local strains in that country. Evidence also suggests that the Gamma variant struggled to compete with other strains in the wild and it never emerged as a major problem outside of Brazil.[91]

Omicron/ B.1.1.529 emerged first in late November 2021 in South Africa and from the outset, this variant was associated with extremely rapid spread. Only one month after it was first detected, Omicron cases had already skyrocketed around the world, completely replacing the Delta variant and resulting in more confirmed SARS-CoV-2 infections than ever seen before. Omicron has multiple spike glycoprotein mutations and these have appeared as subvariants, first BA.1, BA 2-1-6, then BA.5, BQ.1, BQ.1.1, XBB.1.5 and now JN.1. The survival benefit of all the Omicron lineages is the ability to evade antibodies from both previous infection and vaccination plus the ability to use an alternative cell entry pathway. Omicron has caused by far the largest global spike in confirmed SARS-CoV-2 infections of all the known variants, including breakthroughs in vaccinated people and re-infections in those with previous, confirmed COVID-19. Omicron SARS-CoV-2 can infect faster and better than Delta in the airways but with less severe infection in the lungs. The clinical pattern of Omicron infection is therefore much less severe with primarily upper airway symptoms.[92,93] Because case numbers are so high, there are still more than expected hospitalizations and deaths due to COVID, predominantly in high-risk and unvaccinated individuals.[94]

The most successful variants of SARS-CoV-2 have all become dominant because of greater transmissibility relative to their immediate predecessors. The evolutionary pressures facing the virus and thus its patterns of adaptive evolution favor variants that gain their transmission advantage from evading immunity so the Omicron variants have become the norm, a pattern we recognize from seasonal influenza. As of this writing in January, 2024, there is a relative COVD 19 surge, with hospital admissions up more than 3% and deaths from the virus up 14%, per CDC data. Measures of COVID-19-related illness requiring medical attention, such as emergency department visit rates, have also increased, but these remain significantly lower than they were at the same time last year. Similarly, the number of COVID-19 hospitalizations is 22% lower than a year ago and the percentage of total deaths associated with COVID-19 is 38% lower than in 2023.[95] The JN.1 Omicron variant remains the dominant strain of COVID-19 in the U.S. and the world. The symptoms of infection with JN.1 are usually mild, similar to a typical upper respiratory infection, with a sore throat, runny nose, fever and muscle aches.

Omicron variants have continued to dominate the SARS-CoV-2 story since January of 2022 as the pandemic evolved towards endemic status. Omicron variants have spread so rapidly on a global scale that they increased immunity very quickly. At the same time, worldwide vaccination efforts were also building immunity. As a result, viral transmission slowed, and the rates of COVID-19 cases stabilized. Despite relatively high case numbers, COVID-19 is likely moving toward endemic status in the United States. The process of transition to endemic status is gradual, influenced by many factors. One of these is the relatively short duration of immunity after SARS-CoV-2 infection or immunization: people who have been infected or vaccinated are still at risk of reinfection and this will delay the transition to endemicity. Even when endemic status is achieved, continued surveillance for potential new variants and/or a rise in cases remains essential.

Overall, however, there has been a steady decrease in COVID-19 cases since mid-2023, and even with seasonal increases along with other respiratory viruses in fall and winter, this appears to be a sustained trend, as shown in Figure 8.5.

The Pandemic Response: Prevention

Vaccine Development

Within months of the original SARS-CoV's emergence early in the twenty-first century, the spike(S) protein was identified as the immunodominant antigen of the virus. When SARS-CoV-2 appeared, research in early 2020 revealed that binding and neutralizing antibodies also primarily target the receptor-binding domain of the S1 spike subunit. Once this target was identified, efforts to develop a vaccine to elicit an effective immune response to SARS-CoV-2 began, focused on including production of neutralizing antibodies, generation of a T-cell response, and avoidance of vaccine-induced/ immune-enhanced disease.[96]

Traditionally, immunization has been achieved by using deactivated viruses, or by using a live, attenuated virus that has been grown in culture to make it far less virulent. Once inoculated with vaccines based on either of these approaches,

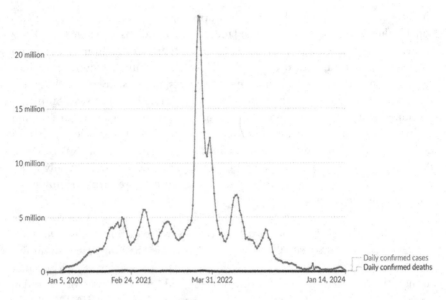

FIGURE 8.5 World confirmed COVID-19 Cases, excluding China, January 5, 2020 to January 14, 2024.

Source: From Our World in Data.org, based on WHO/COVID-19 Dashboard. All visualizations, data and code produced by Our World in Data are completely open access under the Creative Commons BY license.

the body's own immune cells synthesize and store antibodies against the proteins expressed on the surface of viral capsules, ready to mount an immune response when a live version of the virus is encountered.[97]

Unfortunately, vaccine development using either of these methods is very time-consuming, typically requiring more than 10 years. In the middle of a global pandemic with exploding case numbers, hospitalizations and deaths all over the globe, much faster vaccine delivery was needed. Serendipitously, an alternate method using messenger RNA (mRNA) for vaccine delivery had just reached clinical trial stage after more than two decades of research. In mRNA vaccines, lipid nanoparticles are used to protect a stabilized S proteinencoding mRNA en route to the intracellular space. The host cell uses the mRNA to make the target S protein, which induces the desired, coordinated immune response. This technique, the result of more than 20 years of research in multiple, international labs, had already been used to begin development of vaccines for other serious viral diseases including Ebola and Zika.[98,99] When the SARS-CoV-2/COVID-19 pandemic emerged, mRNA scientists and biotechnology labs were ready.[100]

Both mRNA vaccines were 95% efficacious in preventing moderate to severe COVID-19.[101,102] Epidemiological factors facilitated the accelerated timeline of the pivotal trials for these vaccines since with little acquired immunity to SARS-CoV-2 and a sustained high incidence of COVID-19 cases in mid-2020 when trials got underway, finding enough subjects to enroll was easy. The trials demonstrated excellent, near-immediate protection against COVID-19 and severe outcomes like hospitalization and death, and these results were confirmed in post-release studies. Subsequent research showed that vaccine effectiveness decreased relatively quickly over time, leading to recommended booster vaccines, particularly for older-aged individuals. Vaccine effectiveness studies found that protection against symptomatic disease was largely maintained against both the Alpha and Delta variants. Unfortunately, the original vaccines were less effective with Omicron and its subvariants, with breakthrough infections and reinfections. In response, bivalent vaccines have been developed with two messenger mRNA coronavirus components, half targeting the original strain and half targeting Omicron subvariant lineages.[104] Clearly, vaccine development will need to evolve to keep pace with this evolving virus.

Two other vaccines against SARS-CoV-2 have also been released in the United States. The J&J vaccine uses an adenovirus vector to deliver a snippet of SARS-CoV-2-DNA which encodes the spike protein and prompts an immune response. The J&J vaccine had only a 70% efficacy rate and because of complications, this vaccine is no longer available in the USA. The Novavax vaccine injects lab-grown copies of the spike protein that resemble a virus to the immune system plus an adjuvant which stimulates the immune response. Large studies in the USA, Mexico and Britain found two doses of the Novavax vaccine were safe and about 90% effective at preventing symptomatic COVID-19.[105] Like the mRNA vaccines, Novavax was released under an emergency authorization by the FDA and is recommended by the CDC. Internationally, many countries including India, China and Russia have developed and implemented their own vaccines against SARS-CoV-2.

With more than 672 million doses of COVID-19 vaccine given in the United States between 12/14/2020 and 3/1/2023, there has been enough time to evaluate for serious adverse health events after vaccination. These have been very rare and guidance for managing complications is widely available. Perhaps the most concerning side effect has been the development of myocarditis and/or pericarditis, seen most commonly in young males. Fortunately, this resolves spontaneously without residua in almost every case; of note, myocarditis and pericarditis occur more frequently with COVD-19 than they do after vaccination.[106]

All in all, the development and delivery of effective vaccines against SARS-CoV-2 is a scientific and medical triumph. Globally, COVID-19 vaccination is estimated to have saved approximately 20 million lives during just the first year of the vaccine rollout. And vaccine research continues: as of May 6, 2022, the WHO reported that more than 300 COVID-19 vaccines were in preclinical or clinical development and ten COVID-19 vaccines, reflecting eight distinct vaccine products, had been approved for global use. However, vaccine inequity is a persistent problem: less than 20% of people in Africa have been vaccinated against SARS-CoV-2, compared with 75% in high-income countries.

The mRNA technology offers untapped potential for vaccine development against many other serious diseases including some like HIV/AIDS for which no successful vaccine has been developed despite decades of research. Moderna, the biotech company that developed one of the two successful mRNA vaccines, announced that it plans to develop and begin testing vaccines targeting 15 of the world's most worrisome pathogens by 2025 and will permanently waive its COVID-19 vaccine patents for shots intended for low- and middle-income countries. The US biotechnology company also said it will make its mRNA technology available to researchers working on new vaccines for emerging and neglected diseases.

Public Health Guidance

The response to SARS-CoV-2 highlights one of the major results of a massive disease outbreak – recognition of the importance of understanding the pathophysiology of the causative virus and applying that knowledge to manage that epidemic. The most striking result of this is the development of effective vaccines, as already described. Another specific example: once it was understood that the main transmission method of the virus was by inhalation of airborne virus, public health guidance could be tailored to address that factor. Rather than a focus on just public spacing and cleaning surfaces, recommendations to avoid crowded indoor settings and to wear masks when this was unavoidable could be made with confidence. In the USA, the CDC also extensively updated indoor ventilation guidance, setting a target of five air changes per hour for private and public spaces. Joseph Allen, director of the Harvard Healthy Buildings Program, says that "although it's easy to see the guidance only in the context of COVID-19, it will help with many other airborne hazards like wildfire smoke, allergens and other infectious diseases, such as the flu."[107] While there has been resistance to adopting these belated recommendations, it was scientific knowledge that made the advances possible.

The Pandemic Response: Treatment

Therapeutics against COVID-19 have advanced at an astounding pace, and clinicians are now equipped with an armamentarium of treatment options for patients across the spectrum of COVID-19 severity, from mild to critical illness. COVID-19 therapeutics investigated to date include therapies for acute hypoxemic respiratory failure, anti-inflammatory agents, antivirals, antithrombotics, and anti-SARS-CoV-2 (neutralizing) antibodies.

The major morbidity and mortality from coronavirus disease 2019 (COVID-19) has been due to acute viral pneumonia that can evolve to acute respiratory distress syndrome (ARDS) so therapeutic advances in this area have been critical. If respiratory symptoms develop, increasing respiratory support begins with supplementary oxygen, escalating as needed to eventually intubation and mechanical ventilation and, ultimately, extracorporeal membrane oxygenation. One therapy that became standard in patients with COVID-19 lung involvement is the use of awake-prone positioning based on evidence from multiple studies of improved oxygenation and a reduced need for intubation compared with supination.[103] In patients with ARDS caused by COVID-19, use of high-flow nasal cannula O2 and helmet ventilation decreases the need for intubation and mechanical ventilation.[104]

Pharmacologic therapies for COVID-19 can be categorized as targeting the host response to infection (including inflammation, thrombosis, acute respiratory distress syndrome) or targeting the virus directly (including direct antivirals and antibody-based therapies).

Immunomodulary

SARS-CoV-2 infection leads to hyperinflammation characterized by abundant circulating levels of pro-inflammatory cytokines such as IL-6. From the early days of the COVID-19 pandemic, hyperinflammation has been shown to have an important role in the pathophysiology of severe COVID-19. Randomized trials have shown that steroid treatment with dexamethasone is beneficial in hypoxic patients but shows no benefit in patients with milder disease.[105]

Selective monoclonal antibody blockers of inflammatory response have also been shown to be effective; as examples, Tocilizumab is an IL-6 blocker and Baricitinib is an oral Janus kinase 1 (JAK1) and JAK2 inhibitor with anti-inflammatory properties; both reduced mortality in critically ill patients receiving respiratory support.[106]

Antiviral

Therapies specifically targeting SARS-CoV-2 include antivirals that disrupt viral replication, affecting different phases of viremia, including the prevention of viral entry into the host cell and the prevention of both viral activation and replication. Remdesivir inhibits viral replication via an adenosine analog that is incorporated into viral RNA, resulting in the inhibition of further viral replication and early termination of the viral cycle. In both inpatients and outpatients, intravenous remdesivir has been shown to reduce symptoms and illness duration when begun early after symptom onset.[107,111] Nirmatrelvir-ritonavir (Paxlovid) and Molnupiravir are oral anti-viral agents which significantly decrease symptoms and illness duration when started within 5 days of symptom onset; Paxlovid is FDA-approved for outpatient treatment of COVID-19.[108] Multiple existing therapies with known in vitro antiviral activity were tested in clinical trials including many widely used agents such as hydroxychloroquine and ivermectin. All were shown to be ineffective COVID-19 therapies when studied in adequately powered randomized trials.

Antibodies have a key role in the adaptive immune response and are crucial to protecting the host from pathogens. Convalescent plasma can be used to transfer pathogen-specific neutralizing antibodies from previously infected patients, a treatment used in the past and one of the earliest treatments attempted with COVID-19. Several large clinical trials, however, showed no conclusive evidence for benefit of convalescent plasma for COVID-19.[109,113]

Passive administration of pathogen-specific polyclonal or monoclonal antibodies (mAbs) has been used to control viral infections, with the goal of neutralizing a virus by targeting it for elimination and preventing its entry into host cells. Recombinant neutralizing mAbs have been the focus of a large number of COVID-19 studies, developed to target the receptor-binding spike protein of SARS-CoV-2, which mediates viral entry into host cells. Four anti-SARS-CoV-2 mAb products (bamlanivimab plus etesevimab, casirivimab plus imdevimab, sotrovimab, and bebtelovimab) received Emergency Use Authorizations (EUA) from the Food and Drug Administration (FDA) for treatment of outpatients with mild to moderate COVID-19 early in the pandemic, when studies showed they were effective in preventing severe disease and death.[110,112,113] However, laboratory studies have found that the activity of anti-SARS-CoV-2 mAbs against specific variants and subvariants varies dramatically and there are none approved for use against the dominant Omicron variant.

Acute COVID-19 infection is characterized by mononuclear cell reactivity, systemic inflammation and pan-endothelial inflammation contributing to a high incidence of thrombosis in large and small blood vessels, both arterial and venous. This is now recognized as a common and potentially catastrophic manifestation of COVID-19. There are specific recommendations for anti-coagulation management at all levels of COVID-19 disease.[111,115]

The Pandemic Response: Public Backlash

From the outset, information delivery to the public about the pandemic was marred by changing guidelines, clumsy communication, poor coordination and overt political division. In the United States, the focus of leadership was rarely on delivery of accurate information and scientists were unable to report the facts or even clarify mis-statements. It is obvious that with a new virus and a rapidly evolving pandemic, the public needed to hear and understand that public health recommendations would change as knowledge about the virus and the disease increased and circumstances changed – unfortunately, this did not happen. The problem was most acute with regard to the information about masking. As the pandemic evolved, it became clear that the virus is airborne and that, virus transmission is far more likely to occur by inhaled aerosols than by droplet spray. In response, recommendations for mask-wearing and improved indoor ventilation appeared, beginning approximately 6 months after the pandemic began, and emphasis on hand washing and surface cleansing decreased. Masks were recommended for all people over age 2 in a public setting, while traveling, or around others in the same household who might be infected. President Donald Trump immediately undercut this message by vowing not to wear a mask himself. Unfortunately, changing guidance for the public to include masking and avoidance of crowded indoor spaces was a difficult step for the WHO and for national public health organizations to make and even more difficult for the public to accept. It took the WHO until October 2020 to acknowledge that aerosols play a part in disease transmission in community settings and updated guidelines on mask use did not appear until months later.[84] This confused messaging seriously undercut delivery of a critically important public health message. Critics say that even two years into the pandemic, the WHO had not clearly communicated the risks from airborne transmission of this virus. And, perhaps as a result, governments around the world spent much of the pandemic focusing on hand washing and surface cleaning, instead of optimized ventilation and protective masking. Changing messages undoubtedly contributed greatly to resistance to masks and other measures.[117]

Politicized information, conflicting messages amplified on social media, and attempted mask and vaccine mandates led many Americans to question *any* recommendations from the Centers for Disease Control and Prevention (CDC) and other federal health agencies. Vaccine hesitancy and vaccine resistance were powerful forces that substantially limited vaccine acceptance with one third of Americans stating they would never get the vaccine. These attitudes were disturbingly prevalent around the world. By July of 2023, only 70% of the world's population had received at least one vaccination. As the pandemic evolved, there was a substantial erosion of trust in all information from public authorities and even a loss of faith in science itself, not just here in the United States but in many other countries as well.[118] This has important ramifications for any future public health emergencies.

In response to criticism of how it handled the coronavirus pandemic, the CDC is reportedly undergoing an overhaul.[119] A baseline review showed that the traditional scientific and communication processes were not adequate to effectively respond to a crisis the speed, size and scope of the COVID-19 pandemic. "For 75 years, CDC and public health have been preparing for COVID-19, and in our big moment, our performance did not reliably meet expectations," CDC then-Director Walensky said in a statement. "My goal is a new, public health action-oriented culture at CDC that emphasizes accountability, collaboration, communication, and timeliness."[114] Alas, Dr. Walensky's subsequent, abrupt departure from the CDC suggests these plans may never be implemented.[118]

The agency and its work culture need to be transformed with the focus on public health action via accelerated development of public health guidance and improved information sharing and communication with the American public. The CDC website must be streamlined to simplify its public health guidance. Release of data and research findings needs to be accelerated and presentation of information needs to be dramatically improved. Staff – existing and newly hired – must be trained to respond immediately to public health emergencies.

A new executive council will hopefully direct the implementation of these priorities and ensure adequate funding, a critical factor since chronic underfunding undoubtedly contributed to the agency's inadequacies.

The World Health Organization was an important player in the COVID-19 pandemic, although its responses were often delayed so long that they appeared after critical milestones in the pandemic.[116] Most concerning was failure to recognize and act on evidence about the virus or the disease as soon as it emerged – a major example was the delay in acknowledgment that the virus was airborne and that transmission was by inhalation. This significantly compromised adoption of masks. The WHO did spearhead several initiatives including the COVID-19 Solidarity Response Fund, to raise money for the pandemic response; the UN COVID-19 Supply Chain Task Force; and the solidarity trial for investigating potential treatment options for the disease. The COVAX program, co-led by the WHO, Gavi and the Coalition for Epidemic Preparedness Innovations (CEPI) accelerated the development and manufacture of COVID-19 vaccines and worked to guarantee fair and equitable access for every country in the world.

In response to feedback, the WHO has already made plans to respond more rapidly and effectively to another global disease outbreak, launching a process to develop an historic global accord on pandemic prevention and preparedness in December of 2021. In July 2022, it was agreed that the new international instrument on pandemic prevention would be legally binding although final decisions would rest with the WHO. In March 2023, the 194 WHO member-states began negotiations on the proposed global accord on pandemic prevention, preparedness and response. In June of 2023, the WHO countries met again to continue negotiations with a view to presenting a draft to the World Health Assembly in May 2024. The pace of this process illuminates the enormous difficulty and complexity of "coordinating the whole world's response to health emergencies, prevention of disease and access to health care." [116]

However difficult, changes like these are essential to address future pandemics and if implemented, could improve the delivery of critical health information and begin to rebuild trust in science. The wave of disinformation that accompanied the spread of SARS-CoV-2 undermined public health policy responses and amplified distrust among citizens all over the world. Agencies like the WHO and the CDC must leverage improved public reporting to counteract disinformation and support policy, beginning with grounding all public information efforts on open and transparent communication principles.

The Public Response: The End of Zero Covid

January 2023 is three years since Beijing instituted the first Wuhan lockdown which eventually became the extremely punitive "zero-COVID" policy. Although this policy did limit cases and deaths at the time, the economic and social price was substantial. In November of 2022, the Chinese people revolted and there were massive public demonstrations against the COVID controls.

Thousands of people defied heavy penalties for political activity to join the most widespread protests China had seen in decades. On December 26, 2022, China finally ended the zero-COVID policy.

Unfortunately, China was unprepared for this abrupt change. China is an aging country, with vaccination and booster rates lagging far behind what is needed to limit severe illness. Only 40% of people over 80 had received booster shots and almost all had received the domestically developed vaccine, which is less effective and long-lasting than Western alternatives. The absence of an aggressive approach to vaccination left the population extremely vulnerable. With this vaccine history and no natural immunity, experts estimated that as many as 2.1 million lives could be lost. Official numbers are not trustworthy but internet postings suggested there were thousands of early deaths every day after zero-COVID ended. The first wave in urban areas was expected to peak in January 2023 but a second, bigger wave would then reach rural areas where health systems are even weaker.

The World Health Organization has repeatedly urged more transparency from Beijing, requesting more data on genetic sequencing, hospitalizations, intensive care unit admissions and deaths, and on vaccinations delivered and vaccination status but no reports have been forthcoming. For years, a fierce system of Chinese controls held SARS-CoV-2 at bay. Alas, the protracted lockdown was not accompanied by a national program to protect the population and prepare the Chinese health care system for a wave of sick patients.

What happened after China abandoned the zero COVID-19 policy is unknown. Reasoning from what is known about how contagious SARS-CoV-2 is in a population without immunity suggests that almost everyone in China would be infected with the virus within months after the end of the zero COVID policy. However, official Chinese statistics report less than 100,000 deaths in the first 3 months after the lockdown. By contrast, several modeling simulations have suggested 600,000 to 1.5 million deaths. The actual number likely lies between these numbers.[117]

Complete data on what happened and what is currently happening in China are needed to evaluate the ultimate benefit of stay-at-home policies to "flatten the curve" and reduce the flood of patients in an overburdened health care system. Given that the whole population was theoretically destined to be infected with SARS-CoV-2, did flattening the curve make any real difference? Accurate and unbiased data from China about what actually happened during COVID-19 could provide critical information for management of future pandemics.

Looking Back :: Moving Forward

The final trajectory of the 2019 SARS-CoV-2/COVID-19 outbreak is still evolving as this chapter is being written but its enormous global impact is already clear. To the date of this writing in the winter of 2023, there have been more than 774,075,000 cases and 7,000,000 deaths. There are still hundreds of thousands of cases every day and death rates still exceed pre-pandemic data but the overall trajectory of the pandemic has slowed significantly over the last year, as shown in Figure 8.4.

There have been triumphant gains. From the outset, the COVID-19 outbreak transformed how scientists all over the world communicated, with a flood of information released and dissected on social platforms and in the media every day.[118] Medical journals created coronavirus information hubs and manuscripts were published initially as preprints without review, expediting the transfer of information. GISAID (Global Initiative on Sharing Avian Influenza Data), a global science initiative and primary source was established in 2008 to provide open access to genomic data of influenza viruses. Since the very beginning of this pandemic, GISAID expanded its mission to include SARS-CoV-2. On January 12, 2020, the first whole-genome sequences of SARS-CoV-2 were made available on GISAID, initiating the global response to the pandemic. Using the GISAID platform, SARS-CoV-2 viral genomes are posted and analyzed by evolutionary biologists all over the world who can share information from phylogenetic analyses directly. The database has become the world's largest repository for SARS-CoV-2 sequences, providing real-time surveillance of the emergence of new COVID-19 viral strains across the planet and allowing modification of existing vaccines.[118]

Research addressing critical needs began as soon as the new virus was identified with use of existing vaccine platforms to facilitate vaccine development with spectacular results – it was a stunning feat when, by December 2020, less than a year after the genetic code of SARS-CoV-2 had been published, vaccines against SARS-CoV-2 had been developed, trialed, and approved for emergency use – a timeline unparalleled in the history of vaccinology. Treatment trials also began as soon as the outbreak began, and with such high patient volumes, early results were promptly shared and implemented to improve patient care. This was the beginning of the development of an array of therapeutics and preventive measures to address COVID-19 in both inpatients and outpatients. An important research focus was the development of consistent, rapid-response, point-of-care PCR testing including novel testing methods outside of usual point-of-care settings, including drive-by testing.[120]

One area that must be improved based on what we've learned in this pandemic beginning with the very first events in Wuhan is the importance of open and transparent scientific communication at every stage – an informed public that understands the risks and the rationale for proposed interventions is much more likely to cooperate.[121] When the first cases appeared, we saw the risks to public health created by official censorship when Wuhan physicians were silenced by the authorities for sharing information about the new disease with colleagues. Delay in communicating important scientific information such as person-to-person transmission – known to occur from the very first cases in health care personnel – critically compromised the initial response to what was a local disease outbreak and allowed the virus to be carried all over the world. Regrettably, China has given no indication that loosening censorship is on its agenda.

In the United States, poor communication of public health information about the virus and the disease – enormously exacerbated by politicization and social media – resulted in a wave of disinformation that augmented the spread of SARS-CoV-2, undermining policy responses and amplifying distrust among citizens all over the world. We need proactive communication by trusted messengers, including acknowledgment of uncertainty and mistakes with plans to address questions as they arise.[122–125] Effective communication is essential for restoration of faith in science and in government, critical requirements for management of every future disease outbreak.

It appears inevitable that SARS-CoV-2 will become an endemic pathogen in the human population and its impact on our health and daily lives will evolve to reflect that status – in fact, in January 2024, that appears to be the current pattern. Governments and public health officials must transition to a long-term strategy of dealing with SARS-CoV-2 with vaccines and outpatient therapeutics as valuable allies in that process. The most successful variants of SARS-CoV-2 so far have evolved greater transmissibility relative to more ancestral variants. Although higher transmissibility will result in more infections, increasing population-level immunity from infections and vaccinations is already decreasing the health impact of these infections. In order to determine an accurate representation of COVID immunity in the U.S., the CDC has been looking at blood donations since July 2020 to estimate the proportion of people that have immunity, either from infection, from vaccination, or both. By the third quarter of 2022, an estimated 96.4% of persons above 16 years of age had SARS-CoV-2 antibodies from previous infection or vaccination, including 22.6% from infection alone and 26.1% from vaccination alone; 47.7% had hybrid immunity.[126] Durability of immunity and emerging variants like Omicron that gain much of their transmission advantage from evading immunity will persist as problems. The population picture may come to resemble the pattern of influenza with seasonal outbreaks of new variants every winter requiring specifically developed vaccines. For now, the likelihood that SARS-C0V-2 will ever cause another pandemic appears low. However, the evolutionary pressures facing the virus, and therefore its patterns of adaptive evolution, may change and ongoing surveillance is essential. As reported by Jennifer Nuzzo, who runs the Pandemic Center at the Brown University School of Public Health: "It's always a changing situation. People are becoming newly susceptible every day. People are aging into riskier age brackets. New people are being born. The work of protecting people from this virus will continue for as long as the virus continues to circulate on this planet, and I don't foresee it going away for the foreseeable future."[124]

The SARS-CoV-2/COVID-19 pandemic has been a terrible experience with unparalleled disease and death on a global scale. The impact on the economy and on society has been grave. School closures in the USA alone took 50 million children out of classrooms for varying lengths of time, a damaging disruption that we know set progress in math and reading back by two decades and widened the achievement gap that separates advantaged and disadvantaged children.

Economists are predicting that with such a significant educational gap, the COVID generation will experience diminished lifetime earnings. In every area, there have been similar, major pandemic residua.

At the same time, this has been a triumphant time – we have witnessed one of the greatest periods in the history of science as the global science community worked together to address this new virus. The tools and technologies developed to address SARS-CoV-2 will enable a better and faster reaction to the next threat – because, make no mistake, there will be another virus and yet another global viral pandemic. Consider this: while COVID was still winding down, we have already experienced a global MPOX outbreak, as described in Chapter 9. As this book is being completed, the H5N1 *avian* flu pandemic is raging. H5N1 is a perfect example of the kind of virus that could lead to another pandemic, having already killed millions of wild and domestic birds on every continent except Australia. Researchers are very concerned that the virus will mutate to readily infect humans and allow straightforward human-to-human transmission. So far, this has not happened, but increasing reports of large H5N1 outbreaks in farmed mammals represent the very situation that optimally promotes viral mutation.[127] Viral disease outbreaks are everywhere and another global pandemic is inevitable.

References

1. Xiong Y, Gan N. Wuhan coronavirus kills doctor who warned of outbreak. *CNN* Updated 8:15 AM ET, Tue February 4, 2020.
2. Kahn J. China Releases the SARS Whistle-Blower. *The New York Times*. July 21, 2004.
3. The doctor who revealed China's SARS cover-up has been under house arrest in the country since 2019. *Isaac Scher. Snapchat*. Feb 10, 2020, 7:44 AM
4. Doctor's death from coronavirus sparks a digital uprising, rattling China's leaders. Available at: www.washingtonpost.com › world › asia.pacific › 2020/02/0. Accessed Feb. 10, 2020.
5. Zhang H. Grief and wariness at a vigil for Li Wenliang, the doctor who tried to warn China about the Coronavirus. *The New Yorker*. Feb. 11, 2020.
6. Huang C, Wang Y, Li X, et al. Clinical features of patients infected with 2019 novel coronavirus in Wuhan, China. *Lancet* 2020. Published online on Jan. 24, 2020. Available at: http:// doi:10.1016/S0140-6736(20)30183-5. Accessed January 28, 2020.
7. Chan JF-W, Yuan S, Kok K-H, et al. A familial cluster of pneumonia associated with the 2019 novel coronavirus indicating person-to-person transmission: A study of a family cluster. *Lancet* 2020 Jan 24; [e-pub]. Available at: https://doi.org/10.1016/S0140-6736(20)30154-9. Accessed Jan. 28, 2020.
8. Tan W, Zhao X, Ma X, et al. A novel coronavirus genome identified in a cluster of pneumonia Cases – Wuhan, China 2019−2020[J]. *China CDC Weekly*. 2020,2(4): 61–62.
9. Zhu N, Zhang D, Wang W, et al. A novel coronavirus from patients with pneumonia in China, 2019. *N Engl J Med* 2020, Published online, Jan 24. Available at: doi: 10.1056/NEJMoa2001017. Accessed 1/28/2020.

10. Xiaodong W. Progress continues in coronavirus trace: Wuhan Market Cultures. chinadaily.com.cn. Updated: 2020-01-26 14:26.

11. Wang C, Horby P, Hayden FG, Gao GF. A novel coronavirus of global health concern. Lancet. Published online January 24,2020. Available at: https://DOI: 10.1016/S0140-6736(20)30185-9 Accessed Feb. 6, 2020.

12. Yi Y, Lagniton PN12.P, Ye S, Li E, Xu RH. COVID-19: what has been learned and to be learned about the novel coronavirus disease. *Int J Biol Sci.* 2020 Mar 15;16(10):1753–1766. doi: 10.7150/ijbs.45134. PMID: 32226295; PMCID: PMC7098028.

13. South China Agricultural University finds pangolin as a potential intermediate host for new coronavirus. Published Jan. 20,2020. Available at: flutrackers.com < -2019-ncov-new-coronavirus > china-2019-ncov. Accessed Feb 7, 2020.

14. Mueller B. New Data Links Pandemic's Origins to Raccoon Dogs at Wuhan Market. *NY Times.* March 16, 2023.

15. Zhao S, Lin Q, Ran J, et al. Preliminary estimation of the basic reproduction number of novel coronavirus (2019-nCoV) in China, from 2019 to 2020: A data-driven analysis in the early phase of the outbreak. *Inter J Inf Dis* 2020. Published online 30 January 2020. Available at: https://doi.org/10.1016/j.ijid.2020.01.050. Accessed 2/8/2020.

16. WHO. Daily media briefing on #2019-nCoV. Feb. 7, 2020. Available at: www.who.int/ Coronavirus disease 2019 › Media resources. Accessed Feb 8, 2020.

17. Li Q, Guan X, Wu P, et al. Early transmission dynamics in Wuhan, China, of novel Coronavirus–infected pneumonia. *N Engl J Med.* Published January 29, 2020. Available at: www.nejm.org/doi/full/10.1056/NEJMoa2001316. Accessed 2/12/2020.

18. Chen N, Zhou M, Dong X, et al. Epidemiological and clinical characteristics of 99 cases of 2019 novel coronavirus pneumonia in Wuhan, China: a descriptive study. *Lancet* 2020. Published January 30, 2020. Available at: https://doi.org/10.1016/S0140-6736(20)30211-7. Accessed 2/11/2020.

19. Wang D, Hu B, Hu C, et al. Clinical characteristics of 138 hospitalized patients with 2019 novel Coronavirus–infected pneumonia in Wuhan, China. JAMA. Published online February 7, 2020. Available at: http://doi:10.1001/jama.2020.1585. Accessed 2/13/2020.

20. Chu DKW, Pan Y, Cheng SMS, et al. Molecular diagnosis of a novel Coronavirus (2019-nCoV) causing an outbreak of pneumonia. *Clinical Chemistry.* Published January 31, 2020. Available at: https://doi.org/10.1093/clinchem/hvaa029. Accessed 2/12/2020.

21. New lab in Wuhan begins testing for coronavirus, China Daily/ANN. Feb.7, 2020.

22. https://twitter.com/luchenhist/status/1220497118755987456

23. Cohen J. The United States badly bungled coronavirus testing – but things may soon improve. A faulty reagent in a test kit and bureaucratic hurdles have slowed testing for the virus that causes COVID-19. *Science.* 28 Feb 2020. doi: 10.1126/science.abb5152.

24. Gallagher GM. Remdesivir being evaluated against novel coronavirus. Feb. 5, 2020. Available at: www.contagionlive.com › news › remdesivir-being-evaluated-against-novel-coronavirus. Accessed Feb 10, 2020.

25. World Health Organization . Twitter: FACT: COVID-19 is not airborne. March 28, 2020. https://twitter.com/who/status/1243972193169616898. Accessed May 26, 2021.

26. Cohen J. Scientists are moving at record speed to create new coronavirus vaccines – But they may come too late. *Science.* Jan. 27, 2020, 6:30 AM.

27. Coalition for Epidemic Preparedness (CEPI) https://search.yahoo.com/search;_ylt=awro8jn2ca9lgtkcwfjxnyoa;_ylu=y29sbwnncteecg9zazeednrpzamec2vja3nj

28. Cohen J. Unveiling "Warp Speed," the White House's America-first push for a coronavirus vaccine. *Science.* May 12, 2020. doi:10.1126/science.abc7056. S2CID 219432336. Archived from the original on November 29, 2020. Retrieved May 16, 2020.

29. Perper R. As the Wuhan virus spreads, doctors in the city say they face a "flooding" of patients and not enough protective gear. *Business Insider,* January 24, 2020. Available at: www.businessinsider.com/wuhan-coronavirus-doctors-wuhan-patients-protective-gear-2020-1

30. www.bbc.com/news/world-asia-china-5122384

31. Li Z, Chen Q, Feng L, et al. Active case finding with case management: the key to tackling the COVID-19 pandemic. *Lancet* 2020: 396: (10243): 63–70. doi:10.1016/S0140-6736(20)31278-2.

32. WHO International Press Briefing. Feb. 11, 2020. Available at: who-audio-emergencies-coronavirus-full-press-conference-11feb2020-final.pdf

33. 2019 Novel Coronavirus (2019-nCoV) Situation Summary | CDC. Available at: www.cdc.gov › coronavirus › 2019-ncov › summary

34. World Pop Project@WorldPopProject. Assessing spread risk of Wuhan novel coronavirus within and beyond China, January-April 2020: a travel network-based modelling study' with Chinese CDC and Bluedot. Available at: MedArXiv. www.medrxiv.org/content/10.1101/2020.02.04.20020479v1. Accessed 2/14/2020.

35. Mahtani S, Berger M, Taylor A, Iati M. Coronavirus cases surge again in China; more than 1,700 medical workers infected. *The Washington Post.* 2/14/2020.

36. Department of Health and Environmental Sciences, XI'AN JIATONG – Liverpool University (XJTLU). Model Predicts Date for Near-End of New, Confirmed 2019-nCoV Cases in China. Available at: www.xjtlu.edu.cn/en/news/2020/02/model-predicts-date-for-near-end-of-new-confirmed-2019-ncov-cases. Accessed 2/11/2020.

37. https://news.sky.com/story/identity-of-man-linked-to-11-british-coronavirus-cases-revealed. 11931336#:~:text=The%20British%20man%20who%20is,on%206%20February%20with%20coronavirus

38. Krever M, Rivers M, Sandi S, Ripley W. U.S is finally evacuating passengers from the Diamond Princess. CNN. Feb.17, 2020. www.cnn.com/2020/02/16/asia/coronavirus-outbreak-diamond-cruise-us evacuation-intl-hnk/index.html

39. The Novel Coronavirus Pneumonia Emergency Response Epidemiology Team. The Epidemiological Characteristics of an Outbreak of 2019 Novel Coronavirus Diseases (COVID-19) – China, 2020 Feb. 17, 2020. CCDC Weekly. http://weekly.chinacdc.cn/fileCCDCW/journal/article/ccdcw/2020/8/PDF/COVID-19.pdf

40. Pan Y, Zhang D, Yang P, et al. Viral load of SARS-CoV-2 in clinical samples. *Lancet Inf Dis.* Published: February 24, 2020 doi: https://doi.org/10.1016/S1473-3099(20)30113-4

41. Ai T, Yang Z, Hou H, et al. Correlation of Chest CT and RT-PCR Testing in Coronavirus Disease 2019 (COVID-19) in China: A Report of 1014 Cases. Radiology. Published Online: Feb 26 2020 doi: https://doi.org/10.1148/radiol.2020200642

42. Shin Y, Berkowitz B, Kim M-J. How a South Korean church helped fuel the spread of the coronavirus. *The Washington Post.* March 25, 2020. www.washingtonpost. com/graphics/2020/world/coronavirus-south-korea-church/

43. Horowitz J. Italy's health care system groans under coronavirus – a warning to the world. *New York Times.* March 12, 2020. www.nytimes.com/2020/03/12/world/europe/12italy-coronavirus-health-care.html

44. WHO Director-General's opening remarks at the media briefing on COVID-19 – 11 March 2020. www.who.int/director-general/speeches/detail/who-director-general-s-opening-remarks-at-the-media-briefing-on-covid-19---11-march-2020

45. La Maestra S, Abbondandolo A, De Flora S. Epidemiological trends of COVID-19 epidemic in Italy over March 2020: From 1000 to 100 000 cases. *J Med Virol.* 2020 Oct;92(10):1956–1961. doi: 10.1002/jmv.25908. Epub 2020 May 12. PMID: 32314804; PMCID: PMC7264625.

46. Dorigatti I, Okell L, Cori A, et al. Report 4: Severity of 2019-novel coronavirus (nCoV). WHO Collaborating Centre for Infectious Disease Modelling, MRC Centre for Global Infectious Disease Analysis, J-IDEA, Imperial College London. Available at: www.imperial.ac.uk › media › medicine › sph › ide › gida-fellowship. Accessed Feb. 11, 2020.

47. Coronavirus Diagnosis in California Highlights Testing Flaws. The NY Times. By Roni Caryn Rabin, Sheri Fink and Knvul Sheikh, Published Feb. 27, 2020. Updated Feb. 28, 2020. www.nytimes.com/2020/02/27/health/coronavirus-testing-california.html

48. Centers for Disease Control and Prevention. Updated Guidance on Evaluating and Testing Persons for Coronavirus Disease 2019 (COVID-19). www.cdc.gov/coronavirus/2019-nCoV/hcp/clinical-criteria.html

49. Policy for Diagnostics Testing in Laboratories Certified to Perform High Complexity Testing under CLIA prior to Emergency Use Authorization for Coronavirus Disease-2019 during the Public Health Emergency. Feb. 29, 2020. www.fda.gov › media › download

50. Coronavirus May Have Spread in U.S. for Weeks, Gene Sequencing Suggests. *The New York Times.* The Coronavirus Outbreak: Live updates. March 1, 2020. By Sheri Fink and Mike Baker.

51. Coronavirus Outbreak: U.S. Is Now the Global Virus Epicenter. Bloomberg News. www.youtube.com/watch?v=5t3cBX_BceA

52. Executive shelter-in-place order. Governor M. Cuomo. PAUSE: "Policies Assure Uniform Safety for Everyone." March 20, 2020. https://ny.curbed.com/2020/3/20/21187022/coronavirus-new-york-shutdown-shelter-in-place

53. First Covid-19 outbreak in a U.S. nursing home raises concerns. STAT. Eric Boodman & Helen Branswell. February 29, 2020.

54. Wu JT, Leung K, Leung GM, et al. Nowcasting and forecasting the potential domestic and international spread of the 2019-nCoV outbreak originating in Wuhan, China: a modelling study. *Lancet* 2020. Published: January 31, Available at: https://doi.org/10.1016/S0140-6736(20)30260-9. Accessed Feb. 2, 2020.

55. Xi Jinping Says China Must Do Better. The NY Times: The Coronavirus Outbreak. Live Updates. 3/1/2020.

56. Dupont A, Rauch A, Staessens S, et al. Vascular endothelial damage in the pathogenesis of organ injury in severe COVID-19. *Arterioscler Thromb Vasc Biol.* 2021; 41:1760–1773. doi: 10.1161/ATVBAHA.120.315595

57. Abou-Ismail MY, Diamond A. Kapoot S, et al. The hypercoagulable state in COVID-19: Incidence, pathophysiology, and management. *Thromb Res.* 2020 Oct; 194: 101–115.Published online 2020 Jun 20. doi: 10.1016/j.thromres.2020.06.029

58. Bonanad C, García-Blas S, Tarazona-Santabalbina F, et al. The effect of age on mortality in patients with COVID-19: A meta-analysis with 611,583 subjects. *J Am Med Dir Assoc.* 2020 Jul;21(7):915–918. doi: 10.1016/j.jamda.2020.05.045

59. Beigel JH, Tomashek KM, Dodd LR, et al. Remdesivir for the treatment of Covid-19 – Final report. *N Engl J Med* 2020; 383:1813–1826. 11/5/2020. doi: 10.1056/NEJMoa2007764

60. Hung I F-N, Lung K-C, Yuk-Keung E, et al. Triple combination of interferon beta-1b, lopinavir–ritonavir, and ribavirin in the treatment of patients admitted to hospital with COVID-19: an open-label, randomised, phase 2 trial. *Lancet* 2020; 395: 1695–1702. doi: https://doi.org/10.1016/S0140-6736(20)31042-4

61. Ivashchenko AA, Dmitriev KA, Vostokova NV, et al. AVIFAVIR for treatment of patients with moderate COVID-19: Interim results of a phase II/III multicenter randomized clinical trial. *medRxiv preprint.*; posted August 5, 2020. doi: https://doi.org/10.1101/2020.07.26.20154724

62. McBane RD, Torres Roldan VD, Niven AS, et al. Anticoagulation in COVID-19: A systematic review, meta-analysis, and rapid guidance from Mayo Clinic. Consensus recommendation. *Mayo Clin Proc* 2020; 95(11):2467–2486. Published: August 31, 2020. doi: https://doi.org/10.1016/j.mayocp.2020.08.030

63. Sterne JAC, Murthy S, Diaz JV, et al. WHO Rapid Evidence Appraisal for COVID-19 Therapies (REACT) working group. Association between administration of systemic corticosteroids and mortality among critically ill patients with COVID-19: a meta-analysis. *JAMA.* 2020;324(13):1330–1341. doi:10.1001/jama.2020.17023

64. Chen WH, Strych U, Hotez PJ, et al. The SARS-CoV-2 vaccine pipeline: an overview. *Curr Trop Med Rep* 2020; 7: 61–64. https://doi.org/10.1007/s40475-020-00201-6

65. Furukawa NW, Brooks JT, Sobel J, et al. Evidence supporting transmission of severe acute respiratory syndrome coronavirus 2 while pre-symptomatic or asymptomatic. *Emerg Infect Dis.* 2020;26. doi: 10.3201/eid2607.201595

66. Feaster M, Goh YY. High proportion of asymptomatic SARS-CoV-2 infections in 9 long-term care facilities, Pasadena, California, USA, April 2020. *Emerg Infect Dis.* 2020 Oct;26(10):2416–2419. doi: 10.3201/eid2610.202694

67. Oran DP, Topol EJ. Prevalence of Asymptomatic SARS-CoV-2 Infection: A Narrative Review. *Ann Intern Med.* 2020 Sep 1;173(5):362–367. doi: 10.7326/M20-3012

68. Meyerowitz EA, Richterman A, Bogoch II, Low N, Cevik M. Towards an accurate and systematic characterisation of persistently asymptomatic infection with SARS-CoV-2. *Lancet Infect Dis.* 2020; 280(7506):717. https://doi.org/10.1016/S1473-3099(20)30837-9

69. Alene M, Yismaw L, Assemie MA, et al. Magnitude of asymptomatic COVID-19 cases throughout the course of infection: A systematic review and meta-analysis. *PLoS One.* 2021 Mar 23;16(3):e0249090. doi: 10.1371/journal.pone.0249090

70. Godfred-Cato S, Bryant B, Leung J, et al. COVID-19-associated multisystem inflammatory syndrome in children – United States, March-July 2020. *MMWR Morb Mortal Wkly Rep.* 2020 Aug 14;69(32):1074–1080. doi: 10.15585/mmwr.mm6932e2

71. Feldstein LR, Rose EB, Horwitz SM, et al. Multisystem inflammatory syndrome in U.S. children and adolescents. *N Engl J Med.* 2020 Jul 23;383(4):334–346. doi: 10.1056/NEJMoa2021680

72. European Centre for Disease Prevention and Control Multisystem Inflammatory Syndrome in Children. www.ecdc.europa.eu/en/publications-data/multisystem-inflammatory-syndrome-children-mis-c

73. Caro-Patón GL, de Azagra-Garde AM, García-Salido A, et al. Shock and myocardial injury in children with multisystem inflammatory syndrome associated with SARS-CoV-2 infection: What we know. Case series and review of the literature. *J Intensive Care Med.* 2021 Apr;36(4):392–403. doi: 10.1177/0885066620969350

74. Belhadjer Z, Méot M, Bajolle F, et al. Acute heart failure in multisystem inflammatory syndrome in children in the context of global SARS-CoV-2 pandemic. *Circulation.* 2020; 142:429–436. doi.org/10.1161/CIRCULATIONAHA.120.048360

75. Son MBF, Murray N, Friedman K, et al. Multisystem inflammatory syndrome in children – Initial therapy and outcomes. *N Engl J Med* 2021; 385:23–34. doi: 10.1056/NEJMoa2102605

76. McCrindle BW, Harahsheh AS, Handoko R, et al. SARS-CoV-2 Variants and Multisystem Inflammatory Syndrome in Children. *N Engl J Med* 2023; 388:1624–1626. doi: 10.1056/NEJMc2215074

77. WHO Fact sheet. 7 December 2022. Post COVID-19 condition (Long COVID). www.who.int/europe/news-room/fact-sheets/item/post-covid-19-condition

78. Perlis RH, Santillana M, Ognyanova K. Prevalence and correlates of long COVID symptoms among US adults. *JAMA Netw Open.* 2022 Oct 3;5(10):e2238804. doi: 10.1001/jamanetworkopen.2022.38804

79. Sudre CH, Murray B, Varsavsky T, et al. Attributes and predictors of long COVID. *Nat Med* 2021; 27:626–631. https://doi.org/10.1038/s41591-021-01292-y

80. Thaweethai T, Jolley SE, Karlson EW, et al. Development of a definition of postacute sequelae of SARS-CoV-2 infection. *JAMA.* 2023;329(22):1934–1946. doi:10.1001/jama.2023.8823

81. Abbasi J. The COVID Heart – One Year After SARS-CoV-2 Infection, Patients Have an Array of Increased Cardiovascular Risks. *JAMA.* 2022;327(12):1113–1114. doi:10.1001/jama.2022.2411

82. Davis HE, McCorkell L, Vogel JM, et al. Long COVID: major findings, mechanisms and recommendations. *Nat Rev Microbiol* 2023; 21: 133–146. https://doi.org/10.1038/s41579-022-00846-2

83. Bramante CT, Buse JB, Liebovitz DM, et al. Outpatient treatment of COVID-19 and incidence of post-COVID-19 condition over 10 months (COVID-OUT): a multicentre, randomised, quadruple-blind, parallel-group, phase 3 trial. *Lancet Infect Dis.* Published online June 8, 2023. doi:10.1016/S1473-3099(23)00299-2

84. Klompas M, Baker MA, Rhee C. Airborne transmission of SARS-CoV-2. *JAMA.* 2020;172(11):766–7. https://doi.org/10.1001/jama.2020.12458

85. Escandón K, Rasmussen AL, Bogoch II, et al. COVID-19 false dichotomies and a comprehensive review of the evidence regarding public health, COVID-19 symptomatology, SARS-CoV-2 transmission, mask wearing, and reinfection. *BMC Infect Dis* 2021; 21: 710. https://doi.org/10.1186/s12879-021-06357-4

86. World Health Organization. Mask use in the context of COVID-19: interim guidance, 1 December 2020. World Health Organization. https://apps.who.int/iris/handle/10665/337199. License: CC BY-NC-SA 3.0 IGO

87. Volz E, Mishra S, Chand M, Barrett JC, et al. Assessing transmissibility of SARS-CoV-2 lineage B.1.1.7 in England. *Nature.* 2021 May;593(7858):266–269. doi: 10.1038/s41586-021-03470-x. Epub 2021 Mar 25. PMID: 33767447.

88. Thorne LG, Bouhaddou M, Reuschl AK, et al. Evolution of enhanced innate immune evasion by SARS-CoV-2. *Nature* 2022; 602: 487–495. https://doi.org/10.1038/s41586-021-04352-y

89. Dhawan M, Sharma A, Priyanka TN, et al. Delta variant (B.1.617.2) of SARS-CoV-2: Mutations, impact, challenges and possible solutions. *Hum Vaccin Immunother.* 2022 Nov 30; 18(5):2068883. doi: 10.1080/21645515.2022.2068883. Epub 2022 May 4. PMID: 35507895; PMCID: PMC9359381.

90. Kläser K, Molteni E, Graham M, et al. COVID-19 due to the B.1.617.2 (Delta) variant compared to B.1.1.7 (Alpha) variant of SARS-CoV-2: a prospective observational cohort study. *Sci Rep* 2022; 12, 10904. https://doi.org/10.1038/s41598-022-14016-0

91. Duong D. Alpha, Beta, Delta, Gamma: What's important to know about SARS-CoV-2 variants of concern? *CMAJ.* 2021 Jul 12;193(27):E1059–E1060. doi: 10.1503/cmaj.1095949. PMID: 34253551; PMCID: PMC8342008.

92. Dhawan M, Saied AA, Mitra S, Alhumaydhi FA, Emran TB, Wilairatana P. Omicron variant (B.1.1.529) and its sublineages: What do we know so far amid the emergence of recombinant variants of SARS-CoV-2? *Biomed Pharmacother* 2022; 154:113522. doi: 10.1016/j.biopha.2022.113522

93. Chen J, Wang R, Benovich-Gilby N, et al. Omicron Variant (B.1.1.529): Infectivity, vaccine breakthrough, and antibody resistance. *J. Chem. Inf. Model.* 2022; 62(2): 412–422. https://doi.org/10.1021/acs.jcim.1c01451

94. Araf Y, Akter F, Tang Y-d, et al. Omicron variant of SARS-CoV-2: genomics, transmissibility, and responses to current COVID-19 vaccines. *J Med Virol.* 2022; 94: 1825–32. doi: 10.1002/jmv.27588. Epub 2022 Jan 23.

95. Lakshmanane P, Segovia-Chumbez B, Jadi R, et al. The receptor-binding domain of the viral spike protein is an immunodominant and highly specific target of antibodies in SARS-CoV-2 patients. *Sci Immunol* 2020;5(48). 26 Jun 2020. doi: 10.1126/sciimmunol.abc841

96. COVID-19 Activity Increases as Prevalence of JN.1 Variant Continues to Rise. January 5, 2024. www.cdc.gov/respiratory-viruses/whats-new/JN.1-update-2024-01-05.html

97. Saleh A, Qamar S, Tekin A, et al. Vaccine development throughout history. *Cureus* 2021; 13(7):e16635. doi: 10.7759/cureus.16635

98. Beyrer C. The long history of mRNA vaccines. Newsletter. Center for Public Health and Human Rights at the Johns Hopkins Bloomberg School of Public Health. https://publichealth.jhu.edu/2021/the-long-history-of-mrna-vaccines

99. Wang F, Kream RM, Stefano GB. An evidence based perspective on mRNA-SARS-CoV-2 vaccine development. *Med Sci Monit.* 2020 May 5;26:e924700. doi: 10.12659/MSM.9247 00. PMID: 32366816; PMCID: PMC7218962.

100. Corbett KS, Edwards DK, Leist SR, et al. SARS-CoV-2 mRNA vaccine design enabled by prototype pathogen preparedness. *Nature.* 2020 Oct; 586(7830):567–571. doi: 10.1038/s41586-020-2622-0. Epub 2020 Aug 5.

101. Polack FP, Thomas SJ, Kitchin N, et al. C4591001 Clinical Trial Group. Safety and efficacy of the BNT162b2 mRNA Covid-19 vaccine. *N Engl J Med* 2020; 383:2603–15. https://doi.org/10.1056/NEJMoa2034577external icon PMID:33301246.

102. Lewis LM, Badkar AV, Cirelli D, Combs R, Lerch TF. The race to develop the Pfizer-BioNTech COVID-19 vaccine: From the pharmaceutical scientists' perspective. *J Pharm Sci.* 2023 Mar; 112(3):640–647. doi: 10.1016/j.xphs.2022.09.014. Epub 2022 Sep 18. PMID: 36130677; PMCID: PMC9482796.

103. Baden LR, El Sahly HM, Essink B, et al. Efficacy and Safety of the mRNA-1273 SARS-CoV-2 Vaccine. *N Engl J Med* 2021; 384 (5): 403–416. doi:10.1056/NEJMoa2035389

104. Kundi, M. Vaccine effectiveness against delta and omicron variants of SARS-CoV-2. *BMJ* 2023; 381 doi: https://doi.org/10.1136/bmj.p1111 (Published 23 May 2023).

105. Heath PT, Galiza EP, Baxter DN, et al. Safety and Efficacy of NVX-CoV2373 Covid-19 Vaccine. *N Engl J Med* 2021; 385:1172–1183. doi: 10.1056/NEJMoa2107659

106. Oster ME, Shay DK, Su JR, et al. Myocarditis cases reported after mRNA-based COVID-19 vaccination in the US from December 2020 to August 2021. *JAMA.* 2022; 327(4):331–340. doi:10.1001/jama.2021.24110

107. Chua EX, Zahir SMISM, Ng KT, et al. Effect of prone versus supine position in COVID-19 patients: A systematic review and meta-analysis. *J Clin Anesth.* 2021 Nov;74:110406. doi: 10.1016/j.jclinane.2021.110406. Epub 2021 Jun 22. PMID: 34182261; PMCID: PMC8216875.

108. Arabi YM, Aldekhyl S, Al Qahtani S, et al. Effect of helmet noninvasive ventilation vs usual respiratory support on mortality among patients with acute hypoxemic respiratory failure due to COVID-19: The HELMET-COVID randomized clinical trial. *JAMA.* 2022 Sep 20;328(11):1063–1072. doi: 10.1001/jama.2022.15599

109. The RECOVERY Collaborative Group. Dexamethasone in Hospitalized Patients with Covid-19. *N Engl J Med* 2021; 384:693–704. Epub 7/7/2021. doi: 10.1056/NEJMoa2021436

110. Ucciferri C, Vecchiet J, Falasca K. Role of monoclonal antibody drugs in the treatment of COVID-19. *World J Clin Cases.* 2020 Oct 6;8(19):4280–4285. doi: 10.12998/wjcc.v8.i19.4280. PMID: 33083387; PMCID: PMC7559676.

111. Beigel JH, Tomashek KM, Dodd LE, et al. Remdesivir for the treatment of Covid-19 – Final report. *N Engl J Med* 2020; 383:1813–1826. 11/5/2020. doi: 10.1056/NEJMoa2007764

112. Hammond J, Leister-Tebbe H, Gardner A, et al. Oral nirmatrelvir for high-risk, nonhospitalized adults with COVID-19. *N Engl J Med.* 2022; 386(15):1397–1408. doi: 10.1056/NEJMoa2118542

113. Sullivan DJ, Gebo KA, Shoham S, et al. Early Outpatient Treatment for Covid-19 with Convalescent Plasma. *N Engl J Med* 2022; 386:1700–1711. May 5, 2022. doi: 10.1056/NEJMoa2119657

114. Takashita E, Yamayoshi S, Simon V, et al. Efficacy of antibodies and antiviral drugs against Omicron BA.2.12.1, BA.4, and BA.5 subvariants. *N Engl J Med.* 2022;387(5):468–470. Available at: www.ncbi.nlm.nih.gov/pubmed/35857646

115. Mucha SR, Dugar S, McCrae K, et al. Update to coagulopathy in COVID-19: Manifestations and management. *Cleveland Clinic Journal of Medicine.* 2021 Jun. doi: 10.3949/ccjm.87a.ccc024-up. PMID: 33323363.

116. Escandón K, Rasmussen AL, Bogoch II, et al. COVID-19 false dichotomies and a comprehensive review of the evidence regarding public health, COVID-19 symptomatology, SARS-CoV-2 transmission, mask wearing, and reinfection. *BMC Infect Dis* 2021; 21: 710. https://doi.org/10.1186/s12879-021-06357-4

117. Lalani HS, DiResta R, Baron RJ, et al. Addressing viral medical rumors and false or misleading information. *Ann Intern Med* 2023; 18 July, 2023. https://doi.org/10.7326/M23-1218

118. Ioannidis JPA, Zonta F, Levitt M. What really happened during the massive SARS-CoV-2 Omicron wave in China? *JAMA Intern Med*. Published online May 15, 2023. doi:10.1001/jamainternmed.2023.1547

119. Sun LH, Diamond D. CDC, under fire, lays out plan to become more nimble and accountable. *Washington Post*. August 17, 2022 at 5:59 p.m. EDT.

120. WHO: Pandemic prevention, preparedness and response accord. June 24, 2023. www.who.int › news-room › questions-and-answers

121. Cheng X, Chen Q, Tang L, Wu Y, Wang H, Wang G. Rapid Response in an Uncertain Environment: Study of COVID-19 Scientific Research Under the Parallel Model. *Risk Manag Health Policy*. 2022; 15:339–349. https://doi.org/10.2147/RMHP.S351261

122. Lenharo M. GISAID in crisis: can the controversial COVID genome database survive? *Nature*. May 04.2023. www.nature.com/articles/d41586-023-01517-9

123. Ramanan M, Stolz A, Rooplalsingh R, et al. An evaluation of the quality and impact of the global research response to the COVID-19 pandemic. *Med J Aust*. 2020 Oct;213(8):380–380.e1. doi: 10.5694/mja2.50790. Epub 2020 Sep 18. PMID: 32946592; PMCID: PMC7536958.

124. Reddy BV, Gupta A. Importance of effective communication during COVID-19 infodemic. *J Family Med Prim Care* 2020 Aug 25;9(8):3793–3796. doi: 10.4103/jfmpc.jfmpc_719_20. PMID: 33110769; PMCID: PMC7586512.

125. Larsen BJ, et al. Counter-stereotypical messaging and partisan cues: Moving the needle on vaccines in a polarized United States. *Sci Adv* 2023; doi: 10.1126/sciadv.adg9434

126. Jones JM, Manrique IM, Stone MS, et al. Estimates of SARS-CoV-2 seroprevalence and incidence of primary SARS-CoV-2 infections among blood donors, by COVID-19 vaccination status – United States, April 2021–September 2022. *MMWR Morb Mortal Wkly Rep*. 2023;72(22):601–605. doi:10.15585/mmwr.mm7222a3

127. Abbasi J. Bird flu has begun to spread in mammals – here's what's important to know. *JAMA*. Published online February 08, 2023. doi:10.1001/jama.2023.1317

Suggested Reading

A.S. Bhalla. *National and Global Responses to the COVID-19 Pandemic: Do Leaders Matter?* Palgrave Macmillan Cham. London. 2023.

David Quammen. *Breathless: The Scientific Race to Defeat a Deadly Virus*. Simon & Schuster. New York. 2022.

Lawrence Wright. *The Plague Year: America in the Time of Covid*. Knopf. New York. 2021.

Matt Ridley, Alina Chan. *The Search for the Origin of COVID-19*. Harper. New York. 2021.

Sarah Gilbert, Catherine Green. *The Inside Story of the Oxford AstraZeneca Vaccine and the Race Against the Virus*. Hodder & Stoughton Edition 1. London. 2022.

Tapas Kumar Koley, Monika Dhole. *The COVID-19 Pandemic: The Deadly Coronavirus Outbreak*. Routledge. London. 2022.

Yasmeen Abutaleb, Damian Paletta. *Nightmare Scenario: Inside the Trump Administration's Response to the Pandemic That Changed History*. Harper Collins. New York. 2022.

9

MPOX

Out of Nowhere All over Again?

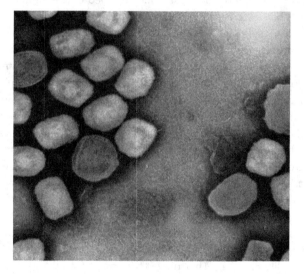

FIGURE 9.1 Mpox/Monkeypox virus.

Source: www.ncbi.nlm.nih.gov

DOI: 10.4324/9781003427667-9

A VISIT FROM THE POX

In the fall of 1998, I was back at Cornell, working as a research assistant and applying to graduate school. I graduated the previous spring, thinking I was going to take some time away from academia. And here I was: back in Ithaca, running statistics and writing essays. It was the first major derailment of my nicely planned life; the first one is always the hardest. And then, suddenly, I had an incredibly painful rash on my left cheek. The welts seemed to be emerging from inside the skin, rather than on top of it. It felt like the line extending from the outside of my eye to my cheekbone was freezing and burning at the same time. I was still only 20 years old so I called my mum – you know, my co-author who went to medical school – in a bit of a quandary. This *hurt*. She said very quickly, "Oh, you have herpes zoster." I didn't hear much past "herpes," but when I was done shrieking like an irate macaque, I heard the second word and then the colloquial, "shingles." We both remembered I had a very light case of chicken pox when I was in kindergarten, so it seemed immensely unfair that my depressed body decided to release that little monster from its box. I started acyclovir and took ibuprofen and stayed home from work for a few days, both because it hurt like the dickens (even air touching it made the nerves fire) and because I looked like a Halloween creature.

Twenty-five years later, monkeypox hit the gay male community of New York City. The very men who survived AIDS and COVID-19 and had just rediscovered the joys of white parties and back rooms were slapped with a painful and humiliating pox. They did not all have physician parents they could call for help: they had something better. They had a network built through the blood and tears of the first decade of AIDS, and it had only gotten stronger in the interim. Most gay male doctors were not publicly out in the early 1980s, and while a few were identified, terrified gay men had almost no place to go with questions about embarrassing genital rashes or confusing symptoms. Now they do. Now they are part of a powerful alliance of activists, lawyers, doctors and politicians who know how to make state governments react, get widespread access to vaccines, and avoid making patients feel like criminals. They proved how powerful a shared experience of terror, pain and loss can make one group of people. Look no further than the more than 900,000 American men who have received the Jynneos vaccine since it became available in 2022.

We all lost something to AIDS, but we gained the knowledge of how much we *can* do when we stand together. In his play *The Normal Heart*, Larry Kramer memorably wrote:

> The only way we'll have real pride is when we demand recognition of a culture that isn't just sexual. It's all there – all through history we've been there; but we have to claim it, and identify who was in it, and articulate

what's in our minds and hearts and all our creative contributions to this earth. And until we do that, and until we organize ourselves block by neighborhood by city by state into a united visible community that fights back, we're doomed. That's how I want to be defined: as one of the men who fought the war.

May we all share that normal heart.

Mpox: Out of Nowhere All over Again?

Monkeypox? It was early May 2022. Weary scientists were still struggling with the emerging Omicron variants of SARS-CoV-2. COVID-19 case numbers and deaths were falling and it almost looked as if there might actually be an end in sight. A new disease outbreak caused by a relatively obscure virus from central Africa was definitely not on the radar. But within only a few weeks, here we were, with dramatically rising numbers from multiple sites all over the world. Ready or not, as shown in Figure 9.2, monkeypox was already a new, multi-nation disease outbreak.[1]

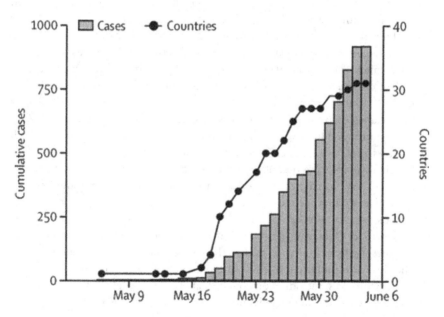

FIGURE 9.2 Cumulative number of confirmed Mpox cases (by confirmation date) since the first reported case in the 2022 outbreak, and cumulative number of countries reporting confirmed cases.

Source: *Lancet Inf Dis* 2022; 22(7): 941–942. Published online: June 8, 2022. doi: https://doi.org/10.1016/S1473-3099(22)00359-0. Reprinted with permission.

The Disease: The Classical Picture

Historically, monkeypox was a disease of young children seen equally in males and females and characterized by the progressive appearance of skin lesions similar to those seen with smallpox, accompanied by fever and malaise. The rash first appeared on the face and quickly spread in a centrifugal distribution over the body. The distinctive pox lesions was initially maculopapular before becoming vesicular and then pustular. Lesions were often present on the palms of the hands and soles of the feet but the rash was not always widespread and could be limited to just a few lesions. Coincident with emergence of the rash was the development of generalized, tender lymphadenopathy. The disease had definite similarities to smallpox but lymphadenopathy is not a characteristic of smallpox and overall, monkeypox disease is much milder.[2]

Symptom severity and disease duration were proportional to the number of skin lesions which were often described as painful until the healing phase when they become itchy. Complications included secondary bacterial infections, broncho- pneumonia, gastrointestinal involvement, encephalitis, myocarditis and ocular infections, which could result in permanent corneal scarring The incubation period was 3–17 days with an average of 10 days during which there were no symptoms. A person with monkeypox – now officially called mpox – was able to transmit the virus to others from the time symptoms started until the rash had fully healed, through direct skin contact with the rash, scabs, or body fluids including respiratory droplets, or by way of contaminated materials like bedclothes of an infected person or animal. Historically, there was no specific treatment and patients were managed with supportive care. Once all scabs had fallen off and a fresh layer of skin had formed, an individual was no longer contagious. Pitted scars and/or areas of lighter or darker skin could remain after scabs had fallen off. Most infected individuals recovered uneventfully within 2–4 weeks but in individuals who had not been vaccinated against smallpox which offers cross-protection, the case fatality rate was reported to be as high as 11%.

Originally, mpox was described exclusively as a zoonosis with cases in humans only found close to tropical rainforests in central Africa which housed potential rodent reservoirs including squirrels, Gambian pouched rats, dormice and different species of monkeys among others. No single reservoir species has ever been identified. Over time, it was recognized that the disease could also be transmitted directly from human to human through contact with body fluids, lesions on the skin or on internal mucosal surfaces, such as in the mouth or throat or respiratory droplets, including on contaminated objects. Outbreaks were usually self-limited with no known epidemics.

The Virus: The Historic Picture

The monkeypox virus (MPXV) is an Orthopoxvirus, a genus that includes smallpox/variola, camelpox, cowpox, and vaccinia viruses. With the eradication of smallpox, MPXV became the foremost Orthopoxvirus affecting humans. At 200–250 nm in size, MPXV is a very large double-stranded DNA virus, about seven times as large as SARS-CoV-2, the coronavirus that causes COVID-19. With electron microscopy, it appears oval and brick- shaped, with characteristic surface tubules and a dumbbell-shaped core (Figure 9.1) The genome is approximately 199 kb of double-stranded linear DNA with approximately 190 non-overlapping open reading frames. Like all orthopoxviruses, the central coding region nucleotide sequence positions in the MPXV are highly conserved and flanked by variable ends that contain inverted terminal repeats. DNA-based viruses like MPXV can correct their own replication errors so they typically collect just one or two mutations per year compared with the much larger number of mutations seen in RNA viruses. Of note, chickenpox, another pox-like disease that displays some similarities in symptomology, is caused by the varicella-zoster virus and is not related to MPXV.

Detection of MPXV DNA by polymerase chain reaction (PCR) is the preferred laboratory test for mpox. The best diagnostic specimens are taken directly from the rash – skin, fluid or crusts. Antigen and antibody detection methods may not be useful as they do not distinguish between the orthopoxviruses.

Until 2022, there were two recognized mpox clades. Clade I was present in the Congo Basin, caused up to 11% human mortality, and was transmitted by rodents with almost no known human-to-human spread. Clade II existed in West Africa and historically, it was associated with milder disease, fewer deaths – mortality less than 1% – and limited reports of human-to-human transmission. The two clades have 95% nucleotide sequence identity.[3]

Epidemiology: The Historic Narrative

The monkeypox virus (MPXV) likely existed for many hundreds of years before 1958 when it was first identified and named for the infected Danish laboratory monkeys in which it first appeared. The first human case was not reported until 1970 in the Congo. Subsequent reported cases were initially rare with just 47 documented over the next decade, scattered through Central and West Africa. As above, the virus was thought to be transmitted from animals to humans but no single, definitive animal source was documented and in four of these earliest reported cases, person-to-person spread was considered to have occurred.[2]

In 1980, global health leaders declared smallpox eradicated and subsequently, MPXV became the most important Orthopoxvirus causing infection in man. Smallpox vaccination (using the vaccinia virus) provides protection against all Orthopoxvirus infections, including monkeypox – these double-stranded DNA viruses are genetically and antigenically very similar, which accounts for this cross-immunity. With elimination of routine smallpox vaccination, there was concern that an increasing proportion of the population in tropical rain forest areas of central and western Africa would lack immunity to monkeypox. It was predicted that the MPXV would continue to be introduced into human communities from animal sources, and that the number of outbreaks would increase as vaccine-derived protection declined in the population. The monkeypox virus was not thought to be transmissible enough to persist in human communities, even in the total absence of vaccination.[4]

Historically, most reports of human monkeypox infections came from West Africa, but after 1981, the majority occurred in the Congo Basin of Central Africa, especially the Democratic Republic of the Congo or DRC. Active surveillance for human monkeypox from 1981 to 1986 in the DRC identified a total of 338 cases, a significant increase over previous reports. The case-fatality rate was 9.8% for persons not vaccinated against smallpox. The secondary attack rate in unvaccinated household members was 9.3%, and 28% of these patients reported an exposure to another case-patient during the incubation period. Transmission chains beyond secondary were rare.[5] A 1987 computer model based on this data predicted that lack of smallpox vaccinations would lead to a substantial increase in new secondary cases over time but none of the simulated models predicted an "explosive" epidemic.[6]

Between 1986 and 2017, sporadic mpox outbreaks continued in sub-Saharan Africa. Over time, these included more annual cases and evidence for person-to-person transmission gradually increased.[5,7] No single animal reservoir was identified but there was still no conclusive evidence that person-to-person transmission *alone* could sustain monkeypox in a population. In a population with low herd immunity, person-to-person transmission plus repeated introduction of the virus from animal reservoirs was considered to be leading to the more frequent and larger clusters of human monkeypox cases in African rainforest areas.

In 2003, a monkeypox outbreak in the US involved 71 confirmed and suspected patients in six states, the majority in Wisconsin. This was the first reported outbreak outside of Africa. Cases were traced to pet prairie dogs who had been housed close to infected small mammals imported from Ghana. At the time, it was unclear whether the virus was transmitted only from animals: while all the infected people had interacted with animals, two also reported coming in contact with lesions or eye fluids from another patient. The virus spread for a little more than a month before dying out. There was no mortality and there has been no recognized recurrence in the USA.[8]

Active, population-based surveillance for monkeypox was conducted in the central DRC between November 2005 and November 2007. Compared with the data in the same health zone from the 1980s, there was a significant, 20-fold increase in human monkeypox cases. The average age of cases was 11.9 years, well above that reported previously; only 3.8% had evidence of previous smallpox vaccination compared with 26.4% of the overall population. Contact with animal reservoir species was still considered to be the major driver of MPXV transmission but again, no single animal reservoir was identified. Based on case histories, increased human-to-human transmission was verified but was not further assessed. With the rising case numbers, the study investigators recommended ongoing, active monkeypox surveillance and more comprehensive assessment of the epidemiology of the disease but this did not occur.[9]

In September 2017, the picture suddenly changed when Nigeria experienced a major monkeypox outbreak with 228 suspected cases, compared with a total of only 3 reported cases in the preceding 18 years. Case findings differed significantly from previous reports of monkeypox where children below 10 years of age comprised 83% of the cases and secondary transmission was rare. Remarkably, the Nigerian outbreak was characterized predominantly by infection in young adult males and by significant person-to-person transmission. Among these infected men, the most common presentation was with genital lesions and concomitant syphilis and HIV infection. Given this striking demography, the investigators considered sexual transmission to be plausible, either through close skin to skin contact during sexual intercourse or by transmission via genital secretions – neither had previously been reported. This possibility was not publicly explored further at that time.[10,11]

In response to this largest documented outbreak of human monkeypox in Nigeria and the striking differences in the demography compared with previous reports, the WHO and the CDC held an informal meeting of experts and representatives from affected countries in 2017. Participants noted that during the past decade, reports of human mpox cases had increased, including in countries that had not reported the disease in several decades. The report from the meeting stated that since 2016, monkeypox cases had been confirmed in the Central African Republic (n=19), the Democratic Republic of the Congo (>1,000 reported per year), Liberia (n=2), Nigeria (n=228), Republic of the Congo (n=88), and Sierra Leone (n=1). The remarkable changes in the affected population and the unique disease presentation noted during the outbreak in Nigeria were alluded to in the report of the meeting but were not part of the final statement which concluded that the emergence of monkeypox had become a global health security concern. In response, the WHO and the CDC were charged to develop "updated guidance and regional training to improve capacity for laboratory-based surveillance, detection and prevention of monkeypox, improve patient care, and outbreak response."[12] Online training courses on monkeypox prevention and control were indeed made available beginning in 2018. From 2018 to 2021, human cases were recognized and confirmed in six African countries; the reemergence and increase in cases resulted in monkeypox being listed in 2019 as a priority disease for immediate and routine reporting through the Integrated Disease Surveillance and Response Strategy in the WHO African region.

During this same time period, eight independent, travel-associated cases of monkeypox were recognized and reported outside of Africa, in persons traveling from Nigeria. The patients were all men aged 30–50 years, and three reported that the rash first appeared in the groin area.[13] Cases included two reports in the UK in 2018. Both had travelled to Nigeria and on return, both presented with genital lesions. Reports do not include sexual history but these cases indicate importation of the MPXV and may represent the beginning of covert circulation of the virus which subsequently burst into the open in 2022.[14]

Thirty years after mass smallpox vaccination campaigns ceased, two important facts about monkeypox emerged from this sequence of case series: human monkeypox incidence had dramatically increased in central African rainforest areas; and human-to-human transmission of the disease, once thought to be very rare, was now an important part of disease transmission. Declining population immunity and rising population numbers could have potentially allowed human-to-human transmission to cross the threshold required for sustained spread of MKPX. Isolated case histories strongly suggested the possibility of sexual transmission. Increasing size and frequency of human monkeypox outbreaks and an evolving epidemiologic picture raised the specter of a potential, major monkeypox pandemic.

May 2022: A Global Monkeypox Pandemic Begins: Epidemiology of the Outbreak

On May 3, 2022, five males with atypical ulcerative skin lesions presented to two different clinics for men who have sex with men (MSM) in Lisbon, Portugal. The lesions appeared predominantly in the genital area (perianal, scrotum and lining of the penis) and evolved with the formation of a central crust. All lesions were at the same clinical stage. Two cases also had papules with similar characteristics on the trunk and limbs, but these were limited, less than 20 papules in total.[15]

Almost simultaneously, a first case of mpox was detected in London on May 6, 2022 in a patient with a recent travel history from Nigeria. On May 16, the UK Health Security Agency reported four new cases with no link to travel. All four of these cases appeared to have been infected in London.

Back in Portugal, multiple differential diagnoses were considered for the 5 presenting cases but on May 16, following an alert from the UK on the European Centre for Disease Prevention platform describing a positive case of monkeypox in an individual with similar genital lesions, laboratory tests for orthopox viruses were conducted. On May 17, real-time PCR results confirmed the diagnosis of MPXV in 3 of the cases in Portugal: by May 27, 2022, 96 cases of monkeypox had been confirmed there. The most common symptoms were the characteristic pox rash but with genital lesions, fever and inguinal lymphadenopathy. A total of 14 cases also had known HIV infection. All tested positive for MPXV DNA by PCR. Preliminary analysis of the virus genome sequence showed that it belonged to the same West African clade identified in the disease cluster in Nigeria.

Meanwhile in the United Kingdom, between May 7 and May 25, 86 additional monkeypox cases were confirmed. Only one of these individuals was known to have travelled to a country where MPXV was endemic. The demographic picture was the same as that seen in Nigeria and in Portugal. Seventy-nine cases with information were male and 66 reported having sex with men. This was the first reported sustained MPXV transmission in the UK, with human-to-human transmission through close contacts, including in sexual networks.[16]

2022–2023: Epidemiology of the MPOX Pandemic

Following these initial reports, mpox case numbers increased dramatically, reported from multiple countries, predominantly in Europe and the Americas but also in Asia, Africa, and Oceania. Belgium, Sweden, and Italy detected their first confirmed MPOX cases on May 19, 2022, followed by France, Germany, the Netherlands and Australia on May 20, 2022. As shown in Figure 9.2, within six weeks, almost 1000 cases had been reported from more than 30 countries all over the globe.[2] (Of note: in this book, an epidemic is a sudden rise in the presence of a disease which is spreading rapidly to many people within a localized community or region. Pandemic refers to an epidemic that has gone international with the disease appearing in other countries and on other continents. By this definition, the 2022 monkeypox outbreak was a pandemic. Throughout, the WHO referred to it as a multi-nation disease outbreak.)

With COVID, involved countries emerged successively, one after another. With monkeypox, cases emerged almost simultaneously in multiple sites all over the world, theoretically fueled by travel of infected individuals, potentially liberated by lifting of COVID-related restrictions on travel and mass gatherings. In response to spiraling case numbers from multiple geographic locations, the Director-General of the World Health Organization (WHO), Tedros Adhanom Ghebreyesus, declared the monkeypox outbreak a "public health emergency of international concern" (PHEIC) on July 23, 2022. By then, there were more than 7000 cases from 60 countries.[17]

In the United States, the first documented case appeared in Boston, Massachusetts, on May 17, 2022. Data from the CDC indicate that 99% of the more than 3000 cases reported between May and July were in men and of those, 94% were among men who had sexual contact with other men. In cases with available information, 41% were also HIV positive. By August 22, monkeypox had spread to all 50 states in the United States, as well as Washington, D.C. and Puerto Rico. By that time, with 5% of the world's population and 25% of the world's cases, the United States had the highest number of monkeypox cases of any country in the world. On August 4, 2022, the US Centers for Disease Control and Prevention declared monkeypox to be a public health emergency.

A similar dramatic rise in cases appeared in close succession in multiple countries all over the world, many of which had never previously reported a single case of monkeypox. Earliest cases occurred in the European Region followed within days by the Americas, especially the United States. The demographic picture first reported in Nigeria in 2017 was reproduced in one country after another, with monkeypox cases overwhelmingly concentrated in networks of men who have sex with men. In every country, the most common reported exposure setting was a sex-on-site event with multiple, anonymous sexual contacts.[17]

This narrative suggested undetected spread of MXPV had likely been occurring in many countries, likely for years. The eight cases with a similar mpox disease pattern who were identified in four countries outside of Africa between 2018 and 2021 after travel from Nigeria supported this hypothesis. These cases may have initiated covert circulation of the virus in multiple sexual networks which subsequently exploded after widespread transmission in the MSM community in the spring of 2022. The COVID pandemic may well have been a factor here, with the enforced reduction in public gatherings and in non-essential travel limiting gatherings and thereby, inhibiting spread of the virus for several years.[13,14]

MPXV outbreaks existed in endemic areas in Africa for many decades where they usually did not extend beyond a few transmission cycles, and person-to-person transmission was rarely reported. By contrast, the 2022 monkeypox pandemic showed sustained transmission among a susceptible demographic group that had not been exposed to smallpox vaccination and therefore lacked cross-protective immunity. A global outbreak almost exclusively involving men who have sex with men suggested extension of an ongoing covert process in a specific demographic group whose behavior put them at special risk. In an interview with the Associated Press, Dr. David Heymann, who formerly headed the WHO's emergencies department, said the leading theory to explain the sudden, accelerated spread of the disease was sexual transmission among gay and bisexual men at international sex parties. "We know monkeypox can spread when there is close contact with the lesions of someone who is infected, and it looks like sexual contact has now amplified that transmission."[18]

And then monkeypox as a global emergency disappeared – almost as rapidly as cases accumulated from May through July, 2022, they fell steadily, beginning in early August.[19] All over the world, new case numbers dropped, as shown in Figure 9.3. The European Region and the Region of the Americas (North and South America and the Caribbean Islands) exhibited the highest number of cases throughout the outbreak and the most rapid decline in new cases. By the end of October 2022, the number of new cases globally had decreased by 40.7% with the maximum decrease in the Region of the Americas (66.9%) and the European Region. The sustained fall in cases continued: by May of 2023, the number of cases over the previous three months had fallen by 90%, compared with the preceding three months and the WHO announced that monkeypox no longer constituted a public health emergency.[20] How this striking decrease occurred is explored below in the discussion of prevention and treatment. As of 8/17/2023, there had been a total of 89,931 mpox cases from 113 countries with 153 deaths.[17]

In November of 2022, the World Health Organization announced a name change: monkeypox was subsequently to be known as mpox. Both names were to be used simultaneously for one year while "monkeypox" was phased out. To reduce any potential stigma related to the location of origin, WHO renamed monkeypox virus variants from the "Congo Basin Central African" as clade one (I) and "West African" strains, clade two (II).

Epidemic curve shown for cases reported up to 07 May 2023 to avoid showing incomplete weeks of data.

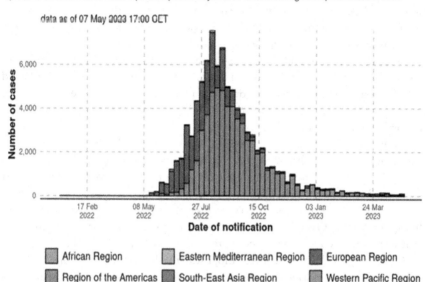

data as of 07 May 2023 17:00 CET

FIGURE 9.3 Global epidemic curve for Monkeypox cases, January 2022–March 2023.

Source: www.who.int/emergencies/situations/monkeypox-oubreak-2022. cdc.gov.

2022–2023: The Disease

Early in the pandemic, an international group of clinicians collaborated to create a global case series describing the presentation, clinical course, and outcomes of PCR–confirmed monkeypox cases.[21] In July 2022, they reported their findings on 528 cases diagnosed between April 27 and June 24, 2022, at 43 sites in 16 countries. The demographics of the infected individuals were in striking contrast to the classic disease picture: 98% were gay or bisexual men, 75% were White, and 41% had HIV infection; the median age was 38 years. In 95% of cases, viral transmission was suspected to have occurred through sexual activity.

Presenting signs and symptoms also differed radically from the traditional clinical picture. Rash without systemic symptoms was the predominant presentation of MPXV infection at diagnosis. Although 95% of infected individuals presented with a vesicular/pustular rash, 64% had less than 10 lesions. In 73% of cases, lesions were in the anogenital area and 10% had only a single genital lesion. Oropharyngeal/ perioral mucosal lesions were also common at presentation. Systemic features preceding or coincident with the rash included fever (62%), lethargy (41%), myalgia (31%) and headache (27%); inguinal lymphadenopathy was reported in 56% of cases. Rectal symptoms were also frequently reported.

Concomitant sexually transmitted infections were present in 29% of those who were tested. Among those with a clear exposure history, the median incubation period was 7 days (range, 3 to 20). Monkeypox virus DNA was detected in 29 of the 32 persons (90%) in whom seminal fluid was analyzed.

Findings from this landmark global case series, emphasized the emergence of a new clinical picture similar to that seen in Nigeria in 2017 – MPXV-infected patients were almost exclusively young men who have sex with men, presenting with oral or anogenital lesions rather than a generalized rash and often with a history of multiple recent sex partners.[21]

Collected over the same time period, a case series of MPXV infection from the same 16 centers described the epidemiological and clinical characteristics of MPXV infection in the much smaller group of 136 women. The cohort comprised 62 trans women, 69 cis women, and five non-binary individuals who were grouped with cis women. Twenty-seven percent of all individuals were living with HIV. Overall, the clinical presentation and course were similar to that seen in males but a third of cis women and non-binary individuals were initially misdiagnosed. Overall, a vesiculopustular rash was the presenting symptom in 93% of cases, described as anogenital in 74%. Mucosal lesions in the oropharynx or eye also occurred in 55% of individuals with available data. MPXV DNA was detected by PCR from vaginal swab samples in all 14 samples tested. All patients recovered with no deaths.[22]

The simultaneous identification of cases in multiple sites outside areas where monkeypox has traditionally been endemic again raised the possibility of ongoing, undetected global spread of the MXPV. The findings in Nigeria in 2017 and as described here in 2022 were confirmed over and over again as cases were reported from all over the world. Within weeks of the first cases, surveillance and testing efforts were initiated and expanded. For example, in the USA, testing capacity grew rapidly, from 6,000 tests per week in June of 2022 to 80,000 per week by July. Most mpox cases recovered without any intervention. Ano-genital lesions were often more painful than the typical skin lesions of mpox and some patients required hospitalization for pain management. However, infected people usually recovered within 3–4 weeks, even without treatment. A minority – roughly 10% – were hospitalized for isolation, pain management, or for complications such as secondary skin infections, abscesses, and/or difficulty in swallowing. Less severe but more common complications included rectal pain, swelling of the penis, and localized, secondary bacterial infections. Serious complications were rare and included epiglottitis, myocarditis, and encephalitis. Sporadic fatal cases were reported with an overall case fatality rate in the 2022–23 outbreak in European countries of less than 0.1%.

An exception was the course of mpox in individuals with advanced HIV infection and low immune cell (CD4+ T cell) counts. In the MPXV pandemic, people living with HIV/AIDS accounted for 38–50% of mpox cases worldwide. A global case series from 19 countries of individuals with CD4 counts less than

350 cells per mm³ included 382 patients, 96% male; at mpox diagnosis, 91% were known to be living with HIV and 65% were adherent to antiretroviral therapy. Severe complications were significantly more common in people with a CD4 cell count of less than 100 cells per mm³ compared with those with counts greater than 300 cells per mm,³ including necrotizing skin lesions, lung involvement, secondary infections and sepsis. Overall, 28% of these patients were hospitalized and one quarter died, all with CD4 counts below 200 cells per mm³.[3,23]

2022–2023: The Virus

Historically, there were two recognized monkeypox virus (MPXV) clades, both associated primarily with disease in young children. Clade I was present in the Congo Basin, was thought to be transmitted by rodents, had limited human-to-human spread but reportedly caused up to 11% mortality; clade II existed in West Africa and had been associated with milder disease, fewer deaths, and more reports of human-to-human transmission. Based on phylogenetic analyses, the 2022–23 MPXV outbreak belongs to the West African clade and is most closely related to the viruses associated with exportation from Nigeria in isolated cases in 2018 and 2019.[24] The multi-country global outbreak appears to have had a single origin, with all sequenced viruses tightly clustered together. However, genome sequencing has revealed some small differences between the current outbreak strains, now classified as clade IIb and clade IIa (previously clade II), and clade I viruses.[25] How these differences contribute to virulence or transmission has not yet been determined.

Knowledge regarding how mpox virus spreads continues to evolve. In laboratory experiments, respiratory transmission of MPXV is inefficient and close skin-to-skin human contact has appeared to be the most important transmission setting. As described, in the current outbreak, the majority of people are thought to have been infected during sexual activity, originally presumed to be due to prolonged intimate contact with infectious mpox lesions on the skin or mucosal surfaces of the mouth, throat, anus, or rectum.[25] However, analysis of semen and vaginal secretions has documented the MPX virus suggesting that true sexual transmission could be part of the pattern of disease spread.[21,22,26,27] The ramifications of classifying monkeypox as a sexually transmitted infection instead of an infection that is transmissible via sex are important and this distinction has not yet been definitively clarified.

Analysis of a large series of MPXV-confirmed cases in the UK indicated that transmission of the virus could occur in pre-symptomatic people, as many as 4 days before symptoms began. This study also suggested that infectious periods were long and that therefore, an isolation period of 16 to 23 days would be required to detect 95% of people with a potential infection. Identification of pre-symptomatic transmission has important implications for infection control globally. As with COVID, relying on identifying and isolating symptomatic individuals will not prevent virus transmission. In addition, postexposure or "ring" vaccination of contacts identified only through individuals with symptoms, will be inadequate so vaccination will need to be extended to high-risk groups.[28]

New pathogens are believed to emerge from animal reservoirs when ecological changes increase the pathogen's opportunities to enter the human population and to generate subsequent human-to-human transmission.[29] The emergence of a disease like mpox as a global pandemic combines two elements: the introduction of the pathogen into the human population; and its subsequent spread and maintenance within the population. Ecological factors such as human behavior influence both of these elements. In the current outbreak, pre-symptomatic spread was documented, monkeypox lesions were relatively few in number, and the disease itself was largely unknown outside of Africa, so failure to recognize the presence of MPXV infection appears likely. In this context, the sexual behavior of young men involving multiple partners could significantly increase the risk of MPXV transmission.

Analysis of the MPXV from the global pandemic is ongoing. Shotgun metagenomics have been used to allow reconstruction and phylogenomic characterization of the first MPXV outbreak genome sequences, showing that this MPXV belongs to clade IIb and that the outbreak most likely has a single origin. The 2022 MPXV clustered with 2018–2019 cases linked to Nigeria but it segregates in a divergent phylogenetic branch suggesting continuous accelerated evolution. An in-depth mutational analysis suggests the action of host APOBEC3 in viral evolution as well as signs of potential MPXV human adaptation in ongoing microevolution.[30] APOBEC3 genes are interferon-stimulated genes whose expression is increased in response to various stimuli. Genetic analyses have shown several mutations which might explain how MPXV has evolved to transmit more readily through sex.[31]

Further evidence from genome sequencing shows that the first cases from 2022 shared 42 single nucleotide differences from the closest MPXV genome sampled in 2018. For a DNA virus, this is an unexpectedly large number of changes within 3 to 4 years and suggests an accelerated evolutionary rate for a poxvirus. Most nucleotide changes were characteristic of the action of APOBEC3 deaminases, as noted above; these host enzymes have a reported antiviral editing function.[32] Taken together, these findings suggest that MPXV was mutating relatively rapidly and that this mutated virus has been circulating in humans since at least 2016. Another study identified multiple introductions of monkeypox viruses of different origins into the USA since 2017, also with evidence of APOBEC3 editing.[33]

Prevention and Treatment

Vaccine

Because mpox was prevented in at least 85% of those vaccinated against smallpox, potential vaccines were available as soon as the 2022 outbreak was recognized.

In addition, historical data collected during the smallpox eradication program had shown that vaccination within 2–3 days of exposure can protect against the emergence of clinical disease, and if given within 4–5 days, can decrease the risk of death.[34]

There are three different smallpox vaccines stored in the US Strategic National Stockpile (SNS), each with distinct implementation considerations: ACAM2000, APSV, and JYNNEOS (also known as Imvamune or Imvanex). ACAM2000 and APSV are live virus vaccines containing the vaccinia virus. With either of these, vaccinia can spread from the vaccination site to other parts of the body or to other people, so vigilant site care is essential from the day of vaccination until the scab falls off, about 14–21 days later. Both are administered as a single dose using the multiple puncture technique developed for administration of the original smallpox vaccine.

Jynneos, the third vaccine, is also a live virus vaccine but it contains a more highly attenuated form of the vaccinia virus which does not cause disease in humans and is non-replicating, meaning it cannot reproduce in humans. It received FDA approval as a preventive vaccine against monkeypox for adults over 18 years of age and for high-risk individuals in September, 2019. Jynneos is administered subcutaneously in two doses separated by 4 weeks for individuals who have never been vaccinated against smallpox. Individuals previously vaccinated against smallpox receive one dose. Full immunity develops 2 weeks after the second dose.[35]

Less than a decade ago, the United States had some 20 million doses of smallpox vaccines in freezers in the Strategic National Stockpile (SNS). Such vast quantities of the vaccine could have slowed the spread of monkeypox as soon as it first emerged in the United States in mid-May. Instead, the SNS had only 2,400 usable doses left in May 2022, enough to fully vaccinate just 1,200 people. The rest of the doses had expired because of plans to replace the liquid form of the vaccine with a freeze–dried version, anticipated to be available in 2023–2024. In response to the emerging pandemic, the FDA authorized emergency use of the Jynneos vaccine and a new, large supply was made available by the end of August 2022, with 1.1 million doses available to states and 6.9 million doses delivered by May 2023.

Other countries in the global north also had vaccine stockpiles. For example, Canada has Imvamune, a non-replicating, third generation smallpox vaccine manufactured by Bavarian Nordic. In the context of the ongoing MPXV outbreaks, Imvamune is currently being provided to provinces and territories for post-exposure and pre-exposure vaccination to individuals/groups at high risk of mpox.

When the mpox outbreak began, the WHO proposed creating a stockpile to equitably share the limited vaccine and drug supplies available worldwide. There is a physical stockpile of smallpox vaccine held at the WHO Headquarters in Switzerland, composed of calf-lymph smallpox vaccines from a variety of sources dating from the final years of the eradication program, estimated to consist of

~2.4 million doses. In addition, there is a pledged stockpile stored by multiple donor countries for use in an international pandemic. Dr. Mike Ryan, the WHO's chief of emergencies, said the global body would work with member nations to create a stockpile from the limited number of available smallpox vaccines to be shared with nations that lack the resources to purchase them. Progress on this is unknown.

Due to the limited supply of vaccines, the World Health Organization recommended prioritizing the vaccination of high-risk groups and in late August of 2022, the USA adopted a new vaccine administration policy, injecting a single, subcutaneous dose of vaccine. This technique was shown to be highly effective and provides 5 doses per vial of vaccine, compared with the previous single dose/vial technique.[36]

At least initially, the vaccine program appeared to be enthusiastically adopted among those at high risk in the US: from September 4–October 1, 2022, a total of 205,504 persons received the second Jynneos vaccine dose. To assess vaccine effectiveness in a real-world setting, mpox incidence by vaccination status was evaluated using surveillance data from more than 9500 vaccine-eligible men aged 18–49 years in 43 US jurisdictions. Among unvaccinated people, mpox incidence was 9.6 times higher than in those who had received 2 vaccine doses and 7.4 times higher among people who had received only one dose. There was no difference in protection between the subcutaneous and intradermal administration routes.[37] In addition to preventing infection, Jynneos was given as postexposure prophylaxis to people with known or presumed exposure to the mpox virus: ideally, vaccination was aimed to occur within 4 days of exposure but since administration up to 14 days after exposure is thought to still provide some protection, delayed vaccine administration was also used.

Vaccination is one of the most important ways to prevent infection. JYNNEOS vaccine effectiveness is reported to be about 75.2% for the single dose and 85.9% for the double dose, consistent with evidence from prior studies.[38] The duration of immunity after vaccination is not known. New cases may still occur in people who have received 2 doses of Jynneos, but symptoms are less severe than in those who have not been vaccinated. Despite the administration of more than 1 million doses of mpox vaccine, the CDC reported that only about a quarter of the defined, at-risk population in the USA have been fully vaccinated.

Public Health Guidance

As already described, since the current global monkeypox outbreak first emerged, the vast majority of cases were in men who have sex with men (MSM), and, in particular, those who have multiple, anonymous partners at venues where knowledge of infection status is often unknown. With an ongoing, global outbreak, providing factual information on where and how the virus was spreading was recognized as critical to help individuals personally lower their risk of exposure. At the same time, it was important to avoid stigmatization and discrimination

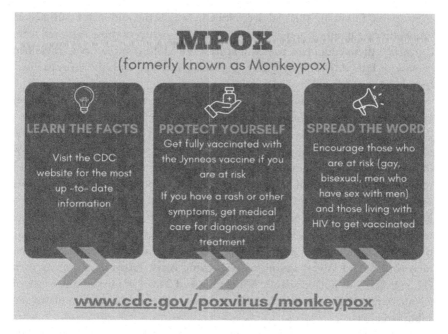

FIGURE 9.4 Poster providing public health guidance on Mpox, summer 2022.

Source: www.cdc.gov

of the communities affected so MSM needed to be involved in solutions for stopping its further spread.

In response to these conclusions, the WHO/Europe recommended that individuals with mpox isolate until the rash has fully healed and a fresh layer of skin has formed, usually 2–4 weeks. Individuals from the MSM community were asked to seriously consider limiting their sexual partners and interactions during the pandemic, as a means to avoid catching and/or spreading monkeypox. Venues for anonymous sex among MSM were asked to participate in efforts to combat the outbreak by disseminating information to those most at risk, informing them about prevention strategies and available health services for testing and treatment. Information about the importance of vaccination and its availability was provided to target populations at highest risk, exemplified in Figure 9.4; vaccination sites were established in MSM recreational venues.

In the USA, the government set up a task force led by Robert Fenton, a logistics expert from the Federal Emergency Management Agency, and Dr. Demetre Daskalakis, director of the CDC's Division of HIV and AIDS Research. Daskalakis is openly gay and sex-positive and the combination of these two leaders was considered to have been an important part of the effective response of the American MSM community to what was characterized an aggressive public health effort. In addition to direct messaging to at-risk individuals, Fenton and Daskalakis used evidence-based guidelines that helped doctors feel comfortable following their advice. Nonetheless, as the outbreak continued to grow – in case numbers and geographical spread – many of those surveyed were concerned there could be a backlash against the MSM community as there had been with HIV/AIDS in the 1980s, with those infected with the virus particularly stigmatized.[39]

Among the known at-risk population in the USA, there was a significant response both to public health messaging and to word-of-mouth information-sharing in the savvy and connected MSM community. A monkeypox-specific follow-up survey completed in August of 2022 by 824 MSM showed that 48% of respondents reported that since learning about the mpox outbreak, they had reduced their number of sex partners and 50% reported reducing one-time sexual encounters and sex with partners met on dating apps or at sex venues. Nearly one in five respondents reported receiving at least one dose of vaccine to prevent monkeypox.[40] There were racial/ethnic and socio-demographic differences in vaccine receipt which was highest among Hispanic/ Latino men (27.1%) and lowest among non-Hispanic Black/ African American men (11.5%); 17.7% of non-Hispanic White men and 24.2% of men of other race or ethnicity received the vaccine. Vaccination was also twice as high in urban and suburban areas.

As in the USA, an online survey in the Netherlands carried out in July and August of 2022 found that 50% of participants reported they had reduced their number of sexual partners and had selected partners more carefully; 66% reported they had avoided visits to gay saunas, sex clubs, and sex parties and were specifically avoiding sexual contacts infected with MPXV. Sex venues and parties in Amsterdam also reported a considerable drop in visitor numbers in July 2022.[41]

And then, suddenly – less than six months after it began – mpox case numbers dropped precipitously in multiple locations. It appears that the virus was controlled through the combination of a behavioral response to public health messaging in the at-risk community, and by adoption of pre-existing smallpox preparedness tools, especially the Jynneos vaccine. In the USA, more than 1 million vaccine doses were administered in 1 year. The emergency outbreak was over.

Despite these congratulatory comments, the fact is that we don't fully understand what drove the global decline since vaccine availability did not occur to any significant degree until after the sharp decline in mpox cases began. In the USA, the vaccine was not available to any extent until early July and a significant number of administered doses was not reported until August, after the steep decline in cases had already begun. In the Netherlands, investigators developed a transmission model fitted to data on mpox cases before July 25, 2022, when the mpox vaccination program started. Data on behavioral changes, namely fewer casual partners and abstention from anonymous sexual contacts were included. When vaccination started, 64% of MSM with very high sexual activity in the model had already been infected.[42] While we do not have a timetable for behavior change, it seems unlikely that this occurred rapidly enough to account for the precipitous decline of cases only three months after the first cases appeared. More likely, significant herd immunity developed in high-risk communities, secondary to the combination of mpox infections (including those that were unrecognized and/or unreported), and post-vaccination immunity, plus behavior change in response to public awareness facilitated by public health messaging. Even with these explanations, the dramatic decrease in cases is remarkable.

Treatment

A crucial factor in controlling the mpox outbreak was the rapid deployment of existing treatments that had been stockpiled for smallpox. After 9/11, the subject of treatment for smallpox was intensively revisited in the USA and globally, and potential vaccines and antiviral medications were identified; this effort is described in Chapter 2. Tecovirimat is an oral antiviral medication for orthopox viruses which inhibits the function of a major MPXV envelope protein required for the production of extracellular virus. In August 2018, the FDA approved TPOXX, a commercially developed version of tecovirimat, to treat smallpox and added two million doses to the American emergency biodefense stockpile. Per that approval, there are specific settings in which TPOXX is recommended: when mpox disease is severe with a large number of confluent or necrotic lesions or severe lymphadenopathy; when there is multi-organ system involvement and associated comorbidities; when pox lesions involve anatomic areas which might result in function-impairing scarring or strictures; or when mpox occurs in immunosuppressed individuals. Although not relevant to this outbreak, TPOXX is also recommended in children, particularly those less than 1 year of age; pregnant or breastfeeding individuals; or those with hemorrhagic disease or integrity-compromising skin conditions. Prescription of TPOXX is prescribed under an expanded access Investigational New Drug protocol and because of this, accessing the drug has been difficult but once approved, it is available from the Strategic National Stockpile at no cost. Through January 2023, 6832 patients with mpox had been treated with TPOXX.[43,44]

Cidofovir (also known as Vistide) is an antiviral agent approved by the FDA for the treatment of cytomegalovirus retinitis in patients with AIDS, and is commercially available as an injection. It has been shown to be effective against orthopoxviruses, in vitro and in animal studies. Data are not available on the effectiveness of cidofovir in treatment of mpox in humans but its use may be considered. Brincidofovir, a prodrug of cidofovir, has an improved safety profile over cidofovir which can cause serious renal toxicity. Brincidofovir is available for treatment of mpox to clinicians who request and obtain an FDA-authorized single-patient emergency use IND for patients with severe mpox who experienced disease progression while receiving TPOXX or have a contraindication for use of tecovirimat.

****

Looking Back :: Moving Forward

The global spread of monkeypox should not have been a surprise. Decades of rising mpox case numbers and of increasing human to human transmission in central and western Africa should have been enough to bring this virus to international attention. And only 5 years before the global pandemic began, there was a large outbreak in Nigeria – a country where mpox was only rarely seen – with a new clinical pattern in a new demographic population that introduced all the elements that subsequently characterized the 2022 global spread. Typically, when a pandemic caused by a novel virus appears, knowledge about the virus is limited and adaptive measures like vaccines and therapeutics are unavailable. This was the scenario with SARS-CoV-2 where even the rapid development of effective vaccines lagged behind the global spread of the virus. But with monkeypox, we knew the potential for this pandemic existed beginning in 1980 when smallpox vaccination ended. The MPXV was well identified and episodic surveillance documented the increasing size and frequency of mpox outbreaks in Africa. The 2017–2018 epidemic in Nigeria clearly demonstrated the evolution of the MPXV and the change in the disease pattern. We even had effective vaccines and putatively effective treatments in global stockpiles.

Out of nowhere? Definitely not.

There are mitigating factors that contributed to the incredibly rapid global spread of this virus. Past epidemics have usually been identified through recognition of an unusual cluster of severe cases. Mpox is not a severe disease and previous outbreaks had occurred almost exclusively in Africa so health care providers in other parts of the world may have had difficulty in recognizing pox lesions, especially when they presented in a new sub-population as occurred with the first mpox cases in 2022. But once those first cases had been diagnosed in multiple locations, failure to immediately recognize and react to the new population in which this outbreak occurred was indefensible. From the very first cases, this pandemic occurred almost exclusively in young men who have sex with men, often involving a history of multiple anonymous partners. There was reluctance to immediately begin public health messaging to this high-risk population because same-sex "amorous relationships" are banned in Nigeria and this group had been stigmatized in infectious disease crises before.[45] While vaccines and potential treatments were theoretically available when mpox went global, there proved to be too few doses of a new and unproven vaccine, treatments were untested and diagnostic tests were limited. And by the time the mpox pandemic began, the whole world was weary of dealing with the COVID-19 pandemic. While we hesitated, the virus spread like wildfire, potentially fueled by the sense of liberation that characterized the end of suppressive measures put in place to prevent the spread of SARS-CoV-2.

As documented in Chapter 11, we have multiple international surveillance systems like ProMED, an official unit of the Infectious Disease Society which links volunteer experts in human, plant and animal disease to subscribers in more than 200 countries who post media reports, online summaries and local observer reports to a public website using email; the Global Public Health Intelligence Network in Canada, which analyzes electronic data to recognize patterns indicative of a possible outbreak; and, the Global Outbreak Alert and Response Network (GOARN), which provides operations and logistics platforms for any WHO response to international public health risks. Combined, these programs coordinate multiple different types of information including electronic case reporting, health care product purchases, work or school absences, presenting symptoms to a health care provider and/or lab test orders to identify a new disease outbreak. The results of optimized, on-the-ground surveillance combined with ongoing internet surveillance from programs like these should allow the earliest possible visualization of potential new disease outbreaks. The information produced through these intensive processes of technological collection is critically analyzed as it emerges and then transmitted to international agencies who are primed to respond immediately. Despite the substantial potential firepower in systems like these, the mpox pandemic emerged almost undetected. It is abundantly clear that viral threats magnify rapidly and easily across geographic boundaries. For the future, we must combine global scan capacity and local preparedness to *immediately* deal with biological health threats as they emerge. Even allowing for the mitigating circumstances that characterized the mpox pandemic, we must do better.

As with all viral infections, progress is also needed in treating monkeypox. Tecovirimat (TPOXX) is an antiviral agent known to have a low resistance barrier since amino acid changes in the MPXV envelope protein that the drug targets can substantially reduce its activity. An ongoing randomized trial is being conducted in 3 sites in the DRC. Initiated in 2018 as part of NIAID DCR's emergency research response which began with the 2018 Ebola outbreak in the Eastern DCR, the protocol was directed at mpox caused by MPXV clade I; it was expanded to include clade IIb at study sites in the US and the United Kingdom when the 2022 outbreak appeared. Results of these trials are pending. Vaccinia immune globulin intravenous (VIGIV) − orthopoxvirus antibodies collected from an immune host − can theoretically be administered on an emergency basis to patients who are severely ill or immunocompromised but so far, there is no evidence that this is effective against monkeypox. There is ongoing research in the development of monoclonal antibodies against mpox and with accelerated development, these could theoretically be available within 3 to 6 months. However, the end of the mpox pandemic means the opportunity to test the safety and efficacy of new treatment methods has been curtailed by a decrease in potential subjects, a major limitation.

Although the Jynneos vaccine provides effective immediate protection against MPXV infection and IgG seropositivity was still present after 2 years, the actual duration of immunity is unknown. Pharmaceutical companies are developing a new vaccine using a norovirus-like particle platform that is designed to target specific antigens rather than the whole virus, and can be produced with simpler machinery. A cheaper and more readily produced vaccine like this should have specific application in Central and Western Africa where MPXV has been endemic for many decades. Though global mpox cases have waned for now, past pandemics have shown that it is essential to be prepared. For the future, efforts must focus on equitable distribution of knowledge and therapies to countries that have dealt with rising case numbers for years and will likely continue to harbor the MPXV and be affected by monkeypox outbreaks.[46]

This book explores the strong evidence that viral zoonoses represent a significant, ongoing threat to global health. The MPXV exemplifies a group of viruses like HIV and Ebola that have emerged from animal reservoirs in the Global South but have only come to attention when they caused a disease outbreak that threatened the global north: the response has been a sudden, panicked struggle to control the outbreak, treat the disease and prevent further cases. With monkeypox, we have no excuse – the progression from localized, self-contained outbreaks in rural Western and Central Africa to increasingly large urban outbreaks with potential for global spread was actually anticipated when smallpox vaccination ended in 1980. The dramatic outbreak which occurred in Nigeria in 2017 exactly predicted the global pandemic which emerged 5 years later. Increased and improved surveillance to detect emerging pathogens is frequently cited as the way to detect an emerging pathogen but here, surveillance *did* effectively identify MPXV and its emergence in a new population as a significant danger to global health. The WHO even addressed the increasing threat of mpox when they held an informal conference in 2018 but they failed to act on the emergence of a new pattern of the disease.[12] Even with substantial prior knowledge and a pre-existing vaccine, the MPXV caused 90,000 mpox cases in 113 countries.

Surveillance alone is not enough – specific methods to rapidly and effectively direct attention and resources to pathogens wherever and whenever they emerge are clearly needed.[47] It is possible that the interposition of COVID-19 which commanded the attention of the entire world was a critical factor in the failure to recognize the emergence of mpox. Nonetheless, we can and must do better to identify emerging disease threats to prevent them from becoming global pandemics.

The emergence of the mpox pandemic even before the COVID-19 pandemic had ended dramatically exposes our global failure to respond effectively to microbial threats. Over the last 120 years, we have seen the emergence of a series of high-impact pathogens which have jumped from animals to infect humans and initiated an accelerating spiral of global viral pandemics. As described with one virus after another in this book, the frequency and intensity of these pandemics has increased, driven by known factors including increasing human population size, urbanization, climate change, environmental degradation and globalized trade and travel.[48] With monkeypox, we must now add a primary and specific focus on the role of human behavior.

****

Addendum: January 2024

While editing this chapter, I found that without fanfare, the WHO had reported a new outbreak of mpox in late November 2023. Reportedly, the DRC has been experiencing its largest, most deadly outbreak of mpox for the last year, with more than 12,000 suspected cases and nearly 600 deaths (a fatality rate of 5.6%) caused by clade I of the MPXV. This far surpasses the death rate from the 2022 *global* mpox outbreak from which there has been only a small stream of confirmed cases since that outbreak was declared officially over in May 2023.

Historically, the dynamics of MPXV clade I transmission in the DRC are not well understood. Cases have been sporadic and the source of infection has been considered to be contact with infected animals or close, skin-to-skin contact between individuals, primarily children. During the 2022 multi-country outbreak, the DRC reported no clade IIb mpox cases but the total number of mpox cases, presumably caused by clade I, was increasing. Between January 1 and November 7, 2023, there has been a dramatic upsurge in cases including – for the first time – well-documented cases of clade I sexual transmission in MSM. In August 2023, mpox cases were reported in Kinshasa, the capital of the DRC, with a median age among confirmed cases of 24 years and a 2:1 ratio of males to females – suggestive of sexual transmission. The rapid rise in case numbers, the fatality rate of 5.6% and the history of sexual transmission are very concerning as is the spread to an urban setting.[47] For the clade IIb virus that spread globally in 2022, genetic analyses showed that several mutations might explain how it had changed to transmit more readily through sex but there is no evidence yet that the clade I virus isolated from these current DRC cases has undergone changes like these.[32,33] Nonetheless, with all these concerning features, the WHO is warning that MPXV clade I could also spread widely among sexual networks. In response, the Ministry of Public Health and Hygiene in the DRC established an Emergency Operations Centre and Incident Management Team in February 2023 but response capacities for mpox remain limited in the country. Stay tuned – with rising case numbers and the introduction of clade I MPXV into international sexual networks, the WHO assesses the risk of international spread to be high.

★★★★★★★★★

HISTORIC PERSPECTIVE: MPOX/MONKEYPOX

MPOX highlights a problem we have historically observed: when a disease is sexually transmitted, we are not very good at preventing it. This is especially true when it is associated with commercial or queer sex. Allan Brandt, in his groundbreaking work on STDs, *No Magic Bullet,* addresses the role of shame, cultural and personal, in the means used to try to prevent soldiers from purchasing sex and acquiring STDs

that would later be transmitted to their wives. One memorable poster designed during WWI warned, "A German bullet is cleaner than a whore." The idea of sex as itself pathological and dangerous persists in our culture, and the association of sex with contagion and risk is also a stubborn one. Look no further than the "bathroom laws" to appreciate the tenacity of our anxieties and our persistent need to control, and even disappear, sexualities that do not gain social approbation. But fear and hatred are not the only reasons that public health institutions might be reluctant to label a disease sexually transmitted. Around the world today, 12 countries impose the death penalty for same-sex sexuality, and six of them consistently apply it. Sixty-five jurisdictions across the world criminalize same-sex consensual sex, many of which specifically identify sex between men in their laws.[49] Institutions like the WHO must walk a gauntlet of educating people about a pandemic associated with a sexually transmitted virus and bringing an active gay community to the attention of a state that would kill them. Mpox, for example, has just appeared again in Nigeria, and in Northern Nigeria, men convicted of having sex with other men can be killed by the state. Should the WHO explicitly name MPXV as a virus most regularly transmitted through male homosexual sex, men with the disease are less likely to seek treatment and thus run the risk of significant complications. Doing so would bring them to the attention of the very authorities they avoid – on penalty of death. They are also less likely to be counted as part of the outbreak, so it will become harder for epidemiologists to map and understand the outbreak – and to respond appropriately. Thus, by only making oblique references to sexual transmission as the route of infection, the WHO is protecting potential targets of state violence. But they are not doing a very good job of getting information to doctors, public health workers, or the people who are likely to become infected.

The gay male community in the global north now has four decades of practice in communicating about the risk of disease. HIV/AIDS came at a time when being gay, even in the relatively liberal countries of North America and Europe, was still barely tolerated in the best cases and persecuted in the rest. When an unknown virus causing the loss of immune function – quickly and unhelpfully labeled GRID (Gay-related immune disease) by the CDC – appeared in San Francisco bathhouses, communication networks – public and underground – emerged to warn gay men of the new threat. Those communication networks morphed into active, resilient and durable powerhouses that insisted that HIV/AIDS research required funding, that patients deserved respectful care, and that the threat of allowing a virus to decimate an entire generation had to take precedence over homophobia. In 1982, in response to the United States government's absolute refusal to discuss HIV/AIDS or fund research into the virus or the disease, Larry Kramer, Nathan Fain, Larry Mass, Paul Popham and Edmund White established the Gay Men's Health Crisis (GMHC). It provided information about the disease through several outlets: establishing a telephone hotline, distributing a printed newsletter that was sent to doctors, libraries, and government officials, and – beginning in 1984 – disseminating guidelines for safer sex. Their informational posters and brochures about condom use appeared in gay clubs and bathhouses, where they reached the people who needed them most. Now the GMHC may best be remembered for its prodigious fundraising efforts on behalf of HIV/AIDS research and patients, and its landmark lawsuits demanding equal protection for AIDS patients. But arguably its most powerful role was using a strong underground social network to educate and inform community members about the risk of unprotected sex. Gay men already navigated the tightrope of discrimination, many staying publicly in the closet to protect themselves and their families, but they knew where the clubs and bars were. And they knew who to ask about a disease that suddenly made their silence even more dangerous. When the GMHC telephone hotline began offering email as an alternative in 2000, a new horizon of communication became available.

Social media might seem an excellent alternative for spreading accurate information about new viruses, modes of transmission, and means of prevention. It is – but because access is limited and tracked under many fascist regimes, it is not a perfect addition. When your online search history can be reviewed at any time, your movement on social media and participation in specific groups or sites tracked, and your online interests criminalized, you might be less likely to participate. The importance of personal communication and known personal networks remains critically important in informing people in persecuted sexual communities about diseases that could kill them.

The immense success of the GMHC-led Mpox vaccine drive reflects the importance and efficacy of institutions like this one. In New York City, which saw epidemic levels of Mpox among gay men during the summer of 2022, thousands of vaccination appointments were filled within hours. The demand for more vaccines and fair treatment for sufferers was supported by the effective and active agents of the GMHC, who demanded that New York State and New York City governments respond without hesitation to this new viral outbreak.

The WHO and other international groups such as MSF would benefit from working through existing social networks and small community-based groups that already serve at-risk groups. Coding their language less obliquely when working with doctors who traditionally treat gay men would also help to educate those at risk of getting and transmitting the disease without putting them at risk of being prosecuted. They are well aware of the risks associated with labeling this a "gay disease," and, in fact, were unable to reach a consensus about labeling mpox as a sexually transmitted disease associated with gay male sex *because* of the threat of perpetuating stigma and inciting violence against gay men. Balancing the risks of stigma and hate crimes against the risk posed by the virus itself is a juggling act requiring tremendous skill. Jason Ciancotto, a vice president of GMHC who was very active in the American movement to educate about mpox, says it perfectly: "We are not going to end HIV, and we're certainly not going to curtail the monkeypox epidemic, by trying to shame people into not having sex or only having certain types of sex with certain people." He adds, "When you equip people with the information they need to make healthy choices for themselves and for their community, and when you help them approach those decisions with self-love and acceptance, it's amazing what the community is able to achieve."[50]

References

1. Kraemer MUG, Tegally T, Pigott DM, et al. Tracking the 2022 monkeypox outbreak with epidemiological data in real-time. *Lancet Inf Dis* 2022; 22(7): 941–942. Published: June 08, 2022. doi: https://doi.org/10.1016/S1473-3099(22)00359-0

2. McCollum AM, Damon IK. Human Monkeypox. *Clin Infect Dis* 2014; 58 (2):260–267, https://doi.org/10.1093/cid/cit703

3. Likos AM, Sammons SA, Olson VA, et al. A tale of two clades: monkeypox viruses. *J Gen Virol* 2005; 86(Pt 10): 2661–2672. www.ncbi.nlm.nih.gov/pubmed/16186219

4. Fine PE, Jezek Z, Grab B, Dixon H. The transmission potential of monkeypox virus in human populations. *Int J Epidemiol*. 1988; 17:643–50.

5. Heymann DL, Szczeniowski M, Esteves K. Re-emergence of monkeypox in Africa: a review of the past six years. *Br Med Bull*. 1998;54(3):693–702. doi: 10.1093/oxfordjournals.bmb.a011720. PMID: 10326294.

6. Jezek Z, Grab B, Dixon H. Stochastic model for interhuman spread of monkeypox. *Am J Epidemiol*. 1987 Dec;126(6):1082–92. doi: 10.1093/oxfordjournals.aje.a114747. PMID: 2825518.

7. Hutin YJ, Williams RJ, Malfait P, Pebody R, Loparev VN, Ropp SL, Rodriguez M, Knight JC, Tshioko FK, Khan AS, Szczeniowski MV, Esposito JJ. Outbreak of human monkeypox, Democratic Republic of Congo, 1996 to 1997. *Emerg Infect Dis*. 2001 May–Jun;7(3):434–8. doi: 10.3201/eid0703.010311. PMID: 11384521; PMCID: PMC2631782.

8. Multistate Outbreak of Monkeypox – Illinois, Indiana, Kansas, Missouri, Ohio, and Wisconsin, 2003. *Mor Mort WR* 2003; 52(27): 642–646.

9. Rimoin AW, Mulembakani PM, Johnston SC, et al. Major increase in human monkeypox incidence 30 years after smallpox vaccination campaigns cease in the Democratic Republic of Congo. *Proc Natl Acad Sci U S A*. 2010 Sep 14;107(37):16262–7. doi: 10.1073/pnas.1005769107. Epub 2010 Aug 30. PMID: 20805472; PMCID: PMC2941342.

10. Yinka-Ogunleye A, Aruna O, Ogoina D, et al. Reemergence of Human Monkeypox in Nigeria, 2017. *Emerg Infect Dis.* 2018; 24(6):1149–1151. https://doi.org/10.3201/eid2406.180017

11. Ogoina D, Izibewule JH, Ogunleye A, et al. The 2017 human monkeypox outbreak in Nigeria – Report of outbreak experience and response in the Niger Delta University Teaching Hospital, Bayelsa State, Nigeria. *PLoS ONE* 2019; 14(4): e0214229. Published April 17, 2019. https://doi.org/10.1371/journal.pone.0214229

12. Durski KN, McCollum AM, Nakazawa Y, et al. Emergence of Monkeypox – West and Central Africa, 1970–2017. *MMWR Morb Mortal Wkly Rep* 2018; 67:306–310. doi: http://dx.doi.org/10.15585/mmwr.mm6710a5external icon

13. McCollum AM, Shelus V, Hill A, et al. Epidemiology of Human Mpox – Worldwide, 2018–2021. *MMWR Morb Mortal Wkly Rep* 2023;72:68–72. doi: http://dx.doi.org/10.15585/mmwr.mm7203a4

14. Vaughn A, Aarons E, Astbury J, et al. Two cases of monkeypox imported to the United Kingdom, September 2018. *Euro Surveill.* 2018;23(38):pii=1800509. https://doi.org/10.2807/1560-7917.ES.2018.23.38.1800509

15. Perez Duque M, Ribeiro S, Martins JV, et al. Ongoing monkeypox virus outbreak, Portugal, 29 April to 23 May 2022. *Euro Surveill.* 2022 Jun;27(22):2200424. doi: 10.2807/1560-7917.ES.2022.27.22.2200424. PMID: 35656830; PMCID: PMC9164676.

16. Vivancos R, Anderson C, Blomquist P, et al. Monkeypox Incident Management Team. Community transmission of monkeypox in the United Kingdom, April to May 2022. *Euro Surveill.* 2022. Jun;27(22):2200422. doi: 10.2807/1560-7917. ES.2022.27.22.2200422. Erratum in: Euro Surveill. 2022 Jun;27(23): PMID: 35656834; PMCID: PMC9164677.

17. WHO Report. World Mpox (Monkeypox) Outbreak – 2022. www.who.int/emergencies/situations/monkeypox-oubreak-2022

18. Heymann D. Monkeypox spread likely "amplified" by sex at 2 raves in Europe, leading WHO adviser says. May 23, 2022 / CBS News Health Watch/AP

19. Khan MR, Hossain MJ, Roy A, Islam MR. Decreasing trend of monkeypox cases in Europe and America shows hope for the world: evidence from the latest epidemiological data. *Health Sci Rep.* 2022;6:e1030. Published online, December, 2022. doi: 10.1002/hsr2.1030

20. Bramswell H. WHO declares end to global health emergency over monkeypox. 2023. www.statnews.com/2023/05/11/who-ends-global-health-emergency-over-mpox/

21. Thornhill JP, Barkati S, Walmsley S, et al. Monkeypox virus infection in humans across 16 countries – April–June 2022. *N Engl J Med* 2022; 387:679–691. doi: 10.1056/NEJMoa2207323

22. Thornhill, JP, Palich R, Ghosn J, et al. Human monkeypox virus infection in women and non-binary individuals during the 2022 outbreaks: a global case series. *Lancet* 2022; 400(103670):1953–1965. Published online, November 17, 2022. doi: https://doi.org/10.1016/S0140-6736(22)02187-0

23. Mitja O, Alemany A, Marks M, et al. Mpox in people with advanced HIV infection: a global case series. *Lancet* 2023; 401: 939–949. Published online: February 21, 2023. doi: https://doi.org/10.1016/S0140-6736(23)00273-8

24. Yinka-Ogunleye A, Aruna O, Dalhat M, et al. CDC Monkeypox Outbreak Team. Outbreak of human monkeypox in Nigeria in 2017–18: a clinical and epidemiological report. *Lancet Infect Dis.* 2019 Aug;19(8):872–879. doi: 10.1016/S1473-3099(19)30294-4. Epub 2019 Jul 5. PMID: 31285143; PMCID: PMC9628943.

25. Americo JL, Earl PL, Moss B. Virulence differences of mpox (monkeypox) virus clades I, IIa, and IIb.1 in a small animal model. *PNAS* 2023; 120 (8) e2220415120. https://doi.org/10.1073/pnas.2220415120

26. Mazzotta AA, Mazzotta V, Vita S, et al. INMI Monkeypox Group. Epidemiological, clinical and virological characteristics of four cases of monkeypox support transmission through sexual contact, Italy, May 2022. *Euro Surveill.* 2022 Jun; 27(22):2200421. doi: 10.2807/1560-7917.ES.2022.27.22.2200421. PMID: 35656836; PMCID: PMC9164671.

27. Peiro-Mestres A, Fuertes I, Camprubi-Ferrer D, et al. Frequent detection of monkeypox virus DNA in saliva, semen, and other clinical samples from 12 patients, Barcelona, Spain, May to June 2022. *Euro Surveill* 2022; 27:2200503.

28. Ward T, Christie R, Paton R S, Cumming F, Overton CE. Transmission dynamics of monkeypox in the United Kingdom: contact tracing study. *BMJ* 2022; 379: e073153 doi:10.1136/bmj-2022-073153

29. Antia R, Regoes R, Koella J, et al. The role of evolution in the emergence of infectious diseases. *Nature* 2003: 426, 658–661. https://doi.org/10.1038/nature02104

30. Isidro J. Borges V. Pinto M, et al. Phylogenomic characterization and signs of microevolution in the 2022 multi-country outbreak of monkeypox virus. *Nat Med* 28, 1569–1572 (2022). https://doi.org/10.1038/s41591-022-01907-y

31. Gao L, Shi Q, Dong X, et al. Mpox, caused by the MPXV of the Clade IIb Lineage, Goes Global. *Trop Med Infect Dis.* 2023 Feb; 8(2): 76. Published online 2023 Jan 20. doi: 10.3390/tropicalmed8020076

32. O'Toole A, Neher R A, Ndodo N, et al. Putative APOBEC3 deaminase editing in MPXV as evidence for sustained human transmission since at least 2016. *bioRxiv preprint.* Posted January 24, 2023. https://doi.org/10.1101/2023.01.23.525187; this version.

33. Gigante CM, Korber B, Seabolt MH, et al. Multiple lineages of monkeypox virus detected in the United States, 2021–2022. *Science.* 2022 Nov 4;378(6619):560–565. doi: 10.1126/science.add4153.

34. Vaccines | Smallpox | CDC. Available at: www.cdc.gov › smallpox › clinicians › vaccines. Accessed on Feb.6, 2020.

35. Desai AN, Malani PN. JYNNEOS vaccine for Mpox. *JAMA.* 2023; 329(22):1995. doi:10.1001/jama.2023.9873

36. Wolff Sagy Y, Zucker R, Hammerman A, et al. Real-world effectiveness of a single dose of Mpox vaccine in males. *Nat Med* 2023; 29: 748–752 (2023). https://doi.org/10.1038/s41591-023-02229-3

37. Payne AB, Ray LC, Cole MM, et al. Reduced risk for Mpox after receipt of 1 or 2 doses of JYNNEOS vaccine compared with risk among unvaccinated persons – 43 U.S. Jurisdictions, July 31–October 1, 2022. *MMWR Morb Mortal Wkly Rep* 2022;71:1560–1564. doi: http://dx.doi.org/10.15585/mmwr.mm7149a5

38. Dalton AF, Diallo AO, Chard AN, et al. Estimated effectiveness of JYNNEOS vaccine in preventing Mpox: A multijurisdictional case-control study – United States, August 19, 2022–March 31, 2023. *MMWR Morb Mortal Wkly Rep,* 2023. doi: 10.15585/mmwr.mm7220a3

39. Perceptions of monkeypox from those most at risk: men who have sex with men having multiple sexual partners. *WHO News Release.* 26 August 2022. www.who.int/europe/news/item/26-08-2022-perceptions-of-monkeypox-from-those-most-at-risk--men-who-have-sex-with-men-having-multiple-sexual-partners

6

40. Delaney KP, Sanchez T, Hannah M, et al. Strategies adopted by gay, bisexual, and other men who have sex with men to prevent Monkeypox virus transmission United States, August 2022. *MMWR Morb Mortal Wkly Rep* 2022; 71:1126–1130. doi: http://dx.doi.org/10.15585/mmwr.mm7135e1

41. Xiridou M, Miura F, Adam P, et al. The fading of the Mpox outbreak among men who have sex with men: a mathematical modelling study. medRxiv preprint, posted February 15, 2023. https://doi.org/10.1101/2023.01.31.23285294

42. Mucker EM, Goff AJ, Shamblin JD, et al. Efficacy of Tecovirimat (ST-246) in Nonhuman Primates Infected with Variola Virus (Smallpox). *Antimicrob Agents Chemother* 2013; 57(12):6246–6253.

43. De Clercq E. Clinical potential of the acyclic nucleoside phosphonates cidofovir, adefovir, and tenofovir in treatment of DNA virus and retrovirus infections. *Clin Microbiol Rev* 2003; 16:569.

44. Dennis Carroll D, Daszak P, Wolfe ND, et al. The global virome project. *Science* 2018; 359: 872–874. doi:10.1126/science.aap7463

45. Treiser R "As monkeypox spreads, know the difference between warning and stigmatizing people." July 26, 2022, www.npr.org/2022/07/26/1113713684/monkeypox-stigma-gay-community

46. Harris E. Global Monkeypox outbreaks spur drug research for the neglected disease. *JAMA* 2022; 328(3):231–233. doi:10.1001/jama.2022.11224 World Health Organization (23 November 2023).

47. Carroll D, Morzaria S, Briand S, et al. Preventing the next pandemic: the power of a global viral surveillance network. *BMJ* 2021; 372: n485. (Published 12 March 2021) doi: 10.1136/bmj.n485

48. Disease Outbreak News; Mpox (monkeypox) in the Democratic Republic of the Congo. Available at: www.who.int/emergencies/disease-outbreak-news/item/2023-DON493

49. humandignitytrust.org/lgbt-the-law/map-of-criminalisation/www.gmhc.org/history/ www.humandignitytrust.org/lgbt-the-law/a-history-of-criminalisation/

50. Cionciotta J. Monkeypox explained: How to protect yourself and what to watch out for. NPR. Monkeypox explained: How to protect yourself and what to watch out for. August 5, 2022.

Suggested Reading

Kimberly Ashby. *Monkeypox: Fact or Fiction*. Self-published. 2022.

Robert Rice. *Monkeypox Virus Disease: A Global Threat to Humanity (An Emergency Call For Survival)*. Self-published. 2022.

Ronald Naresh. *The Monkeypox Virus: An In-Depth Expose on Outbreak Causes, Symptoms, Prevention, and Effective Treatment*. Self-published. 2022.

Tracy J Larsen. *The Curious Outbreak of Monkeypox Virus: The Origin, Outbreaks in the U.S., Transmission, Symptoms, Prevention and Treatment*. Self-published. 2022.

Zdeněk Jezek, Frank Fenner. *Human Monkeypox*. S. Karger AG. 1988.

10

A LOOK BACK

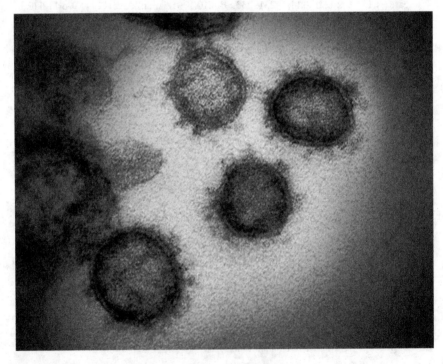

FIGURE 10.1 Electron micrograph of SARS–CoV-2.

Source: Photo courtesy of NIAID.US.gov

DOI: 10.4324/9781003427667-10

DAYS GONE :: DAYS TO COME

This book examines the disease narratives of viral pandemics, beginning with smallpox and yellow fever and extending right through until 2024, with the global pandemic of HIV/AIDS still ongoing, with MPOX/monkeypox just behind us, and the COVID-19 pandemic still on the wane. Even a casual read reveals the dramatic increase in frequency, severity and extent of global disease outbreaks caused by viruses over the last half-century. Epidemiologists, virologists, medical historians and health care providers all over the world are contending with a disturbing new stream of contemporary viral epidemics. In writing this book, we have combined an explanation of the biology of viral epidemics with an exploration of the global context in which they occurred and a description of the corresponding response of science and medicine. The book has followed the chronologic history of viral pandemics, examining each in order.

In these last two chapters, the Doctors Kavey take a different approach. The first chapter – A Look Back – is written by Allison and critically evaluates the response to COVID-19 in the context of the long history of global pandemics. In the last chapter – A Way Forward – Rae-Ellen creates a composite picture of the state of viral infectious disease outbreaks by integrating the biological and environmental factors that emerged as critical in the analysis of the pandemics in the book. It is our hope that by combining the lessons of the past and the present, we can potentially see how to best achieve more timely and effective responses in the future.

A Look Back

As you have read, the history of pandemics provides a specific perspective on the history of the twentieth century. The previous chapters have lauded the scientific achievements and advances in medical practice that resulted from viruses originally understood only as causes of death. The discovery of specific viruses and development of vaccines, in particular, has marked a significant achievement in human comprehension of and ability to withstand viruses. But we still have a great deal to learn, and this chapter takes the opportunity to better understand COVID-19 and our public health responses to it through the lens of the history of our responses to pandemics. By reviewing the development of public health as a field and learning why it continues to rely on a few, traditional approaches to tackling epidemics, we can better understand where we went wrong with COVID-19 and how we can do better when we face the next viral pandemic.

****

I am a historian. Furthermore, I am an early modern historian, which means my expertise reaches back several hundred years before influenza, to a time when all epidemics were defined by the plague, which had fundamentally altered the population and social structure of western Europe between 1348 and 1351 and continued to intermittently explode well into the seventeenth century. At that time, inoculation was practiced regularly in only a few areas (largely the Ottoman East, including Turkey) and was attacked for potentially intervening divine will and causing new pandemics. People did not trust the apparent gift of scientific knowledge that could save them if they were meant to die or kill them by mistake. Urbanization was increasing, but the mortality rate due to starvation, accidents, and diseases of all kinds often exceeded in-migration rates. Disease was believed to result from divine punishment, a curse, miasma or bad water, or just bad luck. Medicine involved treatment intended to restore humoral balance either through sympathetic or antipathetic approaches, herbal remedies, patent medicines sold in trade fairs, and amulets (protective or curative) made or purchased to ward off or cure disease. Medical practitioners came from a variety of backgrounds and classes, were often very expensive, about equally ineffective, and frequently mistrusted as money-grubbing charlatans. Competing belief systems defined the ways in which people understood disease, the authorities they trusted, and the lengths to which they would go to combat a pandemic. They also determined who had the power to force others to comply. In all the epidemics in Europe, for example, for which Jews were scapegoated for poisoning Christians, there are no stories of Jews blaming Christians for disease in their quarters. Sects within Catholicism blamed other Catholic sects or Protestants (and vice versa) for causing epidemics by angering God, but they rarely turned that idea on their own communities. Finally, for many people, the idea of moving beyond a 100-mile radius of the town in which they were born was both unimaginable and unnecessary, and people who looked, believed or behaved differently were utterly frightening and inherently dangerous. The world of disease was very different and so was the response to it.

But, perhaps for the first time ever, my graduate training is perfectly relevant to a modern problem because our response to COVID-19 was not solely grounded in rational, scientific thinking. Should you be wondering to what I refer, let me list the following. The American president at the time, Donald Trump, loudly promoted the use of ivermectin, traditionally used for the treatment of roundworms, as an effective treatment. He also trumpeted the utility of hydroxy-chloroquine, a treatment for malaria. In 2024, Tractor Supply still has warning signs up telling customers not to take ivermectin as a treatment for COVID-19. There is some research supporting the use of ivermectin in treating mild cases of COVID-19, and its broad availability throughout the world has caused some researchers to recommend its use.[1] That does not make it a replacement for the vaccine or for effective anti-retroviral medications. Furthermore, at the time that Trump was promoting its use, there was minimal evidence that it had any effect. Much like the charlatans and mountebanks who capitalized on the terror surrounding the plague by selling amulets and religious icons, Trump and others sold promises they could not keep.[2]

Religious practice and beliefs also changed in the face of the virus. At a time of increasing secularization in the Global North, religious belief strengthened in response to a pandemic that seemingly affected everyone. As it has done for so many historical crises that challenged the human desire to make sense of an unpredictable and frightening world, religious belief offered an explanation for the inexplicable. Furthermore, religious practice offered a set of things to do in the face of tragedy: the ritual of religious practice can provide comfort and a feeling of doing something, when there is little to be done.[3,4] The cultural tools we have to cope with a frightening, destabilizing and fatal disease have not changed much since 1348.

As I write this, the United States is once again experiencing a post-holiday COVID-19 surge, which could be equal to or even greater than the one experienced with the arrival of the Omicron variant. At the same time, very few people are changing their activities, staying home, or even wearing masks. If, as *The Washington Post* claims, stay-at-home restrictions were only ever intended to "flatten the curve … to prevent a surge of patients who were critically ill with an unfamiliar pathogen from overwhelming hospitals," then we are counting on some degree of immunity and the previous deaths of those with pre-existing conditions to accomplish that task. The efficacy of this strategy could be better than you might think, at least if you have some risk tolerance: 35,000 people were hospitalized for confirmed cases of COVID-19 during the week of December 30, 2023, as opposed to 44,000 at the peak last year.[5] If our primary concern is limiting strain on hospitals, then we might be getting there without further public health measures. But before we do what the majority of people wish for – wave goodbye forever to pandemic restrictions and shortages and get back to our lives (though perhaps not our offices) – I think it is worth taking a few minutes to consider what we did not learn from the pandemics that preceded COVID and how they influenced our approach to this pandemic. We need to acknowledge the mistakes we made this time around; placing them in historic context helps to demonstrate their impact. We also made some new mistakes, and it is important to understand what we can do better. Because the next pandemic will be here soon, and we need to be better prepared.

Public Health and Vaccine Development: A Review of Approaches and Conclusions

Quarantine

We have already discussed the development of the public health system and reviewed its reactions across various viral pandemics. But the virus-by-virus approach taken in this book is not always the best way to appreciate the development of a system that took centuries yet still has only three options for dealing with outbreaks of contagious disease: quarantine/containment; prevention through vector identification and elimination – usually accomplished through improved sanitation or behavior change; and vaccination development and provision. Here is a short and important review: the bubonic plague in 1348 formalized the use of quarantine to keep infected individuals and vessels separate from uninfected populations. Quarantine is difficult to enforce, even in 1348, and it assumes no infection is present when no individuals are actively symptomatic, which turns out to be inaccurate for many diseases. But it is a good start for limiting the spread of highly contagious diseases spread by direct physical contact or aerosols. It would be the standard approach throughout the early modern period, with uneven application according to social class – the English aristocracy tended to leave London for the countryside when "the sweat" hit the city, but some were already affected and brought it with them, while the poor were forced to continue working to survive and frequently earned extra money by selling the clothing, shoes, and jewelry taken from corpses. Contact with those corpses obviously increased mortality rates among that population. Quarantine is a good and effective approach to regulating disease spread only when it is effectively enforced across all socioeconomic strata and it is a hard thing to accomplish since it must begin before anyone infected leaves the original geographic region hit by the disease. Since most viruses are not immediately symptomatic and certainly not all are immediately distinguishable from similar but less dangerous diseases, quarantine almost always is a reaction that starts too late to prevent contagion from spreading.

Sanitation

Starting in the late eighteenth century, cholera provided a second outlet for efforts to control disease. John Snow was able to define the cause of a cholera outbreak by mapping cases and determining that they all used water from one pump. By turning off that pump, he effectively turned off the epidemic. He accurately deduced that this meant the water from that well was infected, which led to the effective next question: how do you prevent water from becoming polluted? It also raised the second question – can you control disease by eliminating the vectors that carry it? The two major founders of urban public health, Edwin Chadwick and Lemuel Shattuck, argued the best way to accomplish this was dual efforts to improve sanitation, especially in urban areas, as a general approach to controlling vectors such as rats, flies, and fleas combined with specific efforts to identify vectors responsible for causing individual viruses. This led to some false starts – many pigs died, for example, during the 1918 flu epidemic which was falsely linked to swine flu, and flies died in huge numbers to prevent polio outbreaks during the 1950s. But it also improved sanitation for millions of urban dwellers over time, and I am sure anyone who has survived a garbage strike has a true and loyal appreciation for the efforts of public sanitation workers.

Vaccination

Edward Jenner, aided by the powerful diplomatic wife Lady Mary Wortley Montague, introduced inoculation to Europe. His story is so well known I will not repeat it here, but the introduction of smallpox inoculation and vaccination fundamentally changed the course of medical history by allowing us to effectively protect people from getting a virus. The prisoners on whom the vaccine was tested foreshadowed the many inmates – of prisons and asylums – who would be test cases for future vaccines, including polio. The local outbreaks of smallpox that occurred because of inoculation foreshadowed future outbreaks of other viruses caused by live virus vaccines, including laboratory mistakes in vaccine preparation. The uneven distribution of vaccine across class lines and international borders continues today. But perhaps the biggest cost of vaccination was that it made us feel safe. From the end of the mid-twentieth century polio pandemics, we have enjoyed remarkable good health because of vaccination. Most children in the global north no longer die of, or are permanently affected by, the specters of the pre-vaccination era childhood infectious diseases: measles, mumps, scarlet fever, and polio. We have grown complacent in this historically unique period, and without the constant fear of childhood epidemics, we have come to question rather than appreciate the benefits of vaccination. There were significant human costs in developing these vaccines, but the gain has been far greater.

Public Health Historical Summary

And so we went on for about a century, improving public health by limiting the movement of infected populations and keeping them separate from asymptomatic ones, improving the quality of the water supply, providing reliable garbage removal, developing public sewer systems rather than allowing open drains and cess pits that ran directly into waterways, and – after Joseph Lister's amazing gangrene research was published in 1867 – aggressively cleaning the homes of anyone who died of or survived an infectious disease with carbolic acid. A few codicils: these efforts were disproportionately applied to urban settings, where epidemic disease was more common and more deadly because of overcrowding; these efforts were not universally employed at all socioeconomic levels, with a greater amount of freedom given to the rich and less to the poor; vaccination was not universally adopted and a significant debate raged about the relationship of divine will to vaccination (did God send the disease to be endured, so that vaccination was hubris or did God provide the knowledge to prevent the disease, thus making it heretical not to do so?); rats and flies are certainly unpleasant, but pest control should have included mosquitoes earlier for better efficacy. These efforts also owed as much to the Hippocratic treatise, "Airs, Waters, Places" and applied observation as they did to what we would now call medicine.

It was only with Koch and the discovery of the tubercle bacillus in the late 1800s that we moved from general public health efforts to specific, body and then cell level understandings of disease, shifting from limiting disease vectors to identifying causes, modes of transmission, and–in the case of viruses, developing vaccines. Tuberculosis, the bacterial infection which in many ways defined the nineteenth-century medical universe and provided symptom to autopsy evidence, was both enlightening and infuriating. It played upon many of the weaknesses our medical system still has, and thus even though it is not viral, I will devote a few lines to it here to better understand those weaknesses. Tuberculosis looks like many other common respiratory infections, it has a long incubation period and, after it is walled off by the body and becomes latent, only arises again when the immune system falters. Patients with active TB are infectious during the first stage of the disease and again after it becomes active. The disease is highly infectious to those sharing air with an infected person, which in the nineteenth century included large numbers of people: for the poor, packed into tiny apartments with poor or no ventilation and working in factories with similar conditions, sharing air was inevitable. The larger homes and better ventilation found in wealthier homes should have helped to prevent disease spread, but many businessmen and their wives infected with tuberculosis continued to work, entertain, serve on charities, and go about in society, thus effectively spreading the disease among their peers, while servants working in the homes of infected individuals carried the disease across class lines. Doctors treating tuberculosis as a public health risk advocated strict control and some even supported mandatory registration for poor TB patients but were unwilling to put such strictures on their wealthy patients, and thus the disease continued to thrive.[6] So, entering the twentieth century and the first of the great modern viral pandemics, we have the following: uneven application of quarantine procedures, uneven application of infrastructure improvement, incomplete understanding of disease causation and transmission, almost complete inability to cope with diseases whose early symptoms belied their severity, mimicked other common diseases, or had lengthy periods between infection and significant symptoms.

Specific Viruses, Specific Lessons

Influenza

It cannot be a huge shock then that the influenza pandemic of 1918 was devastating. The incredible thing about our response to that virus, however, was the efficacy of thoughtful and rigorously enforced local interventions. Individual cities that employed clear quarantine procedures and maintained strict rules about public gatherings demonstrated the potential of these seemingly simple protocols.[7,8] A rich historiography compares the local approaches taken in many different cities and demonstrates how a coherent, rapid and aggressive response helped to contain mortality rates in St Louis.[7] On the public health level, influenza left us with stronger local infrastructure in some places and a better knowledge of how quickly interventions need to be applied to be effective. The role of the American Red Cross – described in Chapter 4 – in enforcing local efforts is an important codicil to the 1918 epidemic.[9] By combining the strengths of local government – a powerful force, especially in smaller cities where government officials are often well known and have neighborhood affiliations as well as institutional power – and NGOs staffed by local and imported workers, well-designed efforts to control viral spread can be made even more effective.[10]

On the virology level, however, that strain of the flu proved frustrating. Many leads resulted in dead ends, and the answers to, "why was that strain of influenza so fatal in otherwise healthy young adults," and "how can we prevent another strain like it from emerging" remain unknown despite decades of work. Research progressed enough to show that the influenza virus is resilient, quick to mutate and highly transmissible, that it can jump from animals to humans (avian flu and swine flu being excellent examples, though the swine flu research during the pandemic proved to be a dead end), medical management of individual cases has inconsistent results, and rapid and aggressive public health responses are critical to containing case spread. You might think we put all of those pieces together and turned to the hard work of creating a national, if not international, approach to controlling respiratory viruses. We should have. But the global depression that followed the First World War defeated such efforts, which were deemed to be unnecessary government expenditures.

Because we were busily looking forwards, we also missed an important demographic fact with significant public health implications. Entering the 1918 pandemic, the United States was characterized by dramatic racial variations in mortality, and one might expect influenza to exaggerate those. Existing racial prejudice permitted the opening of white-only clinics throughout the nation, and medical care remained out of reach for many people – especially the poor and African Americans. An increase in racial mortality was certainly the case for the more recent pandemics of HIV/AIDS and COVID-19. It was not the case for the 1918 influenza pandemic, and it would not be for polio either although with polio, the urban poor – African Americans and immigrants – were scapegoated.[11] But ironically, poverty and poor sanitation protected the poor and African American communities from both viruses since early exposure promoted immunity.

Polio

If the influenza pandemic showed the limitations to traditional public health responses such as quarantine and the elimination of public gatherings, which are only as effective as they are enforced, polio showed the racial and socioeconomic biases inherent in our understanding of disease. We did not travel very far from the 1894 tuberculosis registration debate referenced above, in which poor people were easily imagined as listable and quarantine-eligible, while the wealthy were considered above such interventions, before polio once again challenged our ideas about how best to handle public health in the face of viral pandemics. Polio was a periodic "visitor" during the first part of the twentieth century, reaching epidemic levels several times – for example, the 1916 outbreak in New York City was responsible for around 2400 deaths, and it is estimated that polio killed or paralyzed about 500,000 people every year on a global scale by mid-century. The traditional story of polio is the medical triumph of identifying the virus and then making an effective vaccine, with the race between Sabin and Salk and the funding provided by the March of Dimes playing defining roles. This scientific victory, which through significant global effort and funding to provide vaccination to every child, saw the 2002 eradication of polio in the Americas and significant declines in case numbers all over the world, paved the way for later attempts to develop vaccines for viruses such as HIV/AIDS and COVID-19. Vaccines were clearly the wave of the future, and at a time when western culture welcomed science the mark of a civilized society and the defining force of a powerful culture, vaccine research joined atomic investigations in defining Western power over the natural world. But vaccines do not operate in a vacuum, and they must be integrated into a public health infrastructure that supports their development, accurately educates the public about virus transmission, enforces crowd limiting efforts, and – once a vaccine is developed – gets "shots into arms." The public health network into which polio plunged before and during vaccine development had significant problems that contributed to morbidity and mortality. An accurate understanding of how the polio virus was transmitted was the first significant problem. Polio was integrated into the "filth disease" understanding of transmission, but the actual mode was misunderstood and the public health information campaign that ensued was inaccurate and exaggerated existing socioeconomic biases while providing a target for middle class, white, suburban anxiety. It scapegoated "the slums" and their inhabitants for poor garbage disposal methods that brought polio to wealthy areas on the wings of flies.[12] Insects frequently are disease vectors, and this research direction did not wane even after fly eradication efforts during the 1916 epidemic showed no significant decrease in cases. The idea was supported by a 1941 study by Sabin and Ward in which flies were collected from Atlanta and Cleveland, where polio was active, and – after being macerated and injected directly into Cynomolgus monkeys – caused a total of four new active cases. It remained strong despite further fly eradication campaigns in 1945 in New Jersey and 1947 in Illinois failed to statistically reduce polio cases. The fly diversion was an expensive mistake, and public health campaigns that championed fly swatting and mass insect eradication continued even after the 1948 trial that demonstrated fly eradication had no effect on the raging epidemic in Hidalgo, Texas.[13]

The fly as vector was just too appealing to dismiss, even among scientists and especially for the public. It provided a scapegoat to focus cultural hysteria regarding this dangerous and mercurial virus, which seemed to randomly cause mild stomach upset in one child and paralysis in another. It also focused middle class terror on a known and recognizable threat: immigrants and the poor, who already challenged ideas about citizenship, "the common good," and American identity.

The second significant error characterizing the public health campaign against polio was the closing of schools and other public gathering places, such as movie theaters and swimming pools, that served children. The poliovirus is introduced by oral-fecal transmission, not aerosols. Teaching correct handwashing technique and enforcing it in school-aged children would have been a much more effective and less costly approach to controlling the virus. The closures of schools, in particular, created an economic and educational deficit that was still present in affected adults.[14] It is possible some cases were prevented through school closures, simply because keeping children – the main carriers of the virus – away from each other would result in fewer cases. It was, however, a blunt and inaccurate weapon for this particular foe.

The real triumph of the public health campaign against polio was the work by the March of Dimes to keep the vaccine effort funded – to a great extent with public donations – and the extraordinary acceptance of the vaccine. 600,000 American parents volunteered their children to be test subjects for Salk's polio vaccine trials in 1954. (For perspective, polio affected an average of 35,000 people per year, with the high point of 60,000 cases in 1952.) The trials proved successful, and school-based vaccination campaigns began in 1955. Despite the Cutter laboratory disaster, in which attempts to kill the virus for the vaccine failed, resulting in 4,000 polio cases among the 200,000 children given that vaccine, of which 200 had some level of paralysis and 10 died, vaccination campaigns continued with great success.

Why? Scholars propose several reasons. First, Americans believed in science in 1955. We had recently witnessed the triumph of medical science in the form of antibiotics, nuclear bombs had helped win the war, and America was a world power because of its scientific and technological prowess. Second, the March of Dimes door to door campaigns and movie theater funding pleas had kept polio as a national issue. The idea of winning the fight with a vaccine that everyone had longed for and helped to fund with their own dimes, made vaccination a longed-for triumph rather than a risk. Finally, FDR made polio a national fight, and refusing to vaccinate would have been seen as unpatriotic as well as foolish. Patriotism was also remarkably high at mid-century, and the American identity was both more consistent and respectful of presidential authority than it is now.

By reviewing this history, which seems painfully familiar by this point in the book, I hope to highlight why the COVID-19 vaccine uptake was not as universally successful as it should have been, despite the scientific breakthroughs that made the remarkable vaccine so quickly and widely available: (1) patriotism no longer means obedience (especially to that president); (2) misinformation and the plethora of internet lies; (3) lack of shared national identity in the face of opposition (no Second World War to unite us); and (4) too long living with the advantages of science without knowledge of it, and thus lost appreciation for the gift of vaccines and great benefits of scientific knowledge.

COVID-19: A New Virus Exposes Old Problems

The WHO declared COVID-19 – the disease caused by SARS-CoV-2 depicted in Figure 10.1 – to be a pandemic on March 11, 2020 and the Trump administration's first move was to restrict travel of non-American citizens coming from or who had visited one of more than 24 nations in the two weeks before arriving. The first presidential order affecting Americans came on March 16, 2020: "15 Days to Slow the Spread," which ordered people to follow their local and state health board guidelines, to not go to work or send children to school if they were symptomatic, to quarantine at home if someone in the household tested positive for COVID-19, and for older people and those with existing health conditions to stay at home and away from other people. They also reiterated CDC advice to wash hands carefully and repeatedly (which was accurate) and to constantly wipe down surfaces (inaccurate).[15] On March 17, 2020 the USA and Canada determined that public health was best served by closing their borders to non-essential travel, and the USA and Mexico made the same arrangement on March 20, 2020. When none of these efforts resulted in the massive slowdown in cases that was hoped for, "Fifteen Days to Slow the Spread" was reiterated and extended on April 1, 2020 to "Thirty Days to Slow the Spread." It was identical to the first order save the addition of working from home whenever possible and choosing takeout or delivery instead of eating in a restaurant.[16] The guidance was backed with the promise that if "everyone did their part" over 1 million lives could be saved.

But the social and economic changes of essentially quarantining the workforce were severe and, for many, life altering. Professors could work from home without much of a struggle, but veterinarians, doctors, farriers, firefighters, police officers, EMTs, nursing home attendants, garbage collectors and many other service sector employees did not have that option. If you were an "essential worker" – a definition combining federal and state guidance and including people working in "energy, childcare, waste and wastewater, agriculture and food production, critical retail (grocery stores, hardware stores, mechanics), critical trades (construction, electricians, plumbers), transportation, and nonprofits and social service organizations."[17] The Cybersecurity and Infrastructure Security Agency issued two memos on this subject, 4.0 and 4.1, which identified key sectors of the workforce that needed to remain working, be first in line for vaccines and PPE, and manage their labor if they are exposed but not symptomatic. Both memos demonstrate the significant breadth of the health care industry and the socioeconomic strata included in this capacious industry:

> workers, including laboratory personnel, that perform critical clinical, biomedical, and other research; healthcare providers, including but not limited to physicians (MD, DO, DPM), dentists, psychologists, mid-level

practitioners, nurses, emergency medical services personnel, assistants and aids., infection control and quality assurance personnel, phleobotomists, pharmacists, physical, respiratory, speech, and occupational therapists and assistants, social workers, optometrists, speech pathologists, chiropractors, diagnostic and therapeutic technicians, and radiology technologists.

The final category reflects the truly massive range of people employed in this industry: Workers required for effective clinical, command, infrastructure, support service, administrative, security, and intelligence operations across the direct patient care and full healthcare and public health spectrum. Personnel examples may include, but are not limited, to accounting, administrative, admitting and discharge, engineering, accrediting, certification, licensing, credentialing, epidemiological, source plasma and blood donation, food service, environmental services, housekeeping, medical records, information technology and operational technology, nutritionists, sanitarians, etc.[18]

There are two levels of effect here: the first is personal. Some professions were much more likely to contract COVID-19 because they were required to work in the world, and for doctors, nurses, health care technicians, long term health care aides, and EMTs, that world was full of COVID-19. Those individuals navigated a minefield of potential infection and risking bringing the virus home, when not all homes are equally viable as partial quarantine facilities. Those living in crowded, small apartments in the winter, when windows were most likely closed, were more likely to infect the people with whom they lived because of stagnant shared air. Essential employees coming home to people of multiple generations were also facing a nearly impossible challenge of continuing to work while protecting themselves and their parents, grandparents, and children – sometimes all in the same small apartment. PPE was the only protection available, and it was inconsistently distributed, of uneven quality, and supplies were limited.

The lack of PPE for health care workers, especially in the months before the vaccine became available, was something we should have considered and addressed before a respiratory viral pandemic. We should not be struck unprepared to that extent ever again. As Cohen and van der Meulen Rodgers put it, "PPE for healthcare workers is a key component of infection prevention and control; ensuring that healthcare workers are protected means more effective containment for all."[19] They identify four critical factors that explain the shortage, and two are infuriating in that they are easily managed: "a dysfunctional budgeting model" encourages hospitals to minimize costs rather than maintaining sufficient stocks of PPE and "the federal government failed to maintain and distribute domestic inventories." These authors cite budget cuts and policy changes by the Trump administration, beginning in 2016, that included "streamlining the pandemic response team" and the trade war with China – a major PPE supplier – as additional factors that affected our supply of PPE.[19] But the problem was not new in 2019 – in fact, the literature indicates that, as early as 2006, the United States government was aware that it did not have sufficient PPE to respond to a major respiratory infectious outbreak.

The Trump administration complicated this problem by refusing to immediately invoke the Defense Production Act (DPA), which would have required private companies to turn their resources to manufacturing PPE and ventilators. It was April 2020 before the DPA was called into action and major corporations such as General Electric, General Motors and Medtronic started manufacturing ventilators and N95 respirators.[20] This might seem like a quick decision, but a faster invocation of the DPA would have resulted in more respirators and PPE available earlier in the pandemic, when it was desperately needed. By starting production in April, the government essentially ensured that shortages defined the first six months of the pandemic response. And since PPE was in short supply, to the extent that doctors and nurses reported reusing N95 masks and seeing Covid patients without adequate protective gear, it is no surprise that health care workers further down the pay and status chain had even less access to the limited supply. Nursing home aides, health care attendants and hospital sanitation workers faced high levels of potential exposure with very limited protection, and they were also more likely to be returning from work to more crowded homes with people from multiple generations with higher concomitant risk factors.

The socioeconomic effect on infection rates among health care workers – and therefore the risk posed to their cohabitants – was not only found at the lowest end of the pay scale. A study examining infection rates among Licensed Nurse Practitioners (requires a high school degree and 1800 hour training program), Registered Nurses (1 year of education beyond high school and 2,100-hour job training program), and Nurse Clinicians (three year bachelor's degree in nursing science) at a nursing home in Montreal, Quebec during the first four months of the pandemic indicates that, controlling for exposure outside the workplace, residential location, age and gender, the nurses who were paid more because of their higher educational attainment were less likely to be exposed and become infected than their colleagues. "Despite the wide differences in educational requirements and wages, all three occupations have overlapping job descriptions and responsibilities." The authors conclude, "since immigrants and visible minorities were disproportionately employed as low-SES nurses, our results may also reflect workplace-based racialized mechanisms." And "that the observed SES-infection gradient was most likely driven by a combination of inadequate pandemic preparedness and worker training, as well as subtle differences in specific job responsibilities and working conditions across groups."[21]

If people in lower-paying positions had less ready access to the already limited PPE supply and were asked to do tasks with a higher risk of infection, it makes sense that they would have a higher overall infection rate. Their need to work overtime to earn more money to survive could, for those earning less per hour, have resulted in fatigue and thus a lack of physical resources to defend themselves against infection. For those lower-income workers, and their neighbors, studies also show that poor and minority people with COVID-19 had worse outcomes.

A study done on admitted cases from March 14, 2020 through April 24, 2020 across the entire Henry Ford Healthcare System, located in Southeast Michigan (a predominantly white state, where Black Americans constitute about 14% of the population but were 37% of total COVID cases and 42% of deaths) demonstrates that race and socioeconomic status were significant determining factors in morbidity and the need for extraordinary measures to recover from this virus. The authors noted, "patients who received IMV (invasive mechanical ventilation) and ICU care lived in neighborhoods with significantly lower median income, educational attainment, and vehicle access, and higher unemployment rates and food insecurity. Black patients lived in significantly poorer neighborhoods than white patients."[22] They confirm that the nature of employment played a significant role in exposing poorer patients to infection: "Frontline employment comprised a plurality of patients under 65 years, though Black and White patients in our cohort had similar employment characteristics."[22] Finally, they reiterate the risk discussed above of frontline workers bringing the disease home to smaller dwellings where self-quarantine and social distancing are much more difficult. "Social distancing and self-isolation are highly effective in reducing transmission but remain difficult for many Black Americans due to housing density, frontline employment, and food deserts, all of which are linked to socio-economic disparities."[22]

Further scholarship indicates that health care workers of color – Black, Latin-x and Asian – had significantly different COVID-19 experiences than their white colleagues. In a study of 24,769 health care workers drawn from the HERO registry between April 10, 2020 and June 30, 2021, the authors determined:

> 1) Black and Asian participants were less likely than White participants to receive COVID-19 viral testing; 2) Hispanic participants were more likely to be diagnosed with COVID-19 than White participants; 3) Black participants reported less daily impacts of the pandemic and less burnout than White participants, despite the concurrent broad societal awakening to social injustice experienced by Black people and added effect of racism experienced in and outside the workplace; 4) Black participants were much less likely to express interest in participating in a COVID-19 vaccine trial, and Black and Asian participants were much less interested in receiving a COVID-19 vaccine under either full or emergency use authorization, consistent with national trends.[23]

All of this is to say that race played a significant role in determining the experiences health care workers had in encountering, contracting, being treated for and making decisions about vaccinating against COVID-19.

Biological sex also played a role in the level of exposure and risk people experienced during this pandemic. Seventy-six percent of people in the health care professions are female, and women are disproportionately represented in the lower paid strata of health care work. For example, women constitute more than

75% of dental hygienists, dental assistants, nursing assistants, medical assistants, licensed vocational and licensed practical nurses, nurse practitioners, veterinary technicians, medical records specialists, dieticians and nutritionists, registered nurses, home health aides, occupational therapists, pharmacy technicians, massage therapists and personal care aides. They are, however, underrepresented among physicians, constituting 44% of that group.[24] Women in health care were disproportionately affected by the virus and by its ripple effects. Scholars note that female health care workers had

> a higher risk of exposure and infection; barriers to accessing personal protective equipment; increased workloads; decreased leadership and decision-making opportunities; increased caregiving responsibilities in the home when schools and childcare supports were restricted; and higher rates of mental ill-health, including depression, anxiety, and post-traumatic stress disorder.[25]

COVID-19: The Uneven Cost of Quarantine

Perhaps one of the most stressful factors accompanying the pandemic that disproportionately affected women and the poor – both rural and urban – was the closing of all schools for the remainder of the 2020 academic year and the intermittent closings that characterized the fall of 2020 and spring of 2021. School closings were perhaps the most coherent, with 47 states closing their public schools in March of 2020. Public schools in Montana, Idaho and Wyoming were given discretion to re-open on a district level, which occurred in 14 rural districts in Montana, while those in other states remained closed until the end of the school year. They were closed in New England and the Mid-Atlantic through the entire 2020 school year.[26] During the following academic year, districts followed local and state guidelines to determine whether they could remain open, with active cases in the schools, community infection rates, and other factors contributing to the decision. The Omicron variant caused many schools to remain closed from Thanksgiving 2020 through early January of 2021, as cases surged across the country.[27]

Several aspects of school closings are worth considering, given the huge numbers of people affected and the potentially long-term effects of the closings. First, the switch to online education had disproportionately negative effects on socioeconomically disadvantaged students, students of color, and students living in rural areas due to their limited internet and technology access. Scholarship concerning educational attainment loss during summer vacations indicates that students from higher socioeconomic brackets have greater parental support for educational continuity and thus learn less, even during these shorter periods. The same was found to be true for the longer distance learning periods experienced during the pandemic. Parental involvement for students doing distance learning during the pandemic was higher for those from wealthier, whiter homes. In dual-parent households with both parents working from home, women were disproportionately responsible for also assisting their children with school work. When one or both parents were essential workers, oversight was often missing.[19] And, in cases where multiple students were attempting to do their school work on a shared device, educational loss was most apparent. Parents who worked from home had more time and ability than essential workers to help their children navigate online platforms and ensure that they were completing their academic assignments. Third, academic oversight fell disproportionately to women, as did the care of children who were suddenly constantly at home. Fourth, teachers also experienced significant negative effects of the switch to online education, exacerbated by socioeconomic factors. A study of K-12 teachers in Utah that fortuitously began right before the pandemic closed schools indicates the barriers teachers encountered in switching to online and identifies the many purposes schools serve – not all of which can be met on Zoom. Teachers noted that 20% of their students disappeared when the schools closed, and many of their responses stressed the critically interpersonal nature of teaching and peer relationships in guaranteeing student success.[29]

Teachers also were frustrated by reopening plans: while they supported returning to the classroom, they wanted minimal guarantees of public health precautions, such as requiring masks, appropriate ventilation systems, and the possibility of social distancing. Partially due to long-term misinformation from the CDC about the importance of surface cleaning and little to no attention paid to the critical need for ventilation and HVAC systems in windowless rooms with relatively high human density, schools concentrated more on hand sanitizers and consistent cleaning efforts and not on other areas. Limited budgets also made major institutional changes, such as the installation of new ventilation systems, impossible. The fight over masks was a political football and the rules depended greatly on where the school was located. Social distancing was a similar struggle, though it was more universally respected than masks. Cutting class sizes and investing in more effective learning technologies marked districts' socioeconomic status – and to some extent, geographic location. Room density reflects urban versus rural divides and sheds light on the frequently overcrowded classrooms found in cities. Teachers wanted to go back to their classrooms, but they did not want to get sick in order to do so – even after vaccinations were widely available. But in retrospect, around 40% of teachers think their schools were closed for too long and that districts could have acted more quickly to plan for a return to in person education once it was determined that COVID-19 was less likely to affect children.[30]

The long-term effects – on educational attainment and social development – of mass school closings remain a question mark, but they certainly did not improve student outcomes. Early outcomes indicate that schools with fewer in-person days and more hybrid or fully online programs demonstrate significant declines in math scores and, though language scores were more consistent, students of color and those from poorer areas showed significant decline in performance.[31] Furthermore, reading rates were at an all time low in the fall of 2021, likely due to students missing pre-k and/or kindergarten during the pandemic. Graduation rates in 2021 were down, and college application numbers for the fall of 2021 were significantly down.[32] The long-term economic ramifications of these statistics are significant: recovering from a 4–6 week shutdown of schools after Hurricane Katrina took two years, and the bounce back from many months to more than a year of in person education for COVID could take more than a decade, if it occurs at all. Missing critical reading and math skills hinders moving forward with educational attainment, and installing and reinforcing those skills requires time. Lacking those skills limits students' overall employment prospects, as well as their potential to attain higher education, which in turn affects their lifetime earned income. "The paper estimates that boys in elementary school during the pandemic-related school closures could face a salary loss of more than $2,600 per year, and girls could lose more than $1,500 per year. Over their working lives, the average present value of lifetime income reduction could be more than $40,000 for boys and almost $21,000 for girls."[33] Unless we begin to aggressively address the educational deficits created by the school closings, the United States – whose schools remained closed longer than those in many other developed countries – could fall even further behind in educational attainment, a loss we can ill afford in a time of increased international tension and competition.[34]

Vaccination

The development of the mRNA vaccines for COVID-19 should have been met with rounds of applause, broad public uptake, and a quick re-entry to regular work. Instead, the rollout was slow, supplies were limited, administration was clumsy, and false information about the vaccine circulated on social media, where it gained support from political groups and anti-vaccination groups and combined with false information about the virus to encourage a miasma of misinformation. Ironically, the very political party that suggested we keep everything open to achieve herd immunity – while overlooking a few million deaths of the elderly and those with concomitant health problems along the way – rejoiced in spreading false information about the vaccine and the virus. Pierri et al found a convincing correlation between vaccine hesitancy and online misinformation and political partisanship. They note, "These two factors alone explain nearly half the variation in state-level vaccination rates, and are themselves moderately correlated."[35] The Children's Heath Defense Fund, an anti-vaccination organization committed to ending perfectly safe vaccination that protects children against measles, mumps, rubella, polio, rabies, and other potentially fatal diseases, provided the most frequently redistributed nonsense on social media.[36]

Vaccine hesitancy was most notable among three groups: people of color – especially African Americans; women – made worse by the misinformation circulating about potential effects on child-bearing; and conservatives. The last group was certainly targeted by the second most popularly circulated misinformation produced by Breitbart, the nonsense mill created by Steve Bannon, whose political residue includes Donald Trump and the former Prime Minister of the UK,

Boris Johnson – the latter lost his job for lying about his Covid quarantine parties. The hydroxychloroquine and ivermectin myths gained their foothold through social media and conservative "news" outlets, which made many people believe they were viable treatments for the virus and caused some deaths. The American president at the time, Trump, supported the use of both of these treatments, falsely stating in interviews that both were successful treatment options. Trump also walked a fine line in attempting to get mainstream political support for "Operation Warp Speed," a $10 billion public-private partnership initiated by the US government to accelerate the development of COVID-19 vaccines. Trump hoped to get credit for the decades-old research that created the mRNA vaccine technology, while simultaneously maintaining his base of conspiracy theorists through the proliferation of anti-vaccination myths and false treatment promises.

Finally, as a historian, I would like to blame centuries of wrongs at the hands of the medical community for African Americans' hesitancy to get the vaccine. After all, in the past they were frequently the test subjects for unproven treatments without their knowledge or consent – and recent studies suggest that our current health care system is also to blame. It is perhaps not surprising that being black means that you receive less good-quality care, but the blatant disrespect paid to people of color by the American health care system is remarkable. A regular drumbeat of articles over the past five years, but especially since COVID, demonstrates that ideas about pain tolerance, false reporting and general distrust remain a significant part of contemporary African American experience with doctors. While Black and white vaccination rates did even out after the first six months of COVID vaccine availability, mistrust of the medical profession and absence of a close relationship with a personal physician remain strong predictors of vaccine hesitancy.[37] All of these factors contributed to slow uptake of the COVID vaccine in all racial/ethnic groups in comparison to our most recent watershed vaccine for polio. By comparison with COVID, the president at that time oversaw the development, distribution, and administration of the polio vaccine and championed it as a uniquely American scientific triumph. Dwight Eisenhower managed to oversee the widespread vaccination of Americans *even after* the Cutter laboratory mistake. He did not use the vaccine as an opportunity to encourage political partisanship, as more recent American politicians have done, by suggesting that the vaccine might not be safe and perpetuating false correlations between vaccinations and autism, or any other long term negative effects. Instead, he spoke rationally about trusting scientific expertise, understanding the limitations of any vaccination, prioritizing vaccine distribution, and accepting the time required to get everyone vaccinated.[38] Would we have had such leadership in the winter of 2020.

Long Covid: It Never Goes Away

There is little – perhaps no – room in American culture for people who have been sick and survived, but remain affected. And one of the things we have come to realize, after reviewing all these viral pandemics, is that viruses leave their mark: a percentage of total cases will be afflicted with a longer-term and often more serious reaction to the disease. The people who survived polio with damage to one or several limbs were told they must learn to walk and behave normally, lest they be seen as "cripples" and "failures." While their achievements in retraining their neuromuscular systems are incredible, the costs they paid were – over time – unbearable. Post-polio syndrome, which affected many polio survivors, demonstrates the excessive strain placed on their muscles and nervous symptoms in the name of satisfying our desire for survivors to be unstained by their disease. The fortunate few who survived the early decades of HIV and bear the scars of permanently compromised immune systems and multiple organ damage from the treatments that were our desperate first line of defense face a similar response to the polio survivors who preceded them. They are encouraged to be grateful for their survival and to not "dwell" on the physical costs they continue to pay. It is perhaps more difficult to be grateful when you are in kidney failure resulting from side effects of medication you took more than three decades ago, but that is t something the medical field can hear or tolerate. You are alive – be grateful. The same is currently true of those affected by long Covid. This syndrome, which encompasses neurologic, cardiac, and other symptoms, is poorly understood and currently has no effective treatment. Overwhelmed by the largest pandemic since HIV, physicians are exhausted and frustrated by the limitations of our existing medical knowledge to help long Covid patients. So individuals with Long Covid have frequently been encouraged to go home and get on with their lives, preferably without mentioning any ongoing deficits they face after infection with SARS-CoV-2. The NIH is now funding multiple studies into long-COVID, but the individual experiences of people now living with the complications of this virus reflect how little we know and how little grace is given to those who continue to suffer from it.[39]

Where Do We Go from Here?

COVID-19 has morphed from a pandemic inciting panic and causing mortality and morbidity rates with which the Western world in particular was unfamiliar. The vaccinations against which many parents now protest based on misinformation designed to pique their anxiety and play upon their fears for their children have shielded the United States and much of Europe from the lived realities of Africa, the Middle East, and Asia. The science and hard-fought magic of vaccination has allowed the Global North to forget polio, measles, rubella and mumps – those old visitors that terrorized, paralyzed and ended lives for centuries. COVID-19 does not respond as well to vaccination as did polio because the SARS-COV-2 vaccine requires boosting while immunity from the oral polio vaccine is lifelong. COVID-19 is more like influenza, and thus the next chapter of this story will look more like the ongoing struggle we have to contain the flu every year, protect our most vulnerable against it, and stay ahead of its efficient mutation cycles. The other story is about those patients left with the sequelae of the original disease. The influenza pandemic of 1918 not only had a high mortality rate, especially among the young-middle aged, a population frequently safe from virus mortality, but also left some survivors exhausted, apathetic, depressed and with odd neurological complications.[40] Polio left many of its survivors permanently affected, from the few souls kept alive in iron lungs to those suffering lifelong paralysis and muscle weakness. We have a model for this now – we call it living with a disease. We are familiar with the concept of living with cancer or living with HIV. For many cancer patients and, at this time, all AIDS patients, there is no cure. There is, instead, a lifetime – an unexpected gift of medical science – of medical management. That management comes complete with side effects, some of which are painful, severe, and ongoing. When polio patients emerged from their rehabilitation programs in the 1950s, there was no such model available. They were expected to return to "normal life" without complaint or any acknowledgment of any remaining effects of the virus. Patients too affected by polio, who could not disguise their weakness with braces under pant legs or shirt sleeves, were to be kept at home where they would not bring down the national mood.[41] And here we are, in 2024, asking long Covid patients to do the same thing. Many people experiencing the long-term complications of COVID-19, which come in a dizzying array of neurological, cardiac, and endocrine symptoms, find medicine unwilling to accept that a respiratory virus could be the cause of such long-term damage. They face accusations of malingering and hypochondria, as well as doubt that their symptoms are real – even when diagnostic tests prove their existence. The identification of distinct blood biomarkers in patients reporting the symptoms of long Covid, in the words of Ziyad Al-Aly, an epidemiologist at Washington University in St. Louis, quoted in the Washington Post. "… provides objective evidence to legitimize the disease and show it is not made up in people's heads."[42] Why are we so reluctant to accept that disease can leave its marks – not just smallpox scars and withered limbs, but tangled neurons and damaged heart valves? We comfortably accept that rheumatic fever can cause heart damage – so why not COVID-19? And why do we insist on putting an end date on pandemics, when they are better conceived as a new way of living? Our bodies will not be the same, and neither will our memories. We have been reminded very harshly of our fragility. Perhaps we should take a moment to think about what we value most before hurtling back onto crowded trains and planes. We have been reminded what we have to lose – and how much we still have to learn.

Conclusions

The world was ill prepared to cope with a highly contagious respiratory virus like SARS-CoV-2. We had insufficient stores of PPE, disorganized and unruly populations reluctant to accept quarantine restrictions, social distancing regulations, and mask mandates, and no coherent plans in place to address production shortages and distribution problems. We reacted using the time-honored strategies of complaint and lament that have governed public health responses to pandemics with little change since the fourteenth century, and we repeated the mistakes that accompanied them. Quarantine makes a lot of sense, as long as everyone within the quarantine is entirely self-sufficient. (When you locate that utopia, please contact me.) It is much less realistic, even in a land of working from home and Amazon – because someone has to make all those electronics people purchased when their couches became offices, and someone has to deliver all those packages. The fact that most of those things we ordered were not made in America meant that they had to be made overseas, shipped here in containers that required unloading, loaded onto trucks, and driven across the nation. While some people worked from home, other people worked harder than ever on the front lines, placing themselves at risk for infection through exposure and exhaustion. Masking and social distancing would have been a much more effective means of controlling the virus and keeping the country at school and at work. But the knowledge that scientists needed to recognize and deliver those highly effective methods was unavailable early in the pandemic and the messages were subsequently undermined by politics and deliberate misinformation.

The early threat to children assumed for the virus was exaggerated and maintained long after they were proven to be neither especially susceptible nor super spreaders. The threat to grandparents at home became justification for keeping millions of kids out of school, at a cost we have not yet come to appreciate. The grandparents were the ones who needed to shelter in place. The kids needed to wear masks, and get back to school. Districts needed to provide appropriate ventilation for classrooms, PPE for teachers, and vaccinations for all staff. The bigger problems – racial and socioeconomic disparity in overall health, access to health care, and trust in the medical profession – remain. If we don't do something to address these, our next pandemic will again disproportionately damage the lives of the poor and people of color. This cannot surprise us, but I am nearly convinced we will do nothing to address it. We haven't yet. Community-level outreach to these communities that took advantage of existing institutions, such as churches, youth organizations and civil rights groups might be a good way to start. Making physicians and nurses a part of those groups and allowing them to act as envoys for their profession would likely encourage trust and a feeling of connection with the medical community that is lacking for many people of color.

We also desperately need to improve scientific education in every public school in America. There should never again be a majority of people misled by social media to believe anti-vaccination nonsense because they cannot differentiate between disinformation and real science. We have the tools to improve every American's understanding of fundamental scientific information and to teach and re-teach the critical analytical thinking skills that allow people to judge the legitimacy of information from different media outlets. The brutal truth is that the nation that so proudly lined up for polio vaccines has shattered along political divides, and our public education system has been dramatically damaged as a result. It is not sufficient to say that America no longer produces the best science and mathematically educated students in the world   that has not been true for decades. But we can no longer even claim to produce competent judges of scientific information because we are allowing political/religious ideology to determine what too many children learn. Finally, if we continue to be divided into "two Americas" along political lines, we cannot expect to coherently face a pandemic. If one side prides itself on calling long established scientific research "fiction" and the other has to beg for educational funding against a wave of book banning, it is unlikely that we will be able to come together to accept a scientific answer for anything, even a fatal pandemic.

Certainly our response to HIV/AIDS was slowed to a crawl by conservatives who believed that gay men deserved to die horribly. May Jesse Helms live in infamy for saying, "The government should spend less money on people with AIDS because they got sick as a result of deliberate, disgusting, revolting conduct." He tied up funding for HIV research for decades because he was a racist homophobe with too much power handed to him by a state with a majority who agreed with his position. I am actually amazed we managed to vaccinate as many Americans against COVID as we did, considering the hysteria surrounding vaccination. We must stop debating the benefit of vaccinations. Our current public health crises of depression, drug overdose and obesity are only gaining attention because vaccinations stopped the fastest killers of children. If we lose herd immunity due to lack of vaccination for these diseases, we will quickly be reminded of the historic power of these viruses.

If public health is to encompass everything, then it must continue to do what it does well: protect people against known diseases through proven strategies, such as vaccination. We cannot expect to face new diseases with any success if we do not understand and trust the tools we have used for decades to fight old ones. Finally – and surprisingly, for those who know me – we need to think more and better about what we mean by human connection. Many people lamented its loss during the social isolation of Covid, and community – whose absence and the concomitant increase in anomie have marked the twenty-first century – has once again become something we intellectually value. But how do we create community in an age increasingly characterized by the decline in power of the institutions that have traditionally defined it? Most Americans no longer regularly attend a religious institution, community-level government is struggling to attract new recruits, and while hobbies are lovely, they cannot take the identity-defining place of some of these bigger, more concrete institutions. Online communities can satisfy our desire to connect with people sharing similar interests, but they do not provide social interaction and it is increasingly clear that humans are inherently social beings. Offices, in fact, supplied a great deal of that interaction, but as some people continue to work from home, the social role of work has also declined. One thing I propose is to spend more time in your community trying to do something you enjoy that benefits others. If you are interested in parks and recreation, work with a group once a week to pick up and beautify your local park. If you don't have one, perhaps there is a group of people interested in helping to establish one. Turn off Netflix. Leave your living room. And *live!* Because there is so much left to do before the next pandemic, and we who survived have the privilege to do it.

References

1. Schwartz E. "Does ivermectin have a place in the treatment of mild Covid-19?." *New Microb New Infect* 2022; 46: 100985. doi:10.1016/j.nmni.2022.100985
2. Baldwin MR. "Toads and Plague: Amulet Therapy in Seventeenth-Century Medicine." *Bull History Med* 1993; 67(2): pp. 227–47. *JSTOR*, www.jstor.org/stable/44444207. Accessed 31 Jan. 2024.
3. Leonhardt ND, Fahmi S, Stellar JE, Impett EA. "Turning Toward or Away from God: Covid-19 and changes in religious devotion, "March 8, 2023, https://doi.org/10.1371/journal.pone.0280775
4. Upenieks L, Ellison CG. "Changes in religiosity and reliance on God during the COVID-19 pandemic: A protective role under conditions of financial strain?." *Rev Relig Res*, 2022; 64(4): 853–881. doi:10.1007/s13644-022-00523-z; "More Americans than People in Other Advanced Economies Say Covid-19 Has Strengthened Religious Faith," January 27, 2021, www.pewresearch.org/religion/2021/01/27/more-americans-than-people-in-other-advanced-economies-say-covid-19-has-strengthened-religious-faith/
5. Nirappil F. "Is this covid surge really the second biggest? Here's what data shows," *The Washington Post*, January 12, 2024; www.washingtonpost.com/health/2024/01/12/covid-surge-january-2024/?utm_campaign=wp_post_most&utm_medium=email&utm_source=newsletter&wpisrc=nl_most
6. "Discussion on the Advisability of Registration of Tuberculosis," *Trans College Phys Philadelphia*, meeting held January 12, 1894; 3(16): 1–27.
7. Kalnins I. "The Spanish Influenza of 1918 in St Louis, Missouri," *Public Health Nurs*, 2006; 23(5): 479–483.
8. Bootsma MCJ, Ferguson NM. "The effect of public health measures on the 1918 influenza pandemic in U.S. Cities," *Proceedings of the National Academy of Sciences*, 2007; 104(18):7588–7593.
9. Jones MM. "The American Red Cross and local response to the 1918 influenza pandemic: A four-city case study: 1918–1919 influenza pandemic in the United States: Lessons learned and challenges exposed," *Public Health Rep* 1974/2010; 125: 92–104.
10. Bootsma MCJ, Ferguson NM. "The effect of public health measures on the 1918 influenza pandemic in U.S. Cities," *Proceedings of the National Academy of Sciences*, 2007; 104(18):7588–7593.
11. Ellerman M, Wrigley-Field E, Felgenbaum JJ, Helgertz J, Hernandez E, Boen CE. "Racial disparities in mortality during the 1918 influenza pandemic in United States cities," *Demography* 2022; 59(5):1953–1979.
12. Rogers N. *Dirt and Disease: Polio Before FDR*. Newark, New Jersey: Rutgers University Press, 1992.
13. Cirillo VJ. "I Am the Baby Killer! House Flies and the Spread of Polio," *Am Entomol*, 2016; 62(2):83–85.
14. Meyers K, Thomason MA. "Paralyzed by Panic: Measuring the Effect of School Closures during the 1916 Polio Pandemic on Educational Attainment," Working

Paper 23890 for the National Bureau of Economic Research, 2017. www.nber.org/papers/w23890

15. https://trumpwhitehouse.archives.gov/articles/15-days-slow-spread/
16. https://trumpwhitehouse.archives.gov/articles/these-30-days-how-you-can-help/
17. www.ncsl.org/labor-and-employment/covid-19-essential-workers-in-the-states
18. US Department of Homeland Security, Cybersecurity and Infrastructure Security Agency (CISA); Advisory Memorandum on Ensuring Essential Critical Infrastructure Workers' Ability to Work During The COVID-19 Response. 3/19/2020. Updated 8/10/2021. www.cisa.gov/sites/default/files/publications/essential_critical_infrastructure_workforce-guidance_v4.1_508.pdf
19. Cohen J, van der Meulen Rodgers Y. "Contributing factors to personal protective equipment shortages during the COVID-19 pandemic," *Preventative Medicine* December, 2020; 141: 106263, 10.1016/j.ypmed.2020.106263
20. Federal Emergency Management Agency. Applying the Defense Production Act" April 13, 2020, www.fema.gov/press-release/20230510/applying-defense-production-act
21. Godofroy R, Lewis J. "What explains the socioeconomic status-health gradient? Evidence from workplace COVID-19 infections," *SSM – Population Health,* 2022; 18: 101124. doi:10.1016/j.ssmph.2022.101124
22. Daniel Q, Luna Wong, Shallal A, et al. "Impact of race and socioeconomic status on outcomes in patients hospitalized with COVID-19." *J Gen Intern Med,* 2021; 36: 1302–1309 (2021). https://doi.org/10.1007/s11606-020-06527-1
23. Lusk JB, Xu H, Thomas LE, et al . on behalf of the HERO Research Program, "Racial/Ethnic Disparities in Healthcare Worker Experiences During the COVID-19 Pandemic: An Analysis of the HERO Registry," *eClinicalMed,* 2022; 45, art. no. 101314.
24. "Percent of women employees in the 25 largest healthcare occupations," US Bureau of Labor Statistics, www.bls.gov/spotlight/2023/healthcare-occupations-in-2022/home.htm
25. Morgan R, et al. "Women healthcare workers' experiences during COVID-19 and other crises: A scoping review." *Int J Nurs Studies Adv,* 2022; 4: 100066. doi:10.1016/j.ijnsa.2022.100066
26. Zviedrite N, Hodis JD, Jahan F, Gao H, Uzicanin A. "COVID-19 associated school closures and related efforts to sustain education and subsidized meal programs, United States, February 18-June 30, 2020. *PLoS One.* 2021; 16(9): e0248925.
27. Tompkins A. "COVID outbreaks have closed 1,400 schools in 35 states," *Poynter,* September 9, 2021.
28. De Gioannis E, Ballarino G, Cartagini D." Parents and teachers' compensatory strategies during COVID-19 school closures: A scoping review," *Int Rev Educ* 2023; 69: 603–623. https://doi.org/10.1007/s11159-023-10011-3.
29. Judd J, Rember BA, Pellegrini T, Ludlow B, Meisner J. "This is not teaching: The effects of COVID-19 on teachers." Social Publishers Foundation. July 2020. www.socialpublishersfoundation.org/knowledge_base/this-is-not-teaching-the-effects-of-covid-19-on-teachers/
30. Peetz C. "Nearly half of educators believe schools were closed too long during the pandemic," *Education Week,* June 20, 2023, www.edweek.org/leadership/nearly-half-of-educators-believe-schools-were-closed-too-long-during-pandemic/2023/06

31. Halloran C, Jack R, Okun JC, Oster E. "Pandemic Schooling Mode and Student Test Scores: Evidence from US States," National Bureau of Economic Research, Working Paper 29497, November, 2021, www.nber.org/papers/w29497

32. Parolin Z, Lee EK. "Large socio-economic, geographic and demographic disparities exist in exposure to school closures," *Nat Hum Behav* 2021; 5: 522–528. https://doi.org/10.1038/s41562-021-01087-8

33. Kamenetz A. "Two years ago, schools shut down around the world. These are the biggest impacts," Morning Edition. National Public Radio, March 15, 2022, www.npr.org/2022/03/15/1086054482/covid-school-shutdown-biggest-impacts

34. Ihsan Ajwad M, Bilo S. "Seen and unseen effects of Covid-19 school disruptions," May 25, 2022. www.brookings.edu/articles/seen-and-unseen-effects-of-covid-19-school-disruptions/

35. Pierri F, Perry BL, DeVerna MR, et al. "Online misinformation is linked to early COVID-19 vaccination hesitancy and refusal," *Sci Rep*, 2022; 12: 5966. https://doi.org/10.1038/s41598-022-10070-w

36. Ober H. "Black Americans' Covid vaccine hesitancy stems more from today's inequities than historical ones," October 27, 2022, https://newsroom.ucla.edu/releases/causes-of-covid-vaccine-hesitancy-among-black-americans

37. Padansee TJ, et al. "Changes in Covid-19 Vaccine Hesitancy Among Black and White Individuals in the US," *JAMA Netw Open*. 2022; 5(1):e2144470. doi:10.1001/jamanetworkopen.2021.44470

38. Eisenhower DD. "Statement by the President on the Polio Vaccine Situation," May 31, 1955.www.presidency.ucsb.edu/documents/statement-the-president-the-polio-vaccine-situation

39. https://covid19.nih.gov/covid-19-topics/long-covid

40. Phillips H. *In a Time of Plague: Memories of the "Spanish" Flu Epidemic of 1918 in South Africa*. Cape Town: Van Riebeck Society. 2018.

41. Fairchild AL. "The Polio Narratives: Dialogues with FDR," *Bull History Med*, 2001; 75:488–534.

42. Sellers FS. "Four years on, long covid still confounds us. Here's what we now know." *The Washington Post* December, 31, 2023. www.washingtonpost.com/health/2023/12/31/long-covid-symptoms-treatment-research/

Suggested Reading

Anne Schuchat. Public Health Response to the Initiation and Spread of Pandemic COVID-19 in the United States, February 24–April 21, 2020. *MMWR Morb Mortal Wkly Rep* 2020; 69:551–556. doi: http://dx.doi.org/10.15585/mmwr.mm6918e2.

David France. *How To Survive a Plague: The Story of How Activists and Scientists Tamed AIDS*. Vintage Reprint. New York. 2017.

George Rosen, *A History of Public Health*. Johns Hopkins University Press. Baltimore. 2015.

Julie K Silver, *Polio Voices: An Oral History from the American Polio Epidemics and Worldwide Education Efforts*. Praeger. New York. 2007.

Ken Dalton, *Polio and Me*. Different Drummer Press. New York. 2016.

Larry Kramer, *The Normal Heart*. Dutton Adult. New York. 1985.

Nancy Tomes. *The Gospel of Germs: Men, Women, and the Microbe in American Life* (Harvard University Press) 1999. A global analysis of COVID-19 intra-action reviews: Reflecting on, adjusting and improving country emergency preparedness

and response during a pandemic. WHO. 30 Sep 2023 https://reliefweb.int/report/
world/global-analysis-covid-19-intra-action-reviews-reflecting-adjusting-and-
improving-country-emergency-preparedness-and-response-during-pandemic

Paul Monette. *Borrowed Time: An AIDS Memoir.* Harper Perennial. New York. 1998.

Randall M Packard. *A History of Global Health: Interventions into the Lives of Other People.*
Johns Hopkins University Press. Baltimore. 2016.

Sean Strub. *Body Counts: A Memoir of Activism, Sex, and Survival.* Scribner. New York. 2014.

11
A WAY FORWARD

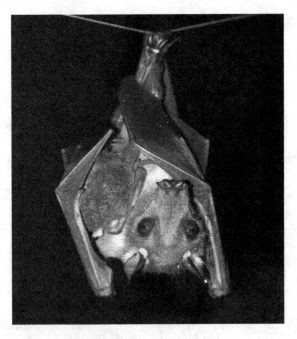

FIGURE 11.1 An adult female hammer-headed fruit bat with attached young in the Republic of Congo. Bats are the natural reservoirs of many viruses.

Source: National Institute of Allergy and Infectious Disease, US National Institutes of Health. www.niaid.gov

DOI: 10.4324/9781003427667-11

A CAUTIONARY TALE: THE ROLE OF GLOBAL TRAVEL

My brother-in-law Chris is an intrepid international traveler – his last two job postings were in Nepal and China and he lived in Africa for years – but even for him, this trip seemed like a bit of a stretch. In order to include his son and family in this year's Christmas celebration, he was flying from Ottawa to Songdo, South Korea for just six days, returning on December 19. The outbound trip was not too bad but the return was a killer – almost 20 hours via Beijing, Vancouver and Toronto before finally reaching home. I admired his commitment but I was glad I was not going with him!

Like many families, our Christmas celebration has become increasingly complex as our children have become grown-ups with families of their own. Home base is my sister's house in Ottawa with the big celebration on Christmas Day. My husband and I usually arrive on the 23rd and leave for home on Boxing Day. My daughter Allison and her partner have a horse farm and take care of all the chores on the 25th so their employees can have the day off, so we have a separate celebration with them – Noel Deux – over New Year's at our place. Chris's two sons and their families are with us roughly every other Christmas, from their homes in South Korea and outside Halifax but neither would be there this year – hence, Chris's trip to Songdo. There were a few added complexities – one of my two nieces, was leaving for Mexico to meet a friend very early on December 26 and the other was flying to Europe on December 27 for a family visit. A modern family in motion ...

One of the joys of my life is the close, easy friendship we have with Sarah and Chris. On Christmas Eve, the four of us ate dinner in front of the fire, sharing a bowl of cheese fondue. This year for the first time they had an artificial tree – an elegant, contemporary metal structure with colored lights along narrow black limbs. I remember thinking how perfectly it suited the modern, vertical design of their townhome. After dinner, we called the Songdo troupe on Skype – the time is 14 hours ahead of us so the kids already had their gifts to show off. Then we ate dark chocolate and drank red wine while we got the stockings ready for the next day.

It must have been about 4am when I heard my sister calling. Chris was ill with severe diarrhea that had started at about one in the morning. I shifted into doctor mode – the stools were liquid, dark brown and very frequent, almost every 15 minutes, reported Sarah. He had cramps but no nausea, vomiting or fever. He had taken one loperamide tablet with no apparent response. Peering up the stairs to their bedroom, he still looked healthy enough and his voice was strong. With his recent trip in mind, I thought it was probably the infamous "traveler's diarrhea" and recommended two loperamide tablets now and a glass of water once every hour and/or every time he had a stool.

By 7am, things were no better. I started Gatorade instead of water plus loperamide every 4 hours and tried to be encouraging – supportive clinical care at its minimal best. It was at this point that our focus shifted to prevention – everyone was scheduled to arrive in the late morning and we needed to minimize any risk of spread. Of course, we could have called off the celebration but no one wanted to do that – it was Christmas after all! We closed the door to the stairs to the master suite – isolating our index case. I felt terrible about shutting Chris away but it had to be done. We agreed that Sarah would be his only physical contact – she would wear disposable gloves and use disinfectant wipes for cleaning. She laundered the bed linens and pj's with bleach – there were multiple trips up and down the stairs to the basement laundry all day long. We stocked all the bathrooms with disinfectant hand wipes and talked with all the guests so they would be aware of the risk and the infection control plan.

As each family arrived, we took them through use of the hand wipes and the strict rule that nothing could be eaten without washing the hands very carefully first. We opened our stockings and scrubbed our hands before we started on the oranges and chocolate and then opened all the gifts. We called Allison and Andy in Millbrook and Chris's other son in Halifax. In the afternoon, Sarah went off to a local hill to see the grandkids with their new sleds and I worked on dinner.

Chris was holding his own. When I checked on him in mid-afternoon, he sounded lonely and discouraged. He said the stool volume was definitely decreasing but they were still completely liquid and very frequent. He was still peeing a fair amount but he never wanted to see Gatorade again. Oh – and could Sarah come up, he had another load of laundry.

Dinner was delicious but it was not the same without Chris, usually the life of the party. We pulled our Christmas crackers and wore paper crowns and read each other's jokes. We drank Prosecco and told stories about turkeys of the past. Full and warm and tired after a long day of people and presents and sledding, the kids were sleepy and they all left soon after dinner with instructions to continue very careful hand washing.

By evening, Chris said he was definitely better – he had been able to sleep for almost 2 hours without racing to the bathroom. We sent up more Gatorade and did the dishes. Then we called Songdo to tell them about Chris and to see if anyone there was sick – all were well with no hint of diarrhea.

The next morning, Chris was downstairs eating applesauce and drinking tea – the diarrhea had ended sometime after midnight. The rest of the group were all well. We made panettone French toast and then headed for home. Over the next few days, we spoke daily – all reports were negative. By New Year's Eve, a week after Chris fell ill with everyone else still well, I felt safe in saying the risk of transmission was over.

The most likely cause of Chris's illness was enterotoxigenic E. coli bacteria. It's hard to say we broke the chain of disease when only one person was infected but traveler's diarrhea is highly contagious. We did follow the basic principles of disease control: early case detection and isolation; community (well, family) education and engagement; supportive clinical care; rigorous infection control; and contact tracing. And looking back on it, without effective infection control, we did have all the ingredients for initiation of a global outbreak with the potential for immediate disease spread on three continents.

Ours was not an unusual situation – for every virus we studied, international travel played an important role in spread of the pathogen: it was international travelers who transported Zika from Asia to Brazil via Yap Island and French Polynesia; international air travelers who carried SARS from China to 40 different countries; local travelers spread Ebola from the DRC to West Africa but international travelers carried it to Nigeria, the United States, the United Kingsom and Spain; the yellow fever virus was transported by West African slaves to the Caribbean where a critical mass of viremic hosts and active vectors in a receptive environment led to centuries of recurrent epidemics throughout the Americas; returning workers carried HIV from the Belgian Congo/ DRC in Central Africa back to Haiti, from Haiti to the United States and from there, all over the world; the polio virus with its long incubation period and predominantly asymptomatic infectious state can travel great distances undetected, entering polio-free areas by land, sea or air travel – a major reason it has still eluded global eradication efforts; smallpox came to Europe from Asia and Africa during the Middle Ages via trade and migration routes and the paths of the crusaders before spreading to the Americas in the ships of Spanish and Portuguese explorers; and the dramatic global spread of the 1918 influenza virus, SARS-CoV-2 and MKPX was accomplished by travelers, albeit by sea in 1918 and by air in 2020 and 2022. International travel played a major role in the spread of all the viral epidemics of the last century that we have studied.

And international travel is dramatically increasing. Based on airline industry data, there is exponential growth in air travel with doubling of passenger-kilometers every 15 years (a passenger-kilometer is equal to moving one person one kilometer). In October of 2017, The International Air Transport Association (IATA) announced industry performance statistics for 2016 showing that system-wide, airlines carried 3.8 billion passengers on scheduled services last year, an increase of 7% over 2015, representing an additional 242 million air trips.

****

In 2011, a University of North Carolina business professor named John Kasarda published a book with Greg Lindsay called *Aerotropolis: The Way We'll*

Live Next. He writes: "The 18th century really was a waterborne century, the 19th century a rail century, the 20th century a highway, car, truck century – and the 21st century will increasingly be an aviation century, as the globe becomes increasingly connected by air." His prediction is reflected in airline industry data: Middle Eastern and Asia Pacific airlines posted their fastest growth in 2017; Latin American and African airlines fly a relatively small proportion of international flight volumes, but both regions saw solid increases. All the major areas of the globe where new viral epidemics have emerged over the last century are areas with increasing air travel.

Travel bans, entry and exit screening and quarantine of returning travelers – all seen repeatedly as the response to disease outbreaks – have not been proven effective but efforts like this are likely to emerge again as they did with SARS-CoV-2. There are many other important factors in the increasing frequency of epidemics over the last century but our Christmas outbreak is a cautionary tale, and a good introduction to a look at global efforts to prevent future pandemics.

A Way Forward

Defining the Enemy: The Virus on Offense

Viruses are formidable enemies. Scientists have only just begun to explore the earth's massive virosphere which comprises the oldest form of life on our planet but we already know there are billions of viruses, more than all other known life forms combined.[1] Despite their tiny size and simple structure, their inability to move, to replicate or to produce energy independently, viruses can control our destiny. The intrinsic ability to mutate allows them to endlessly evolve into new forms with enhanced capacity to parasitize, replicate and cause new disease that can sweep through whole populations, leaving utter devastation behind. As Nobel-prize winning biologist Joshua Lederberg wrote: "The single greatest threat to man's continued dominance on our planet is a virus."[2]

In this book, we concentrate on the viruses which have caused pandemics since the beginning of the twentieth century. We have seen that emerging and re-emerging viruses are causing increasingly frequent disease outbreaks (Figure 11.1). In this chapter, we create a composite picture of the state of viral infectious disease outbreaks by integrating the biologic and environmental factors that emerged as critical in this progression through analysis of the pandemics in this book. We begin by looking at a biogeographic analysis of a 33-year dataset of all 12,202 human disease outbreaks which occurred between 1980 and 2010.[3] In Figure 11.2, the results of the analysis show the total number of outbreaks increased exponentially, with the greatest increase in viral pathogens and significant increases in zoonotic diseases and in both vector-borne and non-vector-borne disease.

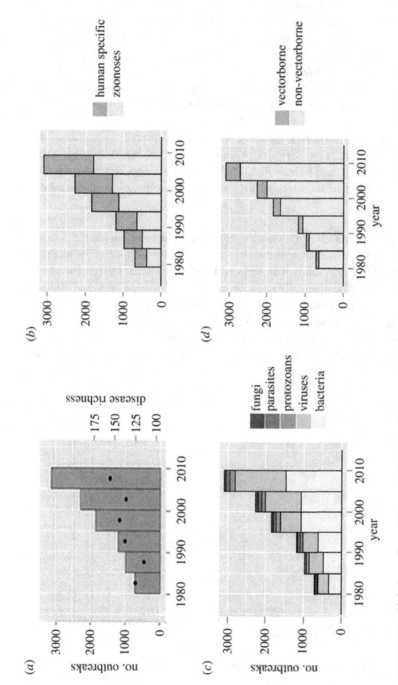

FIGURE 11.2 Global number of human infectious disease outbreaks, 1980–2010. Outbreak records are plotted by: (a) total # of global outbreaks (left axis, bars) and total number of diseases causing outbreaks per decade; (b) host type; (c) pathogen taxonomy; (d) transmission mode.

Zoonoses constitute more than 60% of the roughly 400 infectious diseases that have been identified since 1940, emerging when a virus spills over from its natural host to infect another species. When that other species is human, an immunologically naïve subject is exposed to a potentially devastating new pathogen. This narrative was the story for several of the pandemics that we explored, including HIV/AIDS, SARS, Ebola and COVID-19.

What are the factors behind this dangerous pattern of evolution? The answer is deceptively simple: we are. Warwick Anderson describes this vision as follows:

> Evolutionary processes operating on a global scale were responsible for the emergence of "new" diseases. As environments changed, as urbanization, deforestation, and human mobility increased, so, too, did disease patterns alter, with natural selection promoting the proliferation of microbes in new niches.[4]

Among the human factors considered predominantly responsible for the global increase in infectious disease outbreaks, one of the most important is increasing population density. As shown in the graph in Figure 11.3, our global population has increased dramatically in recent centuries. Between 1900 and 2000, the increase in world population was three times greater than during the entire previous history of humanity – from 1.5 to 6.1 billion in just 100 years.[5]

The latest projections from the United Nations estimate that the world's population will reach 9.6 billion people by mid-century, and 11 billion by 2100.

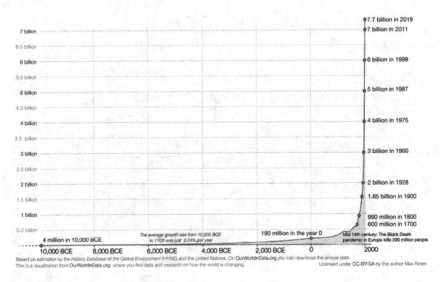

FIGURE 11.3 World population over the last 12,000 years.

Source: Data from the United Nations.[5] Graph from: "Our World in Data." All free: open access and open source.

Disease pathogens spread more easily and quickly when people live in close proximity. Population growth has been most rapid in areas where disease outbreaks occur most frequently, especially where limited health system infrastructure can also facilitate disease spread. For example, in the last 70 years, the population of Sub-Saharan Africa has been increasing at more than twice the rate seen in the high-income countries in the Global North.

Contact rates and behavior patterns within a geographic area drive the transmission of pathogens and the higher the population density, the greater the contact between and among people and pathogens. Because many viruses cannot survive for long outside a host environment, close proximity of hosts, or hosts and vectors, is essential for disease transmission. This is optimized in densely populated areas where interactions with animals and ecosystems are also enhanced, an important factor in the rising prevalence of zoonotic diseases.[6] Zoonotic viruses are the most frequent newly emerging human pathogens, constituting 85% of all pathogens discovered since 1980. Increasing global population density brings wild animal and human populations into closer and more frequent contact, maximizing the emergence of new infectious disease threats with wildlife origins. RNA viruses with their high rates of mutation via nucleotide substitution plus their limited mutation error-correction ability, can easily adapt to new hosts, and therefore represent a major threat for cross-species infection. Reservoir hosts are also encouraged by proximity to potential disease hosts: viruses cannot survive independently but some can be sustained in asymptomatic animal hosts who represent an ongoing source of infection and genetic material for the emergence of new zoonotic pathogens.

Increasing urbanization parallels increasing population density. Only 3% of the world's population lived in urban areas in 1800; this proportion had risen dramatically to 56% by 2020 and is predicted to steadily increase.[7] In urban areas, more frequent contact between more individuals drives infection with directly transmitted disease pathogens. In addition, urbanization increases the preferred habitat for anthropophilic disease vectors like *Ae.aegyptii* and *Ae.albopictus*, the mosquito vectors for the Zika and yellow fever viruses. Increasing vector capacity increases potential disease transmissibility.

High population density and/or urbanization played significant roles in all the epidemics we have studied. One impressive example is the 1918 influenza pandemic where close proximity of military recruits and soldiers during training, transport and engagement in the First World War contributed significantly to global disease spread. The human immunodeficiency virus, HIV, is another good example: the virus is known to have originated in nonhuman primates in Central and West Africa early in the twentieth century. As described in Chapter 6, these original viruses are thought to have crossed over into humans sporadically for many decades, most likely related to hunting and butchering monkeys and chimps, but they never spread enough to cause a disease outbreak because the population of humans in the area at that time was so low. It was only when the virus traveled to Kinshasa, the capital of the Democratic Republic of the Congo, at a time of explosive population growth that the HIV/AIDS epidemic began. Another example: the West Nile virus pandemic (described in Chapter 7) exploded in NYC when large populations of immunologically naive people, reservoir birds and vector mosquitoes were unfortunately clustered together.

Deforestation is another important factor in the global increase in infectious disease. The human activities that drive deforestation – logging, slash and burn commercial agriculture, mining, logging for firewood, subsistence farming and road construction – all bring forest/ jungle animals and people closer together. Deforestation forces wildlife of all kinds, from insects to giant apes, to find new habitats, inevitably, closer to human civilization. Guinea, where the 2014 EBOV outbreak began is a good example: it has lost 20% of its forests since 1990. Loss of primary forest can also lead to changes in the microclimate with enhancement of vector capacity. Zoonotic risk has consistently been shown to be elevated in forested tropical regions experiencing land-use changes.[8]

Global travel and migration are among the most important factors amplifying viral disease spread in the last century. In our highly mobile world, more than half a million travelers are in the air at any one moment. As described in the essay that opens this chapter, travelers carry disease pathogens with them and global travel is increasing exponentially. Higher travel speed and increasing frequency mean that outbreaks that might otherwise have been contained can instead move rapidly into uninfected regions, carried by infected people. The establishment of new travel routes between previously unconnected areas allows direct pathogen spread where none existed. Travel – both local and international – played a major role in the historic spread of all the viral pathogens of the last century but nowhere was this more impressive than with the global spread of SARS-CoV-2 as described in Chapter 8. While Chinese officials were still refusing to certify person-to-person spread of the virus in the month after the first cases appeared, SARS-CoV-2 had already traveled to Thailand, Hong Kong, Vietnam, Malaysia, Singapore, Taiwan, Japan, South Korea, Nepal, Australia, France, the United States, and Sweden – at least 13 countries and four continents. The frequency and speed of contemporary air travel have exponentially increased global connectivity and dramatically exacerbated the spread of viral disease outbreaks.

Finally, climate change plays an important role in enhancing disease spread. As temperatures increase, the mosquito and tick vectors of diseases like malaria, Zika and yellow fever expand their range, moving into regions where they previously could not survive. Seasonal behavior of birds is altered by rising temperatures with loss of normal winter migration in some; in others, migration paths are moving as global temperatures rise, increasing the area for potential disease spread. Changes in the behavior of bird populations are important ongoing factors in the global spread of influenza and West Nile fever. Increases in extreme weather events – an established element of global warming – may also lead to increases in infectious disease outbreaks as seen in the wake of natural disasters, associated with displaced and crowded populations, ideal for virus transmission.

Severe rainfall or flooding with secondary standing water is particularly effective at creating environments suitable for the transmission and propagation of the vectors of viral infectious diseases. Increased variation in weather patterns can result in changes in human and animal interactions, increasing the potential for zoonotic pathogens to move from animals into human populations. For example, food scarcity brought about by drought may lead to increased bushmeat hunting, the original virus transmission event from animals to humans for HIV, and often the initiating event for recurrent outbreaks of Ebola.[9]

We are now entering the Anthropocene era in which human activity is the dominant influence on our planet's climate and ecosystems – changes to the environment have already impacted and will continue to impact human health with an especially strong case for the importance of environmental factors in viral disease spread.

But in this book, we tell the stories of eleven viruses whose unique disease narratives were determined *primarily* by the characteristics of the viral pathogen itself, against this backdrop of scientific, societal and environmental change. As one striking example, influenza, the mercurial, ever-changing virus that caused a true global pandemic a hundred years ago, is the model of an evasive pathogen. It was more than 30 years after the 1918 global pandemic before the importance of the capacity of the virus for constant mutation was recognized as a critical part of its pathogenicity. Decades more were needed to recognize that water birds are natural reservoirs for the virus. Carried by these birds, a newly mutated influenza virus can travel anywhere global flyways go. The combination of a stable but mobile reservoir, multiple animal hosts, and the capacity for endless mutation means global populations are repeatedly unprotected from a novel influenza virus infection. Another example: the human immunodeficiency virus – HIV – has caused the longest continuous pandemic in world history, directly reflecting the complex biopathology of this virus. Its capacity to lie hidden in host cells allows progressive destruction of the body's immune system before the clinical disease, AIDS, emerges. This asymptomatic carrier state allowed the pandemic to expand exponentially before it was even recognized; it was also a critical factor in the delayed development of effective treatment. The extremely rapid mutation rate of the virus continues to frustrate vaccine development efforts. Enormous progress has been made with antiretroviral treatment but there remains a major biologic barrier to HIV eradication: the persistence of integrated replication-competent viral reservoirs in memory CD4+ T cells which emerge whenever antiretroviral treatment is stopped. To this time, these remarkable characteristics of the human immunodeficiency virus have prevented eradication.

The narratives of every virus we describe in this book show us just how dangerous viruses can be. They show us doctors and scientists battling to respond to invisible enemies they are struggling to understand. These are stories of devastating illness and miraculous scientific breakthroughs, amid ongoing efforts to end diseases that emerge and re-emerge to cause devastating losses all over our interconnected planet. Time and again, the viruses themselves challenge our best efforts to subdue or erase them. The pathogenic characteristics of viruses combined with critical environmental and societal factors have fueled a steady increase in the frequency and severity of viral disease outbreaks over the last century. With unprecedented increases in population density and global mobility, climate change and deforestation, novel viral pathogens are increasingly widespread, mobile and transmittable. Ever-increasing global connectedness means no nation is immune to the threat posed by an outbreak caused by an unknown virus in any part of the world, however remote. Vigilant and effective health systems are needed to allow countries to detect and respond to these pathogens and prevent an infectious disease outbreak from becoming a pandemic.

The Defense: Resources for Global Viral Pandemic Response

The World Health Organization (WHO)

As the designated health branch of the United Nations, the WHO is the guardian of global health and security, empowered by its constitution since 1948 to prevent the international spread of disease. Until 1995, this role was confined to management of outbreaks of cholera, yellow fever and the plague, as defined by the original International Health Regulations (IHR). With ongoing emergence of new international disease threats – especially HIV/AIDS – the Forty-eighth World Health Assembly in 1995 belatedly called for a substantial revision of the Regulations. The SARS pandemic in 2002–2003 caused further pressure for IHR reform which finally resulted in the revised International Health Regulations (IHR)/2005) which became effective in 2007.[10] The revised regulations aimed to "prevent, protect against, control and provide a public health response to the international spread of disease." They include specific measures to limit the spread of health risks to neighboring countries while minimizing travel and trade disruption. The IHRs include an algorithm for assessment of events that might constitute a Public Health Emergency of International Concern (PHEIC), defined as "an extraordinary event which is determined ... to constitute a public health risk to other States through the international spread of disease; and, to potentially require a coordinated international response."[10]

Compared with the previous relatively narrow focus on specific diseases, the 2005 IHRs define disease very broadly as "all illnesses or medical conditions, irrespective of origin or source that could present significant harm to humans" – a major increase in the WHO's scope of responsibility, intended to initiate global cooperation in disease preparedness. According to the legal scholar David Fidler, the 2005 IHR revision was "one of the most radical and far-reaching changes in international law on public health since the beginning of international health co-operation in the mid-nineteenth century."[11] Unfortunately, this substantial increase in responsibility was not accompanied by any sustained source of additional funding.

The process for declaration of a PHEIC was entirely new and unfamiliar, and its first implementations – for the H1N1 flu in 2009 and for poliomyelitis in 2014 – received highly critical responses from the international community. But it was the 5-month delay in declaration of the 2014 Ebola outbreak in West Africa as a PHEIC – consistently identified by independent reviewing bodies as an important failure – that led to an intensive review of the WHO response to an international disease outbreak. That review identified failure to ensure development of the IHR core capacities in member states and the absence of a funded emergency response network as additional critical WHO failings in the Ebola epidemic.[12] Theoretically, the new broadened scope and required national, health care infrastructure core capacities defined in 2005 gave the WHO the opportunity to lead a well-equipped global public health team. The deficiencies of the Ebola performance, however, made it clear that the WHO was not prepared to respond to a major pandemic. Critical reviews underlined the divide between what the global community expected the WHO to do in every health crisis and what it was able to do with its current organizational and financial constraints.

In response, the WHO developed a comprehensive plan to address the identified inadequacies, beginning with development of a separate Health Emergencies(WHE) program with defined organization-wide guidelines for infectious hazard management, organization and assessment of member state preparedness and emergency information management, supported by rapidly accessible financial support.[12-14] Led by an Executive Director, the WHE Program was intended to handle operations for *all* emergencies. As part of the program, the WHO would work to create a global health workforce to provide surge support to national health systems through their Regional Organizations, delivering clinical care to emergent disasters and outbreak-affected populations.

Disease surveillance was identified as a critical inadequacy so future in-country surveillance activities of member nations were to be integrated with national health care systems so that data collection and analysis were immediately available. To achieve this, innovations in data collection were to be introduced, potentially including geospatial mapping, mHealth communications, and platforms for self-monitoring and reporting. Stronger collaboration between private and public sector actors was planned to take this forward.

Finally, there had been a significant discrepancy between Member States' financial contributions and their expectations of the WHO emergency response. The result had been a constant struggle to mobilize resources in light of simultaneous, competing priorities. Going forward, the WHO proposed to work with the World Bank to develop a Pandemic Emergencies Fund to be used to facilitate the response to large-scale crises due to high-risk infectious threats.

The WHO's response to discovery of the limitations uncovered by the Ebola epidemic was potentially transformative.[12-14] In theory, if these sweeping new global operational responsibilities were fully implemented, they could significantly improve WHO's epidemic responsiveness at both the global/macro-operational and member nation levels. In addition to its traditional role of coordinating the international response to containing disease outbreaks and providing effective relief and recovery to affected people, the WHO would now work directly with countries on development of the health care infrastructure necessary for surveillance, case detection, patient care and disease preparedness. Progress was to be monitored by a UN-based Independent Oversight and Advisory Committee. At the 70th World Health Assembly in 2016, the Committee reported that the WHO was "making efforts at all levels to transform itself into an operational organization in emergencies."[15]

****

COVID-19 Arrives: Response of the World Health Organization

Four years later, the devastating SARS-CoV-2/COVID-19 pandemic presented an unwelcome emergency opportunity requiring intensive WHO performance. No country in the world was spared from COVID-19 as within weeks an existential pandemic threat became a catastrophic reality. How did the WHO respond to this overwhelming global pandemic?

As described in the preceding chapter, the Chinese outbreak response began quietly when on December 31, 2019, the Municipal Health Commission in Wuhan, China announced an outbreak of pneumonia of unknown etiology and alerted the WHO. A week later, Chinese scientists identified and sequenced the virus responsible for the illness and determined that it was a novel coronavirus, very similar to the original SARS-CoV, with shared, high-sequence identity with bat-derived SARS-like coronaviruses, suggesting a zoonotic origin. The remarkably rapid sequencing of the virus and the public release of this information turned out to be very rare, accurately reported events in the Chinese response to the disease outbreak. For the next 2 weeks, local health officials continued to erroneously assure the public that there were no new cases in Wuhan and no cases at all outside the city. An expert team from the Chinese Ministry of Health visited Wuhan in early January and reported incorrectly that there was no person-to-person transmission and that the outbreak was well controlled. At this critical turning point, the Chinese authorities put secrecy and order ahead of openly confronting the growing crisis and risking public alarm or political embarrassment – portraying the outbreak as a well-managed situation, completely under control.

Meanwhile, in response to the initial announcement of the disease outbreak, the WHO initiated a series of measures typifying the institutional response to what they described as a localized outbreak, including technical guidance on how to address potential cases based on what was known from China about the virus at the time. This information was sent to member states via the standard IHR methods with no specific communication at the national leadership level. Infection and prevention control guidance to protect health workers followed with recommended droplet and contact precautions; masks were only recommended for aerosol-generating procedures in health care settings. On January 13, WHO officials confirmed a case of COVID-19 in Thailand, the first recorded case outside of China – despite the obvious importance of this event, there was no additional, official response. On January 14, WHO's technical COVID lead noted in a press briefing that there *may* have been limited human-to-human transmission of the coronavirus, and therefore, there was a risk of a possible wider outbreak – no official statement addressed this. From January 20–21, WHO experts from its China and Western Pacific regional offices conducted a brief field visit to Wuhan and then issued a statement reporting that there was evidence of human-to-human transmission in Wuhan but more investigation was still needed to understand its full extent. The WHO Director-General convened an Emergency Committee (EC) meeting on January 22–23 to assess whether the outbreak constituted a public health emergency of international concern (PHEIC) with no consensus achieved. Five days later, a senior WHO delegation led by the Director-General traveled to Beijing to meet China's leadership, to learn more about China's response and offer technical assistance.

Meanwhile, while meetings and press briefings continued, the virus was spreading rapidly throughout and beyond China, exacerbated by Lunar New Year travel. Knowledge of the virus was limited at that time, especially the fact that a large proportion of people infected with SARS-CoV-2 have no or minimal symptoms although this information had already emerged in Wuhan by mid-January. While the WHO was advocating for the traditional epidemiologic approach of identification and isolation of symptomatic, infected individuals with tracing and quarantine of their contacts, the outbreak was expanding all over the world. Aware of their own escalating case numbers, Chinese authorities abruptly placed a complete lockdown on Wuhan on January 23, eliminating all forms of transportation and effectively sealing off the city. Other cities across Hubei Province rapidly instituted their own travel restrictions, putting much of the province of 59 million people in a de facto lockdown. By then, an estimated five million people had already left the city for the Lunar New Year holiday. As described in Chapter 8, there was a prompt, sustained fall in Chinese case numbers while these increased in every other country. Early suppression of evidence about the virus and the outbreak by Chinese authorities aided by the cautious WHO response squandered a critical early window of opportunity when isolation of an informed Wuhan populace could potentially have limited the virus's spread.

It was not until January 30 that the novel coronavirus outbreak was declared a PHEIC. On that day, there were already 7818 total confirmed cases worldwide, the majority in China plus 82 cases reported in 18 countries outside China. In retrospect, the deliberately suppressed public response in China and the slow and deliberate pace of the response of the WHO projected to the world the impression that the outbreak was relatively minor with no cause for an urgent response.

In subsequent reviews, February 2020 is described as a "lost month" for the global reaction to COVID-19 as individual nations developed their own responses to the epidemic with no international leadership and little apparent sense of urgency. In the United States, for example, then-President Trump focused exclusively on preventing entrance of travelers from China. This resulted in an advisory against travel to China and quarantine of US citizens and permanent residents returning to the USA from China plus barring the entry of other foreigners with recent travel to China. Despite the already known spread of the virus, there was no effort to address travel to other countries nor potentially infected travelers arriving from other countries. More importantly, there were major unaddressed problems with testing for the virus: guidelines from the US Center for Disease Control and Prevention (CDC) strictly limited testing for SARS-CoV-2 to only individuals who had been potentially exposed by travel to Wuhan, China, or by close contact with recent Chinese travelers. This made identification of COVID cases presenting with the clinical picture of pneumonia of unknown etiology impossible, and ignored potential infections by travelers arriving from other countries. The restricted testing situation supported the false impression that the USA had only a handful of COVID-19 cases and this persisted – unchallenged – until the beginning of March. Internationally, there was similar, limited, public health action to address the spread of the virus beyond partial closure of borders with China by adjoining countries and by reduced or suspended service to China by many international airlines. Failure to aggressively alert nations of the gravity of this disease as a major, international outbreak was a significant failure of the WHO response.

The measured pattern of the WHO response continued in February, beginning with finalization of a "Strategic, Preparedness and Response Plan" on February 4 – while case numbers rose all over the world, the WHO's efforts centered on a theoretical plan to improve the capacity to respond to a disease outbreak. On February 4, the WHO Director-General did ask the UN Secretary-General to activate the UN crisis management policy but the official focus remained on a response to a local disease outbreak in China.

WHO meetings and publications continued but by mid-February, some sense of urgency began to appear. When the WHO Director-General spoke at a Security Conference in Munich, he expressed concern at the global lack of urgency in funding the response. A WHO/China Joint Mission began that same week: 25 national and international experts, co-led by the WHO and the China National Health Commission, were tasked with assessing the seriousness of this new disease, its transmission dynamics, and the nature and impact of China's control measures, via field visits to Beijing, Guangdong, Sichuan and Wuhan. The Joint Mission issued a report of its findings on the last day of February, warning that "much of the global community is not yet ready, in mindset ... (nor) materially, to implement these measures."[16] The Report still stressed that to reduce the scope of COVID-19, near-term readiness planning must embrace large-scale implementation of the traditional public health measures, specifically case detection and isolation, contact tracing and monitoring/ quarantining via community engagement. In other words, the focus was unchanged.

The original WHO official statement on prevention of infection with SARS-CoV-2 was flawed and this was sustained for the first 9 months of the pandemic while case numbers increased exponentially Based on the similarities between the original SARS coronavirus and SARS-CoV-2, the WHO announced that the principal mode by which people are infected with SARS-CoV-2 was through exposure to respiratory droplets carrying infectious virus. For this reason, maintaining a distance of 6 feet between people was recommended as the primary measure needed to prevent direct infection. Because it was reportedly also possible for people to be infected through contact with contaminated surfaces or objects (fomites), rigorous surface cleansing efforts and strict handwashing were also recommended. There was a definitive statement that the virus was not airborne so masks were specifically *not* recommended. This turned out to be a major error, not addressed until many months had passed.

In retrospect, many of the efforts of the WHO in January and February 2020 seem remarkably traditional and passive: essentially futile actions in the face of a rapidly emerging catastrophe. It was not until March 11, 2020, when there were already more than 118,000 known cases of COVID-19 in 114 countries with 4,291 deaths, that the WHO finally declared COVID-19 to be a pandemic. The timing of this declaration reflects the cautious, reactive state of the WHO's initial response to COVID-19.

****

After this slow start, the WHO did develop important measures specific to COVID-19 including:

- Establishment of a global network of specialized referral laboratories with expertise in the molecular detection of coronaviruses to support national labs performing diagnostic tests in their own countries.
- Creation of global availability of testing and personal protective equipment, sending 250,000 coronavirus tests to more than 70 laboratories around the world, as well as 500,000 masks, 350,000 pairs of gloves, 40,000 respirators, and nearly 18,000 isolation gowns to 24 countries.[13]
- Launch of the Global Collaboration to Accelerate the Development, Production and Equitable Access to New COVID-19 Diagnostics, Therapeutics and Vaccines as a G20 initiative.[17] This ground-breaking effort was designed to accelerate the global development, production and delivery of SARS-CoV-2/COVID-19 tests, treatments, and vaccines, while ensuring equitable access. A critical component of the collaboration was COVAX, the COVID-19 Vaccines Global Access.
- Support of the WHO Coronavirus (COVID-19) Dashboard and the Coronavirus Resource Center at Johns Hopkins which combined to provide continuously updated sources of COVID-19 data, displaying cases and deaths in tables and maps. The dashboard began reporting on January 22 as the first global map to track COVID-19 cases and deaths.

- Establishment of the WHO Hub for Pandemic and Epidemic Intelligence in Berlin with the foundational investment of the Government of the Federal Republic of Germany in September 2021 to support countries, regions, and global actors in averting and managing public health threats efficiently. Through 2022, the WHO Hub was a center of innovation and excellence in public health surveillance, filling an important support function for public health engagement in its projects and external programs.
- Introduction of a global collaboration, the International Pathogen Surveillance Network,[18] to harness pathogen genomics to improve disease surveillance and identify and respond to disease-causing agents before they become epi/pandemics. The Network connects representative members from different countries, aiming to improve sample collection and analysis to facilitate public health decision-making. Pathogen genomics involves analyzing the genomes of viruses, bacteria, and other contagions to understand their infectivity, deadliness, and transmission and using this information to improve the global response to disease outbreaks.

Other International Health Organizations

Multiple international health organizations have collaborated to optimize the response to biological threats like SARS-CoV-2, including the Global Health Security Agenda (GHSA),[19] a joint effort of the CDC, Department of Defense, and the US Agency for International Development (USAID) which facilitates collaborative efforts to improve the competence of existing national health care infrastructure for detection and control of disease outbreaks through a partnership of nearly 70 nations, international organizations, and non-governmental stakeholders; the National Public Health Institutes (NPHI),[20] works with the CDC and GHSA to support achievement of the WHO/IHR core capacities for infrastructure development; and the United Nations Children's Emergency Fund (UNICEF), a major player in international health initiatives, prioritizing the needs of the world's most vulnerable children in areas of critical unrest. UNICEF delivered diagnostics, therapeutics and vaccines to millions of children and families affected by the COVID-19 pandemic.

Non-governmental humanitarian groups (NGOs) are also a critical component of the response to disease outbreaks. A subset of NGOs focus their efforts exclusively on medical support. Chief among these is Medecins Sans Frontieres (MSF) (Doctors Without Borders), the medical aid group that has been providing emergency assistance since 1971, in response to natural disasters and major disease outbreaks all over the globe. Across multiple projects including COVID-19, MSF teams have implemented infection prevention and control measures and provided access to protective equipment, COVID-19 tests, oxygen and drugs for supportive care and treatment as COVID-19 spread in countries without access to these tools.

Surveillance/Disease Outbreak Detection

Surveillance for outbreak detection means identifying and verifying an increase in the frequency of a disease above its background occurrence, a critical first response to a disease outbreak.[21] Traditionally, surveillance has been relatively passive, based on accumulated case reports of diseases, or by clinicians and laboratories who identified disease clusters and alerted public health officials. If you remember, this was how the first stage of the influenza pandemic was identified in 1918 and how the first clinical cases of AIDS were reported in 1981. This is also the way the COVID-19 pandemic presented, as a cluster of cases of pneumonia of unknown etiology in Wuhan, China. To be most effective, surveillance systems must be accurate, timely and complete – all significant challenges in resource-poor areas.[22] Effective, ongoing surveillance was a critical absence to Ebola in Guinea, Sierra Leone and Liberia where delayed disease recognition allowed exponential spread through the three countries. In a review of emerging infectious disease threats, Director Anthony Fauci from the National Institute of Allergy and Infectious Disease identified optimization of global surveillance to detect outbreaks early as a number one priority.[23]

An enormous amount of valuable information about infectious diseases is found in web-accessible sources: disease reporting networks, news outlets and social networking sites hold tremendous potential to provide real-time epidemic intelligence, complementary to traditional surveillance sources. Newer surveillance systems can analyze electronic data and recognize early patterns suggestive of a possible outbreak. More than 60% of initial outbreak reports now come from unofficial informal reports, including sources other than the electronic media. As an example, the Epidemic Intelligence from Open Sources (EIOS)[24] initiative of the WHO Health Emergencies Program is a collaboration of multiple public health stakeholders around the globe that uses publicly available information from new and existing networks to provide public health intelligence and allow early detection of public health threats.

By using EIOS, the WHO systematically captured mainly unstructured information (e.g. media articles, listservs, community-based reporting) to follow the pandemic in real time, as it evolved. This included recognizing epidemiological trends to supplement the information available through indicator-based surveillance, identifying the emergence of viral variants, surges in cases, hospitalizations and deaths at sub-national levels. Triaging the unprecedented high volume of information was managed by information sharing with collaborating organizations including: ProMED mail[25] which links experts in human, plant and animal disease to volunteer subscribers in more than 200 countries who post media reports, online summaries and local observer reports to a public website using email. Global moderators screen reports to highlight the most important events, 24/7/365, identifying an average of eight outbreaks per day; the Global Public Health Intelligence Network (GPHIN)[26] developed by Health Canada, a secure Internet-based early-warning tool that continuously searches global media sources to identify information about disease outbreaks and other international public health events by analyzing more than 20,000 online news reports in nine languages every day to provide potential signals of emerging public health events which are then reviewed by a multilingual, multidisciplinary team. GPHIN initially detected signals of what would become the COVID-19 pandemic on December 30, 2019, and distributed this the following morning in their Daily Report; HealthMap[27] is an American multi-stream real-time surveillance platform that continually aggregates reports on new and ongoing infectious disease outbreaks and displays them on a global map. Updating 24/7/365, the HealthMap system monitors, organizes, integrates, filters, visualizes and disseminates online information about emerging diseases in nine languages, utilizing online informal sources for real-time surveillance of emerging public health threats; the Global Outbreak Alert and Response Network (GOARN)[28] provides operations and logistics platforms for any WHO response to international public health risks by electronically uniting more than 100 existing networks through a computer-driven tool for real-time gathering of disease intelligence. When a significant public health event is identified, GOARN provides event-based surveillance, rapid risk assessment and communication, and critical information platforms for response coordination. This evolution of public health intelligence activities using multiple sources illustrates the future directions in which these methodologies can be developed and used.

Several programs address surveillance capacity at the local level including the Emerging Threats Program (ETP)[29] within USAID which draws on expertise from across animal and human health sectors to build regional, national and local capacities for early disease detection, laboratory-based disease diagnosis, rapid response and containment and risk reduction. In October 2023, USAID launched the "Localize Global Health Security Project," a 5-year contract that will work with local organizations to strengthen their capacities to prevent, detect and respond to emerging health threats in 15 countries through Africa, Asia, Latin America and the Caribbean. The CDC developed the Frontline Field Epidemiology Training Program (FETP)[30] in response to the Ebola epidemic as a 3-month, accelerated training program in field epidemiology that specifically targets the district level. FETP-Frontline has trained more than 1354 graduates in 24 countries, the majority in Africa and southern Asia.

Finally, in response to COVID-19, the US State Department established a new Bureau of Global Health, Security and Diplomacy in August 2023. The Bureau will integrate global health security as a core component of US national security and foreign policy.[31]

The results of optimized, on-the-ground surveillance combined with ongoing Internet surveillance from programs like these integrated with real-time information on geography and travel patterns allows the creation of global maps that allow the earliest visualization of potential new disease outbreaks. Surveillance systems provide routine data to multilateral, multinational agencies which can analyze and disseminate information on disease trends at regional, national and global levels. These agencies also share data from other countries when the impact of a public health event crosses national borders, a standard of practice codified by the 2005 International Health Regulations (IHR 2005). Use of Internet and digital surveillance methods combines the classic "shoe leather," on-the-ground epidemiologic techniques first implemented by John Snow with high-level informatics to forecast disease outbreaks and prevent future pandemics. With COVID-19, the initial outbreak was identified simultaneously by these global surveillance systems with subsequent tracking as the pandemic evolved.

Pathogen Identification and Definition

Complete epidemiologic, microbiologic, pathophysiologic and molecular bio-logical knowledge of a disease pathogen is crucial for management of any infectious disease outbreak. Definitive scientific investigation of the infecting pathogen must be an early and ongoing goal in any outbreak, allowing a focus on the discovery and production of diagnostics, therapeutics and vaccines. With a new pathogen, gaps in knowledge about the infectious agent can delay all aspects of the response to a disease outbreak. There is no substitute for sound, complete knowledge of the biology of a disease pathogen.

An obvious example: as the HIV/AIDS pandemic unfolded, engagement of the scientific community lagged behind, related to politically-driven decreases in national funding for scientific research and societal bias against homosexu-ality.[32] As described in Chapter 6, the pandemic had been in full swing for at least 5 years before it was recognized that infected individuals had asymptomatic latent disease for an average of 10 years before the overt AIDS picture emerged. Once it was understood that progressive destruction of the immune system was ongoing during all this time, research could be directed at an effective approach to treatment – albeit, 15 years after the first cases. Definitive scientific investiga-tion and understanding of the infecting pathogen is a critical early and ongoing priority in any disease outbreak.

There are important positive consequences of this knowledge, as seen with the SARS-CoV-2 /COVID pandemic. Only a week after the first cases were reported, genetic sequencing of the virus had been completed. Research in the next few months confirmed that binding and neutralizing antibodies pri-marily target the receptor-binding domain of the S1 spike subunit on SARS-CoV-2.[33,34] These critical pieces of information allowed immediate initiation of efforts to develop a preventive vaccine. Already available for potential evaluation in humans were candidate vaccines developed for other coronavirus pathogens, SARS-CoV and MERS-CoV. Working with the vaccine-maker Moderna, the Vaccine Research Center at the US National Institute of Allergy and Infectious Diseases (NIAID) developed a vaccine protocol based on the gene sequence of the virus reported by Chinese researchers and a novel messenger RNA platform previously shown to trigger an immune response in animals. Using this method-ology, Moderna had developed a vaccine for MERS-CoV that had already been tested in animals. Incredibly, Moderna created a trial SARS-CoV-2 vaccine just 42 days after the genetic sequence of the virus was described. The first batch had already been shipped to NIAID for phase I human testing as early as April, 2020 with simultaneous efficacy testing in an animal model followed by large human trials – these were relatively easy to accomplish with thousands of new cases emerging every day. It was a spectacular achievement when, by December 2020, less than a year after the genetic code of SARS-CoV-2 had been published, vaccines against SARS-CoV-2 had been developed, trialed and approved for emergency use – a timeline unparalleled in the history of vaccinology.[35]

In the USA alone, from December 2020 through November 2022, the COVID-19 vaccination program is estimated to have prevented more than 18.5 million additional hospitalizations and 3.2 million additional deaths. Without vaccination, there would have been nearly 120 million more COVID-19 infections. The SARS-CoV-2 vaccine experience is a model for aggressive development of future viral vaccines and demonstrates just how critical knowledge of a pathogen can be in guiding the scientific response to a disease outbreak.

Health Care Infrastructure and Community Involvement

Disease outbreaks typically erupt at the community level and communities are key drivers in the persistence and transmission dynamic of infectious diseases. In a global pandemic, the most vulnerable communities are often located in isolated, remote areas so the local health care system is the first line of defense. Unfortunately, most serious disease outbreaks have occurred in resource-poor areas without a strong health care infrastructure. The 2014–2015 Ebola epidemic in West Africa exemplifies this situation.[36]

As described in Chapter 7, the index case occurred in a very small village with no electricity and no reliable communication system. The health care pathway started with a single community health worker in a nearby village who lacked any knowledge of Ebola. In the absence of a functioning health system with a network of laboratories, Ebola spread rapidly, undiagnosed, for almost 4 months. When patients did encounter health care workers, they were completely unprepared to control the spread of infection so the disease spread within clinics and hospitals. Health care workers were among the first to contract the disease and die. For frightened patients, existing health services became associated with disease and death. Ten months after the EVD pandemic began, the CDC described the overall state of health services as completely lacking with "no personal protective equipment, no training in infection control and no surveillance system."[36] Despite efforts to stabilize the situation by providing doctors, nurses, medication, supplies and temporary isolation units, case numbers and deaths continued to rise, reflecting the difficulty of adapting to an unknown cultural setting with sustained resistance from terrified communities.

Among all the concerns raised in this desperate situation, one of the most important was the lack of trust between communities and health care workers because epidemic management depends on community engagement for case identification and isolation, contact tracing, quarantine, clinical care and infection control. Sustained engagement with local community groups builds trust and confidence in response efforts, optimizing necessary social mobilization. When health care workers are seen as dangerous aliens – something that can easily occur when groups of white strangers arrive in full hazmat gear with face guards and masks – it is easy to see how fear and mistrust can develop. Community members need culturally appropriate education so they can cooperate with infection control measures. In an intense disease transmission setting, community engagement is essential for this to occur.[37] During the 2014–15 Ebola outbreak, early efforts at public communication tried to generate behavioral change by emphasizing the need to cooperate because of the disease's high fatality rates and the absence of a cure. Rather than encouraging the infected to come forward, this messaging drove suspected cases to avoid testing and led families to hide their sick members. Over time, a focus on reaching out to communities and trying to understand the cultural context of the crisis gradually resulted in community buy-in. Once established, education about the danger of traditional burial methods and the importance of alternate methods was effectively conveyed along with the need for immediate isolation of symptomatic individuals, the importance of contact tracing and the reasons for quarantine of community contacts. For all the sophisticated international efforts that Ebola engendered, it was these community engagement efforts that finally ended the epidemic.[38]

The post-Ebola position of the WHO addresses this clearly, identifying a country's existing health care infrastructure as the critical first line of disease defense.[39] Even when health infrastructure is excellent, trust in the public health system and community engagement are important. The complicated response to COVID-19 shows how fragile this connection can be when overwhelming case numbers combined with increasing distrust in public health delivery to overwhelm health care systems in one highly developed country after another.

In the past, the response to a major global pandemic involved emergency efforts directed and administered by foreign aid groups aimed almost exclusively at stopping the spread of disease. Emergency aid workers have been like firefighters arriving at a monstrous forest fire: they are there to put the fire out! Once the fire is out – once the chain of disease transmission has broken – emergency aid groups go home. The goal has been a rapid response to an emergency situation, not the development of a sustainable health care system. As described by Randall Packer in "A History of Global Health," some of this crisis mentality is a residua of colonial times when groups like the Rockefeller Foundation created International Health Commissions to stamp out diseases like yellow fever in Cuba, Panama and West Africa. The colonial past of global health often involved providing "disease-focused interventions … over the development of basic health services."[40]

Even now, we can see this crisis mentality in some international medical humanitarian responses where global efforts can focus on providing specific, emergency interventions like the vaccines provided in the recent yellow fever outbreak in Angola or medications to treat HIV infection in sub-Saharan Africa. By contrast, supporting the development of health care systems is a long-term effort coordinated with the population of a country, requiring sustained resources of money and personnel and time. The new plan calls for the WHO to work directly with countries on development of the necessary health care infrastructure to support all aspects of the response needed to prevent local infectious disease outbreaks from becoming global pandemics. The newly established Global Health Security Agenda (GHSA) is partnering with multiple countries, international organizations, and non-governmental stakeholders to accelerate this process by supporting achievement of the WHO core capacities of health care infrastructure. The CDC's Frontline Field Epidemiology Training Program trains staff members from the local Ministry of Health to provide community-based disease surveillance, capable of providing real-time disease data at the very outset of an outbreak.[41] A initiative supported by the WHO and the United Nations provides technical support for training of 2 million new community health workers (CHWs) across Africa to identify unusual health events in their communities and report these by mobile phone to the nearest health center for further investigation.[42-45] CHWs can function as the first level of a comprehensive national early warning and response system for new disease events. If achieved, these proposed changes could combine to transform the ground-level response to a disease outbreak.

A third option for promotion of community engagement is involvement of the public in disease detection. Public participation in science dates back thousands of years but extension into disease detection is relatively recent. Now called citizen scientists, individuals all over the world are engaged in a wide array of disease outbreak projects including vector detection and surveillance.[46-49] Efforts like this can help to restore confidence where trust in the public health system has been compromised.

Lessons learned from past pandemics support the development of strong national health care infrastructure and an adequate number of trained workers for surveillance, detection, treatment and control of disease outbreaks. Including community-based systems and public participation as essential components of health care delivery will optimize communication, engagement, education and outbreak response.

Financial Support

Responding to all the requirements of a global response to major disease crises requires major financial support. There have long been calls for increased global cooperation and international funding support for the development of pandemic preparedness and response capabilities worldwide, but no *sustained* funding mechanism has been initiated. Public health and the appropriate provision of health care infrastructure have been considered the sovereign responsibility of individual countries: unfortunately, the means to fulfill this responsibility have consistently been inadequate. Increasingly, global disease outbreaks require international collective action, and effective and efficient governance of the global health system.[50] Critical health care inadequacies are typical in resource-poor countries like those of West Africa where the Ebola epidemic arose, in sub-Saharan Africa where 70% of people living with HIV/AIDS worldwide now reside, or in northeastern Brazil where the 2015 Zika epidemic emerged. At the WHO, funding is a critical priority for improved epidemic preparedness but historically, member states have been reluctant to provide the UN organization with adequate core funding – much of its income has been tied to specific projects, giving it less flexibility. Going forward, adequate funding for the WHO agenda and for all the agencies that support global health security is essential.

International humanitarian aid has been effective as a crisis-based response but this is neither sufficient to address basic health care inadequacies nor sustainable beyond the short-term. PEPFAR – the President's Emergency Plan for AIDS Relief – is an example of the power of national humanitarian aid when appropriately deployed.[51] Development of highly effective combinations of antiretroviral medications(ART) that suppressed the replication of HIV transformed the lives of HIV-infected people in resource-rich countries beginning in the mid-90s. However, more than 90% of all HIV infections were occurring in resource-limited countries, particularly sub-Saharan Africa, where patients had little or no access to antiretroviral medications. In response, US President George W. Bush launched PEPFAR in May of 2003 in 14 countries in Africa and the Caribbean that, collectively, accounted for nearly 20 million HIV-infected men, women, and children. Originally, PEPFAR provided $15 billion over 5 years, targeted for prevention of 7 million new HIV infections, treatment of 2 million HIV-infected persons, and care for 10 million HIV-infected people. Continuously funded with bipartisan support since its inception, PEPFAR-funded programs have treated 13.3 million HIV-infected men, women, and children with anti-retroviral therapy. The program has also supported the development of sustainable health system capacity by investing in the critical infrastructure of laboratories and training more than 220,000 health care workers. As of September 30, 2022, PEPFAR has enabled more than a dozen countries to control the spread of HIV and/or reach the Joint United Nations Program on HIV/AIDS 2025 95-95-95 HIV targets: 95% of all people living with HIV know their HIV status, 95% of those with diagnosed HIV infection are receiving sustained antiretroviral therapy (ART), 95% of all those receiving ART have achieved viral suppression by 2025. Even without a vaccine or a cure, PEPFAR has supported substantial global progress toward achieving the UN Sustainable Development Goal of ending the AIDS pandemic as a public health threat by 2030. PEPFAR demonstrates the power of well-funded, targeted support in the global health arena.[52]

Many private philanthropic organizations play a critical role in funding responses to disease outbreaks independently or as part of private-public partnerships. As an example, the Bill & Melinda Gates Foundation's Emergency Response Program has been intensively involved in vaccine development, especially the efforts to eradicate polio and malaria. They also collaborate with other foundation programs to develop and introduce innovative products and approaches that can save lives and build community resilience before an emergency occurs. The emergencies they have responded to have included the Ebola virus outbreak in West Africa, cholera outbreaks in Cameroon, floods and landslides in Kashmir and Nepal, Typhoon Haiyan in the Philippines, and conflict and displacement in the Central African Republic and South Sudan.[53]

The World Bank's International Development Association (IDA), established in 1960, has provided grants and low to no-interest loans for projects and programs that boost economic growth, reduce poverty, and improve people's lives in the world's 77 poorest countries, 39 of which are in Africa. In response to the Ebola epidemic, a scaled-up IDA commitment was initiated to improve pandemic preparedness in at least 25 countries over 3 years by funding an integrated series of projects supporting health care infrastructure development and strengthening the capacity for regional disease surveillance and response.[54] The Pandemic Emergency Financing Facility (PEF) is a quick-disbursing financing mechanism that provides a surge of funds to enable a rapid and effective response to a large-scale disease outbreak of a pre-identified group of diseases including pandemic influenza, SARS and MERS-CoV, Ebola, Marburg and Crimean Congo hemorrhagic fever, Rift Valley fever, and Lassa fever. The PEF functions as insurance for pandemic risk, offering coverage to all low-income countries eligible for financing under IDA. International organizations and NGOs supporting response efforts in affected countries are also eligible to apply for these emergency funds which are grant-based and do not need to be repaid. The costs of insurance premium payments for the first 3 years are already committed by donors.[55]

Unfortunately, the global devastation that has resulted from COVID-19 revealed that these existing efforts were inadequate. In response, the World Bank launched a new global, multilateral financing mechanism known as the Pandemic Fund (PF) whose specific purpose is to provide sustained financing to help countries build their capacity to prevent, prepare for, and respond to epidemics and pandemics.[56] The primary objective of the Fund is to provide a dedicated stream of long-term funding supporting existing capacity-building efforts. The PF encourages new funding from domestic governments and the private sector in support of pandemic preparedness activities rather than re-directing existing government donor financing to global health security. By March 2023, more than 100 countries had already submitted proposals for funding, totaling over $7 billion. As of May 22, 2023, 26 donors (including countries, philanthropic foundations, and non-profit organizations), the total amount received from donors and available for use is reported as $1.1 billion, $300 million of which is dedicated to funding projects resulting from the first call for proposals. It remains to be seen how well funders and funding mechanisms will respond to this new opportunity to support the development of pandemic preparedness.[56]

One area that will require specific funding is support for research and development of diagnosis, prevention and treatment methods for pathogens that have the potential to initiate a major disease outbreak. In the past, research has not often focused on rare diseases in resource-poor countries. Ebola is an excellent example of this – the virus had caused more than 20 outbreaks since its identification almost 40 years ago but no vaccine had been developed by the time the 2014–15 epidemic exploded. Pharmaceutical companies have focused their research efforts on diseases that affect societies whose citizens are able to pay for new products. Research should be focused on infectious pathogens with the potential for epidemic spread, with vaccines, therapeutics and diagnostics developed to the stage where they can be rapidly tested and produced in the event of an outbreak. As an example, twenty years of research led up to availability of the mRNA vaccine platforms which were used to develop the SARS-CoV-2 vaccines. Dedicated funding is urgently needed to expand this kind of anticipatory research. Funding mechanisms could include public or private grants, research prizes, advance market commitments, or subsidization of basic research efforts. Funds for emergent research and development in direct response to a rapidly evolving outbreak will also be needed.

Robust and sustained investment like that intended by the new PF is essential to establish an effective system to prevent and respond to disease outbreaks. Ensuring adequate preparedness by supporting the development of appropriate health care infrastructure in resource-limited countries, establishing a comprehensive system of early disease detection and response, and targeting research to support these efforts requires substantial, sustained financing. The investments needed are small compared to the significant costs imposed by pandemics, measured in lives lost and foregone economic growth.

★★★★★★★★

The stage is set. On one side is a vast army of emerging and re-emerging viruses, armed with inherent biologic characteristics that make them the most formidable of all enemies. On the other are an extensive armory of global resources, from international organizations to governmental programs supporting scientific research to pharmaceutical industry developments. The backdrop is a constellation of critical, contemporary societal and environmental factors. It is only a matter of time until yet another virus emerges with the right combination of high infectivity, ready transmissibility and high mortality in a globally connected area, primed to initiate another global pandemic. The impact of COVID-19 transcended all existing standards and made it clear that to mount an effective response to the looming threat of viral disease outbreaks, a whole planetary response will be required.

Looking Back :: Moving Forward

The last century has seen a steady increase in the frequency, diversity and severity of viral disease outbreaks like those we describe in this book. The viruses that caused these outbreaks, most of animal origin, exemplify the variability and rapid mutability that make them so dangerous. In many outbreaks, it is the characteristics of the viral pathogen itself that initiate the outbreak and promulgate the expansion from outbreak to pandemic in the current scientific, medical, societal and environmental context. Pandemics like HIV/AIDS, SARS, Ebola, Zika and COVID-19 underscore – dramatically and tragically – what we already know: in a world as interconnected as ours, outbreaks anywhere, even in the remotest corners of the planet, can impact the whole world.

In this chapter, we review the power inherent in viral pathogens, the current environment that supports global disease spread and the many systems that have already been developed to respond to disease outbreaks. All are well-intentioned, designed with proven ability to detect a disease outbreak anywhere in the world. Detection is the critical first step in outbreak control but evaluation of many of these pandemics showed that the response to the evolution of a viral outbreak can be ponderous and convoluted, encumbered by politics and policies at multiple levels, with tragic consequences. We have seen how delay in acting on critical scientific evidence that emerged early in a disease outbreak can result in dangerous exponentiation of the problem. With COVID, for example, it was clear from the very first weeks of the outbreak that the virus was transmitted directly from one person to another and that infected individuals were often asymptomatic. As leaders of the global response, the WHO was theoretically engaged in managing the outbreak from the beginning but they failed to act on this critical information for months, allowing the virus to spread all over the globe. With monkeypox, a localized disease outbreak in Nigeria in 2017 signaled a dramatic change in the pattern of MPXV infection and transmission. This information was delivered to international epidemiologists within months but failure to act allowed the virus to spread unremarked over the next 5 years to more than 100 countries. All the scientific ability, all the medical knowledge, all the advanced technologies at our disposal are useless if we do not acquire and act on critical evidence that emerges about a virus and a disease as an outbreak unfolds.

The pandemics we have studied have often been characterized by a patchwork of reactions with each involved nation-state developing its own response. In today's complex world, a fragmented response like this is completely ineffective. To deal decisively with what will certainly be future pandemic threats will require nations and their governments to respond together within an inclusive, interactive, coordinated framework. A model for this kind of response is the Independent Panel for Pandemic Preparedness and Response in the United Kingdom, created by the WHO Director-General. He recommended establishment of a "Global Health Threats Council" led by international Heads of State, representative of all the world's regions.[57] To be effective, the Council would have immediate access to essential scientific expertise and financial resources. Such a Council could develop a universal algorithm outlining an organized and appropriate response to be used to address any global disease outbreak. A recognized international voice of authority with regional, national and global representatives like this would provide the leadership needed to address the multiple problems inherent in a global pandemic as they appear, including responses to new evidence and management of misinformation before the endless cycle of transmission and re-transmission by social media networks begins. An essential element for such a Council would be a mandatory schedule of objective evaluation of pandemic management at defined intervals, like the stopping guidelines used for monitoring of clinical trials; this would allow early recognition of failing responses so that important changes can be implemented as problems are recognized. Limitations in basic health care infrastructure at the national level in under-resourced countries can significantly compromise all efforts to contain a dangerous, fast-moving viral outbreak and these must be addressed. The World Health Organization has set a deadline of May 2024 to agree on a new pandemic accord and on amended International Health Regulations describing instruments which can ensure that all people, in all countries, are protected from public health emergencies of international concern.[57] The kind of panel proposed here would be coordinated with but not managed by the WHO, and would provide an independent international voice of authority to address the multiple problems inherent in a global pandemic as they appear. The world has changed – an authoritative, inclusive, coordinated global response network like this is now essential.

While the exact source and virulence of the next emerging pathogen are difficult to predict, there is a significant risk that the next outbreak could be even more severe than any we have experienced. Known factors like high population density, increasing proximity between animals and people, extreme climate events, environmental destruction, and increasingly rapid and extensive global travel maximize the potential for viral mutations to spill over from animals to humans and be rapidly transmitted all over the world. Emergence of another virulent strain of a highly transmissible airborne virus could result in millions more deaths. The impact of a novel virus like a new strain of influenza or SARS-CoV-2 could far outreach existing gold standards for viral pandemic tragedy. At this moment the emergence of another such pathogen feels almost inevitable.

With time, commitment and financing, we can study each new viral pathogen so that knowledge of every aspect of a virus informs our response to diagnosis, prevention and treatment; we can create faster, smarter response capabilities by further strengthening global surveillance systems integrated with web-based disease reporting systems; we can expand local disease response by supporting the development of effective health care infrastructure and maximizing community engagement and front-line disease reporting; we can develop stand-by emergency epidemic response teams, ready for mobilization whenever the call comes; and, we can create stable ongoing sources of financial support. With conviction and commitment, all these responses are within our reach. Will this be enough?

We must try. Ultimately, the odds that a given virus will cause an outbreak depend on the virus itself, the animals that host it, the people who are at proximate risk for infection, and the environment in which all of us live. Too often, global panic about an epidemic has been followed by complacency and inaction – I sense this happening now while COVID-19 is still with us. We cannot let that happen. Development of appropriate health care infrastructure and comprehensive, coordinated disease detection and response capacities, particularly in "hot spot" areas like central Africa and Southeast Asia where a confluence of risk factors contribute to the emergence of novel viruses, is our best option – our only option – for urgent and immediate disease containment and interruption of transmission of a new viral pathogen. Because while we are analyzing previous epidemics and developing new strategies and trying to envision and finance the ultimate pandemic response system, viruses are continuing to emerge and endlessly evolve into new forms with ever greater capacity to transmit, parasitize, replicate and mutate, causing new and more devastating global pandemics.

References

1. Crawford DH. *Viruses. A Very Short Introduction..* New York, NY: Oxford University Press Inc. 2011. Pg. 16.
2. Smolinski MS, Hamburg MA, Lederberg J. *Microbial threats to health: emergence, detection, and response.* Washington, DC: National Academies Press. 2003.
3. Smith KF, Goldberg M, Rosenthal S, et al. Global rise in human infectious disease outbreaks. *J R Soc Interface* 2014; 11:20140950. http://dx.dol.org/10.1098/rsif.2014.0950
4. Anderson W. Natural histories of infectious disease: Ecological vision in twentieth century bioscience. *Osiris* 2004;19: 39–61.
5. United Nations World Population Prospects, Deutsche Stiftung Weltbevolkerung. www.knowledge.allianz.com
6. Jones KE, Patel NG, Levy MA, et al. Global trends in emerging infectious diseases. *Nature* 2008; 451: 990–994.
7. Rocha LE, Thorson AE, Lambiotte R. The non-linear health consequences of living in larger cities. *J Urban Health* 2015;92(5): 785–799. doi: 10.1007/s11524-015-9976-x.
8. Murray KA, Daszak P. Human ecology in pathogenic landscapes: two hypotheses on how land use change drives viral emergence. *Curr Opin Virol.* 2013; 3(1): 79–83.
9. Global Management of Infectious Disease After Ebola. Edited by Sam F. Halabi, Lawrence O. Gostin, Jeffrey S. Crowley. Oxford University Press. 2017. Pg. 1–2.
10. WHO. International Health Regulations (2005); www.who.int/ihr/publicati ons/9789241580496/en/
11. Fidler D. From international sanitary conventions to global health security: the new International Health Regulations. *Chinese J Int Law* 2005; 4(2): 326.
12. WHO Ebola Response team. After Ebola in West Africa – unpredictable risks, preventable epidemics. *N Engl J Med* 2016; 375:587–596.
13. WHO. Global Policy Group Statement on reforms of WHO work in outbreaks and emergencies. 30 January 2016. www.who.int/about/who_reform/emergency-cap acities/emergency-programme/en
14. WHO. Progress Report on the Development of the WHO Health Emergencies Programme. 30 March 2016. https://extranet.who.int/.../progress-report-developm ent-who-health-emergencies-programme
15. WHO | Independent Oversight and Advisory Committee for the WHO Emergency Capacities Reform. www.who.int/about/who_reform/emergency-capacities/oversi ght-committee/en

16. The WHO-China Joint Mission Final report. www.who.int/docs/default-source/coronaviruse/who-china-joint-mission-on-covid-19-final-report.pdf

17. WHO Press Release: Launch of a landmark collaboration to accelerate the development, production and equitable global access to new COVID-19 essential health technologies. www.unicef.org/rosa/press-releases/global-leaders-commit-further-support-global-equitable-access-covid-19-vaccines www.who.int › news › item

18. International Pathogen Surveillance Network (IPSN). www.who.int › initiatives › international-pathogen-surveillance-network

19. Global Health Security Agenda: Home www.ghsagenda.org/

20. Fitzmaurice AG, Mahar M, Moriarty LF, et al. Contributions of the US Centers for Disease Control and Prevention in Implementing the Global Health Security Agenda in 17 Partner Countries. *Emerg Infect Dis* 2017; 23: S15–S24. www.cdc.gov/eid

21. Thacker SB, Lee LM. The Cornerstone of Public Health Practice: Public Health Surveillance, 1961–2011. *MMWR Suppl.* 2011 Oct 7;60(4):15–21.

22. Kluberg SA, Mekaru SR, McIver DJ, et al. Global capacity for emerging infectious disease detection, 1996–2014. *Emerg Infect Dis.* 2016; 10. http://dx.doi.org/10.3201/eid2210.151956

23. Paules CI, Eisinger RW, Marston HD, Fauci AS. What recent history has taught us about responding to emerging infectious disease threats. *Ann Intern Med* 2017;167:805–811.

24. The Epidemic Intelligence from Open Sources (EIOS) Initiative. www.who.int/initiatives/eios

25. Carrion M, Madoff LC. Pro-MED mail: 22 years of digital surveillance of emerging infectious diseases. *Int Health* 2017; 9:177–183.

26. Mykhalovskiy E, Weir L. The Global Public Health Intelligence Network and early warning outbreak detection: a Canadian contribution to global public health. *Can J Public Health.* 2006 Jan-Feb;97(1): 42–44.

27. HealthMap. www.healthmap.org/

28. Heymann DL, Rodier GR. the WHO Operational Support Team to the Global Outbreak Alert and Response Network. Hot spots in a wired world: WHO surveillance of emerging and re-emerging infectious diseases. *Lancet Infect Dis* 2001; 1: 345–53.

29. US Agency for International Development (USAID): Pandemic Influenza and Other Emerging Threats. www.usaid.gov/.../pandemic-influenza-and-other-emerging-threats/programs

30. Andre AM, Lopez A, Perkins S, et al. Frontline Field Epidemiology Training programs as a strategy to improve disease surveillance and response. *Emerg Inf Dis* 2017(Suppl):23:S166–S173.

31. Inside the New Bureau of Global Health Security and Diplomacy. www.thinkglobalhealth.org/article/inside-new-bureau-global-health-security-and-diplomacy

32. Shilts R. *And the Band Played On: Politics, People, and the AIDS Epidemic.* New York, NY. St. Martin's Press. 1987.

33. Marston HD, Paules CI, Fauci AS. The critical role of biomedical research in pandemic preparedness. *JAMA* 2017; http://jamanetwork.com/. Accessed 10/04/2019.

34. Huang, Y., Yang, C., Xu, Xf, et al. Structural and functional properties of SARS-CoV-2 spike protein: potential antivirus drug development for COVID-19. *Acta Pharmacol Sin* 2020; 41, 1141–1149. https://doi.org/10.1038/s41401-020-0485-4

35. Jackson LA, Anderson EJ, Rouphael NG, et al. An mRNA Vaccine against SARS-CoV-2.*Preliminary Report. N Engl J Med* 2020; 383:1920–1931. doi: www.nejm.org/doi/full/10.1056/nejmoa2022483

36. Shoman H, Karafillakis E, Rawafi S. The link between the West African Ebola outbreak and health systems in Guinea, Liberia and Sierra Leone: a systematic review. *Glob Health.* 2017; 13: 1. Published online Jan 4 2017.

37. Schoch-Spana M, Nuzzo JB, Usenza C. On behalf of the working group on community engagement in health emergency planning. Community engagement: leadership tool for catastrophic health events. *Biosecur Bioterror* 2007; 5(1): 8–25.

38. WHO | Community engagement and social mobilization. Available at: www.who.int/csr/disease/ebola/training/community-engagement/en/

39. Dong W, Fung K, Chan KC. Community mobilization and empowerment for combating a pandemic. *J Epidem Comm Health* 2010; 84(2):182–183.

40. Packard RM. *A History of Global Health. Interventions Into the Lives of Others.* Johns Hopkins University press. Baltimore, MD, 2016

41. André AM, Lopez A, Perkins S, et al. Frontline Field Epidemiology Training Programs as a Strategy to Improve Disease Surveillance and Response. *Emerg Inf Dis* 2017; 23(Suppl): S166–S173.

42. Health workforce requirements for universal health coverage and the Sustainable Development Goals. 2016, World Health Organization: Geneva.

43. Protecting Humanity from Future Health Crises. Report of the U.N. High-level Panel on the Global Response to Health Crises. 25 January 2016. www.un.org/.../2016-02-05_Final_Report_Global_Response_to_Health_Crises.pdf

44. Källander K, Tibenderana JK, Akpogheneta OJ, et al. Mobile health (mHealth) approaches and lessons for increased performance and retention of community health workers in low- and middle-income countries: a review. *J Med Internet Res* 2013 Jan 25; 15(1):e17

45. Freifeld CC, Chunara R, Mekaru SR, et al. Participatory epidemiology: use of mobile phones for community-based health reporting. *PLoS Med* 2010 Dec 7;7(12):e1000376

46. Smolinski MS, Crawley AW, Olsen JM, et al. Participatory disease surveillance: Engaging communities directly in reporting, monitoring, and responding to health threats. *JMIR Public Health Surveill* 2017; 3(4):e62.

47. Palmer JB, Oltra A, Collantes F, et al. Citizen science provides a reliable and scalable tool to track disease-carrying mosquitoes. *Nat Commun* 2008; 8: Article number: 916. doi:10.1038/s41467-017-00914-9

48. Susampao P, Chanachai K, Petra P, et al. Digital functions in a participatory One Health surveillance initiative aiming for pandemic averting. *Int J Inf Dis* 2016; 53(Suppl):S-32.

49. Karimuribo ED, Mutagahywa E, Sindato C, et al. A smartphone app (afyadata) for innovative one health disease surveillance from community to national levels in Africa: Intervention in disease surveillance. *JMIR Public Health Surveill* 2017; 3(4):e94. doi: 10.2196/publichealth.7373

50. Sands P, Mundaca-Shah C, Dzau VJ. The neglected dimension of global security – a framework for countering infectious-disease crises. *N Engl J Med* 2016; 374(13):1281–1287.

51. Eisinger RW, Fauci AS. PEPFAR Zero to 15 years and counting lives saved. *N Engl J Med* 2018; 387:314–316.

52. The United States President's Emergency Plan for AIDS Relief. Dec. 1, 2023. www.pepfar.gov

53. Bill & Melinda Gates Foundation. Homepage. www.gatesfoundation.org/

54. International Development Association (IDA) – World Bank Group ida.worldbank.org/

55. Pandemic Emergency Financing Facility – World Bank Group. www.worldbank.org/en/topic/pandemics/brief/pandemic-emergency-financing-facility

56. The Pandemic Fund – World Bank Group. www.worldbank.org/en/programs/financial-intermediary-fund-for-pandemic-prevention-preparedness-and-response-ppr-fif

57. COVID-19: Make It the Last Pandemic. The Independent Panel for Pandemic Preparedness and Response. Co-Chairs: Helen Clark & Ellen Johnson Sirleaf. theindependentpanel.org

Suggested Reading

Andreas Sing, Ed. *Zoonoses - Infections Affecting Humans and Animals: Focus on Public Health Aspects.* Springer Netherlands. 2014.

Emerging Viral Diseases: The One Health Connection. Institute of Medicine, Board on Global Health, Forum on Microbial Threats. 2015.

Gerald T. Keusch. *Achieving Sustainable Global Capacity for Surveillance and Response to Emerging Diseases of Zoonotic Origin.* National Academies Press. 2009.

Linda Chelan Li. *Facts and Analysis: Canvassing COVID-19 Responses.* City University of Hong Kong Press. 2021.

Marcos Cueto, Casa de Oswaldo Cruz, Theodore M Brown, Elizabeth Fee. *The World Health Organization: A History.* Routledge. May 2019.

Warren A Andaman. *Animal Viruses and Humans, a Narrow Divide: How Lethal Zoonotic Viruses Spill Over and Threaten Us.* Paul Dry Books. 2018.

INDEX

Printed in the United States
by Baker & Taylor Publisher Services